LABORATORY DIAGNOSIS

OF

KIDNEY DISEASES

LABORATORY DIAGNOSIS
OF
KIDNEY DISEASES

Compiled and Edited by

F. WILLIAM SUNDERMAN, M.D., Ph.D., Sc.D.
Director, Institute for Clinical Science
Director of Education, Association of Clinical Scientists
Clinical Professor of Medicine, Jefferson Medical College
Philadelphia, Pennsylvania

and

F. WILLIAM SUNDERMAN, JR., M.D.
Professor and Head
Department of Laboratory Medicine
University of Connecticut School of Medicine
Hartford, Connecticut

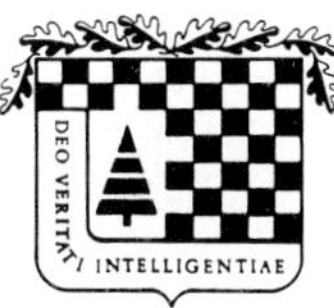

WARREN H. GREEN, INC.
St. Louis, Missouri, U.S.A.

Published by

WARREN H. GREEN, INC.
10 South Brentwood Blvd.
St. Louis, Missouri 63105, U.S.A.

Library of Congress Catalog Card No. 73-76164

Printed in the United States of America
3-B   (147)

Seminar Faculty

DIRECTOR OF SEMINAR
F. WILLIAM SUNDERMAN, M.D., Ph.D., Sc.D.
Institute for Clinical Science
Philadelphia, Pennsylvania

ERNEST C. ADAMS, JR., Ph.D.
Ames Research Laboratory
Elkhart, Indiana

GONZALO E. APONTE, M.D.
Jefferson Medical College
Philadelphia, Pennsylvania

ROBERT W. BERLINER, M.D.
National Heart Institute
NIH, Bethesda, Maryland

GEORGE P. BLUNDELL, M.D., Ph.D.
Oscar B. Hunter Memorial Laboratory
Washington, D.C.

JOSEPH S. BURKLE, M.D.
York General Hospital
York, Pennsylvania

ROBERT CADE, M.D.
University of Florida
College of Medicine
Gainesville, Florida

F.A. CARONE, M.D.
Northwestern University
Medical School
Chicago, Illinois

SIDNEY CASSIN, Ph.D.
University of Florida
College of Medicine
Gainesville, Florida

HERBERT DERMAN, M.D.
City of Kingston Laboratory
Kingston, New York

MONO J. DOSHI, M.S.
Miami Valley Hospital
Dayton, Ohio

KURT M. DUBOWSKI, Ph.D.
University of Oklahoma
School of Medicine
Oklahoma City, Oklahoma

GEORGE H. FETTERMAN, M.D.
Children's Hospital
Pittsburgh, Pennsylvania

MARVIN FORLAND, M.D.
University of Texas Medical School
San Antonio, Texas

AFRED H. FREE, Ph.D.
Ames Research Laboratory
Elkhart, Indiana

HELEN M. FREE, B.S.
Ames Research Laboratory
Elkhart, Indiana

ERVIN A. GOMBOS, M.D.
New York University
School of Medicine
New York, N. Y.

FRANCESCO DEL GRECO, M.D.
Northwestern University
Medical School
Chicago, Illinois

FARID I. HAURANI, M.D.
Jefferson Medical College
Philadelphia, Pennsylvania

ROBERT H. HEPTINSTALL, M.D.
Johns Hopkins Hospital
Baltimore, Maryland

PETER B. HERDSON, Ph.D.
University of Auckland
Medical School
Auckland, New Zealand

HOWARD C. HOPPS, M.D.
Armed Forces Institute
of Pathology
Washington, D. C.

BENJAMIN N. HORWITT, Ph.D.
Bio-Science Laboratories
Van Nuys, California

J. DE LA HUERGA, M.D., Ph.D.
Northwestern University
Medical School
Chicago, Illinois

ROBERT B. JENNINGS, M.D.
Northwestern University
Medical School
Chicago, Illinois

FRANK B. JOHNSON, M.D.
Armed Forces Institute
of Pathology
Washington, D. C.

BERNARD J. KATCHMAN, Ph.D.
Miami Valley Hospital
Dayton, Ohio

GEOFFREY KENT, M.D., Ph.D.
West Suburban Hospital
Oak Park, Illinois

P. A. KHAIRALLAH, M.D.
Cleveland Clinic Foundation
Cleveland, Ohio

PATRICK KNIGHT, M.D.
University of Arkansas
School of Medicine
Little Rock, Arkansas

WILLIAM T. KNIKER, M.D.
University of Texas
Medical School at San Antonio
San Antonio, Texas

LEOPOLD G. KOSS, M.D.
Memorial Hospital
New York City, New York

MICHAEL LUBRAN, M.D., Ph.D.
University of Chicago
College of Medicine
Chicago, Illinois

JOHN T. McCALL, Ph.D.
The Mayo Clinic
Rochester, Minnesota

MEYER M. MELICOW, M.D.
College of Physicians & Surgeons
New York City, New York

AUGUST MIALE, Jr., M.D.
Georgetown University Hospital
Washington, D. C.

MANFORD D. MORRIS, Ph.D.
University of Arkansas
School of Medicine
Little Rock, Arkansas

F. K. MOSTOFI, M.D.
Armed Forces Institute
of Pathology
Washington, D. C.

ROBERT C. MUEHRCKE, M.D.
West Suburban Hospital
Oak Park, Illinois

J. M. BRIAN O'CONNELL, M.D.
Georgetown University Hospital
Washington, D. C.

RODGER PALMER, M.D.
University of Florida
College of Medicine
Gainesville, Florida

EDMUND A. PETRUS, M.D.
Passavant Memorial Hospital
Chicago, Illinois

PIN H. PU, M.D.
University of Florida
College of Medicine
Gainesville, Florida

HOWARD QUITTNER, M.D.
University of Arkansas
School of Medicine
Little Rock, Arkansas

IRENE E. ROECKEL, M.D.
University of Kentucky
School of Medicine
Lexington, Kentucky

SEYMOUR ROSEN, M.D.
Beth Israel Hospital
Boston, Massachusetts

JOHN SAVORY, Ph.D.
University of Florida
College of Medicine
Gainesville, Florida

GEORGE E. SCHREINER, M.D.
Georgetown University Hospital
Washington, D. C.

CHARLES O. SENNETT, JR. M.D.
U. S. Naval Medical School
Bethesda, Maryland

JOSEPH C. SHERRICK, M.D.
Passavant Memorial Hospital
Chicago, Illinois

LYNWOOD H. SMITH, M.D.
Mayo Clinic
Rochester, Minnesota

BENJAMIN H. SPARGO, M.D.
University of Chicago
College of Medicine
Chicago, Illinois

F. WILLIAM SUNDERMAN, JR., M.D.
University of Connecticut
School of Medicine
Hartford, Connecticut

JENO E. SZAKACS, M.D.
St. Joseph's Hospital
Tampa, Florida

BETTY VOGH, Ph.D.
University of Florida
College of Medicine
Gainesville, Florida

FREDERICK I. VOLINI, M.D.
Northwest Community Hospital
Arlington Heights, Illinois

EARL B. WERT, M.D.
Mobile Infirmary
Mobile, Alabama

J. HENRY WILKINSON, D.Sc., Ph.D.
University of Pennsylvania Hospital
Philadelphia, Pennsylvania

ROBERT E. ZIPF, M.D.
Miami Valley Hospital
Dayton, Ohio

Preface

This book contains the edited proceedings of an Applied Seminar on the Laboratory Diagnosis of Kidney Diseases, held in Washington, D.C., under the auspices of the Association of Clinical Scientists. In organization and format, this volume is similar to the published proceedings of eight previous seminars.

Never in the history of civilization has scientific knowledge advanced with such rapidity as it does now. Compared to the last century, the advancements during this century represent a great upheaval. In recent years, one of the most striking changes in clinical science is the accelerated rate of change itself. The Applied Seminars of the Association of Clinical Scientists are designed to cope with these changing times so that the dissemination of knowledge in clinical science may keep pace with the acquisitions.

The furtherance of clinical science depends in large measure upon developments in methodology. It is for this reason that a number of procedures are included in this volume which are not currently undertaken in many clinical laboratories; nevertheless, in our opinion these procedures may play increasingly important diagnostic roles in future years. It is our hope that clinical scientists will find the chapters on methodology helpful in initiating newer procedures in their laboratories. It is also our hope that the chapters pertaining to fundamental considerations and clinical interpretations may be useful in applying the current concepts of renal diseases to patients at the bedside.

Our grateful appreciation is expressed to the lecturers who have generously contributed their time and energies to the success of the Applied Seminar and to the preparation of these proceedings. Our thanks are given to our publisher, Mr. Warren H. Green, and his staff for their gracious cooperation.

Contents

LABORATORY DIAGNOSIS
OF
KIDNEY DISEASES

Chapter 1

Anatomy and Ultrastructure of the Kidney

JENO E. SZAKACS, M.D.

INTRODUCTION

The kidneys are vital excretory organs that regulate the internal environment of the body. In adult man, they weigh 120 to 150 gm each and through their vascular tree flows approximately 1200 ml of blood per minute, some 25% of the total cardiac output. The vascular and epithelial elements form special functional units, the nephrons, consisting each of a *glomerulus* and a *tubule.*

The special apposition of blood vessels and tubules gives a characteristic gross appearance to the kidney and this organization assures the required degree of function. A renal cortex and medulla can be differentiated on a cut surface of the mammalian kidney, and the demarcation is usually enhanced by the arcuate arteries, though not in all species. The cortex contains all glomeruli and the convoluted tubules. The medulla contains some or all of the parallel descending and ascending segments of the renal tubules, called the loops of Henle, and the collecting ducts. The schematic diagram (Fig. 1) from Pitts (13) illustrates the organization of the different layers of the kidney. In man, most nephrons are cortical and only 1/8 of the nephrons are juxtamedullary, with long thin loops

of Henle extending into the renal pyramids, while in desert animals most or all nephrons are provided with long thin loops of Henle that allow them to conserve water by concentrating the urine to a high degree. Pitts' diagram also illustrates the relationship of blood

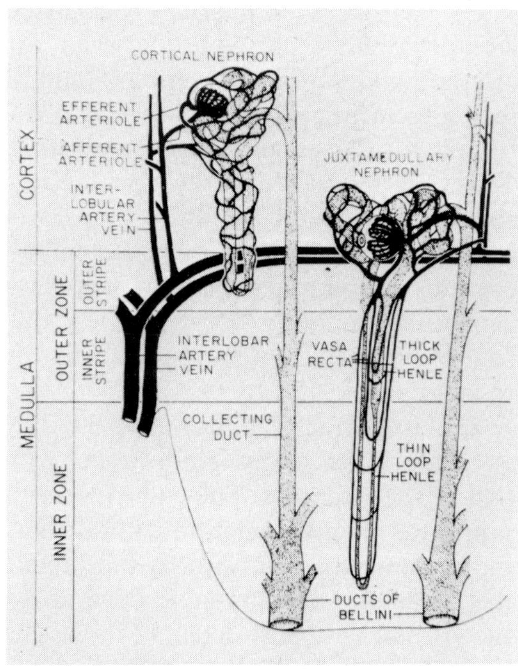

Fig. 1. Distribution of nephrons in the different layers of the kidney. Drawing from Pitts (13).

vessels to the nephron. Blood is carried through interlobar branches of the renal artery to the arcuates, interlobular arteries and afferent arterioles to the renal glomerulus. It leaves the glomerulus via the efferent artery which provides branches to form vascular loops around the convoluted tubules, and the vasa recta to parallel the loops of Henle. The venous blood is emptied into the interlobular veins and returns to the renal veins by vessels paralleling the similarly named arteries.

The following is a brief illustrated description of the salient points and of the more recent information about renal structures, including that obtained by electron microscopy. Much has been written on this subject. Classical histologic techniques culminated in the works of Möllendorff (20) and Goormaghtigh (4) in the 1930's. More recently, classical chapters on the ultrastructure of the kidney were written by Rhodin (16), Spargo (18), and Latta (10).

THE RENAL GLOMERULUS

The structure of the renal glomerulus has been studied extensively and our understanding of its function is better than that of the tubules. The identification of the anatomical site where each of the physiological processes takes place is the great challenge of our time.

The renal glomerulus is a specialized arterial capillary network between the afferent and efferent arterioles, and it serves to form about 180 liters of ultrafiltrate per day in an average adult man. The two arterioles form the vascular pole and from there the capillary loops project into Bowman's capsule. Bowman's capsule surrounds the entire capillary glomerulus and gives origin to the proximal convoluted tubule opposite to the vascular pole.

The glomerular capillaries are lined by an endothelial layer continuous with that of the arterioles. The endothelium is supported by a basement membrane and the mesangium. Opposite to the lumen, the basement membrane is covered by the visceral epithelial cells. At the vascular pole, this epithelial layer and the basement membrane reflects to form Bowman's capsule. The epithelium becomes flattened and is referred to as the parietal epithelium of the glomerulus (Fig. 2).

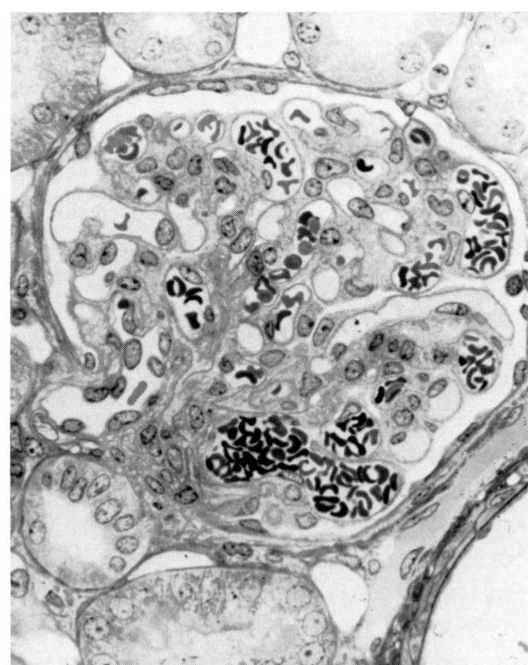

Fig. 2. Photomicrograph of the renal glomerulus. Note the vascular pole, macula densa and lacis. The basement membrane at the macula densa is ill defined and continuous with the fibrils of the lacis. Only the afferent artery is in the plane of section. The capillary basement membrane, endothelial and epithelial cells are easily identified at the periphery of the lobules. (x 500)

Silver impregnation and thin sectioning permitted the light microscopist to visualize the capillary basement membrane with its reflections and continuity with that of Bowman's capsule, but only electron microscopy allowed resolution of the fine structure of the mesangium between the capillaries. The mesangial space between two or three capillary loops is filled by cells and intercellular matrix and it is enclosed by the endothelial side of the basement membrane. The mesangium provides points of attachments for the basement membrane (Bohle and Herfarth (1)).

The Capillary Endothelium. The capillary wall is supported by the basement membrane at the periphery and by the mesangial cells between capillary loops. Endothelial cells line the entire capillary lumen covering the basement membrane and at the mesangium they are directly apposed to the mesangial cells. The nucleus is usually in the mesangial area and is surrounded by cytoplasm containing most of the cellular organelles: The Golgi apparatus, mitochondria, some rough endoplasmic reticulum and the centriole. The remaining cytoplasm is attenuated, forming a thin layer covering the peripheral portion of the capillary. On cross-section the attenuated endothelium appears discontinuous with interruptions at regular intervals. Tangential sections reveal round or elliptical openings about 1000 Å in diameter. The apparent openings are referred to as endothelial "fenestrae." High resolution electron micrographs reveal the fenestrae to be closed by a thin diaphragm (Rhodin, 1962 (14)). According to Ito (1964) (8), this diaphragm is formed by two outer protein layers of the plasma membrane, while the inner protein and lipid layers reach only to the edge of the

fenestration. This protein-mucoprotein diaphragm is considered by Rhodin to provide the kidney's filtering action,— thus permitting small molecules to pass through while retaining larger ones. In addition, large molecules were shown to be actively transported through the endothelium (Meneffe (11)), from the lumen both to the basement membrane and to the mesangium or juxtacollicular region in a form of modified phagocytosis. Pinocytotic vacuoles are seen as well as a complex system of vacuoles in the endothelial cytoplasm close to the mesangium. These participate in the transport of fluids and several other particles including those experimentally marked, such as globin.

Glomerular Basement Membrane. The basement membrane envelopes the capillary loops together with the mesangium much the same way as the mesentery envelopes the intestinal tract. The reflections of the basement membrane are well illustrated in Figures 2, 3 and 4. The illustrations also show that in preparations stained with uranyl acetate and lead hydroxide the basement membrane is resolved into three layers—a central dense layer and an inner and outer electron lucent layers. The thickness of the basement membrane varies from species to species. In man, it measures 3500 Å. Electron micrographs of fixed material reveal a fibrillar substructure that impressed many investigators by its similarity to filters. It was thought that the basement membrane could form a filtration barrier, but more recent evidence indicates that the basement membrane is a thixotropic gel. This would explain diffusion of small molecules through the basement membrane and retention of some larger ones while large aggregates would produce enough mo-

 Laboratory Diagnosis of Kidney Diseases

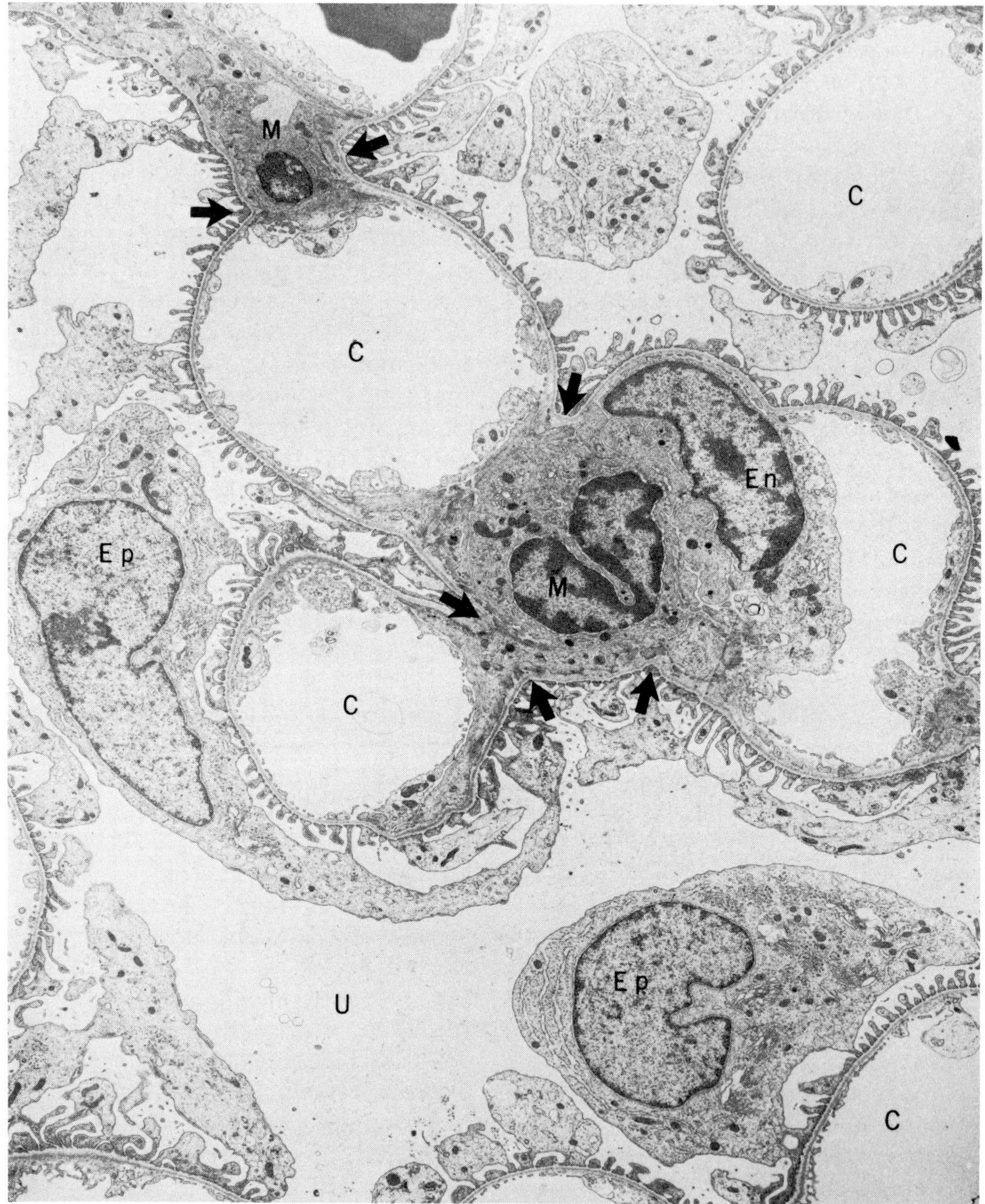

Fig. 3. Electron micrograph of glomerular capillaries. A mesangial cell (M) is seen between three capillaries (C) in the center. The basement membrane is attached to the mesangium and its reflections are marked by arrows. The lumen is lined by attenuated endothelium. The nucleus and cell body of one endothelial cell (En) are covering the mesangial portion of the capillary. Visceral epithelial cells (Ep) are shown wrapped around the outside of the capillary wall. (U) urinary space. (x 16,000)

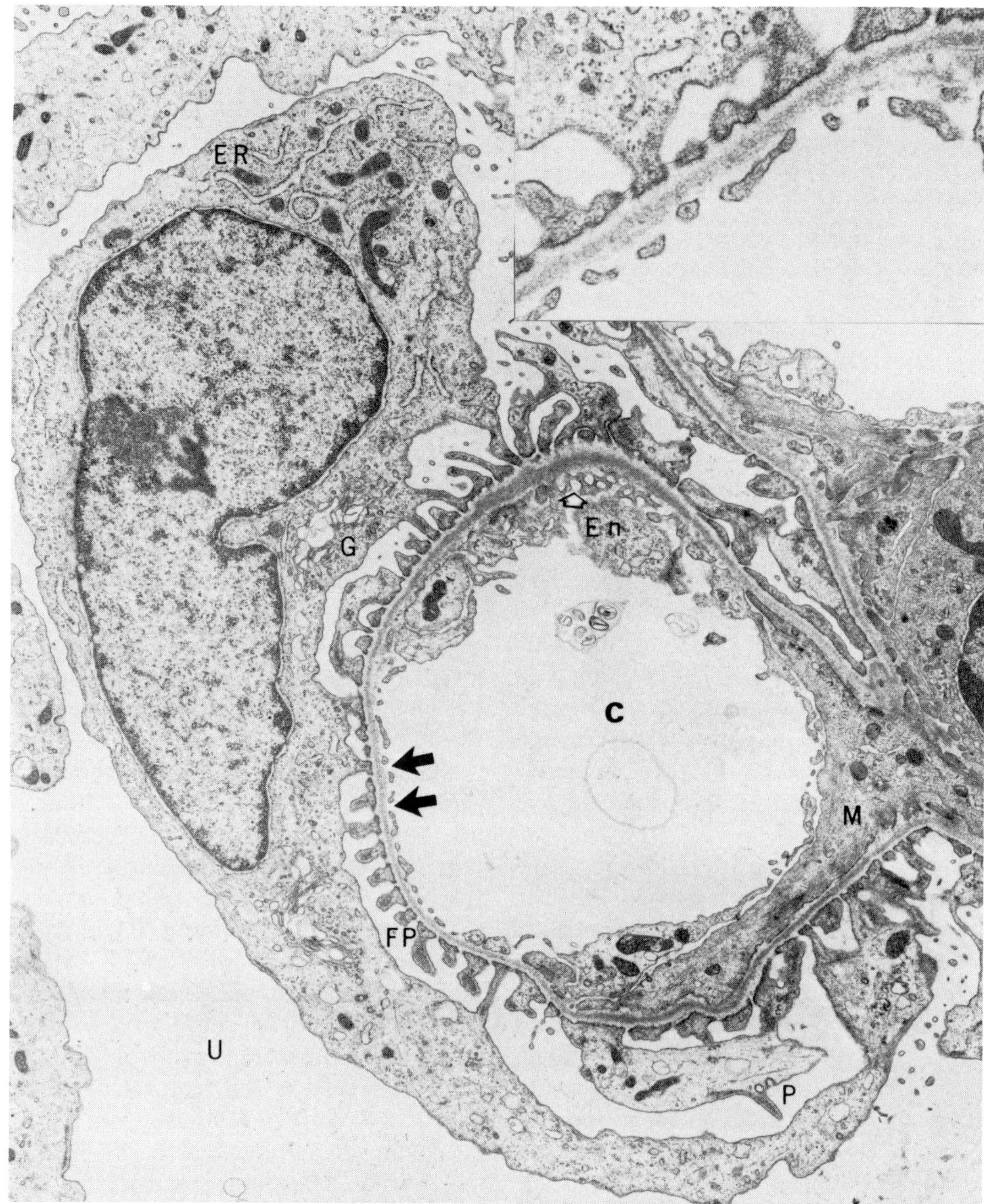

Fig. 4. Glomerular capillary. The endothelium (En) shows fenestrae sectioned both tangentially *(open arrow)*, and across *(solid arrow)*. The cytoplasmic organization of the epithelial cell is well illustrated. There are rough endoplasmic reticulum (ER) and mitochondria above the nucleus. Note the Golgi complex at G and the numerous small vescicles. The epithelial cytoplasm in addition contains prominent microtubules. Pinocytic vescicles are present at P. A mesangial cell process (M) is seen insinuated between endothelium and basement membrane. (x 33,000)

The insert illustrates the organization of the basement membrane into three layers: the inner light layer below and the outer light layer above the dense central layer. Foot processes above the basement membrane are connected to each other by a thin slit pore membrane represented by a narrow black line. (x 44,000) lecular pressure to liquify momentarily the membrane and force their way through (Meneffe (11)) (Figs. 3, 4).

Glomerular Epithelial Cells. The visceral epithelial covering of the glomerular capillaries consists of highly specialized cells. They are formed of a large flat cell body that gives origin to a cytoplasmic extension divided into many processes that intertwine with those of neighboring cells and cover the entire capillary surface. The cells are also called podocytes and the cytoplasmic processes foot processes as they attach to the basement membrane by an enlarged portion. There is a narrow slit between the foot processes of a rather uniform size covered by a thin membrane referred to as the "filtration slit membrane" (Yamada, 1955 (19)) (Fig. 4). The cell body contains in abundance cytoplasmic organelles and a large irregularly shaped nucleus. Epithelial cells take an active role in glomerular filtration. Water and small molecules passing through the basement membrane are absorbed by the epithelial cells and transported into the urinary space. Pinocytosis and confluent vacuoles were observed during transport of ferritin (Farquhar and Palade, 1960) (2) hemoglobin and other proteins. Globin, on the other hand, is not taken up by the epithelial cells, it passes between the epithelial slit processes displacing the slit membrane. This was taken as evidence for selective absorption of materials by the epithelial cells (Meneffe (11)).

At the vascular pole the capillary epithelial lining is continuous with the parietal epithelium covering Bowman's capsule. The parietal epithelial cells are flattened pavimentous cells forming a single layer, without the structural complex differentiation of the visceral epithelium.

The Mesangium. Between capillary loops a third type of cell is seen in electron micrographs (3), the mesangial cell, and the region between capillaries enclosed by basement membrane and endothelial cells is referred to as the mesangium or axial region (Figs. 3, 5).

Mesangial cells have irregular contours and may have cytoplasmic processes that extend beneath the endothelium to cover a considerable segment of the capillary circumference, or they may appear in the capillary lumen penetrating through the endothelial fenestrae. In the many invaginations of the plasma membrane, an extracellular material similar to the basement membrane is seen, and referred to as mesangial matrix. There is a complement of cytoplasmic organelles in the mesangial cell and characteristically small bundles of intracellular fibrils.

Mesangial cells serve to anchor the capillary basement membrane, as it does not completely surround the capillary. When mesangial cells are selectively destroyed with Habu snake venom (Sakaguchi and Kawamura, 1963 (17)) the glomerulus is transformed into a blood filled sac of basement membrane covered by epithelial cells.

Another function ascribed to the mesangial cells is the removal of filtration residues to prevent clogging of the basement membrane, based on demonstration of phagocytic activity of the mesangial cells (Farquhar and Palade, 1962 (3)).

JUXTAGLOMERULAR APPARATUS

The juxtaglomerular apparatus includes the vascular hilus of the glomerulus with the afferent and the efferent arterioles forming a wedge-shaped space closed at its base by a specialized

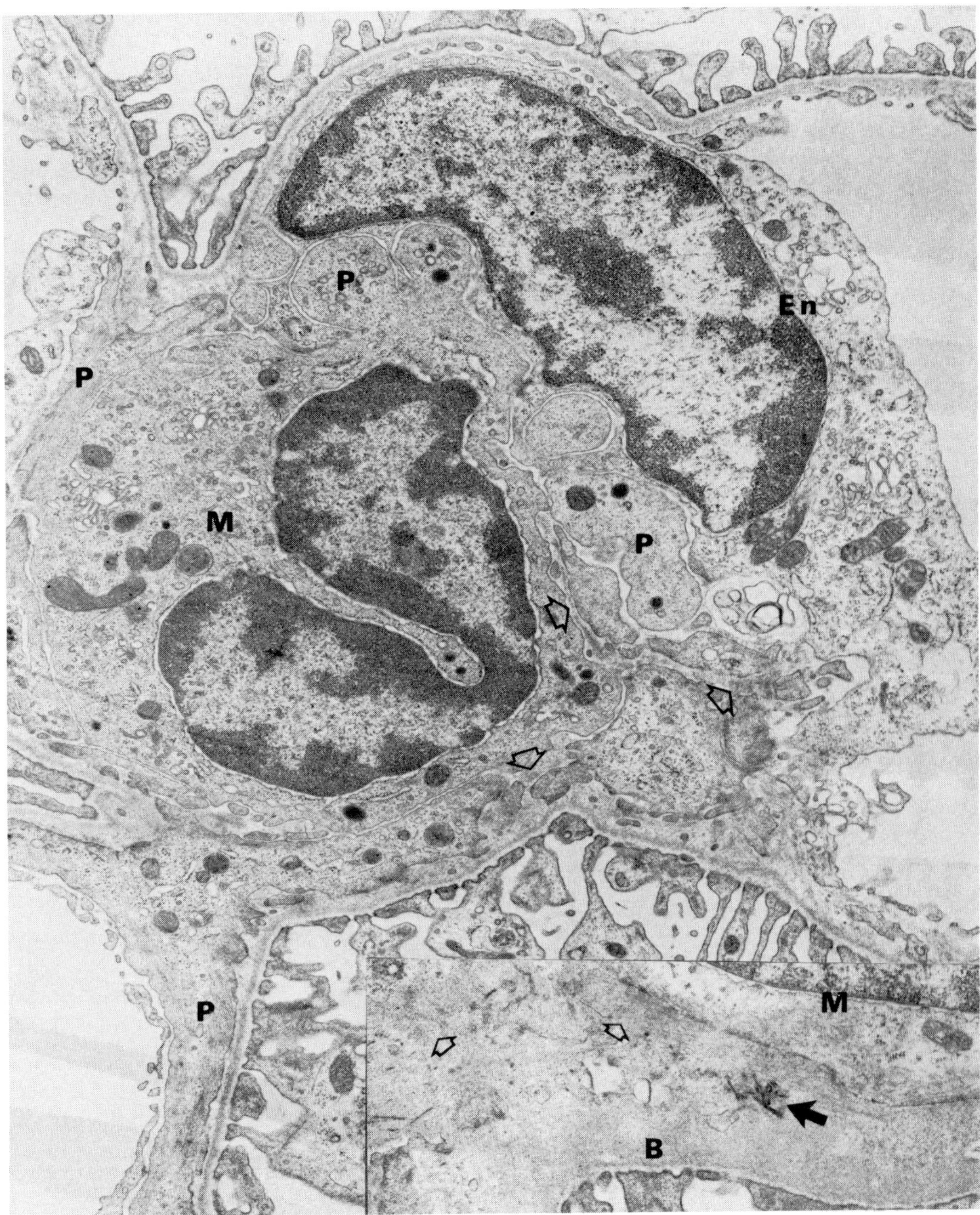

Fig. 5. Mesangial region. The mesangial cell (M) extends many cytoplasmic processes (P) and it is surrounded by a fibrillar material *(open arrow)* resembling the basement membrane (B) and referred to as mesangial matrix. In some species collagen fibers are also present in this location. Rhesus monkey kidney is shown in the insert, the solid arrow pointing to collagen fibrils. (x 40,000. Insert, x 16,500)

portion of the distal tubule of the glomerulus, the macula densa. This space is filled by a number of fusiform cells supported by a dense mesh of basement membrane (Fig. 6).

The smooth muscle cells of the afferent arterioles in this region differentiate to form cells containing a number of endocrine granules. Such granules are not ordinarily seen in the wall of the efferent arteriole. The granules are osmiophilic rounded or elongated and are limited by a single membrane. In addition to the granules, a few myofibrils

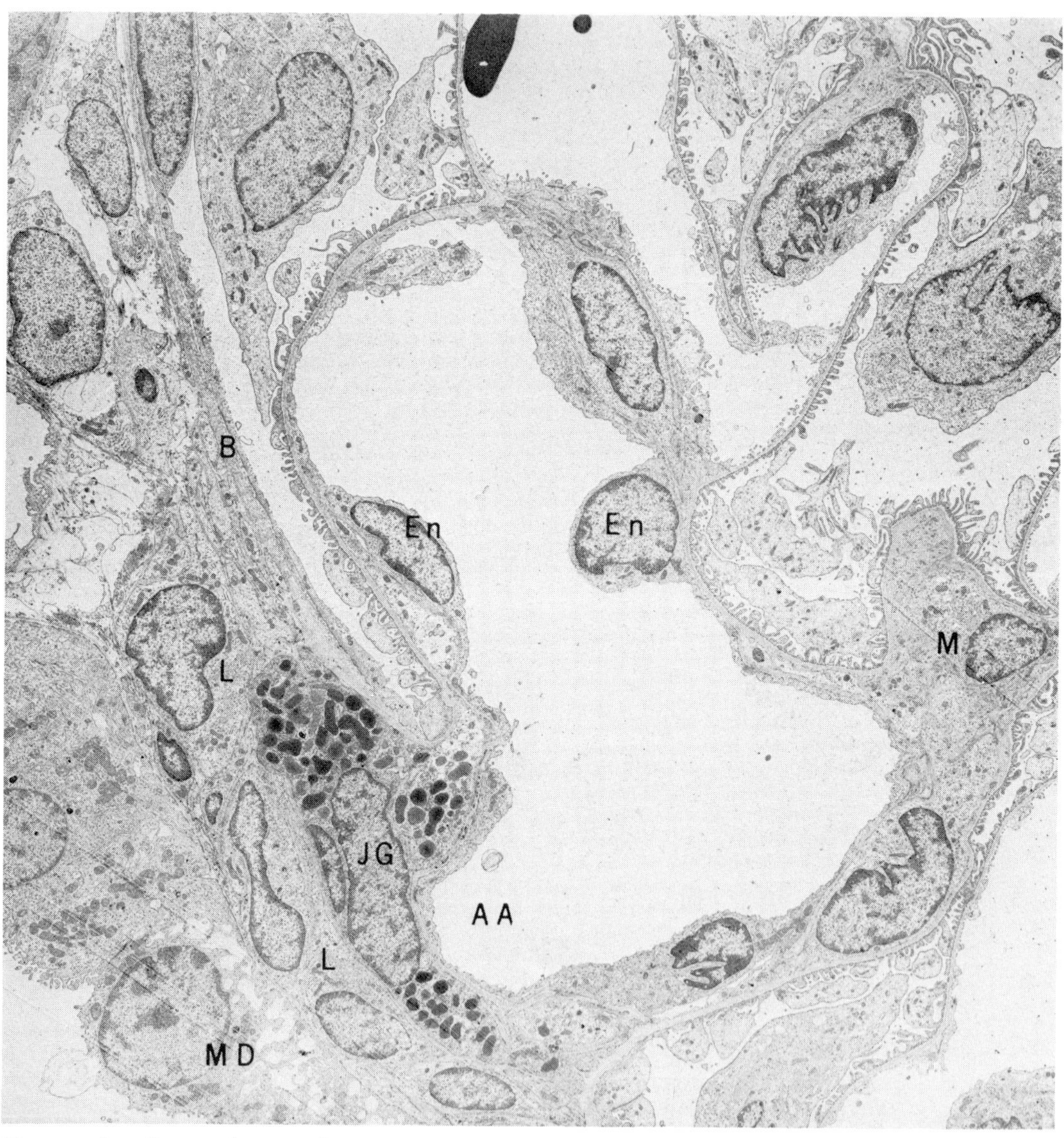

Fig. 6. Juxtaglomerular apparatus. Myoepithelial cells (JG) with secretory granules are seen in the media of the afferent arteriole (AA) entering the glomerulus. The lacis (L) is formed of undifferentiated elongated cells surrounded by basement membrane and is in contact with the macula densa (MD). Bowman's capsule (B) is seen to reflect at the vascular pole where it is continuous with the basement membrane of the glomerular capillary tuft. Endothelial cells are marked En and mesangial cells M. (x 4,000)

may be seen in these cells designated as "myoepithelial" cells. The functional cycles of the myoepithelial cells were studied in great detail by Hartroft (5, 6) and others (7). Hyperactivity is characterized by increased granulation and occurs on sodium-free diets, following adrenalectomy and in mercurial poisoning. Unilateral renal ischemia also causes hypergranulation in the affected kidney and degranulation in the opposite one, when it is intact and the ischemia is not so severe as to cause atrophy of the affected organ. Usually, hypergranulation is present during the first three weeks of ischemia.

The function of the myoepithelial cells as baroreceptors is questionable,

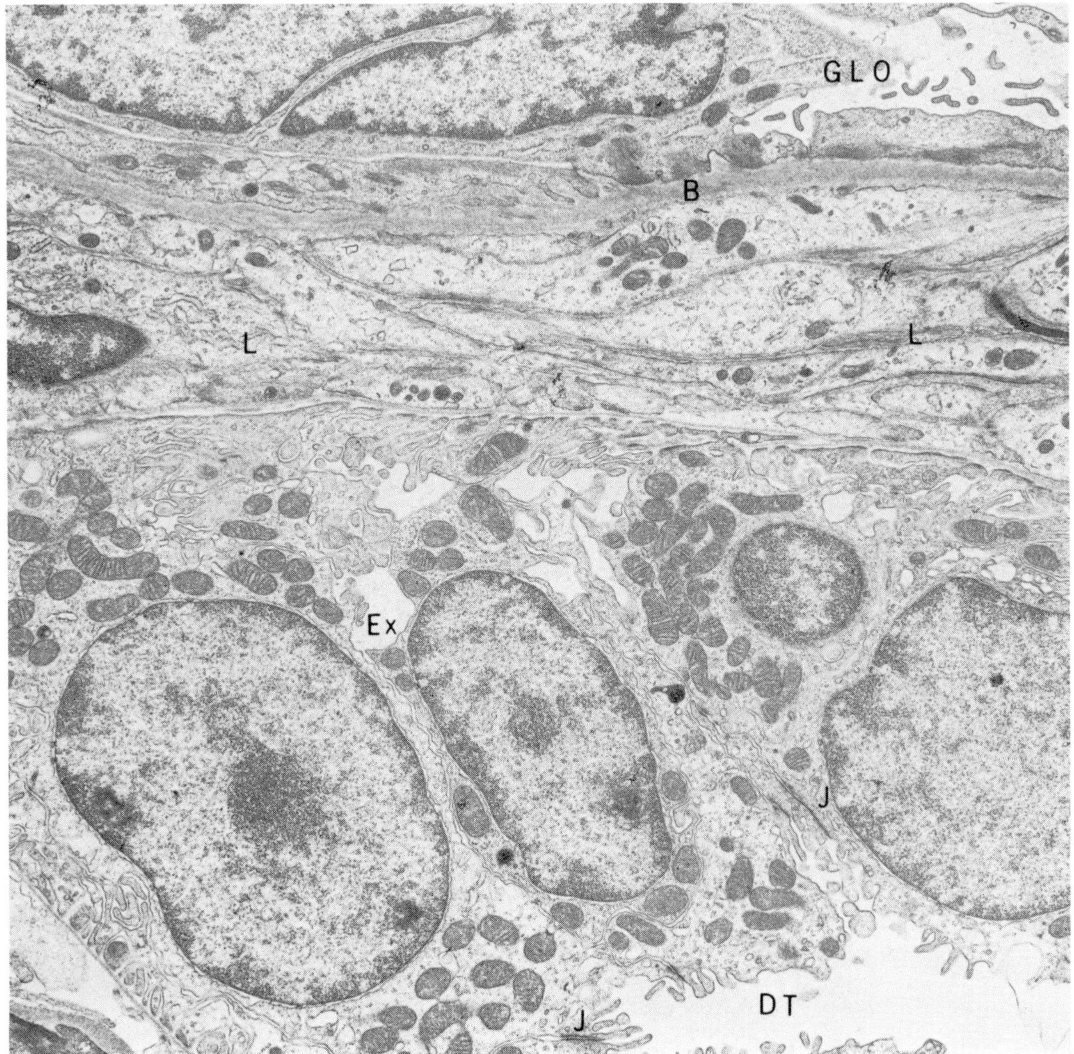

Fig. 7. Macula densa. The lumen of the distal tubule (DT) is surrounded by cells with apical microvilli. The plasma membranes form tight intercellular junctions (J) at the lumen, but large extracellular spaces are seen between cells (Ex). The basilar plasma membrane shows complex infoldings. The upper half shows part of the glomerulus (Glo) with Bowman's capsule (B) and portion of the lacis (L). (x 13,000)

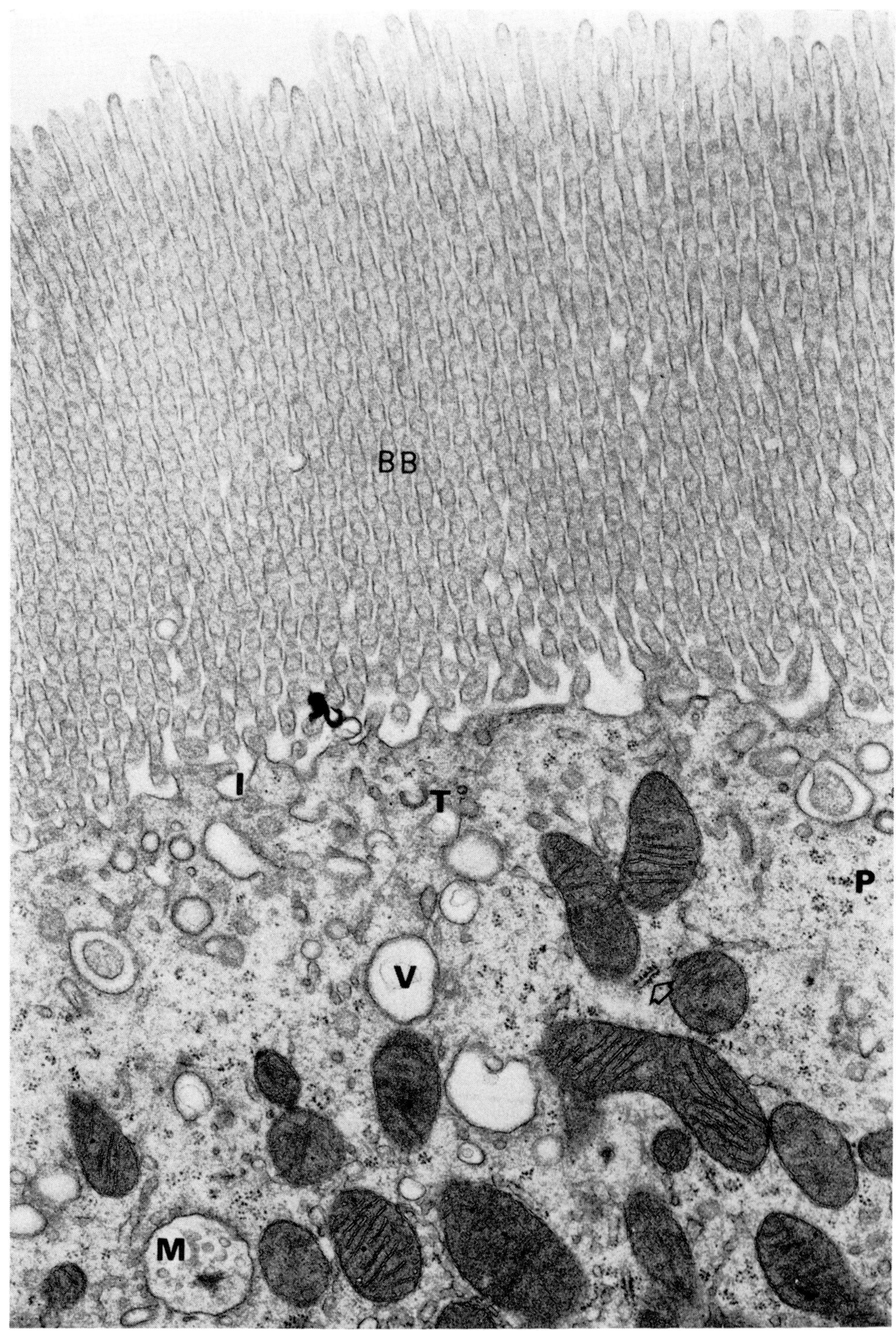

Fig. 8. Proximal tubule, apical portion. Prominent long microvilli form the brush border (BB) and are characteristic of the proximal tubule. The plasma membrane invaginates (I) between villi and gives rise to thick walled vescicles (V). In addition, tubular structures, the dark apical tubules (T), are seen in this area. Polyribosomes (P) and membrane bound ribosomes (open arrow) are seen. Mitochondria are large and abundant. At M there is a multivesciculate body. (x 28,000)

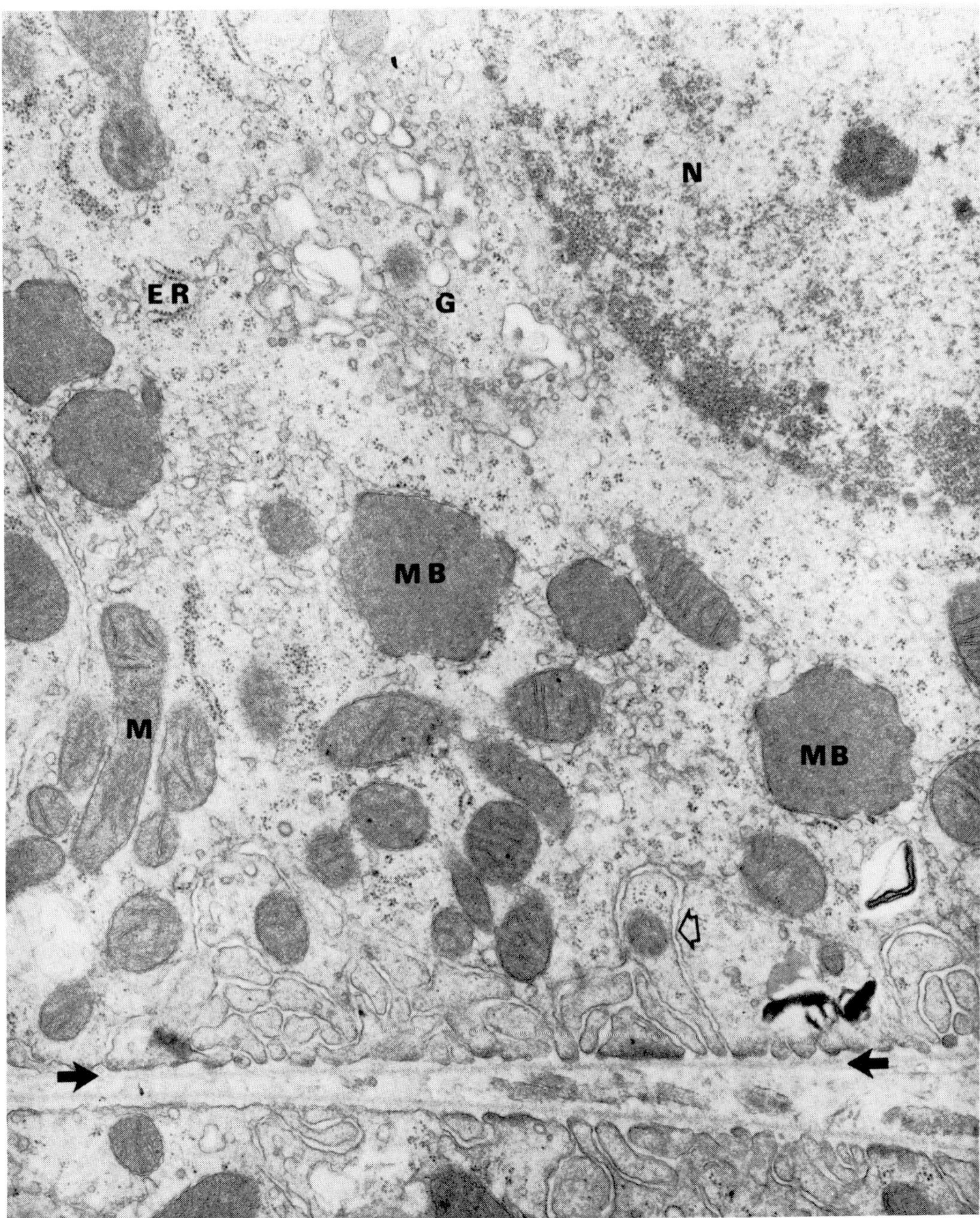

Fig. 9. Proximal tubule, basal portion. Note the well formed Golgi complex (G) next to the nucleus (N). There are complex membrane structures, some associated with ribosomes (ER). There are numerous membrane bound microbodies (MB) present that may show considerable variation of structure. Note the basilar infoldings and interdigitation of the plasma membrane *(open arrow)*. The basement membrane is straight *(solid arrow)* and does not follow the plasma membrane. (x 28,000)

but their response to plasma sodium levels is well established and their function in this respect parallels that of the adrenal cortex. Hatt suggests that the juxtaglomerular apparatus may be an intermediary between the kidney and the adrenal cortex which regulates sodium balance through release of aldosterone (7).

The macula densa is a specialized portion of the distal tubule with the epithelial cells supported directly by the lacis. The differentiation (see Figs. 6, 7) suggests that this area is osmotically sensitive, but if it has an active regulative role due to its strategical location is not established at this time, and it is indeed questioned.

THE RENAL TUBULES

The structure of the renal tubules varies considerably along their length and even within segments.

The proximal tubules are lined by tall columnal epithelial cells with a promin-ent brush border. The ultrastructure of these cells is very complex. The cell wall is formed of a 90 Å thick plasma membrane which at the base and lateral margin of the cell divides the cytoplasm into interdigitating processes (Figs. 8, 9). The brush border in addition to the plasma membrane is covered by an amorphous layer.

At the base of the microvilli, there are invaginations that are considered to be sites of pinocytosis. Deeper in the cytoplasm are vacuoles with light content. These vacuoles are varying in size and enlarge in osmotic diuresis. In addition, tubular structures, the dark apical tubules, and rough endoplasmic reticulum are seen in the apical portion of these cells. Mitochondria are numerous as are other organelles. Close to the nucleus is a prominent Golgi complex, rough and smooth endoplasmic reticulum and characteristic microbodies of somewhat heterogeneous structure, that correspond to the light microscopist's cytoplasmic granules or hyaline droplets. They may or may not be limited by a membrane,

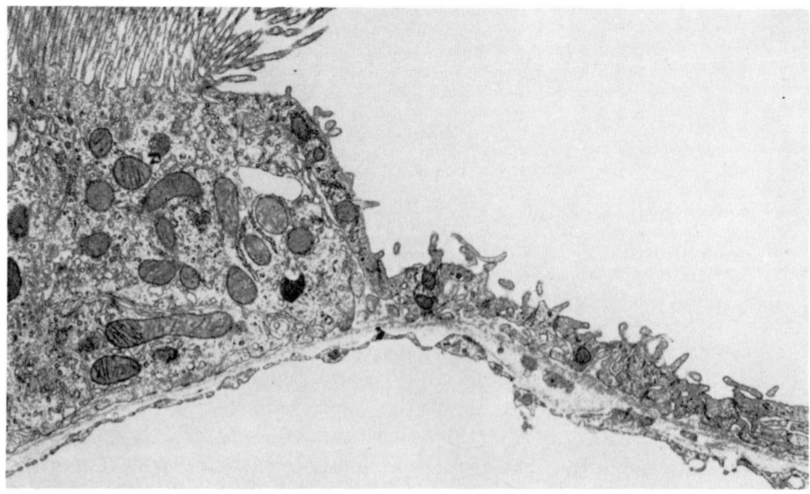

Fig. 10. Transition between proximal tubule and descending thin limb of Henle's loop. (From: Osvaldo L., and Latta, H.: With permission of the authors and of Academic Press, New York (12).)

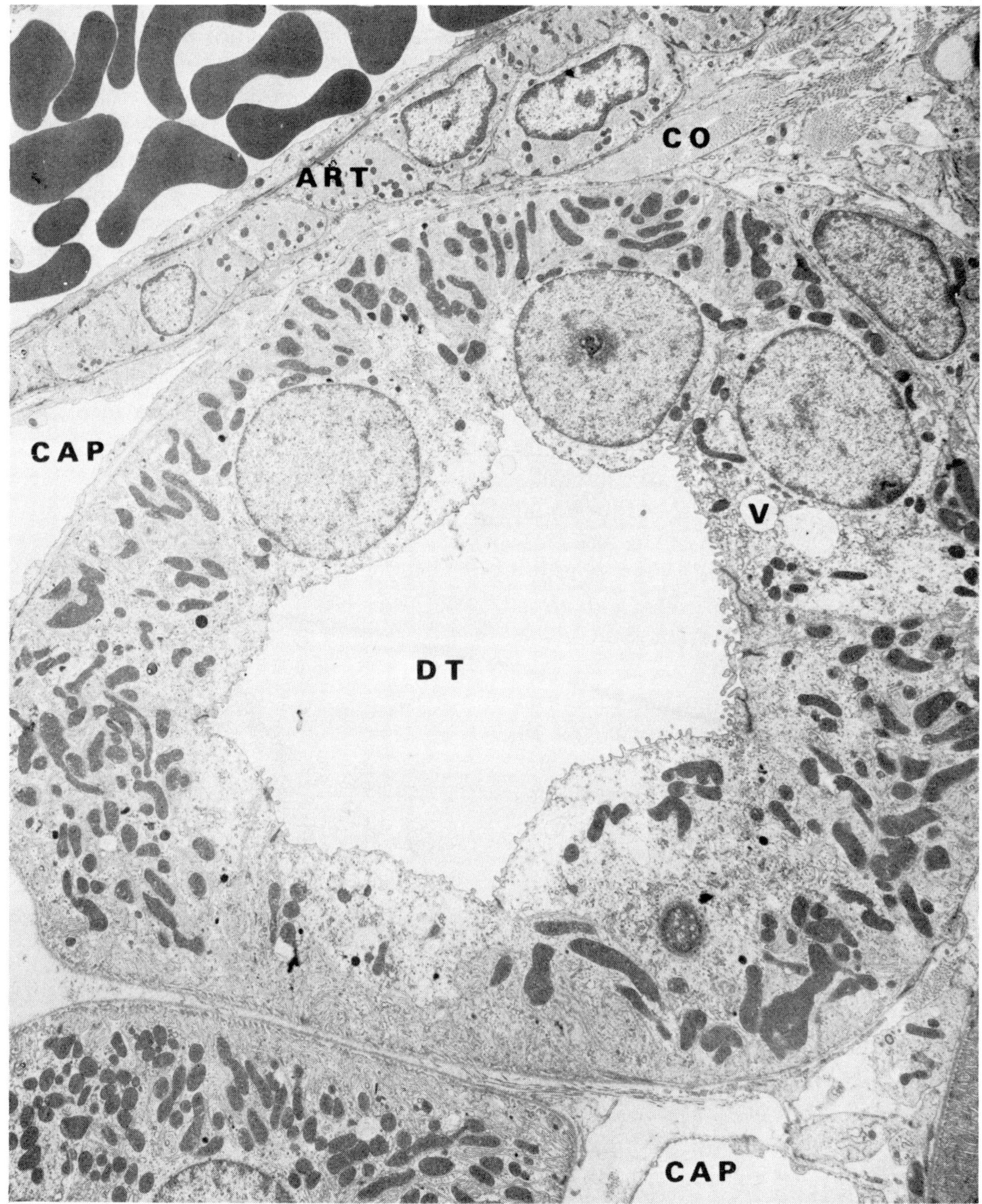

Fig. 11. Distal tubule (DT). Short irregular microvilli are present. The apical cytoplasm shows vacuolization (V). The basal plasma membrane forms deep infoldings. Note also artery (ART), capillaries (CAP) and collagen fibers (CO). (x 7,000)

and may or may not contain acid phosphatase (Mannsbach (9)). In addition, multivesicular bodies with amorphous or crystalline inclusions may be present.

The epithelial cells are supported by a well formed basement membrane and are in close contact with capillaries at their base. Between cells, the plasma membrane forms prominent attachment zones, the zonula adherens, and small tight junctions known as zonula occludens. These attachments prevent leakage of tubular fluid into the intercellular space. The large number of complex membranes and organelles is an anatomic expression of the high rate of metabolic activity that takes place in the proximal tubules. Here, 80 to 85% of the glomerular filtrate is reabsorbed. This requires the active transport of Na and to a limited extent of glucose, phosphate and other compounds.

Differences in distribution of apical vacuoles and microbodies, in the size of the mitochondria and in the development of the basal and lateral infoldings of the plasma membrane are known to occur in parts of the convoluted tubule and between the convoluted and straight portion of the proximal tubule, with the straight portion showing fewer or smaller of these organelles and membranes.

The transition between straight portion and thin segment of Henle's loop is abrupt. It is illustrated by Osvaldo and Latta in Figure 10 (12). The microvilli at the luminal surface and interdigitating projections of the plasma membrane at the basilar and lateral surfaces are characteristic of the descending thin loops, and are absent in the ascending portions.

The distal tubule includes the thick ascending segment of the loop of Henle and the distal convoluted part.

A special area is the macula densa where the convoluted part begins. This forms part of the juxtaglomerular apparatus. The cells are taller and closer together with large elliptical nuclei and are in direct contact with the lacis (Fig. 7). Between cells and cytoplasmic processes, extracellular compartments may be prominent and this is considered an indication of the great osmotic sensitivity of the area.

The intercalated part forms the large cortical portion of the distal convoluted tubule (Figs. 11, 12). Characteristic of the convoluted tubule is the basilar plasma membrane with deep infoldings

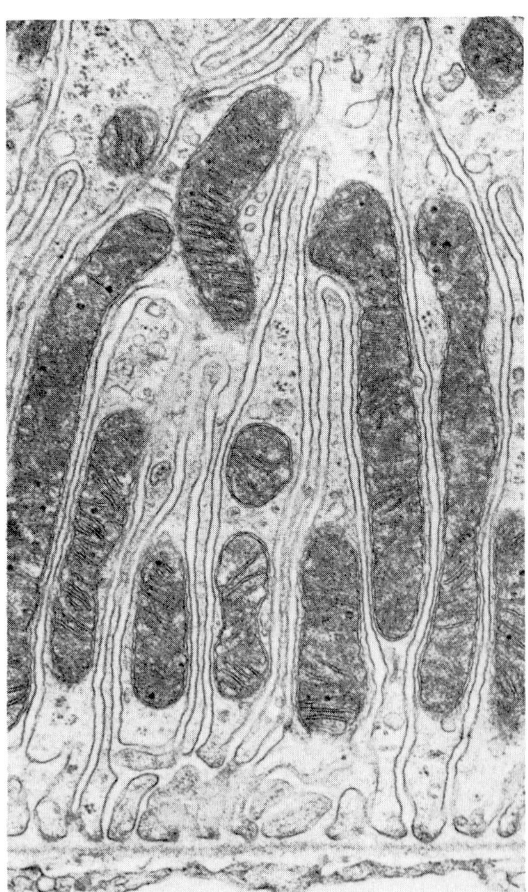

Fig. 12. Distal tubule. Enlargement of basal part to illustrate the complex course of the basilar plasma membrane and its close relation to the mitochondria. (x 33,000)

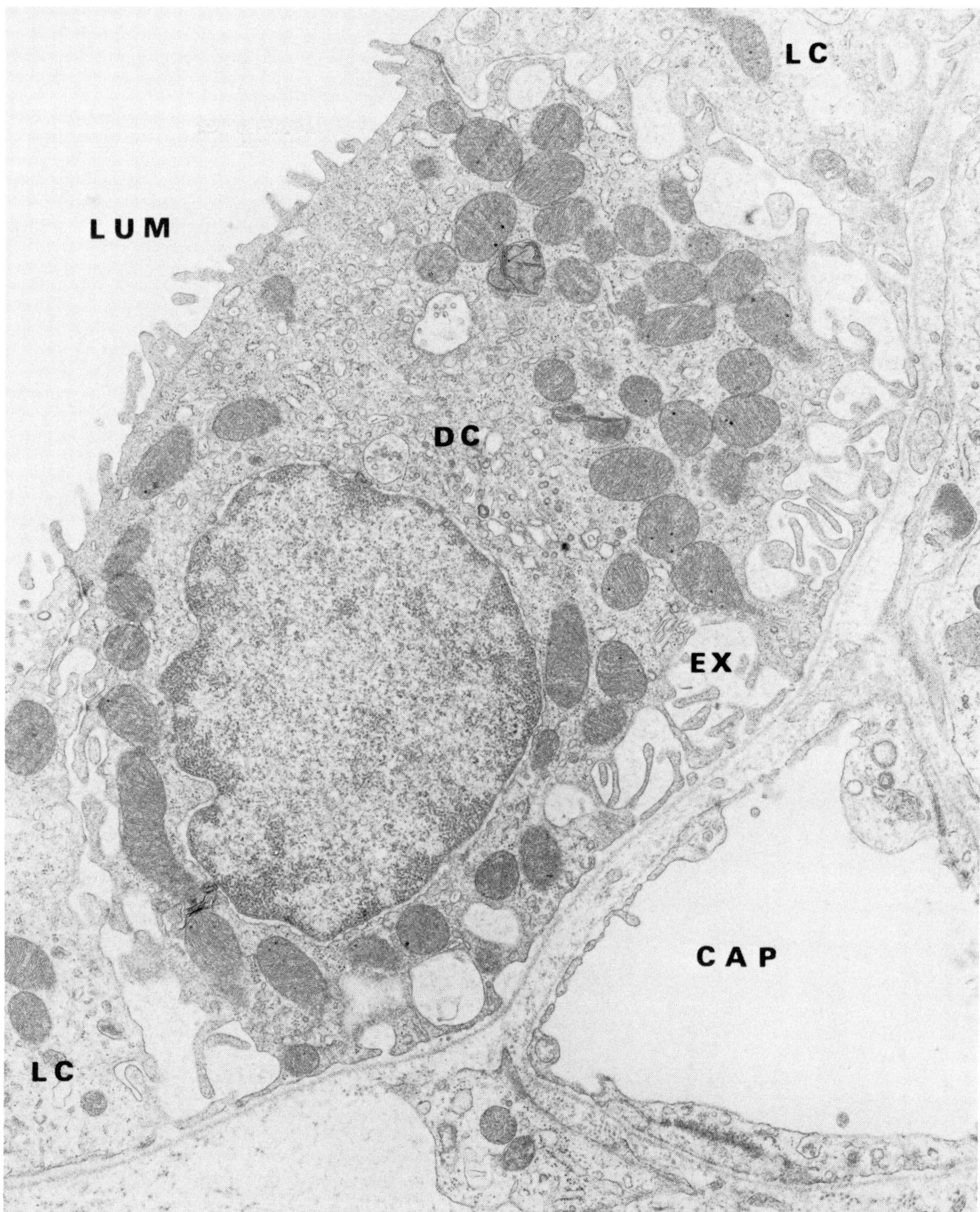

Fig. 13. Dark cell (DC) of medullary collecting tubule. Note the large extracellular compartment (EX). Compare the dense crowded cytoplasm with that of the light cells (LC) on the sides. The capillary endothelium is fenestrated with the diaphragm visible as a dark line. The capillary basement membrane is thin and it closely parallels that of the tubule. (x 26,000)

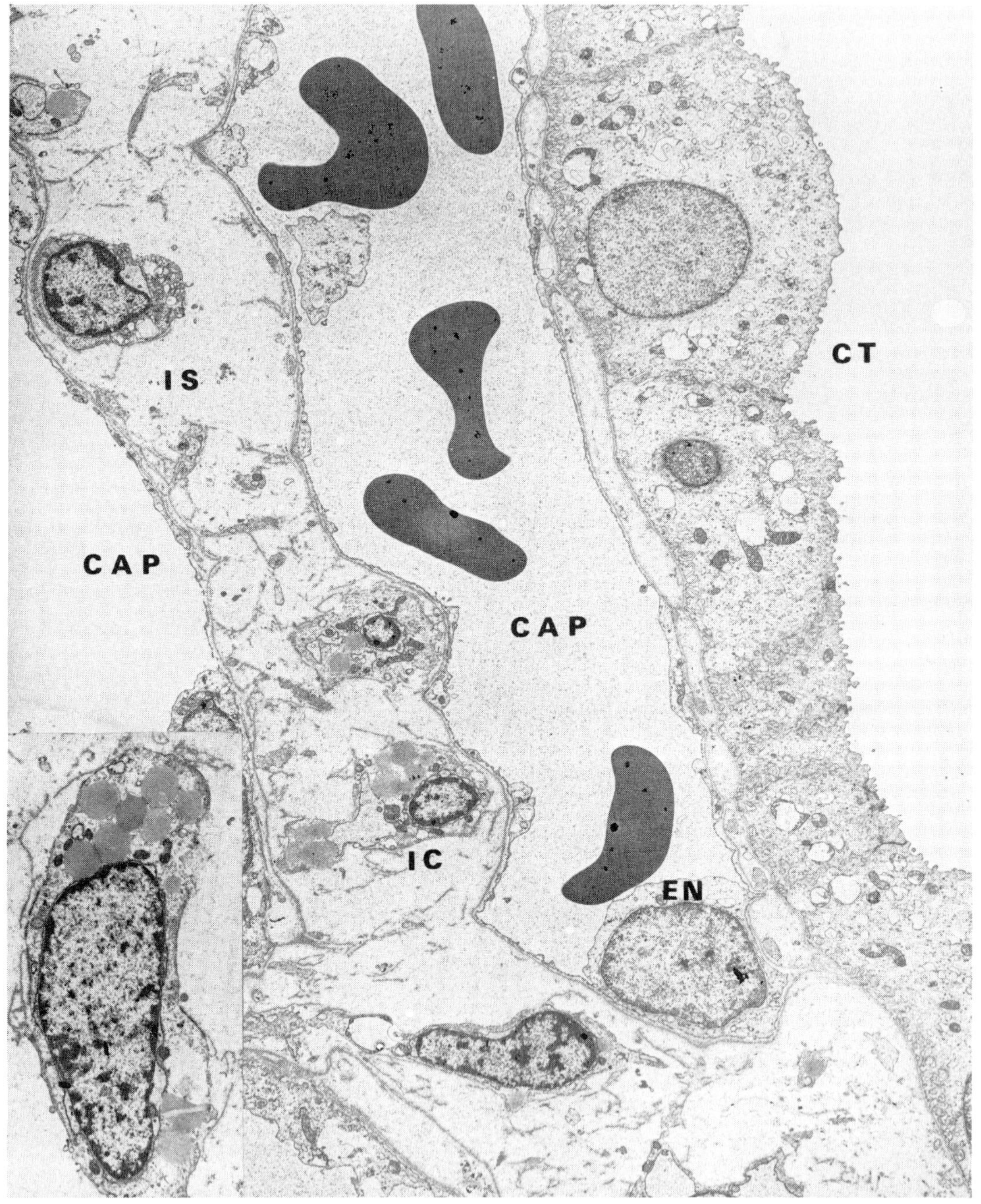

Fig. 14. Inner layer of medulla. The illustration shows a collecting tubule (CT), capillaries, (CAP), and interstitial space (IS) with interstitial cells (IC). Note the endothelial cell (EN) and its attenuated fenestrated portion that lines the capillaries. An interstitial cell is seen in the insert. (x 5,000. Insert, x 8,250)

and the close relationship of mitochondria to these membranes. The apical portion of the cells shows few irregular microvilli and vacuoles are seen in the cytoplasm.

The collecting tubules have a cortical and a medullary portion. The epithelium is formed of low cuboidal cells, rather light in appearance with few single cells with dark cytoplasm. These dark cells show microvilli and basilar infoldings (Fig. 13). The cytoplasmic matrix is denser and more organelles are present in these cells. Dark cells become less numerous in the medullary collecting tubules.

The Medulla. Functional anatomy of the medulla is best understood when the tubules, blood vessels and interstitial tissue are studied in an integrated manner. The thin loops of Henle, medullary collecting tubules and the capillaries have a parallel course to each other, with interstitial cells oriented perpendicular to their direction (Fig. 15). There is, in addition to the well known change in osmotic gradient which increases from the base to the tip of the renal papillae, an oxygen gradient with increasing anoxia toward the tip of the papillae. The entire blood supply of the medulla as it is emphasized by Spargo is carried in thin walled loops of capillaries from the cortico-medullary junction where afferent and efferent vessels may be in contact to favor countercurrent exchange.

The capillary endothelium is attenuated in both afferent and efferent branches but the efferent capillary endothelium is fenestrated. There is a thin basement membrane but no capillary pericyte to support these vessels. The interstitial cells bridge the space from capillary basement membrane to that of the tubules suspended in a space largely filled by fluid (Fig. 14).

Fig. 15. Photomicrograph of the renal papilla, inner layer. Note the thin loop of Henle and its relationship to the capillaries, collecting tubule and interstitial cells. (x 500)

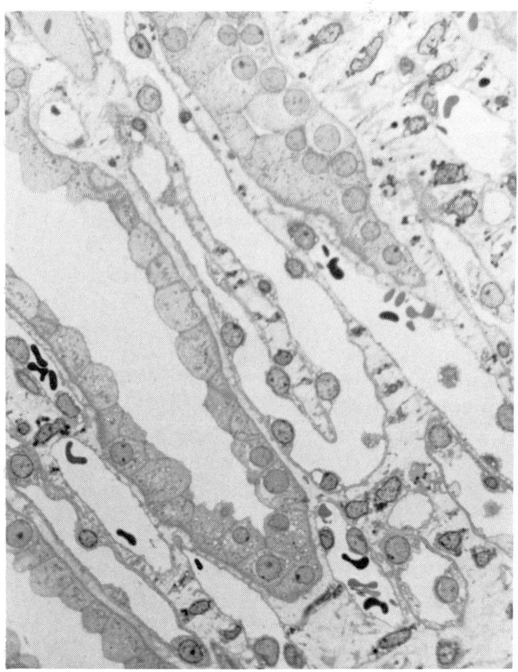

It should be stated in conclusion that the contribution of many investigators to the current knowledge of ultrastructural anatomy of the kidney could not be mentioned in this short description although their findings were fundamental. The information is already of practical significance. The renal glomerules, for example, undergo diagnostic morphologic changes under many pathologic conditions and early changes may be detected by electron microscopy long before they become evident by the classical histologic methods. Thus, study of ultrastructure has direct applications to patient care, and it is indispensable in elucidating normal functions of the kidney and pathogenesis of renal disease.

Diseases primarily affecting the renal tubules are currently being investigated and with modern techniques of fixation and sectioning it is hoped that early lesions will become detectable by electron microscopy, enlarging again by a step the scope of laboratory diagnosis.

The assistance of Joseph T. Blake in preparation of illustrations is gratefully acknowledged.

REFERENCES

1. Bohle, A., and Herfarth, C.: Zur Frage eines intercapillarien Bindegewebes im Glomerulus der Niere des Menschen. Arch. Pathol. Anat. Physiol., *331*, 573-90.
2. Farquahar, M. G., and Palade, G. E.: Segregation of ferritin in glomerular protein absorption droplets. J. Biophys. Biochem. Cytol., 7:297-304, 1960.
3. Farquhar, M. G., and Palade, G. E.: Functional evidence for the existence of a third cell type in the renal glomerulus. J. Cell Biol., *13*:55-87, 1962.
4. Goormaghtigh, N.: La fonction endocrine des arterioles renales. Louvain, Librairie Fonteyn, 1942.
5. Hartroft, P. M., and Hartroft, W. S.: Studies on renal juxtaglomerular cells. I: Variation produced by sodium chloride and desoxycorticosterone acetate. J. Expl. Med., *97*:415-427, 1953.
6. Hartroft, P. M., and Newmark, L. N.: Electron microscopy of renal juxtaglomerular cells. Anat. Rec., *139*:185-199, 1961.
7. Hatt, P. Y.: The juxtaglomerular apparatus. In Dalton, A. J., and Haguenau, F. (eds): Ultrastructure of the Kidney. New York, Academic Press, 1967.
8. Ito, S.: The surface coating of enteric microvilli. Anat. Rec., *148:*294 (abstract).
9. Maunsbach, A. B.: Electron microscopic observations of cytoplasmic bodies with crystalline patterns in rat kidney proximal tubule cells. J. Ultrastructure Res., *14*:167-189, 1966.
10. Latta, H., Maunsbach, A. B., and Osvaldo, L.: The fine structure of renal tubules in cortex and medulla. In Dalton, A. J., and Haguenau, F. (eds.): Ultrastructure of the Kidney. New York, Academic Press, 1967, pp. 1-56.
11. Menefee, M. G., and Mueller, C. B.: Some morphological considerations of transport in the glomerulus. In Dalton, A. J., and Hagnenan, F. (eds.): Ultrastructure of the Kidney. New York, Academic Press, 1967.
12. Osvaldo, L., and Latta, H.: The thin limbs of the loop of Henle. J. Ultrastructural Res., *15*:144-168, 1966.
13. Pitts, R. F.: Physiology of the Kidney and Body Fluids. Chicago, Year Book, 1963.
14. Rhodin, J. A. G.: The diaphragm of capillary endothelial fenestrations. J. Ultrastructure. Res., *6*:171-185, 1962.
15. Rhodin, J. A. G.: An Atlas of Ultrastructure. Philadelphia, Saunders, 1963, 222pp.
16. Rhodin, J. A. G.: Structure of the kidney. In Strauss, M. B., and Welt, L. G. (eds.): Diseases of the Kidney. Boston, Little, Brown, 1963, pp. 1-29.
17. Sakaguchi, H., and Kawamura, S.: Electron microscopic observations on mesangiolysis. The toxic effects of "Habu Snake" venom on the renal glomerulus. Keio J. Med., *12*:99-106.
18. Spargo, B. H.: Structure of the kidney. In Mostofi, F. U., and Smith, D. E. (eds): The Kidney. Baltimore, Williams and Wilkins, 1966, pp. 17-59.
19. Yamada, E.: The fine structure of the renal glomerulus of the mouse. J. Biophys. Biochem. Cytol., *1:551-566, 1955.*
20. von Mollendorff, W.: Der Exretionsapparat. In von Mollendorff, W. (ed.): Handbuch der Mikroscopischen Anatomie des Menschen, 7, Part 1, 1-328. Berlin, Springer, 1930.

Chapter 2

Correlations of Renal Function and Morphogenesis in the Embryo and Neonate

BETTY VOGH, PH.D., and SIDNEY CASSIN, PH.D.

Since 1881, when a Frenchman named Bar (34) injected ferrocyanide into 24-day rabbit fetuses, work has been underway to understand renal function before birth. Structure and function have usually been studied as separate entities, and even today it is unusual for a single investigator to look at both. Correlations must be made from the work of many.

Pioneering studies of human fetal and neonatal function date from 1945 to 1955 largely and have tended to develop a nearly universal belief that renal function at birth is "immature." The word "immature" has not been rigorously defined, and we should like to distinguish between inability to perform adult functions and rate of performance or functional capacity. That certain differences between newborn and adult renal capacities do exist seems unquestionable; but the blanket application of the concept "immaturity" to the whole of renal function at and following birth seems unwarranted.

Considerations in this chapter are confined largely to data on human kidney, but with occasional digressions to draw supportive evidence from other species. Attention is directed to the following categories of renal function: 1) physical development; 2) osmotic function and filtration; 3) secretory function; 4) transport of electrolytes, and 5) acidification.

The human embryo, in contrast to lower vertebrates, does not develop a clearly defined pronephros. The mesonephros develops from the lower cervical and upper thoracic portions of the so called "intermediate cell masses" which fuse to become the nephrogenic cord (19, 36). First to form is the mesonephric duct which enters the cloaca. Then primitive tubules arise, and each tubule elongates to contact a newly formed glomerlus and to join into the mesonephric duct. The 4mm human fetus has a functioning mesonephros (2, 31). The mesonephros develops maximally between the fourth and ninth weeks (2, 31), gaining more and more nephrons, with each glomerulus fed by a glomerular artery directly off the embryonic aorta (19).

Both light and electron microscopy by de Martino and Zamboni (31) verifies that in the mesonephros each glomerlar artery arranges itself into an afferent and an efferent vessel on either side of a dense capillary tuft. The efferent vessel gives off a branch to the interstitium. Electron microscopy shows that the afferent and efferent vessels contain no myoepithelial cells, nor do they come into juxtaposition. There is no juxta-glomerular apparatus. The vessels are filled with immature blood cells. Glomerular capillaries are surrounded by endothelial cells and visceral epithelial cells just as in the adult, but both layers are thicker than in the adult kidney. A well developed basal membrane underlies the endothelium. The visceral epithelium extends foot processes of variable sizes over the basement membrane. Fenestrations in the endothelium are few in number but very similar to those in adult (31). Foot processes of the visceral layer of the human fetus are unlike adult in that no trabeculae with slits between are seen.

The capsular spaces of the glomeruli are continous with the tubules. Proximal portions of the tubules are lined with microvilli. Between the microvilli, invaginations leading to intracellular vesicles are frequent. Nuclei are basally placed, and the abundant cytoplasm contains numerous granules and organelles. Distal tubules are connected to proximal tubules by a short, but not thin, segment of cells which are transitional in morphology. Distal tubular cells contain few or no organelles in the apical portions but basal portions contain a high concentration of mitochondria around the nucleus.

Since the work of Gersh in 1937, the mesonephros has been known to be capable of secretion and filtration (18). The low net filtration pressure, thick cell layers and dearth of fenestration lead us to believe that filtration per glomerulus would be low, but in the absence of measurements we could as well argue that none of these structures is rate limiting and that, given the filtration pressure, fetal and adult rates would be comparable. It is unknown whether the major route of transfer is direct secretion into the tubule or glomerular filtration (20).

Figure 1 is a drawing adapted from Haines and Mohuiddin (19) and Torrey (31). It depicts rather schematically the mature mesonephros, degenerating rostrally, still forming caudally. The mesonephros functions until the end of the fourth gestational month, producing a fluid which is hypoosmotic. Near the end of this time, a diverticulum or metanephric bud forms where the mesonephric duct enters the cloaca. Around the bud, the lumbar and sacral portions of the nephrogenic cord gather to form a blastema. The inset in Figure 1 shows the beginning of the elaboration of the metanephros or adult kidney from the bud and blastema. The bud subdivides and elongates, one end of the elongated portion becoming the renal pelvis with collecting ducts, the other the ureter. From within the blastema, new nephrons form and open into collecting ducts.

From these details, it can be seen that the earliest human kidney is quite similar in structure to the adult kidney. Each nephron has, however, far less total tissue than a nephron from an adult so that its overall function might be limited.

The task is now to describe how nearly complete the development of the metanephros is in late gestation and early postnatal life. To this end, it will be useful to consider the concept of renal development favored by Torrey (36) the concept of the holonephros. Torrey regards the pronephros of lower

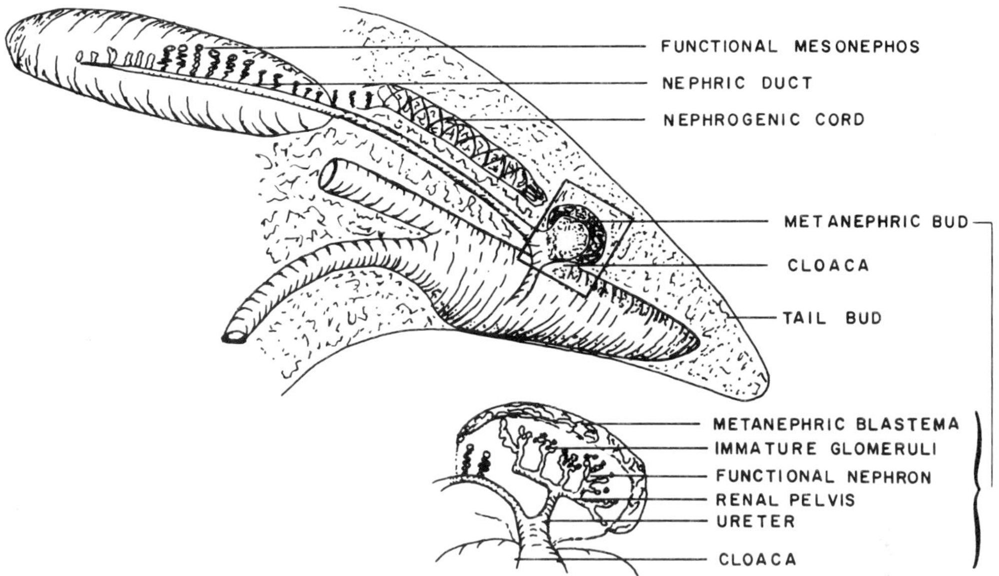

Fig. 1. Schematic representation of the mesonephros and beginning metanephros of the human embryo. Note the presence of defunct nephrons of simple structure in the rostral mesonephros at the same time nephrons having convoluted tubules are functioning in the mid-portion. New nephrons are shown still forming in the caudad mesonephros and, below these, the metanephric bud is beginning to develop. The inset shows the early nephrons, pelvis and ureter forming from the metanephric bud. Drawing adapted from Haines and Mohuiddin (19) and Torrey (35). The authors thank Mr. Arthur Ellison for preparing this drawing.

mammals, the mesonephros and the metanephros as parts of a functional and morphological continuum. As seen in Figure 1, there is a gross morphological continuum, but this alone is not sufficient to support Torrey's concept. Many structures are emerging or disappearing in the embryo. But, it is significant that although the earliest mesonephrons are very simple in form, their fine structure differs hardly at all from the fine structure of the adult kidney in man (31) and in other mammals which have been studied (23). It is likewise significant that cellular transport of weak acids (16, 18, 22) in the three stages of embryonic kidney is qualitatively alike.

Gersh did not study human embryos, but his 1937 paper deserves attention.

His experiments cover a wide phylogenetic range: cats, rabbits, pigs, opossums, and chicks. His paper reviews the work of men whose technically less perfect experiments he set out to improve. Although his results are only qualitative, they confirm elimination from the embryo of ferrocyanide primarily by glomerular filtration, and of phenol red primarily by secretion in all stages of mesonephric and metanephric development in all species tested. Secretion of phenol red is present as soon as proximal tubular cells have differentiated. At least in rabbit and chick this precedes the beginning of glomerular filtration. [Secretion of phenol red has since been shown in pro- and mesonephrons of flounder and frog to be competitive with para-aminohippurate and penicillin (16, 22).] The secretory processes employ phosphate bond energy derived from anaerobic metabolism (16, 22). The beginning of filtration does not appear to correlate with any light-visible histologic changes. Gersh (18) also showed that the aging mesonephros may functionally overlap a developing metanephros, the two performing as one. Thus, when the rostro-caudad degeneration of the mesonephros proceeds at a rate greater than the development of the metanephros, a decrease in renal enzyme activity (7, 11) or phenol red (18) secretion takes place. Gersh (18) found that at a variable interval after glomerular and tubular functions have become established, water reabsorption (as evidenced by increase in dye concentration) begins to occur in the loops of Henle. This is seen only in tubules in which the cells in the transitional zone between proximal and distal tubules have become thin envelopes of cytoplasm barely covering the nuclei, structure typical of adult loops.

If one applies Gersh's morphological criteria for secretion and water reabsorption to the human embryo, then this embryo should begin to secrete when it is 32 mm long (at which time about 15 nephrons can be seen) and should reabsorb water in the loop of Henle at 81 mm (about 13 weeks gestational age). Recent dissections of human tubules by Osathanondh and Potter (32) indicate that loops of Henle become thin as soon as the tubules to which they belong elongate to lie caudal to the glomerular structure, i.e., in the 8 to 9 week fetus of 25 to 30 mm. At this stage, 12 to 20 nephrons are attached to the mesonephric duct. Before elongation each tubule lies in an S-shaped coil above its glomerulus. It seems reasonable to conclude from Gersh's data and from later work as well (16, 22, 35) that urine is being formed in the adult pattern in all stages of embryonic development and that the age differences in renal function are differences in degree rather than kind.

Studies of renal enzyme activities as clues to renal maturity have been pursued with enthusiasm. The phosphatases have received a major share of attention both as possible initiators of differentiation processes and as energy suppliers for active transport, but despite careful studies (9) conclusions in this area are largely speculative.

Efforts to correlate excretion of nitrogen as ammonia, urea or uric acid with dominance of pro-, meso- or metanephros could not be confirmed (8). Enzyme activity associated with production of uric acid in chicks' urine correlated with the number of functioning nephrons. Similar correlation with the number of functioning nephrons has been found for other enzymes (7). Enzyme changes are still being sought which might be causally related to induction of differentiation. To date, the lactic dehydrogenase isozymes are the only group of enzymes which have a correlation between concentration of various forms of the enzyme and age of the fetal kidney. This relationship has been studied mostly in chicks (30) and mice (11).

It may be asked whether or not the neonatal kidney is prepared to handle a solute load or a water load or an acid load. To answer this, more must be known about the loop of Henle and the renal papilla, as well as something about the way in which loads and responses to loads are expressed, and a little about the body fluid compartments.

The loops of Henle and portions of

the distal tubules are the sites of renal concentrating and diluting mechanisms. The length of a loop in the metanephros depends to a large extent on the age of the nephron (32), for all portions of the tubules grow until the tubules reach the renal pelvis, and thereafter growth is chiefly an elongation of the thin portion. For early-formed tubules, the distance from nephrogenic zone to pelvis is short and the time remaining for elongation of the thin segment is great. At birth, all but 7 to 20% of the tubules have extended below the corticomedullary junction (14, 32). However, only about one-eighth of all the nephrons in the kidney of an adult have a long ascending and descending loop of Henle. Those nephrons originating in the final days of nephrogenesis (usually 34th week, sometimes after delivery at term), would not be expected to develop loops, for their tubules would not reach the pelvis before growth ceased. Nephrons control concentration or dilution of urine by virtue of their ability to reabsorb sodium and to concentrate it and urea in the papilla, and by their response to antidiuretic hormone. Whether the response is one of dilution or concentration will depend on the amount of change in body salt or water content, the fluid volume into which the change is distributed, the sensitivity of volume and osmoreceptors to the concentration changes and the sensitivity of the tubules to hormones such as antidiuretic hormone and aldosterone. It should be kept in mind that the total body water as per cent of body weight falls throughout fetal life and at birth is about 10% higher than the adult value (17). Of this water, a larger proportion is extracellular than intracellular. This relationship reverses by about the third postnatal month as more and more soft tissue and bone is

laid down. A water load or a solute load calculated on a body weight basis must be thought of as distributed into a proportionately much larger volume in the newborn than in the adult. It would then cause less change in concentration and less stimulation to volume or osmoreceptors. These receptors may be innately less responsive at birth than later.

It has been pointed out that although each differentiated cell has adult or adult-like functions, the total mass of cells is quite small at birth as compared to adulthood. A newborn kidney may weigh 30 gm (28). An adult kidney will weigh about 300 gm (34). In order to discuss how this small kidney functions for its age, its function should be related in some way to the size of the tissues it serves. In most investigations of postnatal renal function, this is done by calculating doses, flow rates, urine volumes, etc., either per kilogram of body weight or per some function of body weight presumed to estimate surface area. Then the final result is expressed as function per 1.73 meter^2, thus extrapolating to the area of the 70 kilogram man. For many years, this has been the accepted practice since no other basis provides such a ready comparison to the adult. The use of surface area and other standards of comparison is discussed in detail by Homer Smith (34). It is possible to alter conclusions about maturation of function by using body weight or some other basis of calculation of results (24, 26, 34).

Rose Ames (3) reported in 1953 a study of the human newborn response to water loading. Her work still stands as authoritative. She gave 30 ml per kg orally to infants and found that the volume excreted in 3 hours varied directly with age, being less than 10% of the load on the first day of life and 100% of load by 1 month of age. Work in dog and rat showed a similar age-correlated decrease in time to peak of diureses and increase in height of flow (1). [But McCance and Taylor (24) found newborn equal to adult reponse when the load was 6% of body water.] Ames (3) then investigated the response to antidiuretic hormone (ADH) and found that term infants less than 3 days of age gave no response although endogenous ADH was present in their urine. Infants 5 days old responded with a brief decrease in diureses when given 5.5 to 7.5 milliunits per meter^2. The conclusion is usually drawn, from probably insufficient evidence, that some immaturity of the renal tubule makes it insensitive to ADH until the fifth day, or that the brevity of the majority of the loops of Henle at birth causes an inadequate osmotic gradient across the tubule.

Upon this latter point, it may be said that the young rabbit and rat have been shown by Yaffee and Anders (43) to have a sodium concentration in the renal papilla equal to that of the adult, hence a sodium gradient equal to adult. Urea, however, is low in the papilla of the newborn. The result for the infant is a maximal concentration of urine to only 500 to 600 mosm per liter during water deprivation unless a high protein diet is fed to the newborn. Urine concentration on a high protein intake can rise to 1200 mosm per liter (12). The infant does not have difficulty diluting urine (retaining salts while excreting free water) but can dilute urine to one-sixth the osmolality of plasma. This matches the adult minimum value (6, 42).

Low glomerular filtration rate (GFR) is often cited as a cause of poor response to water loading (12, 39). According to Adolph, GFR shows no relationship to

diuretic response (1). That the GFR is low is widely accepted as fact. Not all glomeruli have reached their maximal development by the time of birth and the capillaries of immature glomeruli are covered by thick cell layers. Figure 2a (40) describes the histology of the newborn pig kidney. The human fetus at about 32 weeks looks very much like this, with two layers of new structures recognizable as glomeruli and a relatively amorphous area between them and the capsule. Whereas this nephrogenic zone usually ceases to function before birth in the human, it persists until about 30 days of age in the pig. At that time, the kidney still shows a paucity of tubular tissue. Figure 2b shows the pig kidney at 30 days. By 65 to 70 days tubular mass

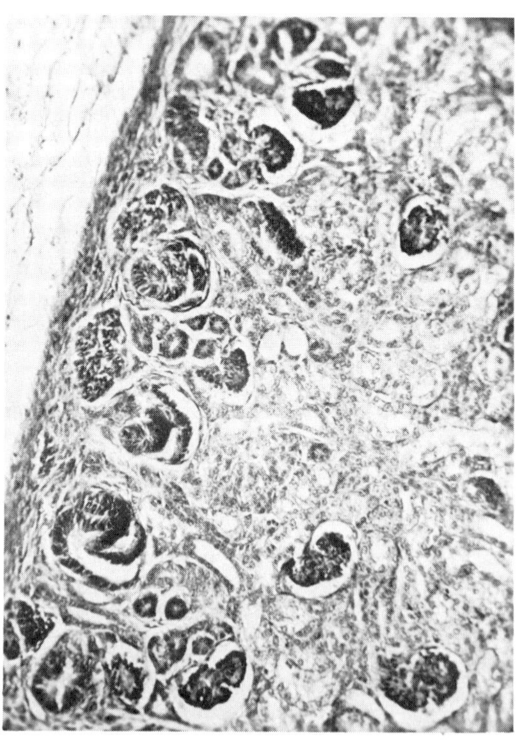

Fig. 2a. Section through renal cortex of a pig 12 hours old. Note the high density of newly formed glomeruli arising from the relatively amorphous nephrogenic zone.

appears to be fully developed. The advent of birth, at least in the human, seems to stimulate the thinning out of the cells that have been assumed to be the physical barriers to filtration. Possibly the rising blood pressure after birth, increasing net filtration pressure, is important in bringing about the change in cell height in the endothelial and epithelial layers of the glomeruli.

Barnett (4), using the 1.73 meter^2 basis, found GFR to be about 50 ml per minute (in contrast to the adult value of 125 ml per minute) while premature infants 49 to 107 days postnatal age but having the same body weights as the term infants had GFR of about 70 ml per minute. Vesterdal (38) and others report lower figures for GFR in infants. The range of values reported by Smith (34) as a composite of values from the work of many investigators is 15 to 65% of adult GFR for the first postnatal month. These data are all calculated on the basis of surface area.

The early appearance of a capacity for secretion of weak acids by proximal tubular tissue has already been discussed. However, the renal blood flow in the newborn has not as yet been considered. Smith gives the clearance of para-aminohippurate (PAH) in infants as 5 to 50% of adult during the first month of life (34). All the work prior to 1960 assumed normal adult extraction of PAH by the nephrons and, as a result, reported immature blood flow. Calcagno and coworkers (5) measured extraction ratios and found them 30% lower in the newborn than in the adult, reaching adult value by the eighth month. It cannot be said whether this low extraction means less transporting structure, less transport energy, incomplete vascular development or lack of juxtaposition of vascular elements to proximal tubules.

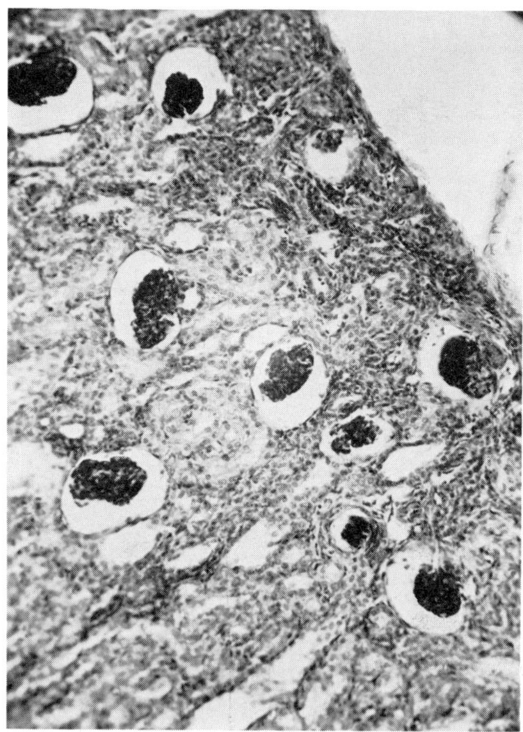

Fig. 2b. Section through renal cortex of a pig 30 days old. No new glomeruli are being formed, but the spacing of those recently formed indicates that only a small amount of the tubular mass has developed for these glomeruli. Both sections are P. A. S. stained and magnified 235 times.

The myth that glomerular function matures faster than tubular function was dispelled when the extraction was determined. Filtration fraction expressed as GFR/clearance of PAH is high, but the fraction GFR/ true renal plasma flow gives the normal adult value of 0.20. This implies equal rates of maturation of the two functions.

Despite the fact that not all of the proximal convolutions are completed, and that the brush border is less dense than later (37), the newborn infant can reabsorb sodium very efficiently (33, 41) and, as has been shown, the medullary concentration of sodium does not appear to be deficient. In fact, the young

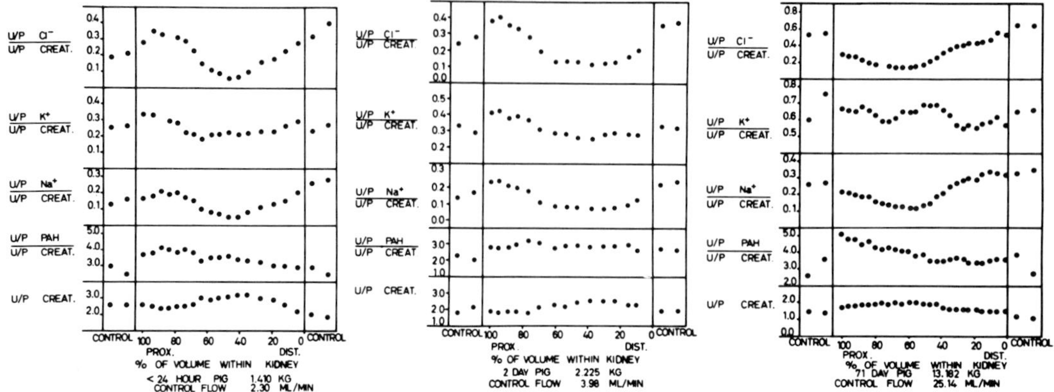

Fig. 3. Comparison of stop flow information from three pigs, one less than 24 hrs., one 2 days and on 71 days after birth. The animals were given 20% mannitol intravenously and water (10 ml/kg at 30 minute intervals) by stomach. Urine flow rates were 1.6, 1.8 and 1.8 ml/kg minute, respectively, prior to ureteral occlusion. Urine was held within the tubules 7 minutes, then serially collected for analysis.

kidney has some difficulty getting rid of a salt load because of its high reasorbative capacity and its low ability to concentrate. In a classic study in 1949, Dean and McCance (10) gave 10% sodium chloride to the extent of 0.8 to 1.4 gm/kg to infants and adults and found that the adults had excreted nearly all the load before the newborn saluresis was at maximal intensity. Here, again, it may be asked whether the load per kilogram provides the same stimulus to systemic and renal mechanisms in newborn as in adult. The newborn and adult responses to salt loading differ in this respect: the adult dilutes his urine from a high osmolality while the newborn elaborates a more concentrated urine than usual. The final product of the two differs but little in osmolality (10). It should be remembered that the load given by Dean and McCance is well beyond normal physiological load. The aldosterone response for the infant is not known (39). As another means of looking at renal function in the newborn quantitatively, stopflow experiments were undertaken (29) on newborn and maturing pigs (40). Figure 3 shows the results from three of these animals. The data are plotted, as for most stopflow data, so as to rule out the effects of water reabsorption by using the ratio: clearance of X/clearance of inulin or creatinine. This ratio is plotted for serial samples of urine collected after release of urine held 6 to 7 minutes within the kidney. Here X is either sodium, potassium, chloride or PAH. Mannitol loading was employed to establish a large diuresis. Allowing for all the possible artifacts which accrue to stopflow experiments, we have never the less shown that when the urine flow per kilogram was approximately equal for the different ages, their stop flow patterns are nearly identical. Values of the ratio greater than 1 indicate net secretion; values less than 1, net reabsorption. These studies provide further evidence that when similarly stimulated to respond, the kidney at different ages elaborates urine in much the same way. The ages shown here cover a range of morphological changes from that seen in Figure 2a to complete maturity.

Control of acid-base balance is not neglected by the newborn kidney. It produces little NH_4^+ before birth but excretes NH_4^+ readily after birth (27). As the total acid excreted increases with age, the fraction excreted as NH_4^+ increases. Titratable acid increases also, limited only by the availability of inorganic phosphate in the diet (25). Breast milk contains less phosphate than cow's milk, and in a breast-fed baby a higher proportion of the total acid will be excreted as NH_4^+ (21). Even though the capacity to lower urinary pH in response to an NH_4Cl load is low at 7 days of age in breast-fed babies (21), urinary pH in the the normal physiological state is as low as for the adult, both in newborn babies fed cow's milk (25, 27, 33) and in infants one month of age (13). The infant may have difficulty handling a sodium bicarbonate load since he does not excrete the sodium excess rapidly, but his renal regulation of plasma bicarbonate level is well developed. The renal threshold for excretion of bicarbonate is a plasma concentration of 21.5 to 22.5mM, lower than the adult threshold. This threshold, which obtains at least throughout the first year of life is the cause of the so-called acidosis of the infant. The maximal reabsorption rate of bicarbonate per 100 ml of glomerular filtrate is identical to the adult value (13).

Vesterdal (39) discussed some func-tional limitations of the newborn kidney and, while maintaining that these were immaturities, he nevertheless adopted the reasoning which McCance and Widdowson (41, p.159) have proposed for years: namely, that the newborn kidney is capable of doing all that it is normally called upon to do. While it may be slow in responding to pathological demands, it has been observed that no normal adult response is completely absent.

There are changes in function, such as the beginning of filtration, and differences in function such as those between some species, for which no morphological explanation exists. Furthermore, no one has isolated any structural feature which can be held responsible for the business of active or carrier mediated renal transport. Forster points out (15) that further study of structures in relation to functions is necessary for an understanding of the mechanism of the dynamic equilibrium which the renal tubular cells maintain. Based upon present information it may be concluded that the newborn renal response as well as the adult is proportional primarily to the mass of functioning tissue when extra-renal factors controlling kidney function are equally operative. The age-dependency of extra-renal stimuli deserves careful consideration in any investigation of prenatal or postnatal renal function.

BIBLIOGRAPHY

1. Adolph, E. F.: Ontogeny of physiology regulation in the rat. Quart. Rev. Biol., *32:*89-137, 1957.
2. Alexander, D. P., and Nixon, D. A.: The foetal kidney. Brit. Med. Bull., *17:*112-118, 1961.
3. Ames, R. G.: Urinary water excretion and neurohypophyseal function in full term and premature infants shortly after birth. Pediatrics, *12:*272-281, 1953.
4. Barnett, H. L.: Influence of postnatal age on kidney function of premature infants. Proc. Soc. Exptl. Biol. Med., *69:*55-57, 1948.
5. Calcagno, P. L., Rubin, M. I., and Bruck, E.: True effective renal plasma flow and filtration fraction in young infants as determined by extraction ratios with renal vein catheterization. Am. J. Dis. Child. *100:*576, 1960.
6. Calcagno, P. L., Rubin, M. I., and Weintraub, D. H.: Studies on the renal concentrating and diluting mechanisms in the premature infant. J. Clin. Invest. *33:*91-96, 1954.
7. Chaube, S.: Hypoxanthine dehydrogenase in the developing chick embryonic kidney. Proc. Soc. Exptl. Biol. Med., *111:*340-342, 1962.
8. Clark, H., and Fischer, D.: A reconsideration of nitrogen excretion by the chick embryo. J. Exptl. Zool., *136:*1-15, 1957.
9. Davies, J.: Correlated anatomical and histochemical studies on the mesonephros and placenta of the sheep. Am. J. Anat., *91:*263-299, 1952.
10. Dean, R. F. A., and McCance, R. A.: Renal responses of infants and adults to administration of hypertonic solutions of sodium chloride and urea. J. Physiol., *109:*81-97, 1949.
11. Ebert, J. D.: Developmental, kinetic and immunological studies of enzymes. Carnegie Inst. Wash., Year Book, *62:*428-437, 1963.
12. Edelmann, C. M., Jr., and Barnett, H. L.: The role of the kidney in water metabolism in young infants. J. Pediat., *56:*154-179, 1960.
13. Edelmann, C. M., Jr., Soriano, J. R., Boichis, H., Gruskin, A. B., and Acosta, M. I.: Renal bicarbonate reabsorption and hydrogen ion excretion in normal infants. J. Clin. Invest., *46:*1309-1317, 1967.
14. Fetterman, G. H., Shuplock, N. A., Philipp, F. J., and Gregg, H. S.: The growth and maturation of human glomeruli and proximal convolutions from term to adulthood. Studies by microdissection. Pediatrics, *35:*601-619, 1965.
15. Forster, R. P.: Kidney cells. In Brachet, J., and Mirsky, A. E., (eds.): The Cell, Vol. 5. New York, Academic Press, 1961. p. 89 ff.
16. Forster, R. P., and Taggart, J. V.: Use of isolated renal tubules for the examination of metabolic processes associated with active cellular transport. J. Cell. Comp. Physiol., *36:* 251-270, 1950.

17. Friis-Hansen, B.: Changes in body water compartments during growth. In Linneweh, F. (ed.): Die Physiologische Entwicklung des Kindes. Berlin, Springer-Verlag, 1959, pp. 197-203.
18. Gersh, I.: The correlation of structure and function in the developing mesonephros and metanephros. Contrib. Embryol. Carnegie Inst. Wash., *26:*33-58, 1937.
19. Haines, R. W., and Mohuiddin, A.: Handbook of Human Embryology. Baltimore, Williams and Wilkins, 1965, pp. 66-71.
20. Hamilton, W. J., Boyd, J. D., and Mossmann, H. W.: Human Embryology. Baltimore, Williams and Wilkin, 1962, p. 269.
21. Hatemi, N., and McCance, R. A.: Renal aspects of acid-base control in the newly-born. III. Response to acidifying drugs. Acta Paediat., *50:*603-616, 1961.
22. Jaffee, O. C.: Phenol red transport in the pronephros and mesonephros of the developing frog *(Rana pipiens).* J. Cell. Comp. Physiol, *44:*347-364, 1954.
23. Leeson, T. S.: The fine structure of the mesonephros of the 17-day rabbit embryo. Exptl. Cell. Res., *12:*670-672, 1957.
24. McCance, R. A.: The correct physiological basis on which to compare infant and adult renal function. Lancet, *II:*860-862, 1952.
25. McCance, R. A.: Development of homeostasis with special reference to factors of the environment. In Symposium of the Czeckoslovak Academy of Sciences, Prague, 1961, pp. 49-54.
26. McCance, R. A., and Widdowson, E. M.: New thoughts on renal function in the early days of life. Brit. Med. Bull., *13:*3-6, 1957.
27. McCance, R. A., and Widdowson, E.: Renal aspects of acid-base control in the newly born. I. Natural development. Acta Paediat., *49:*409-444, 1960.
28. McKay, E. M.: Kidney weight, body size and renal function. Arch. Int. Med., *50:*590-594, 1932.
29. Malvin, R. L., Wilde, W. S., Vander, A. J., and Sullivan, L. P.: Localization and characterization of sodium transport along the renal tubule. Am. J. Physiol., *195:*549-557, 1958.
30. Markert, C. L., and Ursprung, H.: The ontogeny of isozyme patterns of lactate dehydrogenase in the mouse. Develop. Biol., *5:*363-381, 1962.
31. de Martino, C., and Zamboni, L.: A morphologic study of the mesonephros of the human embryo. J. Ultrastruct Res. *16:*399-427, 1966.
32. Osathanondh, V., and Potter, E.: Development of human kidney as shown by microdissection. IV. Development of tubular portions of nephrons. Arch. Path., *82:*391-411, 1966.
33. Royer, P.: Renal elimination of electrolytes in the newborn. In, Linneweh, F. (ed.): Die Physiologische Entwicklung des Kindes. Berlin, Springer-Verlag, 1959, pp. 220-226.

34. Smith, H. W.: The Kidney. Structure and Function in Health and Disease. New York, Oxford University Press, 1951, pp. 495-496, 500-501, 543.
35. Sperber I.: Abstract in XVII International Physiol. Congress. at Oxford, July 21-25, 1947. p. 217.
36. Torrey, T. W.: Morphogenesis of the vertebrate kidney. In De Haan, R. L., and Ursprung, R. (eds): Organogenesis, New York, Holt, Rinehart and Winston, 1965, pp. 559-579.
37. Vernier, R. L.: Current concepts of renal development. Pediatric Clin. N. Amer., *11:*759-766, 1964.
38. Vesterdal, J.: Glomerular filtration and renal water excretion. In Linneweh, F. (ed.): Die Physiologische Entwicklung des Kindes. Berlin, Springer-Vergal, 1959, pp. 204-211.
39. Vesterdal, J.: Endocrine control of the water balance in the newborn. Biolog. Neonat., *10:*66-75, 1966.
40. Vogh, B., and Cassin, S.: Stopflow analysis of renal function in newborn and maturing swine. Biol. Neonat., *10:*153-165, 1966.
41. Widdowson, E. Chemical structure, functional integration, and renal regulation as factors in the physiology of the newborn. In Josiah Macy, Jr. Foundation Conference on the Physiology of Prematurity. Lanman, J. T. (ed.): Madison, N. J., Madison Printing, 1959, pp. 97-172.
42. Wojnarowski, M.: Maturation of osmotic function of the kidney. Polish Medical Sci. and Hist., Bull., *9:*89-91, 1966.
43. Yaffee, S. J., and Anders, T. F.: Renal solute content in young rabbits Am. J. Dis. Child., *100:*558, 1960.

Chapter 3

Microdissection of the Nephron: The Method and Its Applications*

GEORGE H. FETTERMAN, M.D., NANCY S. FABRIZIO, B.S., and FRANCES M. STUDNICKI, B.S.

INTRODUCTION

Most of the methods utilized in the study of renal morphology before and during Bowman's time can best be described as preliminary forms of the modern techniques of microdissection. With the introduction of the histologic section and staining methods in the mid-eighteen hundreds, the attention of morphologists was diverted to the wealth of cellular detail provided by the newer technique, so that by the turn of this century, Peter of Greifswald (1) and Huber (2) in this country were among the few who still used the older method of microdissection in their investigation of renal structure.

Peter's studies (1) delineated the architectonic patterns of the normal kidneys of various species as composed of *nephrons,* a term which was later introduced by Braus in 1924 (3). In 1915 Oliver (4) and von Mollendorf (5) independently demonstrated the first functional gradient to be recognized in the nephron by the use of vital staining.

In 1939, Oliver, in *The Architecture of the Kidney in Chronic Bright's Disease,* (6) described the transformation of the architectonic pattern which occurs in the kidney in chronic renal disease, and the numerous and varied alterations that take place in the individual nephrons. Oliver's observations were accomplished by means of microdissection amplified by differential staining of the isolated nephrons, thus revealing their cellular structure. Microinceration was also applied for the localization of mineral metabolites (7). Sir Robert Platt, in 1952, expressed the change in attitude which has evolved in the study of renal disease by his statement, "We must think in terms of nephrons rather than kidneys" (8).

The method of microdissection has retained and expanded its usefulness because it is the one technique that permits the study of the nephron in its continuity, an essential datum in the understanding of its functional activities.

---

*Aided by grants from National Institute of Child Health and Development and from the Richard King Mellon Foundation.

SOURCE MATERIAL FOR TECHNIQUE

The method to be described is the Oliver technique for microdissection of the nephron (9, 10) This technique is practiced in the Renal Research Unit at CIBA, Summit, New Jersey (11), and in the Microdissection Laboratory of Children's Hospital of Pittsburgh. The method is used with slight modifications by Dr. E. M. Darmady in the Microdissection Division of the Central Laboratory, Portsmouth, England.

Principle

With this technique, renal tubules and, indeed, whole nephrons may be dissected out and examined. The tubules of the collecting system are also susceptible to such study. Thus, information as to the distribution and exact localization of lesions in the kidney may be obtained.

The method also provides an opportunity for microscopic examination of renal structure at a low magnification, bridging the gap between gross examination and the magnifications ordinarily used for the study of histologic slides by light microscopy.

Either qualitative or quantitative studies are feasible.

The method thus provides an approach to the study of renal disease not duplicated by any other technique.

Material Suitable for Microdissection

The method is applicable to both necropsy and biopsy material from man or animals. For some unknown reason, kidney tissue that has been in formalin for at least 4 or 5 weeks lends itself to dissection better than blocks fixed for lesser periods of time. Formalin-fixed material that has been in fixative for many years is suitable for dissection.

Reagents, Stains, Solutions and Supplies

10% neutralized formalin
Concentrated HCl
HCl, 0.1 Normal
10% Ferric chloride, aqueous
0.25% Ferric chloride, aqueous
1% Hematoxylin, aqueous
Distilled water
75 x 25 mm Microscopic slides
25 mm sq. Coverslips
Vaseline Petroleum Jelly
3¼" x 4¼" Kodak Panatomic-X film
Appropriate developing, stop-bath and acid-fix solutions
Glossy photographic paper, various grades of contrast
Dry mounting tissue
Strathmore drawing board, 2 ply with smooth surface, size 23" x 29"

Equipment

Widefield binocular dissecting microscope, with illumination
Stender dishes, 60 x 35 mm
Fume hood
Needle holders
Sewing (beading) needles
Filar eyepiece micrometer
Camera lucida attachment
Map measure
Leitz Aristophot photomicrographic apparatus
Dark room setup with developing tanks, etc.
Contact printing equipment
Print drying machine
Electric iron (for dry mounting)
Map cabinet (for filing large mosaic photomicrographs)

Procedure

Maceration

Maceration is one of the most difficult steps of the procedure in that it takes considerable experience to know when the optimum stage of maceration has been reached.

A block of formalin-fixed kidney tissue is selected and trimmed so that, if possible, it includes portions of cortex, medulla, and papilla (Fig. 1-A) An average block might measure 2.0 x 1.2 x

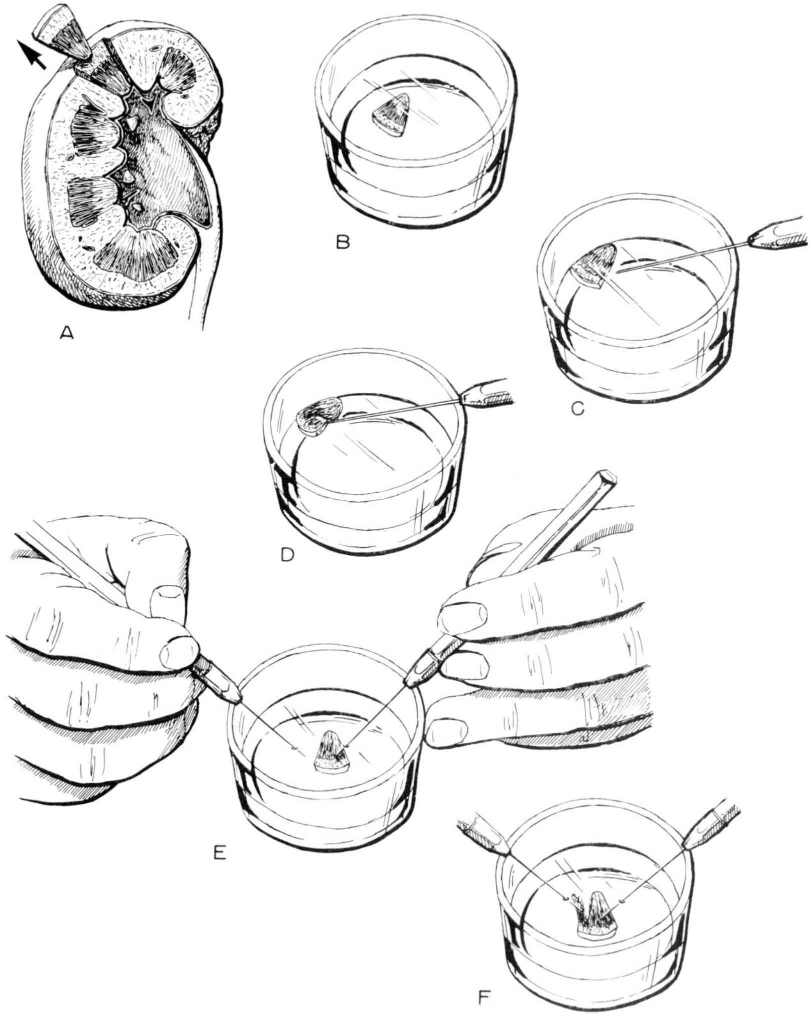

Fig. 1-A.   To show selection and removal of block from a formalin-fixed piece of kidney. In most instances, the kidney will have been divided into slices before fixation.

Fig. 1-B.   The block is shown, covered with acid, in a Stender dish.

Fig. 1-C.   The dissector is about to test the stage of maceration of the block, which has been in the HCl for 24 hours.

Fig. 1-D.   Slight pressure of the needle causes indentation of the block, suggesting that maceration is at or near optimum stage. When pressure of needle is removed, the dent disappears.

Fig. 1-E.   To show the dissecting needles, as the dissector begins to separate a piece from the main block. The block has been washed and is in the third wash of distilled water, to which a drop or two of N/10 HCl has been added.

Fig. 1-F.   A piece is being detached from the main block. The small piece will now be dissected, beginning at the edge where separated from main block.

0.2 cms. The block is rinsed in tap water and then placed in a small Stender dish. Sufficient concentrated HCl is added to cover block completely, as shown in Figure 1-B. With lid on, the dish is placed in a fume hood and kept at a constant temperature of 70° F (21°C)±2.

It usually requires from 24 to 40 hours in the acid for the optimum degree of maceration to occur. The block of tissue becomes soft and compressible as the proper stage of maceration is approached. One may, with practice, gauge the proper degree of maceration by touching the block with a dissecting needle or applicator stick, as it lies in the acid (Figs. 1-C and 1-D).

If not sure whether or not the proper degree of maceration has been reached, a tiny fragment of the block may be teased off with dissecting needles and transferred to a Stender dish filled with distilled water. This sample is placed in an oven at 55°C for 15 minutes. It is then removed, and an attempt at micro-dissection made. If the sample is soft enough so that tubules may be separated, the main block of tissue is sufficiently macerated and may be washed. If, however, the sample of tissue is hard and brittle, the degree of maceration is insufficient and the main block of tissue should be allowed to remain in the acid for 3 to 5 hours longer.

When proper maceration has been effected, the acid is poured off carefully.

The block, left in the Stender dish, is then washed 3 times with distilled water, dripping the water gently into the dish until full, and pouring off carefully. The final wash water, to which one or two drops of N/10 HCl have been added,* is left in the dish and the block, in dish, is

stored in refrigerator until needed. The macerated block will keep in the refrigerator for 2 to 4 days.

When macerated tissue is first placed in water, it will stiffen, but it should soften in one hour at 70°F or 15 minutes at 55°C. If tissue coming from the acid is soft enough to tease out at once, it is probably overmacerated, the tubules will be swollen and the tissue will not keep.

The dissection is performed in a Stender dish under a widefield binocular dissecting microscope. A dark stage is preferable. Lighting is direct. Magnifications in a range from 10X to 45X are found useful.

Dissection

Ordinary needle holders are used, fitted with long, thin, sewing needles. We prefer to use "beading needles," as suggested by Bialestock (12).

The dissector sits in a comfortable chair, with body still and arms supported on the bench or table. The fingers do the work (Fig. 1-E).

The first portion of the block to be dissected is separated from the main block (Fig. 1-F). This fragment may or may not be transferred to another Stender dish, in distilled water to which a few drops of N/10 HCl have been added.

Using the needles, the tissue is pulled apart carefully. One may start at capsule, at lateral edge of block, or perhaps in its center. A convolution may present at surface of block and serve as a beginning point. One can try to separate interesting convolutions from the maze of tubules by gentle manipulation. (The needles must be kept clean, as tubules tend to stick to dirty or corroded needles.) A distal tubule may be found coiled in the mesh formed by the convoluted portion

---

*Unless water is acidified, nephrons tend to adhere to dish or needles.

of the proximal tubule. The distal tubule will often adhere to the glomerulus.

Tubules may break. The broken portions of a particular tubule may be mounted on the same slide. Small pieces of tubule can be saved for practice in mounting.

With experience, one should become able to isolate and mount complete nephrons. In the beginning, attempt to get out complete proximals with the corresponding glomeruli. Practice isolating and mounting any portions of nephron or collecting system is helpful.

As dissection progresses, considerable unwanted material accumulates which tends to litter the dissecting field and cause unnecessary confusion. This debris may be drawn up in a dropper and discarded. It is well to keep the dissecting dish clean!

Comment

There is usually no problem in recognizing the point of demarcation between proximal tubule and descending limb of Henle, because of the abrupt narrowing of the proximal tubule at that point. In some of the tubules, at term and later infancy, the narrowing is more gradual. Here, the change in cell density and pattern may be useful in gauging the line of demarcation. If in doubt, staining of the tubule may be helpful (13).

Mounting

Coverslips are prepared by putting a thin line or streak of petroleum jelly on two opposing edges. The streaks of petroleum jelly usually measure something less than 1 mm in thickness before coverslip is applied. The coverslip is then placed on the bench with vaseline side up.

The isolated tubule is placed in the center of the dish, leaving undissected material on the right (if right handed).

With the left hand, a microscopic slide is introduced into the dish at a 45° angle until it touches bottom. With needle held in the right hand, the tubule is raised in the water and brought to the slide (Fig. 2-G). The tubule usually adheres to the slide on application, and the slide, with tubule, may be raised out of the water. The tubule or nephron should then remain in place.

The slide is then inverted and gently applied to the prepared coverslip (Fig. 2-H), the vaselined edges matching the long edges of the slide. One end of the slide and one end of the coverslip are flush. The nephron now is enclosed in a chamber that is open at two ends. Using a dropper, the chamber is carefully and slowly filled with water taken from the dissecting dish.

The tubule or nephron, as now mounted, may be studied at once, may be measured if desirable, may be photographed unstained, may be stained and then photographed or may be stored in a covered Petri dish in the refrigerator until appropriate methods are applied.

The nephron is preserved in water in any case, as ordinary clearing and mounting techniques cause unacceptable shrinkage and distortion. Many abnormalities in the nephron may be detected in unstained specimens. In most of our studies in normal or diseased kidneys, only a small percentage of the nephrons or collecting tubules isolated and studied are stained or photographed.

Measurement

Measurements are made on unstained material. Measurement of nephrons or portions of the collecting system may be indicated in certain types of studies. Details of these steps are well covered in reports by Oliver (10) and the present authors (14).

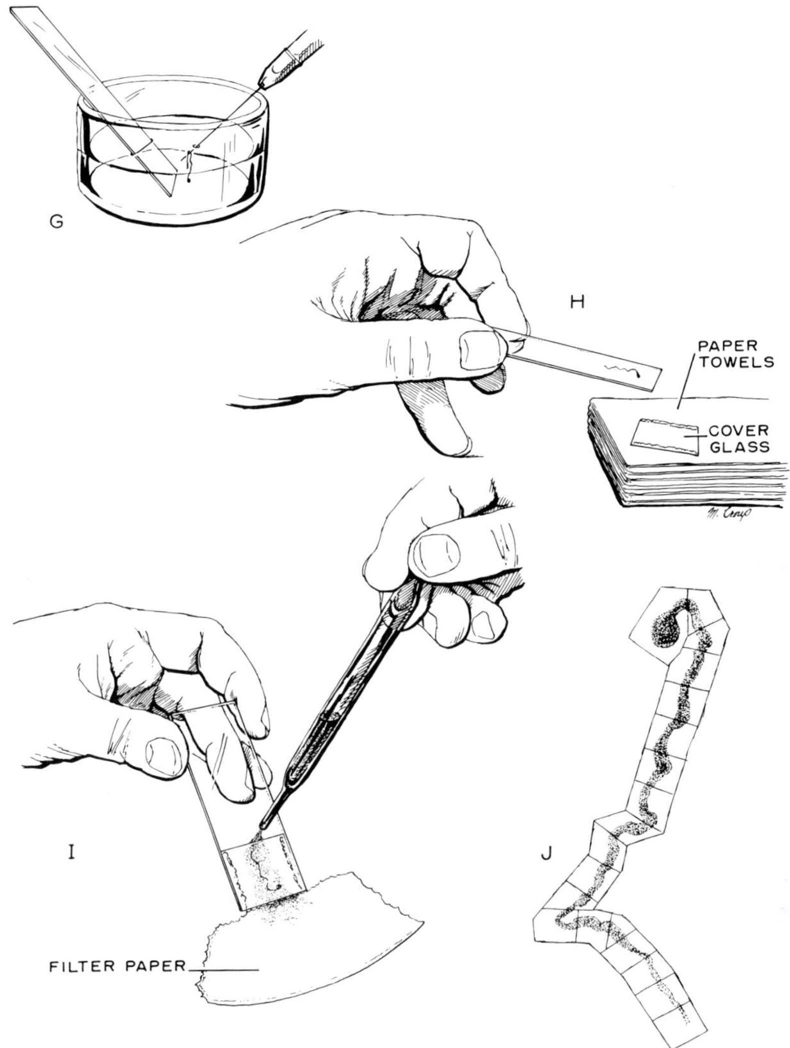

Fig. 2-G. A stage in the mounting process. A proximal tubule, with glomerulus, is being brought up to slide. Although not shown, the slide is being held by thumb and forefinger of left hand.

Fig. 2-H. The slide with proximal tubule attached is being inverted over the specially prepared cover glass.

Fig. 2-I. Showing a step in the staining process. A staining solution is being introduced into one end of the chamber by means of the dropper, and fluid is being removed at other open end of chamber by the application of a fragment of filter paper.

Fig. 2-J. A diagrammatic representation of a mosaic photomicrograph. In a finished mosaic, the boundaries of the units of the mosaic are not as distinct as shown in this diagram.

In brief, glomerular and tubular diameters are obtained by use of a filar eyepiece micrometer. The length of tubules is ascertained by making camera lucida drawings and then measuring them with a map measure. The final values for lengths and diameters are obtained by the use of appropriate conversion factors.

To achieve uniformity and consistent accuracy in measurements, kidney tissue from each individual is sampled at least three times. This means that separate blocks are taken from the kidney and macerated and dissected on different occasions. If possible, the samples from any one subject are dissected by at least two different workers.

The measurements of normal human nephrons has been found to be practically interchangeable in the three laboratories mentioned in the *Introduction*.

Staining

A number of staining methods may be utilized.

For cytological investigation, iron hematoxylin, fat and iron stains (15) are all of value.

It is likely that a variety of other staining methods might be applied.

Vital staining procedures (4, 16) have also been used with success.

Staining with iron hematoxylin will be described.

Staining solutions are introduced by dropper into the chamber containing the nephron and drawn through the chamber by filter paper applied at the opposite end of the chamber (Fig. 2-I). The steps are as follows:

1. 10% ferric chloride — 2 minutes
2. Rinse with tap water
3. 1% hematoxylin — 5 seconds
4. Rinse with distilled water

5. Differentiate with 0.25% ferric chloride
   (This step should be controlled under the microscope. Usually takes 20-30 seconds.)
6. Wash thoroughly with distilled water

The Appearance of Nephrons Stained with Iron Hematoxylin

There is considerable cellular detail in a well stained nephron, particularly if the original formalin-fixation was prompt. Nuclei appear as unstained vesicles, but a surprising amount of cytoplasmic detail is apparent. For a more detailed description of the appearance of dissected nephrons stained with iron hematoxylin, the report of Oliver, MacDowell and Tracy (9) should be consulted.

Comment

In staining in step 3, MacDowell prefers to apply hematoxylin for 30 seconds, or until tubule is a deep velvety black. This, of course, means that differentiation is more time-consuming.

If solutions or water are moved through the chamber too quickly or too vigorously, the nephron may become detached and be lost.

The top of coverslip should be kept clean during the staining process.

Don't press down on coverslip or nephron may become flattened.

Other staining methods may be used, such as a Sudan type for fat, or one of the stains utilizing the Prussian blue reaction for iron.

Photography of Stained Nephrons

Since the nephrons mounted in water are perishable and the stain fades within a few days, photomicrography, if essential, should be accomplished promptly.

Details of photography are not included in these instructions, except those involving special adaptations for photography of microdissected material.

The Mosaic Photomicrograph

The large size of many of the nephrons or tubules makes it impossible to obtain any detail in a single photomicrograph of the entire structure. Accordingly, multiple overlapping photomicrographs are taken of a tubule or nephron, and contact prints of these are joined in a mosaic similar to an aerial map (Fig. 2-J). Sufficient overlap is allowed so that adjoining prints may be cut on the bias. The overlapping negatives should be numbered in continuity as they are exposed, to make the subsequent assemblage of the mosaic photomicrograph easier.

For tubules or nephrons of ordinary size, a magnification of 200X is used. This means that the final mosaic photomicrograph is usually quite large and must be mounted on a large cardboard measuring 23" x 29". If prints are needed for publication, a single photograph may be taken of the entire mosaic photomicrograph. This results usually in a reduction of magnification to 40X to 80X, with some loss of detail.

When nephrons to be photographed are enormous in size, the original overlapping photomicrographs should be taken at a lower magnification, such as 40X, if the mosaic photomicrograph is to be handled with any degree of convenience.

The overlapping glossy contact prints, whether of 200X or 40X magnification, are assembled in continuity on heavy cardboard with masking tape, or pinned in place by thumb tacks. While in place, they are trimmed with an X-acto knife or razor blade. The mosaic is then permanently secured to a large cardboard, usually 23" x 29", with dry mount tissue.

Comment

The overlapping photomicrographs are best taken by the research associates who have performed the actual microdissection, mounting and staining of the nephrons. On many days, 200 to 300 pictures will be exposed and developed. The microdissectors also make the contact prints, and assemble them into mosaics.

The photography department of the institution is only called upon to take the pictures of the completed mosaic photomicrographs which are to be used for publication.

The original mosaic photomicrographs are large and require special arrangements for filing and storage.

Discussion

Proficiency in and understanding of the microdissection technique depend greatly upon the operator's powers of concentration and patience. At least two-thirds of the persons who have studied microdissection technique in our laboratory have displayed promise or have actually developed skill in the technique. Some of these were physicians, some were medical students and some were biologists or medical technologists.

The three steps, procedures or areas which cause greatest difficulty in the procedure are: control of maceration, mounting of dissected material and interpretation of results!

The technical excellence of preparation is an indispensable feature of this field. Artefacts due to poor fixation, overmaceration, inadequate or overstaining must all be viewed with discrimination, as they may cause errors in interpretation. The principal investigators and research associates must be able to distinguish between the truly thin or atrophic neck of a proximal tubule and one that has been stretched and "pulled out" by the stress of mounting.

Sources of Error

It is important that tissue to be dissected be well fixed and properly macerated if reliable observations are to be made. Overmaceration must be guarded against, as the artefacts resulting therefrom may be interpreted improperly.

Swelling of tubules may take place during or following dissection as the result of overmaceration or because of too long storage at room temperature.

In quantitative studies, when accurate measurements are required, care in the prevention of tubular swelling is essential.

Range of Values

Normal quantitative values for size of human nephrons at various stages of development have been published (10, 14), but need not be listed here in a treatise concerned almost exclusively with technique.

Applications and Clinical Interpretation

Many lesions of nephrons and collecting tubules which are visible by light microscopy in histologic preparations are also demonstrable by microdissection. This supplementary method enables one to determine just where in the nephron or collecting system a structural change exists.

A classical application of the method made by Oliver (9) in the study of the pathogenesis of acute renal failure, deserves mention. Lesions were consistently demonstrated in not only the "lower nephron" but also the proximal tubule. The nature of the lesions, the timing of regeneration, if the lesion was reversible, were found, along with clinical chemical observations, to explain the bizarre chain of clinical events in the syndrome.

A fruitful and fascinating application of renal microdissection has been in relation to renal tubular micropuncture studies in experimental animals (17, 18, 19, 20). It was by means of microdissection that the Wearn-Richards procedure on the readily visible nephron of the amphibian was extended to the mammalian nephron (17). In these studies the method is used to identify the punctured tubule and locate the exact site of puncture within the tubule. Evidence is also provided as to the presence or absence of structural change, such as necrosis, in the tubule.

Darmady has used the method, with modification, in the study of nephrons in certain examples of inborn errors of metabolism (21, 22). Notable among these studies was the demonstration of the peculiar deformity, shortening and atrophy of the proximal tubule in cystinosis. This proximal tubular change is readily correlated with a number of the clinical renal aberrations of the disease.

Darmady has also used autoradiography with microdissection to determine the absorption and localization of various labelled substances within the nephron in experimental animals (23).

The method is valuable in the study of normal development (24, 25), as well as developmental abnormalities of the kidney. A number of authors have applied the method to the study of cystic kidneys (24, 26, 27, 28, 29).

Quantitative studies involving measurements of glomeruli and proximal tubules have been pursued (10, 14). These have been of special interest in obtaining anatomic correlates of glomerulotubular balance.

Examples of Diseased Nephrons as Visualized by the Microdissection Technique

Mosaic photomicrographs of nephrons or portions thereof as prepared by the methods described in this chapter are illustrated in figures 3 to 6.

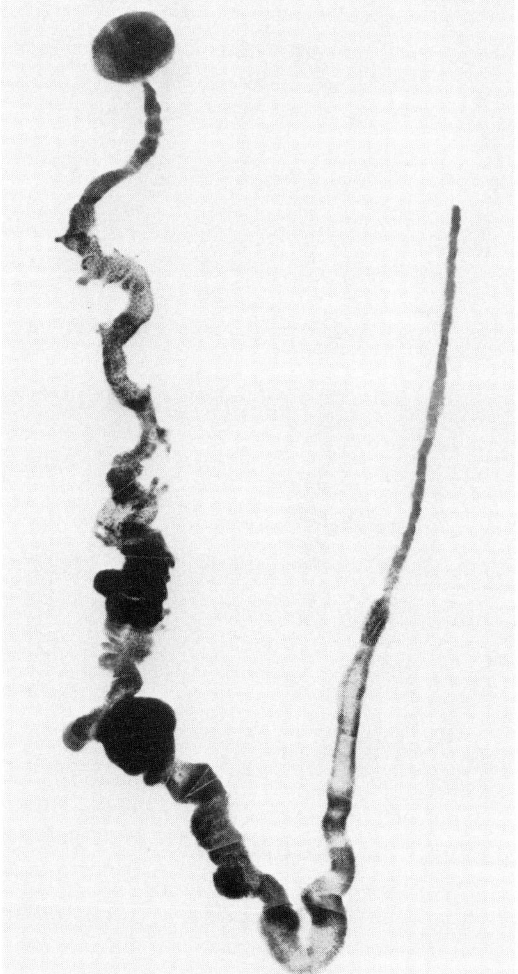

Fig. 3. Mosaic photomicrograph of a deformed proximal tubule from kidney of 13-month-old boy with renal dysplasia. The miniature diverticula of convoluted portion are striking. Reduced to X46 from X200.

Renal Dysplasia

A proximal tubule from a dysplastic kidney is shown in Figure 3. The tubule is shortened, deformed and presents many tiny diverticula. Both kidneys of the 13-month-old child from whom this nephron was obtained presented islands of cartilage and primitive ducts.

Fanconi's Syndrome with Cystinosis

In Figure 4, eight proximal tubules from the kidneys of 5 children succumbing of cystinosis are shown. The children ranged in age from 2-7/12 to 12-1/2 years. Each of the tubules presents the "swan neck" lesion in its first portion. In addition, each of the tubules is shortened and deformed. The incidence of "swan neck" lesions in the population of nephrons sampled from each of these 5 cases varied from 36% to 89%. In a sixth case, not illustrated here, no "swan necks" were found, but nearly every tubule examined was markedly narrowed along its entire length.

Familial Juvenile Nephronophthisis (30, 31, 32)

In kidneys from at least several examples of this syndrome, diverticula of a number of the descending limbs of Henle have been encountered (31, 33). In Figure 5, portions of nephrons, including descending limbs in which this diverticulous change is striking, are shown. These are from the kidney of a 7-year-old boy.

The resemblance between and perhaps the identity of juvenile familial nephronophthisis and medullary cystic disease has attracted considerable attention recently (34, 35, 36)

Hereditary Nephritis (Alport's Syndrome)

The marked hypertrophy and lengthening which may occur in many of the

 Laboratory Diagnosis of Kidney Diseases

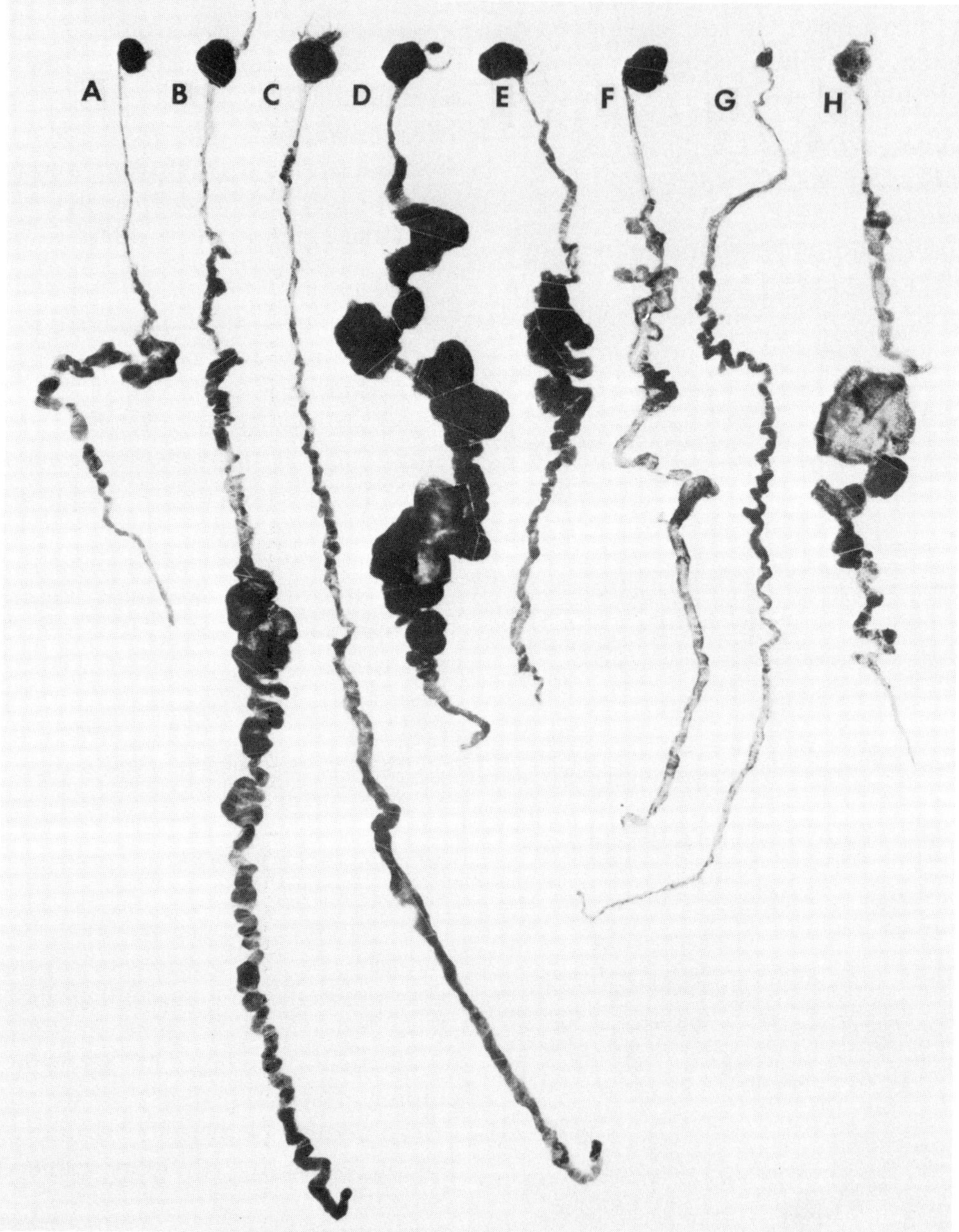

Fig. 4. Mosaic photomicrographs of 8 proximal tubules from 5 patients with cystinosis. They are arranged in order of age, from left to right. All present "swan neck" lesions. Reduced to X36 from X200. (Originally published in Proceedings of the Third International Congress of Nephrology, Washington, 1966, Basel, S. Karger, 1967, Vol. 2.)

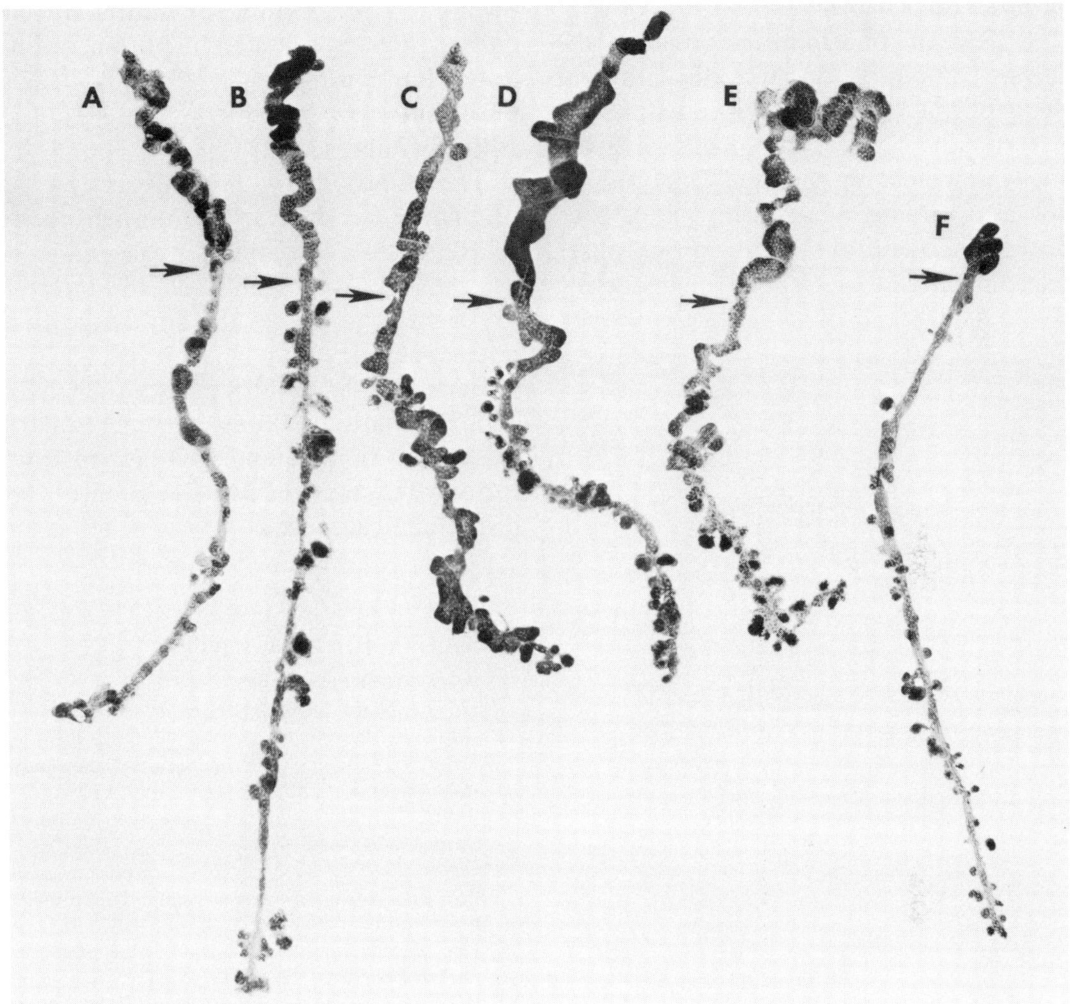

Fig. 5. Mosaic photomicrographs of portions of 6 nephrons from case of nephronophthisis. Each includes all or part of the descending limb of Henle, Note the many diverticula. The arrows mark the line of demarcation between proximal tubule and descending limb of loop of Henle. Reduced to X54 from X200. (Originally published in Proceedings of the Third International Congress of Nephrology, Washington, 1966, Basel, S. Karger, 1967, Vol. 2.)

proximal tubules in chronic parenchymal disease of the kidney is illustrated in Figure 6. Here, a complete nephron from the kidney of a 15-year-old boy in the end stage of hereditary nephritis is seen. This tubule is representative of the hypertrophied nephrons in this kidney. The proximal tubule measures 41.94 mm in length, the mean proximal tubular length of an age control being 13.90 mm. The disparity between the volume of this hypertrophied proximal tubule and the mean proximal tubular volume of the age control is striking, the volume of the diseased proximal tubule being .227 cu mm; the mean volume of control, .029 cu mm.

Modifications of the Method

A few of the modifications of the Oliver technique for microdissection of the nephron should be mentioned.

Darmady (21) has made certain changes which, in the final analysis, do not alter findings, but in his hands have proved expeditious. His group uses micromanipulators to hold the dissecting needles. They mount nephrons differently. They do not stain nephrons ordinarily but bring out detail in their photomicrographs by the use of phase contrast microscopy.

The method of microdissection as originated by Hayward, requiring special fixation and employing collagenase as the macerating agent, is of interest (37, 38). It possesses the advantage that nuclear staining may be achieved.

Bartman has modified both the Oliver and Hayward methods of renal microdissection in attempts to demonstrate various enzymes (39) in the nephron by histochemical means.

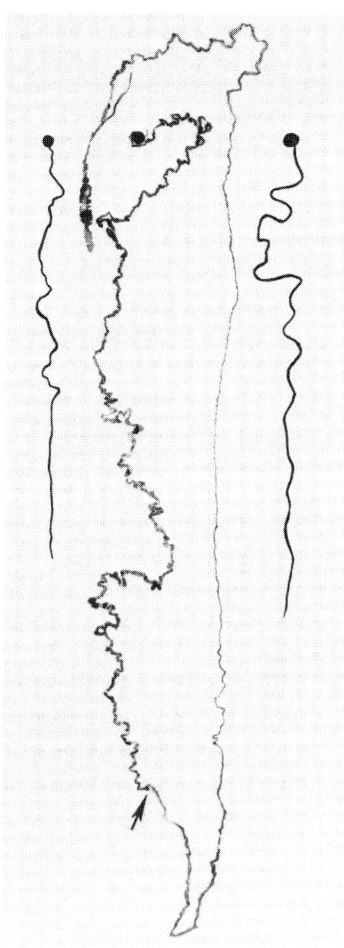

Fig. 6. Mosaic photomicrograph of complete nephron from kidney of patient with end stage hereditary nephritis. The proximal tubule is enormous. The arrow marks end of proximal tubule. The silhouette at left represents an average proximal tubule from age control (15 years), the one at right an average proximal tubule from a normal adult kidney. Reduced to X6.5 from X200.

BIBLIOGRAPHY

1. Peter, K.: Untersuchungen über Bau and Entwicklung der Niere. Jena, G. Fischer, 1909-1927.
2. Huber, G. C.: On the development and shape of uriniferous tubules of certain of the higher mammals, Amer. J. Anat., *4* (Suppl) :1-98, 1905.
3. Braus, H.: Lehrbuch der Anatomie. Berlin, J. Springer, 1924, Bd. 2.
4. Oliver, J.: The histogenesis of chronic uranium nephritis with especial reference to epithelial regeneration. J. Exp. Med., *21*:425-451, 1915.
5. von Möllendorff, W.: Die Dispersität der Farbstoffe, ihre Beziehungen zu Ausscheidung and Speicherung in der Niere. Ein Beitrag zur Histophysiologie der Niere. Anat Hefte, *53*:87-323, 1915.
6. Oliver, J.: Architecture of the Kidney in Chronic Bright's Disease. New York, Paul B. Hoeber, 1939.
7. Oliver, J.: An essay toward a dynamic morphology of the mammalian nephron. Am. J. Med., *9*:88-101, 1950.
8. Platt, R.: Structural and functional adaptation in renal failure. Brit. Med. J., *1*:1313-1317, 1952.
9. Oliver, J. MacDowell, M., and Tracy, A.: The pathogenesis of acute renal failure associated with traumatic and toxic injury. Renal ischemia, nephrotoxic damage and the ischemuric episode. J. Clin. Invest., *30*:1307-1351, 1957.
10. Oliver, J., and MacDowell, M.: The structural and functional aspects of the handling of glucose by the nephrons and the kidney and their correlation by means of structural-functional equivalents, J. Clin. Invest., *40*:1093-1131, 1961.
11. MacDowell, M.: Personal Communication, 1958.

12. Bialestock, D.: Personal Communication, 1960.

13. Darmady, E. M.: Correlation of renal function and structure. J. Clin. Path., *18*:493-499, 1965.

14. Fetterman, G. H., *et al:* The growth and maturation of human glomeruli and proximal convolutions from term to adulthood. Studies by microdissection. Pediatrics, *35*:601-619, 1965.

15. Oliver, J.: New direction in renal morphology: "A method, its results and its future. In, The Harvey Lectures, Harvey Society of New York, 1944-45, Series 40. Lancaster, Pa., Science Press, 1945. pp. 102-155.

16. Oliver, J., Bloom, F., and MacDowell, M.: Structural and functional transformations in the tubular epithelium of the dog's kidney in chronic Bright's disease and their relation to mechanisms of renal compensation and failure. J. Exp. Med., *73*:141-160, 1941.

17. Walker, A. M., and Oliver, J.: Methods for the collection of fluid from single glomeruli and tubules of the mammalian kidney. Amer. J. Physiol., *134*:562-579, 1941.

18. Walker, A. M. ,*et al:* The collection and analysis of fluid from single nephrons of the mammalian kidney. Amer. J. Physiol.,*134*:580-595, 1941.

19. Oliver, J., and MacDowell, M.: Studies by microdissection and micropuncture of the abnormal kidney; the structural aspect. In proceedings of the Second International Congress of Nephrology, Prague, 1963. Excerpta Medica International Congress Series No. 78. Amsterdam. Excerpta Medica Foundation, 1964, pp. 13-20.

20. Biber, T. U. L., Mylle, M., and Gottschalk, C. W.: Micropuncture study of kidney function in rats with experimental tubular necrosis. In, Proceedings of the Second International Congress of Nephrology, Prague, 1963, Excerpta Medica International Congress Series No. 78. Amsterdam, Excerpta Medica Foundation, 1964, pp. 21-27.

21. Darmady, E. M., and Stranack, F.: Microdissection of the nephron in disease. Brit. Med. Bull., *13*:21-26, 1957.

22. Darmady, E. M., *et al*: The proximal convoluted tubule in the renal handling of water. Lancet, *2*:1254-1256, 1964.

23. Darmady, E. M., *et al*: Location of ^{131}I pitressin in kidney by autoradiography. Clin. Sci., *19*:229-241, 1960.

24. Oliver, J.: A new look at the development of the nephrons and the kidney and their relations to renal cystic disease. In, Glomerulare and Tubulare Nierenkrankungen (Internationales Nierensymposion, Wurzburg, 1960). Stuttgart, Georg Thieme Verlag, 1962, pp. 29-33.

25. Osathanondh, V., and Potter, E. L.: Development of human kidney as shown by microdissection. (3 articles.) Arch. Path., *76:271, 1963.*

26. Baxter, T. J.: Morphogenesis of renal cysts. Amer. J. Path., *38*:721-731, 1961.

27. Bialestock, D.: Microdissection study of nephrons and cysts from an infant with pyelonephrities. Aust. Ann. Med. 7:93-101, 1958.

28. Heggo, O., and Natvig, J. B.: Microdissection studies of structural changes in cystic disease of the kidneys. Lancet, *2*:616-617, 1963.

29. Osathanondh, V., and Potter, E. L.: Pathogenesis of polycystic kidneys. (6 articles.) Arch. Path., *77:459, 1964.*

30. Fanconi, G., *et al* :Die familiare juvenile Nephronophthise (Die idiopathische parenchymatöse Schrumpfniere), Helv Paediat. Acta 6:1-49, 1951.

31. Ivemark, B. I., Ljungqvist, A., and Barry, A.: Juvenile nephronophthisis, Part II. A histologic and microangeographic study. Acta Paediat., *49*:480-487, 1960.

32. Royer, P., *et al*: Les nephropathies tubulo-interstitielles chroniques idiopathiques de l'enfant. Ann Pediat., *10*:620-633, 1963.

33. Fetterman, G. H., Fabrizio, N. S., and Studnicki, F. M.: The study by microdissection of structural tubular defects in certain examples of the hereditary nephropathies. In, proceedings of the Third International Congress of Nephrology, Washington, 1966. Basel, S. Karger, 1967, Vol. 2, pp. 235-250.

34. Herdman, R. C., Good, R. A., and Vernier, R. L.: Medullary cystic disease in two siblings. Amer. J. Med., *43*:335-344, 1967.

35. Mongeau, J. G., and Worthen, H. G.: Nephronophthisis and medullary cystic disease, Amer. J. Med., *43*:345-355, 1967.

36. Strauss, M. B., and Sommers, S. C.: Clinical and pathological identity of medullary cystic disease and familial juvenile nephronophthisis. Amer. Soc. Nephrology, Los Angeles, Oct. 18-19, 1967. Abstracts, p.63.

37. Hayward, N. J.: Collagenase maceration in renal microdissection: Preservation of nuclear staining, Brit. J. Exp. Path., *45*:68-74, 1964.

38. Thompson, M. E., Shuplock, N. A., and Fetterman, G. H.: Collagenase method of microdissection: Preservation of nuclear staining. Arch. Path., *78*:568-571, 1964.

39. Bartman, J., and Dixon, J. F.: Histochemical analysis of microdissected nephrons: Enzyme stains. Stain Techn., *41*:229-233, 1966.

Chapter 4

Patho-physiology of Renal Concentrating Defects

F. A. CARONE, M.D.

In this chapter, the mechanism by which urine is normally concentrated, including recent studies on the possible role of renal lymphatics, will be presented briefly and then functional and structural correlations will be made in several renal diseases in man where loss of concentrating ability is a prominent feature. The mammalian kidney is faced with the problem of salvaging the enormous quantity of fluid delivered to the tubules by the glomerular filtrate, which in man amounts to approximately 180 liters per day. This is accomplished largely by isoosmotic reabsorption of glomerular filtrate by the tubules especially the proximal tubule. In addition, to conserve as much water as possible, the mammalian kidney has developed a concentrating process which operates as a countercurrent multiplier and can make the urine several times more concentrated than plasma. Urine concentration occurs in the renal medulla, an area of the kidney with unique functional and morphological features.

It is generally accepted that the renal concentrating mechanism depends upon active transport of sodium salts out of the relatively water impermeable ascending limbs of Henle and that counter current flow in Henle's loops multiply this effect in the direction of the papilla (1, 2) (Fig. 1). This creates an increasing osmotic gradient from outer medulla to papillary tip. In Figure 1 impermeability of the ascending limb to water is indicated by a heavy solid line. Figure 1 shows that in the ascending limb, active reabsorption of sodium reduces the osmolality of early distal tubular fluid to 100 mOsm and that the osmolality of interstitial, tubular, and vascular fluids increase from 300 to 1300 between the outer medulla and the papillary tip. During dehydration, a high level of antidiuretic hormone greatly increases the permeability of distal tubules and collecting ducts to water. This causes tubular fluid to become isotonic with plasma along the distal tubule. The urine, then, becomes concentrated by fluid in the collecting ducts attaining osmotic equilibrium with the hyperosmotic interstitium in the medulla so that the final urine has an osmolar concentration equal to that of interstitial fluid at the tip of the papilla.

The blood vessels in the medulla (vasa recta), which also form hairpin loops, play an important role in preserving the osmotic gradient in the medulla by acting as counter current exchangers and removing interstitial water of tubular

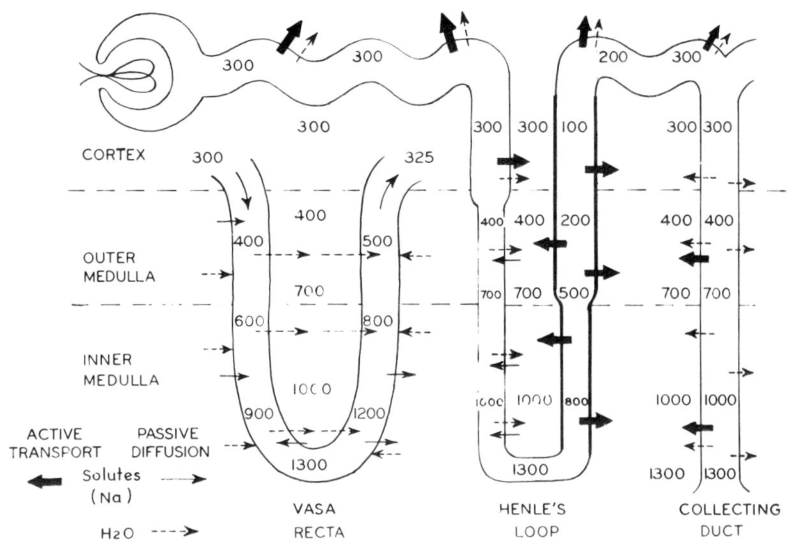

Fig. 1. Summary of active and passive transport of water and solute in the nephron and vasa recta during the elaboration of a concentrated urine. Osmolality of tubular, vascular, and interstitial fluid is expressed as mOsm per Kg H_2O; impermeability of the ascending limb of Henle's loop to water is represented by a darker line. (Adapted from Pitts (1).)

origin. As shown in Figure 1, as blood flows down the medulla, water diffuses out and permeable solutes diffuse into the blood. As the blood ascends, the reverse occurs. This process tends to retain highly permeable substances within the medulla and to short-circuit significant quantities of water across the top of the loops so that effective blood flow is reduced and solute washout due to blood flow is kept to a minimum. Thus, in Figure 1, blood flowing into the vasa recta has an osmolality of 300 m Osm while that flowing out has an osmolality of only 325 mOsm indicating that loss of solute from the medulla is quite small. Without countercurrent flow and exchange in the vasa recta, blood flowing through the medulla would exit with a very high osmolality and result in considerable loss of solute and depletion of the high osmolality within the medulla. Another function of the vasa

recta vital to the concentrating process is removal of water from the medulla (3). Significant amounts of water are transported into the medullary interstitium from the descending limbs of Henle's loops and the collecting ducts (Fig. 1). Lack of an efficient means to remove this water would result in loss of the medullary osmotic gradient and impairment of the concentrating process. Since vasa recta blood is postglomerular and has an increased oncotic pressure on account of glomerular filtration, the vasa recta can transport significant quantities of water from the medulla (indicated by the outer arrows in Fig. 1) so that vascular outflow in the medulla could exceed inflow by an amount comparable to glomerular filtration fraction, i.e., about 20%.

Recent experiments performed by Dr. Stolarczyk and myself, suggest that the renal lymphatics play a role in the concentrating process. The acute effects of completely occluded or increased lymph flow on renal function, particularly concentrating ability, were investigated in rats. Lymph flow from the left kidney was either blocked by ligating the lymphatics or increased by partially occluding the left renal vein. The right kidney served as a control in both groups of animals. Complete occlusion of renal lymphatics caused more than a 3 fold increase in urine flow and solute excretion (Table I). Total solutes in the renal papilla (an indication of tissue osmolality) and urine osmolality were moderately increased. On the other hand, an increase in renal lymph flow due to partial renal vein occlusion had the opposite effects. Urine flow, and urine solute excretion were markedly reduced (Table I). Total tissue solute in the papilla and urine osmolality, as would be expected, were greatly decreased. In agreement with the latter findings are the observations that a number of conditions that increase lymph flow in the

kidney such as water or solute diuresis (4), increased renal vein pressure (5), lower urinary tract obstruction or stop-flow procedures (6) result in depletion of medullary hyperosmolality and impairment of concentrating ability. Thus, occlusion of renal lymph flow can increase medullary osmolality and urine concentrating ability while increased lymph flow has the opposite effect. These findings suggest a role for the renal lymphatics in the concentrating mechanism which probably is related to the degree of movement of water and solute through the medullary interstitium and out the lymphatics. Consideration of such a role requires an understanding of the morphology and function of certain structures in the medulla. As discussed previously, in the medulla the loops of Henle and the vasa recta are looped structures and act as countercurrent exchangers which tend to retain highly permeable substances within the medulla. The collecting ducts and lymphatics, however, are not looped

TABLE I—EFFECTS OF OCCLUDED OR INCREASED LYMPH FLOW
ON COMPOSITION OF THE URINE AND RENAL PAPILLA

	Urine Volume ml/2 hrs	Solute Excretion μOsm/2 hrs	Total Solute, Papilla mEq	Urine Osmolality mOsm
Normal	.165 ±.024	.133 ±.014	868.3	806 ±46.4
Occluded Lymph Flow	.554 ±.038	.709 ±.056	972.1	1280 ±56.3
p*	<0.01	<0.01	<0.05	<0.01
Normal	.223 ±.021	.233 ±.019	764.6	1046 ±41.3
Increased Lymph Flow	.112 ±.014	.066 ±.008	584.2	595 ±24.6
p*	<0.01	<0.01	<0.01	<0.01

Figures represent means ± S.E.
* Derived from paired comparison analysis of 8 animals.

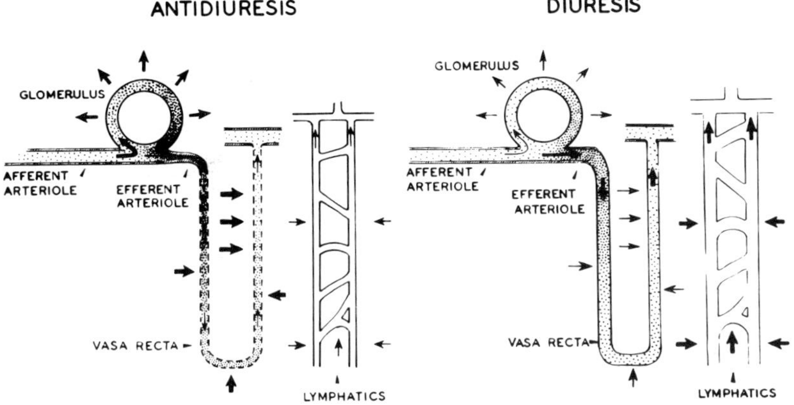

Fig. 2. Proposed role of medullary vessels and lymphatics in the concentrating process. Arrows indicate direction and magnitude of water or fluid transport while the dark stippling within vessels indicates protein concentration or oncotic pressure. During antidiuresis and high antidiuretic hormone activity, constriction of efferent arterioles of juxtamedullary glomeruli decreases flow, diverts more blood through the glomeruli and increases filtration pressure and filtration fraction so that oncotic pressure in increased maximally. In creased permeability of vasa recta permits greater exchange of water from descending to ascending limbs, especially in the outer medulla. The combined effects are a slow blood flow in the medulla with a high oncotic pressure which results in minimal solute washout and maximal removal of interstitial water. This, in turn, would greatly diminish loss of fluid and solute into lymphatics and maintain the medullary osmotic gradient at a high level. The reverse changes would occur during periods of diuresis and low antidiuretic hormone activity.

and represent direct exits for water or solute. It is known that water and solute are transported into the medullary interstitium from collecting ducts (7), but there is little evidence that the reverse occurs. Thus, only the lymphatics represent a direct route for the escape of excess water or solute accumulating in the medulla. It should be stressed that the lymphatics can function only passively and that lymph flow would be determined by the degree of water and solute movement between the medullary interstitium and the renal tubules and vasa recta. During diuresis or antidiuresis, the quantity of water and solute transported into the medullary tissues by the loops of Henle and the collecting ducts probably does not vary greatly (7). On the other hand, it has been shown that medullary blood flow is significantly reduced during dehydration or high ADH activity and greatly accelerated during water or osmotic diuresis (8). Furthermore, net transport of water into the medullary interstitium from the tubules is largely removed by the vasa recta (3, 7). This would suggest that the magnitude of lymph flow in the medulla is mainly dependent upon the functional activity of the vasa recta.

In Figure 2 are shown, diagramatically, the proposed interrelated roles of the lymphatics and the vasa recta in the medulla. Note that afferent and efferent arterioles of juxta medullary glomeruli form continuous channels from which the glomerular capillaries arise as side branches. Arrows indicate the direction and magnitude of water or fluid transport while the dark stippling in the vessels indicates plasma protein concentration or oncotic pressure. In this proposal, it is postulated that antidiuretic hormone (ADH) induces vasoconstriction and increases the permeability of vasa recta to water. During antidiuresis and high levels of ADH activity, constriction of the efferent arteriole diverts more blood through the glomerulus and increases filtration pressure and filtration fraction so that plasma protein content and oncotic pressure are increased in the vessels. Increased permeability of vasa recta to water indicated by the interrupted lines, would permit greater exchange of plasma water from descending to ascending limbs, especially in the outer medulla. The combined effects would be a slow blood flow in the medulla with a high oncotic pressure. This would result in minimal solute washout and maximal removal of interstitial water of tubular origin by the vasa recta. This, in turn, would greatly diminish lymph flow and loss of fluid and solute by this route, so that the medullary osmotic gradient would be maintained at a high level. On the other hand, during diuresis and low levels of ADH activity, vaso-dilatation of the efferent arteriole would enhance flow to the vasa recta, but diminish flow to the glomerulus. Thus, filtration fraction and oncotic pressure in the vessels would decrease. Diminished vascular permeability to water with less exchange of plasma water across the limbs of the vasa recta would not significantly decrease blood flow. A rapid flow of blood with a lower oncotic pressure in the medullary vessels would result in a greater washout of solute and less removal of interstitial water from the medulla. Consequently, lymph flow with solute loss would increase and the combined effect would

be to lower medullary osmolality and concentrating ability. Intermediate changes would allow the kidney to regulate water excretion over a wide range of physiologic activity.

Knowledge of the concentrating mechanism, which has been gathered largely from studies in animals, can be helpful in clarifying the nature of concentrating defects in certain renal diseases in man. In many renal diseases, there is progressive diffuse destruction and scarring of the renal parenchyma, so that various renal functions, such as glomerular filtration rate and concentrating ability, are reduced roughly in parallel. Other disorders, that involve chiefly the cortex, such as diffuse glomerular diseases, generally spare concentrating ability during their early stages. On the other hand, some renal disorders cause specific structural alterations in the medulla and are characterized by a disproportionate loss of concentrating ability. These cases offer us the unique opportunity to study the concentrating process in man. Such a case that we studied (9) was a 37-year-old man with chronic osteomyelitis who died from a carcinoma of the lung. He had a long history of polydypsia, polyuria and nocturia. A Hickey-Hare test showed that he excreted a urine more dilute than plasma, since following 14 hours of dehydration, urine osmolality was only 200 m Osm compared to 290 for plasma. After the intravenous infusion of 300 ml of 3% NaCl, urine volume dropped but urine osmolality remained essentially unchanged. Similarly, vasopressin had no effect on urine osmolality indicating that diabetes insipidus in this case was nephrogenic in type. At post mortem, the kidneys showed amyloidosis with extensive involvement of medullary structures but only minimal deposits in the cortex.

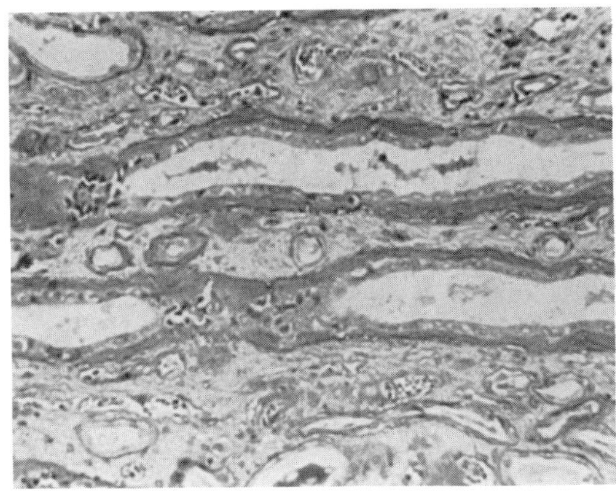

Fig. 3. Renal amyloidosis. Thick collars of amyloid deposited on the inner aspect of the basement membranes of two collecting ducts in the renal papilla. X 300

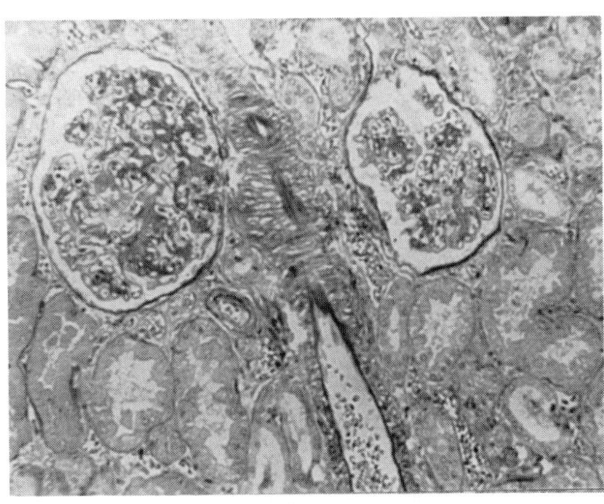

Fig. 4. Renal amyloidosis. Renal cortex showing minimal amyloid deposition in glomeruli and small arteries. X 300

By microdissection, the deposits of amyloid were localized chiefly in thick cuffs surrounding the collecting ducts (9). Amyloid formed thick collars within the basement membranes of collecting tubules which was most prominent in the inner medulla (Fig. 3) and gradually diminished in the outer medulla. Amyloid also involved the vasa recta and the medullary interstitium to a lesser degree. There was only minimal amyloid deposition in the cortex involving the glomeruli and occasional arteries (Fig. 4). Loss of concentrating ability in this patient may be explained by 3 possible mechanisms: 1) the thick cuffs of amyloid restricted the diffusion of water out of the collecting ducts into the medullary interstitium; 2) impaired reabsorption of sodium or other ions from the collecting ducts resulted in a lower osmolar concentration in the medulla, and 3) amyloid involvement of the vasa recta impaied the removal of interstitial water and thereby increased lymph flow and loss of medullary solutes. This case, then, represents an unusual experiment

of nature and underlines the role of the collecting ducts and probably the vasa recta in the production of a concentrated urine in man.

A second example is medullary cystic disease, a rare disorder occuring equally in males and females and most commonly seen in the first two decades of life (10). The medulla, as the primary site of disease, is suggested by a long history of polydypsia and polyurea. Clinical investigations of these patients reveal no antecedent history of kidney disease. There is always a dilute urine, and inability to concentrate the urine. Laboratory studies reveal a negative urine sediment, little or no proteinuria, no bacteruria in most cases, limited ability of the kidneys to alter hydrogen ion or bicarbonate excretion, a salt losing syndrome in 1/2 of the cases and a normal or slightly elevated blood pressure. The insidious onset of progressive uremia and anemia generally lead to death at an early age. It is becoming increasingly clear that what is called nephronophthesis in the European literature and medullary cystic disease in the American literature are one and the same disease (11).

Pathologically, the characteristic finding, consists of multiple small cysts localized almost entirely in the medulla. Grossly, their number and size vary markedly from one medulla to another (Fig. 5). Generally, they are quite small and therefore, can be easily overlooked. They vary in size from being barely perceptible by naked eye up to about one centimeter in diameter (Fig. 5). Microscopically, the cysts are lined by flat or low cuboidal epithelium and are located in the renal medulla except for a rare cyst in the cortex (Fig. 6). Another typical alteration in the medulla is a prominent increase in the connective tissue framework of the medullary interstitium (Fig. 7) which in some cases is infiltrated with lymphocytes, occasional

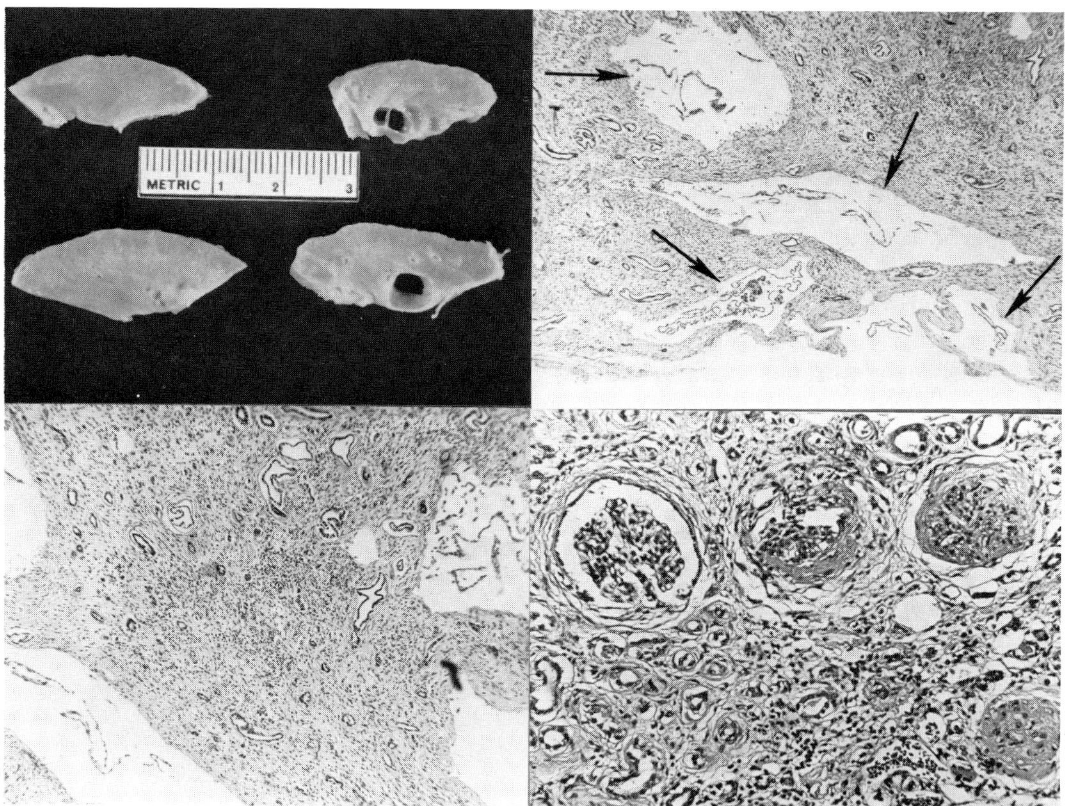

Fig. 5. *(upper left)* Medullary cystic disease. Four renal medullae from the same kidney showing the marked variation in the number and size of cysts from one medulla to another.

Fig. 6. *(upper right)* Medullary cystic disease. Four cysts (arrows) in the renal papilla with marked interstitial fibrosis and tubular destruction and atrophy. X40

Fig. 7. *(lower left)* Medullary cystic disease. Marked increase in connective tissue of the medullary interstitium with round cell infiltration. There is evidence of atrophy, dilatation and loss of tubules. X 80

Fig. 8. *(lower right)* Medullary cystic disease. Renal cortex showing marked tubular atrophy, interstitial fibrosis and glomerular hyalinization. The glomerulus in the upper left corner appears normal. X 200

TABLE II—CORRELATIONS IN MEDULLARY CYSTIC DISEASE

Pathological Changes	*Clinical Findings*
Medullary Cysts and Fibrosis with Tubular atrophy and obstruction	Loss of Concentrating ability Low specific gravity Polyuria, polydypsia
↓ Intrarenal hydronephrosis ↓	
Dilatation, atrophy and Fibrosis of cortical tubules	Inflexible handling of NA^+, H^+ "Salt losing nephritis"
↓ Glomerular hyalinization	Uremia-anemia O-Trace albuminuria, negative sediment
No or slight vascular disease	Normal or slightly increased B.P.

plasma cells and large mononuclear cells. The fibrous reaction often forms dense collars of hyaline collagenous tissue around the cysts or tubules. The cysts and fibrosis impinge upon normal medullary structures and cause marked obstruction, atrophy, and replacement of the tubules, especially collecting ducts. This, in turn, results in extensive atrophy and fibrous replacement of tubules and glomeruli in the cortex (Fig. 8). The unaffected glomeruli appear normal, i.e., there is no hypercellularity, basement membrane thickening, necrosis, exudation, crescent formation, etcetera (Fig. 8). The few functioning nephrons show marked hypertrophy which can be seen in the form of enlarged glomeruli and enormous dilatation of occasional proximal convolutions. There is no evidence of primary disease involving the tubules, interstitium or blood vessels of the cortex. The cortical arteries are normal or may show the early changes of sclerosis. Microdissection studies, currently in progress in our laboratory, have shown that the medullary cysts are not isolated structures but occur in collecting ducts as localized out pouchings of the tubules and Fetterman *et al.* (12) have demon-

strated that diverticulous alterations of the Loops of Henle is a striking feature of the disease. There is evidence that the cysts enlarge with time and cause progressive tissue damage since in one of our cases, a 42-year-old woman, one kidney was congenitally hypoplastic, and had only tiny cysts in the medulla, while the other kidney showed compensatory hypertrophy, and had greatly enlarged cysts along with the other morphologic features of the disease.

In Table II, a correlation is proposed between the structural changes and the functional and clinical features of the disease. The primary changes affect the medulla with gradual disruption of its structural architecture and functional capacity. Since this is the site of the urine concentrating process, loss of concentrating ability and polyuria as early manifestations of the disease are understandable. Enlargement of the cysts and the increasing fibrosis of the medullary interstitium gradually replace, destroy and obstruct tubules and cause intrarenal hydronephrosis which, in turn, leads to damage of cortical tubules and glomeruli and results in diminished tubular and glomerular function. Involvement of collecting ducts greatly accelerates all of these changes since one terminal collecting duct drains approximately 10,000 nephrons.

A final example, which presents another unique opportunity to study the renal concentrating process in man, is sickle cell anemia. Most patients with this disease cannot concentrate their urine above 450 mOsm. In children with the disease, exchange of the defective red cells with normal red cells returns renal concentrating ability to normal, indicating that the primary defect does not reside in the kidney. Perillie and Epstein (13) have shown that the red cells in this disease sickle when they are immersed in hypertonic salt solutions. They postulate that in the kidney, the red cells sickle within the vessels upon entering the hypertonic medulla. This would reduce medullary blood flow and the supply of oxygen available to the tubular cells of Henle's loop. Less sodium would be actively reabsorbed into the interstitial space and medullary osmolality and concentrating ability would drop. Our studies on the role of renal lymphatics suggest another mechanism to account for the concentrating defect in this disease. A marked reduction in blood flow due to sickling of the red cells would greatly decrease the amount of water removed from the medullary interstitium by the vasa recta. This would correspondingly enhance the flow of lymph and loss of solute. Since the lymphatics are direct channels out of the medulla, a greatly increased flow of lymph would dissipate the osmotic gradient in the medulla and result in impaired concentrating ability.

In conclusion, the mechanism by which the mammalian kidney concentrates urine is well established and is based largely on observations in laboratory animals. Correlation of structural and functional changes in certain renal diseases in man where loss of concentrating ability is the primary defect, indicates that the urine concentrating process in man is similar to other mammals.

REFERENCES

1. Pitts, R. F.: Physiology of the Kidney and Body Fluids, Chicago, Year Book, 1963.
2. Jamison, R. L., Bennett, C. M., and Berliner, R. W.: Countercurrent multiplication by the thin loops of Henle. Am. J. Physiol., *212*:357, 1967.
3. Carone, F. A., Everett, B. A., Blondeel, N. J., and Stolarczyk, J.: Renal localization of albumin and its function in the concentrating mechanism. Am. J. Physiol., *212*:387, 1967.
4. Mayerson, H. S.: The lymphatic system with particular reference to the kidney. Surg., *116*:259, 1963.
5. LeBrie, S. J., and Mayerson, H. S.: Influence of elevated venous pressure on flow and composition of renal lymph. Am. J. Physiol., *198*:1037, 1960.
6. Jaenike, J. R., and Bray, G. A.: Effects of acute transitory urinary obstruction in the dog. Am. J. Physiol., *199*:1219, 1960.
7. Ullrich, K. J., Kramer, K., and Boylan, J. W.: Present knowledge of the countercurrent system in the mammalian kidney. Progr. Cardiovasc. Dis., *3*:395, 1961.
8. Thurau, K., Deetjen, P., and Kramer, K.: Hämodynamik des Nierenmarkes. II. Mitteilung. Pflügers Arch. ges. Physiol., *270*:270, 1960.
9. Carone, F. A., and Epstein, F. H.: Nephrogenic diabetes insipidus caused by amyloid disease. Evidence in man on the role of the collecting ducts in concentrating urine. Am. J. Med., *29*:539, 1960.
10. Strauss, M. B.: Clinical and pathological aspects of cystic disease of the renal medulla: an analysis of sixteen cases. Ann. Int. Med., *52*:373, 1962.
11. Strauss, M. B., and Sommers, S. C.: Medullary cystic disease and familial juvenile nephronophthesis. New Eng. J. Med., *277*:863, 1967.
12. Fetterman, G. H., Fabrizio, N. S., and Studnicki, F. M.: The study by microdissection of structural tubular defects in certain examples of the hereditary nephropathies. Proceed. 3rd Inter. Congr. of Nephrology Vol. 2, pp. 235-250. New York, S. Karger, 1967.
13. Perillie, P. E., and Epstein, F. H.: Sickling phenomenon produced by hypertonic solutions: A possible explanation for the hyposthenuria of sicklemia. J. Clin. Invest., *42*:570, 1963.

Chapter 5

The Control of Renal Excretion of Sodium

ROBERT W. BERLINER, M.D.

Until a few years ago, most of those who had considered the problem of sodium excretion continued to assume that changes of sodium excretion could be explained by some combination of changes in the rate of glomerular filtration and in the secretion of salt-active steroids by the adrenal cortex. The inherent errors in the measurement of glomerular filtration rate made it difficult to be certain that changes in sodium excretion were not produced by changes in filtration too small to measure. And in case one had doubts about these, there were always possible changes in aldosterone secretion to take up the slack. While there were many observations that could be interpreted this way only by straining credulity, it is nevertheless true that the idea did not really catch on until the experiments of de Wardener *et al.* (4). Although a number of other aspects of the response to the infusion of isotonic saline were investigated in their studies, the key observation that seems to have put investigation in this field back on the track was a very simple one. de Wardener and his associates gave dogs large doses of salt-retaining steroids and vasopressin, so that suppression of the endogenous secretion of these hormones could not significantly affect events subsequently observed. They then infused isotonic saline solution and at the same time tightened a constricting clamp on the aorta so as to reduce renal arterial pressure and glomerular filtration rate. Despite the large amounts of steroids and the reduced filtration rate, a marked increase in sodium excretion occurred.

The essential features of this experiment have been confirmed by a number of subsequent studies (1, 5, 13, 19) and, in some of these, several of the more obvious changes caused by infusion of saline, such as dilution of the plasma proteins and distortion of the anion pattern of the blood, have been excluded as important factors in the diuretic response.

There has been considerable speculation and some differences of opinion concerning the mediation of this response to the infusion of saline. de Wardener and his associates thought that there was probably some hormone responsible, most likely a hormone released in the saline-infused dog that depressed sodium reabsorption although it could not be excluded that the hormone was one that promoted sodium reabsorption, release of which was suppressed by infusion of saline. In quest of the hypothetical hormone, they cross-circulated blood between dogs infused with saline and normal hydropenic recipients. Although there was some increase in salt excretion in the recipients, the experiments were interpreted as essentially negative because the increase in salt excretion was 3 to 10 times greater in the saline-infused donors than in the recipients of their blood. Nevertheless, de Wardener *et al.* did not abandon the idea of a humoral agent, suspecting, instead, that it might have too short a half-life to achieve an effective concentration in the recipient dogs.

Others have attempted, in rather similar studies, to demonstrate a humoral agent in the blood of saline-infused animals. Davis and his colleagues (9) reported what they interpreted as positive results although they had the same differences in salt excretion between donor and recipient that had led de Wardener's group to consider their experiments negative. On the other hand, Levinsky has carried out massive cross-circulations between salt-infused and hydropenic dogs and could find nothing he was willing to interpret as suggesting the presence of a humoral agent (12).

In an attempt to avoid the dilution of any humoral agent in the blood of the recipient, which must occur when cross-circulation is performed, there have been several studies in which isolated kidneys have been perfused with blood from saline-infused animals. Both de Wardener and his associates (4) and Lichardus and Pearce (15) found that sodium excretion increased when the kidneys were perfused with blood from animals undergoing diuresis. However, such perfused kidneys are known to deteriorate with time, the changes observed were rather

small, and there was no return to perfusion with the blood of hydropenic animals to show that the increase of sodium excretion was not simply a consequence of the passage of time. Consequently, these studies do not appear to be entirely convincing.

Meanwhile there are some who have stressed the role of changes in the flow and composition of the blood in the kidney as a major factor in the diuresis of saline infusion. Notable among these have been Earley and his associates (6, 7) who have carried out extensive experiments to examine the relationship between pressures and flows in the renal capillary circulation and the excretion of sodium. They have shown that salt excretion is increased when vasodilation is produced in the kidney and there is a striking further increase when blood pressure is then raised. Furthermore, they find that when plasma oncotic pressure is reduced sodium excretion increases and when plasma protein concentration is raised, salt excretion falls. Dr. Earley is inclined to relate the changes in sodium reabsorption to changes in renal interstitial volume in accord with a suggestion of Lewy and Windhager (14).

Whatever the mediation of the change in salt excretion, the immediate renal mechanism seemed to be clear up to 6 or 8 months ago. Several years ago, Drs. Dirks and Cirksena in our laboratory had found, in micropuncture studies in dogs, that when saline was infused there was a marked depression of the fraction of the glomerular filtrate reabsorbed in the proximal tubule (5). This depression persisted even when glomerular filtration rate was reduced 50% or more by partial clamping of the renal artery, so that it appeared clearly to be due to a decrease in the reabsorptive activity of the proximal tubules. It appeared that this depressed reabsorption was responsible for the increased excretion of salt, especially since the amount of extra sodium that was calculated to escape reabsorption in the proximal tubule was larger than what actually appeared in the urine. That is, reabsorption in the remainder of the tubule appeared to be actually increased.

This change in reabsorption in the proximal tubule with saline infusion was confirmed in the rat by Landwehr, Klose and Giebisch (11), by Cortney *et al* (3), and by Rector and his associates (18). In addition we showed that dogs with constrictions on the thoracic segment of the inferior vena cava, which do not have a diuresis when infused with saline, also had no decrease in reabsorption in the proximal tubule (2).

In addition to the mechanism by which reabsorption in the proximal tubule is depressed, findings first reported by Rector and Seldin and their associates are both exciting and disappointing (16). They used the shrinking drop method devised by Gertz to measure the reabsorptive activity of the proximal tubule (8). In this procedure a segment of proximal tubule is filled with colored castor oil and the oil column is then split by the injection of a droplet of isotonic saline. As the sodium is reabsorbed from the saline, the drop shrinks and the ends of the oil column approach each other. This process is recorded photographically and the length of the drop is measured in each photograph. When these lengths are plotted semilogarithmically against time they describe a straight line, the slope of which is a measure of the rate of sodium transport. Rector and his colleagues have used this technique as an assay system for factors that depress reabsorption in

the proximal tubule and found that reabsorption is depressed when rats are infused with the plasma of dogs infused with saline while plasma from hydropenic dogs has no effect. The material in the dog's blood is dialyzable and when the dialysate is used as the saline for the shrinking drop, reabsorption is depressed. They further report that the material is more concentrated in internal jugular blood than in peripheral blood and is absent in rats with lesions of the median eminence (17). It thus appeared that the material might be the agent responsible for regulating reabsorption of sodium by the renal tubule. However, this turns out not to be the case because when rats are injected with this material and show depressed reabsorption in their proximal tubules, they do not have an increase in sodium excretion. Obviously, something more must be involved. This conclusion had already been reached on the basis of certain studies in our laboratory. In an attempt to determine what part of the extracellular fluid volume was most critical in the response to saline infusion, Drs. Knox, Davis, Wright and Howards injected dogs with concentrated human serum albumin, thus expanding plasma volume at the expense of the remainder of the extracellular fluid (10). Reabsorption in the proximal tubule was depressed to an extent similar to that observed with saline infusion. Unlike the latter, however, the increase in sodium excretion with the albumin was trivial. Thus, depressed proximal reabsorption is not enough to guarantee increased sodium excretion; reabsorption in more distal segments must also be limited. Therefore, the so called "third factor" appears to be at least third and fourth and possibly additional factors as well.

REFERENCES

1. Blythe, W. B., and Welt, L. G.: Dissociation between filtered load of sodium and its rate of excretion in the urine. J. Clin. Invest., *42*:1491-1496, 1963.
2. Cirksena, W. J., Dirks, J. H., and Berliner, R. W.: Effect of thoracic cava obstruction on response of proximal tubule sodium reabsorption to saline infusion. J. Clin. Invest., *45*179-186, 1966.
3. Cortney, M. A., Mylle, M., Lassiter, W. E., and Gottschalk, C. W.: Renal tubular transport of water, solute, and PAH in rats loaded with isotonic saline. Am. J. Physiol., *209*:1199-1205, 1965.
4. de Wardener, H. E., Mills, I. H., Clapham, W. F., and Hayter, C. J.: Studies on the efferent mechanism of the sodium diuresis which follows the administration of intravenous saline in the dog. Clin. Sci., *21*:249-258, 1961.
5. Dirks, J. H., Cirksena, W. J., and Berliner, R. W.: The effect of saline infusion on sodium reabsorption by the proximal tubule of the dog. J. Clin. Invest., *44*:1160-1170, 1965.
6. Earley, L. E.: Influence of hemodynamic factors on sodium reabsorption. Ann. N. Y. Acad. Sci., *139*:312-327, 1966.
7. Earley, L. E., and Friedler, R. M.: The effects of combined renal vasodilation and pressor agents on renal hemodynamics and the tubular reabsorption of sodium. J. Clin. Invest., *45*:542-551, 1966.
8. Gertz, K. H.: Transtubuläre Natriumchloridflüsse und Permeabilität für Nichtelektrolyte im proximalen und distalen Konvolut der Rattenniere. Pflugers Arch. ges. Physiol., *276*:336-356, 1963.
9. Johnston, C. I., and Davis, J. O.: Evidence from cross circulation studies for a humoral mechanism in the natriuresis of saline loading. Proc. Soc. Exper. Biol. & Med., *121*:1058-1063, 1966.
10. Knox, F., Davis, B., Howards, S., Wright, F., and Berliner, R. W.: The effect of infusion of hyperoncotic albumin solution on sodium reabsorption by the proximal tubule of the dog. Fed. Proc., *26*:547, 1967.
11. Landwehr, D. M., Klose, R. M., and Giebisch, G.: Renal tubular sodium and water reabsorption in the isotonic sodium chloride-loaded rat. Am. J. Physiol., *212*:1327-1333, 1967.
12. Levinsky, N. G.: Nonaldosterone influences on renal sodium transport. Ann. N. Y. Acad. Sci., *139*:295-303, 1966.
13. Levinsky, N. G., and Lalone, R. C.: The mechanism of sodium diuresis after saline infusion in the dog. J. Clin. Invest., *42*:1261-1276, 1963.
14. Lewy, J. E., and Windhager, E. E.: Micropuncture study of the effect of partial renal venous occlusion on proximal tubular fluid reabsorption in the rat nephron. Fed. Proc., *26*:375, 1967.
15. Lichardus, B., and Pearce, J. W.: Evidence for a humoral natriuretic factor released by blood volume expansion. Nature, *209*:407-409, 1966.
16. Martinez-Maldonado, M., Kurtzman, N. A., Rector, F. C., Jr., and Seldin, D. W.: Evidence for a hormonal inhibitor of proximal tubular reabsorption. J. Clin. Invest., *46*:1091-1092, 1967.
17. Rector, F. C., Jr., Martinez-Maldonado, M., Kurtzman, N. A., and Seldin, D. W.: Site of formation of the natriuretic hormone. Abstracts, The American Society of Nephrology, 1st Annual Meeting, Los Angeles, California, Oct. 18-19, 1967, p. 55.
18. Rector, F. C., Jr., Sellman, J. C., Martinez-Maldonado, M., and Seldin, D. W.: The mechanism of suppression of proximal tubular reabsorption by saline infusions. J. Clin. Invest., *46*:47-56, 1967.
19. Rector, F. C., Jr., Van Giesen, G., Kiil, F., and Seldin, D. W.: Influence of expansion of extracellular volume on tubular reabsorption of sodium independent of changes in glomerular filtration rate and aldosterone activity. J. Clin. Invest., *43*:341-348, 1964.

Chapter 6

Mechanisms for the Renal Excretion of Phosphate and Calcium

FRANK A. CARONE, M.D.

A. MECHANISM OF RENAL EXCRETION OF PHOSPHATE

There is no conclusive evidence on the mode of phosphate excretion by the mammalian kidney or the site of action of parathyroid hormone on the renal tubule. This subject has been reviewed by Bartter (1) and more recently by Arnaud, Tenenhouse and Rasmussen (2). It has been shown that certain lower forms, such as fish with aglomerular nephrons and the alligator, secrete phosphate through the renal tubules (1, 2). Moreover, the studies of Levinsky and Davidson (3), have established that the renal tubule of the chicken secretes phosphate and that parathyroid extract delivered to the kidneys through the portal circulation increases phosphate excretion. Using standard clearance methods, a number of studies in dogs and cats suggest a tubular secretory mechanism for phosphate however as discussed by Bartter, the data from these studies cannot be interrupted with certainty (1). On the other hand, standard renal clearance studies in dog and man (1) and two separate stop-flow studies in the dog (4, 5) suggest that filtration and reabsorption are the only processes involved in the excretion of phosphate

and that parathyroid hormome increases phosphate excretion by decreasing tubular reabsorption rather than stimulating tubular secretion of phosphate.

Renal micropuncture techniques would offer a direct approach to this problem. In the following experiments, performed in our laboratory, phosphate was determined at an ultramicro level by a modified molybdate method in which ascorbic acid develops a stable reduced color complex (6). The method is 7 to 8 times more sensitive than standard molybdate procedures if the samples are read at a spectrophotometer setting of $820\ m\mu$. Determinations were made on a final volume of $20\ \mu l$ in Lowrey-type microcuvettes which have a light path of 10 mm.

In order to study the mechanism for the renal excretion of phosphate and the mode and site of action of parathyroid hormone in rats, micropuncture experiments were done in the following groups of animals: 1) normal; 2) normal-phosphate loaded; 3) parathyroidectomized; 4) parathyroidectomized-phosphate loaded, and 5) parathyroidectomized before and after the administration of highly purified parathyroid extract.

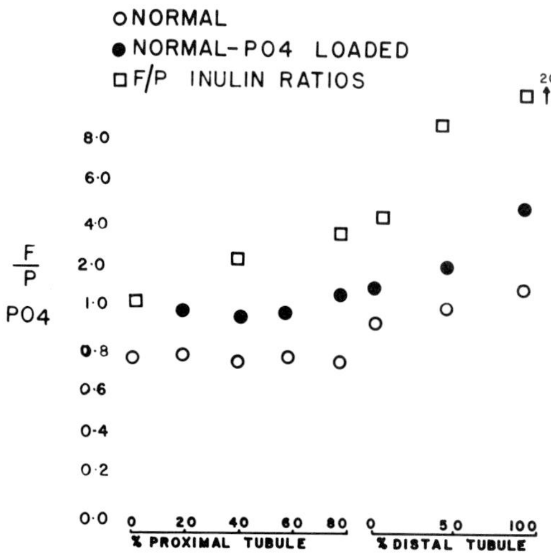

Fig.. 1. Mean phosphate and inulin concentration ratios (tubular fluid to plasma, F/P) in normal and normal phosphate-loaded rats expressed as a function of tubular length.

In Figure 1 are shown the results of micropuncture experiments in normal and phosphate loaded rats. The horizontal axis shows puncture sites along the nephron as a percentage of overall tubular length and the vertical axis tubular fluid to plasma (TF/P) phosphate ratios. Open circles are from normal animals and solid circles from normal animals given a phosphate load intravenously. The open squares are corresponding tubular fluid to plasma inulin ratios which are an index of water reabsorption. The figures are mean values from a large number of experiments. Five micropuncture samples of glomerular filtrate from normal animals had a mean fluid to plasma phosphate ratio of 0.81 indicating that 19% of inorganic plasma phosphate is not filterable. In normal rats, TF/P phosphate ratios averaged approximately 0.80 along the proximal tubule indicating proportionate reabsorption of phosphate and water by the proximal tubule and varied between 0.9 and 3.8 in the distal tubule.

Phosphate loading induced an enormous phoshaturia and yielded higher TF/P ratios both in proximal and distal tubules, being as high as 8.5 in the latter.

In these experiments, TF/P inulin ratios were always significantly higher than corresponding phosphate ratios, both in the proximal and distal tubule (Fig.1) indicating that the tubules at any particular site reabsorbed more water than phosphate. Therefore, the rise in phosphate concentration could be accounted for entirely by water reabsorption, even in phosphate loaded animals. Thus, evidence for tubular secretion of phosphate is lacking. These findings suggest that renal excretion of phosphate in normal and phosphate loaded animals is due solely to glomerular filtration and tubular reabsorption.

In Figure 2 are shown the results in parathyroidectomized and phosphate loaded parathyroidectomized rats. The open circles are values from animals that were only parathyroidectomized. In these animals, phosphate ratios fell progressively along the proximal tubule and averaged 0.16 in the late proximal, 0.12 in the distal and 0.4 in the urine. Note that phosphate concentration remained essentially unchanged from the late proximal tubule to the urine indicating that phosphate was reabsorbed in amounts roughly equal to that of water. The low concentration of phosphate in tubular fluid, following parathyroidectomy, constitutes strong evidence that phosphate reabsorption is an active process. It has been postulated that the electrical potential within tubular cells is more negative than the tubular lumen and that the phosphate concentration in cellular water greatly exceeds that of plasma (7). Therefore, the net transport of phosphate out of the tubules and into the cells occurs against a combined electrochemical gradient which requires the expenditure of energy. Thus, these findings show that proximal, distal, and collecting tubules can reabsorb phosphate by an active process. Since the tubules of parathyroidectomized animals are maximally reabsorbing phosphate, phosphate loading in such animals should demostrate a tubular secretory mechanism for phosphate if one exists. The solid circles (Fig. 2) show the results of phosphate loading in parathyroidectomized animals. TF/P phosphate ratios increased and averaged 1.1 in the proximal tubule and between 1.5 and 8.4 in the distal tubule. These values, however, were always considerably lower than corresponding inulin TF/P ratios, which are not shown on Figure 2. This indicates that water reabsorption by the tubules always exceed phosphate reabsorption, so that the increase in phosphate concentration could be accounted

for entirely by water reabsorption. Thus, there is no need to postulate a tubular secretory mechanism.

In Figure 3 is shown the effect of parathyroid hormone on renal tubules. Samples of tubular fluid were taken from the same puncture site in parathyroidectomized rats before and after the administration of parathyroid hormone. The open circles, below, are TF/P phosphate ratios in parathyroidectomized animals while the solid circles, above, are values from the same puncture sites after the intravenous administration of parathyroid hormone. The open triangles are corresponding tubular fluid to plasma inulin ratios and the values on the right are urine to plasma phosphate ratios. As above, following parathyroidectomy, phosphate concentration decreased along the nephron and remained at low values. After the administration of parathyroid hormone, there was a significant increase

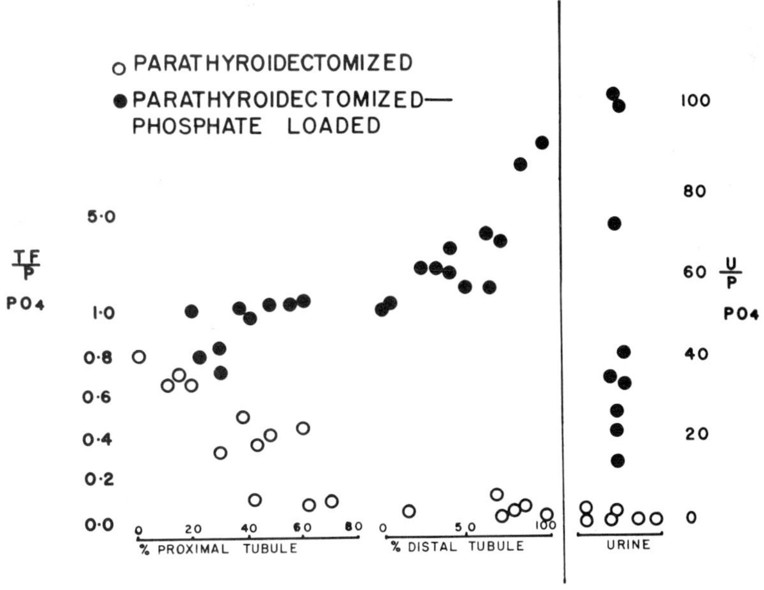

Fig. 2. Summary of phosphate concentration ratios in tubular fluid (TF/P) and urine (U/P) in parathyroidectomized and parathyroidectomized phosphate-loaded rats expressed as a function of tubular length.

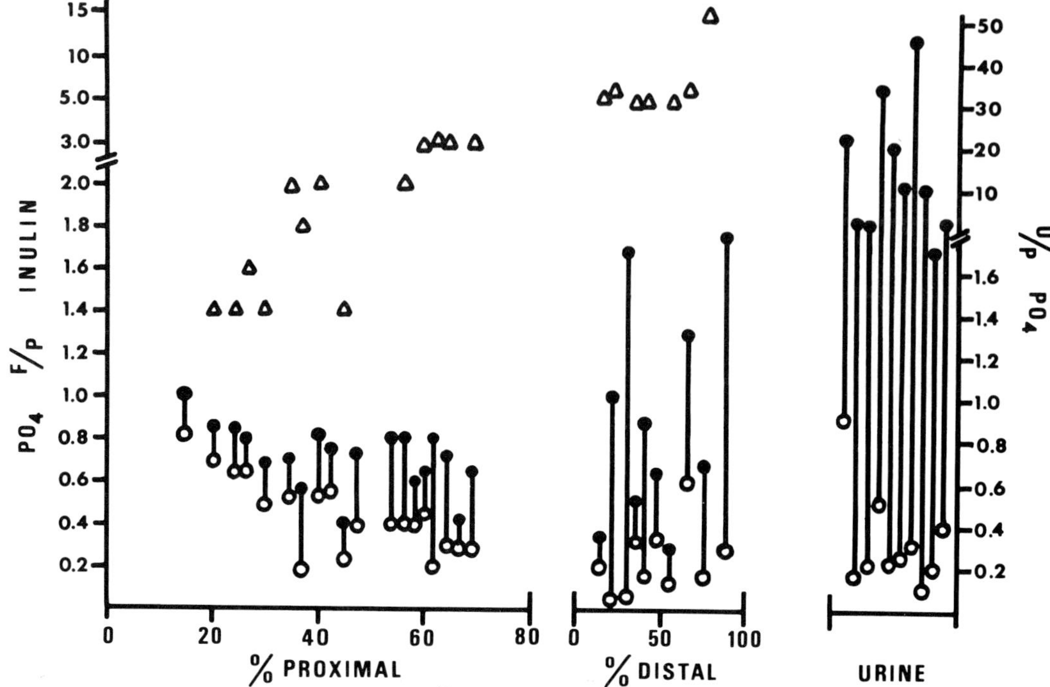

Fig. 3. Summary of phosphate concentration ratios (F/P) in the same tubular puncture sites and in urine (U/P) in acutely parathyroidectomized rats before (O) and after (●) the intravenous infusion of parathyroid hormone and corresponding inulin concentration ratios (F/P).

in the phosphate concentration of all tubular samples and, correspondingly, a marked increase in the excretion of phosphate in the urine. Note again, that TF/P inulin ratios were always considerably higher than phosphate ratios, even after the administration of parathyroid hormone, indicating greater water than phosphate reabsorption by the tubules. These findings show that parathyroid hormone has a direct effect on the renal tubules and that it produces phosphaturia by suppressing tubular reabsorption of phosphate rather than stimulating a secretory mechanism.

To summarize, these studies employing direct micropuncture methods in the rat show that phosphate excretion in the mammalian kidney is due to glomerular filtration and active tubular reabsorp-

tion; there is no evidence for a tubular secretory mechanism. Parathyroid hormone has a direct effect on the renal tubules and enhances phosphate excretion by decreasing tubular reabsorption.

B. MECHANISM OF RENAL EXCRETION OF CALCIUM

Standard renal clearance studies in the dog suggest that calcium excretion by the mammalian kidney involves glomerular filtration and subsequent reabsorption of most of the filtered calcium (8). Data from stopflow studies in the dog indicate that reabsorption of calcium in the distal nephron is an active process (9). Lassiter, Gottschalk and Mylle (10) studied the mechanism of calcium excretion in rats and hamsters by micropuncture methods using ^{45}Ca and found active reabsorption of calcium by all parts of the nephron, with the bulk of filtered calcium being reabsorbed by the proximal tubule. They also found that the pattern of calcium reabsorption by the tubules was similar to that of sodium, suggesting that the two are related. The studies of Walser (11) on calcium and sodium clearances show that these ions are reabsorbed and appear in the urine in about the same proportions that they are present in the plasma. From this data, he suggests that the renal tubular cells maintain a constant ratio of sodium to calcium ions in the tubular fluid due to competitive binding of sodium and calcium at the cell membrane.

There is no evidence available to suggest that calcium is secreted by the mammalian nephron. The complexing of ionized calcium by inorganic or organic anions greatly decreases tubular reabsorption of calcium and may increase calcium excretion from a few percent of the filter load up to 80%. This suggests that only ionized calcium is actively reabsorbed by the tubules and that complexed calcium is largely excreted in the urine. The studies of Kleeman *et al* (12) in dogs and man indicate that parathyroid hormone contributes to the homeostatic regulation of the tubular reabsorption of calcium, since they found in a number of experimental or clinical conditions that parathyroid hormone causes a decreased excretion and, presumably, an increased tubular reabsorption of calcium.

Using micropuncture methods, the renal excretion of calcium has been

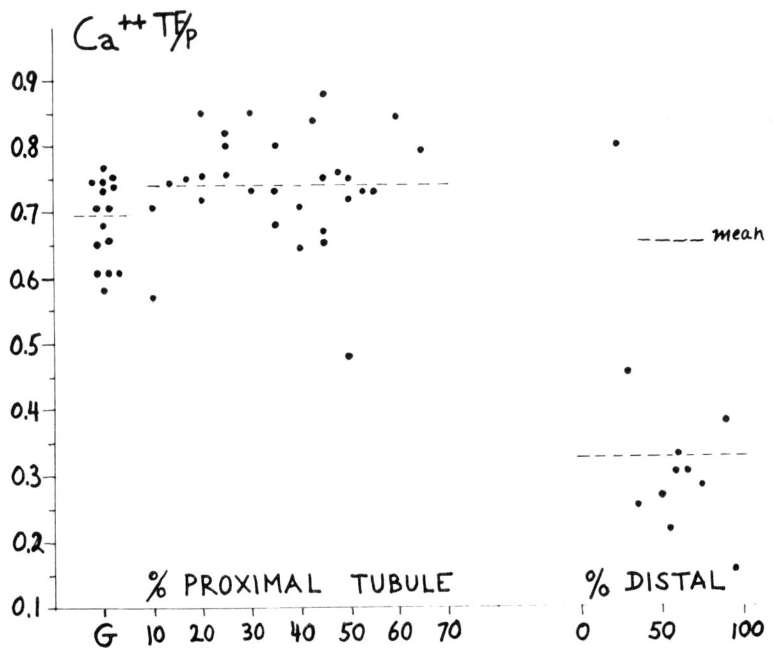

Fig. 4. Summary of calcium concentration ratios in glomerular filtrate (G) and tubular fluid (TF/P) in normal rats expressed as a function of tubular length.

TABLE 1—AVERAGE TUBULAR FLUID TO
GLOMERULAR FILTRATE RATIOS OF CALCIUM
AND INULIN IN NORMAL RATS

Site	Calcium	Inulin	% Calcium Reabsorbed $100 - (\frac{\text{Calcium}}{\text{Inulin}} \times 100)$
Early Proximal	1.0	1	0
Late Proximal	1.06	3	64.7
Early Distal	0.72	5	85.6
Late Distal	0.44	21	97.9
Urine	1.03	588	99.8

investigated in our laboratory in normal rats.* An ultramicro colorimetric method using the dye Arsenazo was developed for the determination of calcium. The test was adapted to an automated microanalytical system for the determination of this element in serum and urine. In Figure 4 are shown the results in 14 normal animals. The fluid to plasma calcium ratios in glomerular samples, labeled "G" in Figure 4, had a mean of 0.69, indicating that roughly 69% of plasma calcium in the normal rat is filterable and that approximately 31% is bound to plasma protein. Calcium tubular fluid to plasma (TF/P) ratios averaged 0.73 in proximal samples, 0.40 in distal samples and 0.71 in the urine. Since the tubular lumen has a negative change, the low calcium TF/P ratios in distal samples indicate active reabsorption of calcium by the distal nephron against a combined electrical and chemical gradient. The micropuncture study of Lassiter and co-workers (10) has shown active reabsorption of calcium by the proximal tubule during mannitol diuresis. The quantity of filtered calcium reabsorbed at various sites along the nephron can be calculated from the data

in Table I. In the first column are recorded average calcium concentrations, expressed as a fraction of the calcium concentration in glomerular filtrate. The second column shows the average concentration ratios for ^{14}C inulin at the same sites, obtained from a similar group of rats. The third column gives the percentage of filtered calcium that is reabsorbed at various sites along the nephron, which is derived by subtracting from 100, the calcium ratio divided by the inulin ratio. It can be seen that approximately 65% of filtered calcium is reabsorbed by the convoluted (surface) segment of the proximal tubule, 21% by the descending pars recta of the proximal tubule and the loop of Henle, 12% by the distal tubule and 2% by the collecting ducts. In this group of animals, only 0.2% of the filtered calcium was excreted in the urine. These data indicate that filtered calcium is reabsorbed by all portions of the nephron, but that the bulk of calcium reabsorption occurs in the proximal tubule.

In summary, these studies show that calcium excretion in the mammalian kidney involves the processes of glomerular filtration and active tubular reabsorption. Although calcium is largely reabsorbed by the proximal tubules, all portions of the nephron including collec-

---

*This work was done in collaboration with Dr. Nicholas J. Blondeel, University of Louvain, Belgium.

ting ducts participate in the active reabsorption of calcium.

In conclusion, micropuncture methods are being employed, more and more, to study directly normal and abnormal renal function. In this discussion, an attempt has been made to show the kinds of information that can be obtained from direct micropuncture experiments on the kidney and to show how this data is interpreted. This knowledge will be of increasing importance in the future in evaluating new observations in renal pathophysiology and in relating this information to clinical problems involving the kidneys.

REFERENCES

1. Bartter, F. A.: The effect of the parathyroid on phosphate excretion. In Greep, R. O., and Talmage, R. V. (eds.): The Parathyroids. Springfield, Thomas, 1961, 338-403.
2. Arnaud, C. D., Jr., Tenenhouse, A. M., and Rasmussen, H.: Parathyroid hormone. Am. Rev. of Physiol., *29:*349-372, 1967.
3. Levinsky, N. G., and Davidson, D. G.: Renal action of parathyroid extract in the chicken. Am. J. Physiol., *191:*530-536, 1957.
4. Lambert, P. P., Vanderveiken, F., DeKoster, J. P., Kahn, R. J., and De Myttenaere, M.: Study of phosphate excretion by the stop-flow technique. Nephron, *1:*103-117, 1964.
5. Samiy, A. H., Hirsh, P. F., and Ramsay, A. G.: Localization of phophaturic effect of parathyroid hormone in nephron of the dog. Am. J. Physiol., *208:*73-77, 1965.
6. Chen, P. S., Jr., Toribara, T. Y., and Warner, H.: Microdetermination of phosphorus. Anal. Chem., *28:*1756- , 1956.
7. Strickler, J. C., Thompson, D. D., Klose, R. M., and Giebish, G.: Micropuncture study of inorganic phosphate excretion in the rat. J. Clin. Invest., *43:*1596-1607, 1964.
8. Chen, P. S., Jr., and Neuman, W. F.: Renal excretion of calcium by the dog. Am. J. Physiol., *160:*623-631, 1955.
9. Howard, P. J., Wilde, W. S., and Malvin R. N.: Localization of renal calcium transport; effect of calcium load and of gluconate anion on water, sodium and potassium. Am. J. Physiol., *197:*337-341, 1959.
10. Lassiter, W. E., Gottschalk, C. W. and Mylle, M.: Micropuncture study of renal tubular reabsorption of calcium in normal rodents. Am. J. Physiol., *204:*771-775, 1963.
11. Walser, M.: Calcium clearance as a function of sodium clearance in the dog. Am. J. Physiol., *200:*1099-1104, 1961.
12. Kleeman, C. R., Bernstein, D., Rockney, R., Dowling, J. T., and Maxwell, M. H.: Studies on the renal clearance of diffusable calcium and the role of the parathyroid glands in its regulation. In, Greep, R. O., and Talmage, R. V. (eds.): The Parathyroids. Springfield, Thomas, 1961, 353-382.

Mechanisms of Diuretics

ROGER F. PALMER, M.D.

Diuresis is defined as an increase of urine flow. Even though flow may be increased by all diuretic agents, the composition of the urine varies widely. An effective diuresis in clinical parlance has come to mean a net loss of water and ions, principally sodium and chloride from the body. Urine flow increases secondary to the increased amount of these ions in the urine. Loss of these substances is desirable in clinical states where edema (an abnormal increase in extracellular fluid) is a problem. The most common edema producing situation is congestive heart failure, which, when sufficiently advanced, results in massive increases in Na^+, Cl^- and water in extracellular spaces. This increase in extracellular water compromises the failing heart by further overloading the left ventricle. Reduction of the volume of extracellular fluid via the kidneys is desirable. Other edema states include cirrhosis, nephrotic syndrome and renal disorders.

The means by which a diuresis can be produced are many. To understand how diuretic agents work requires an understanding of how urine formation proceeds. Approximately one fourth of the cardiac output of blood flows through the kidneys. A portion of the plasma is filtered through the glomerulus. All substances of low molecular weight (usually less than 30,000) and some protein appear in the proximal tubule. Large molecular weight proteins and formed blood elements remain. The contents of the filtrate are then reabsorbed by the tubules to a more or less extent by a variety of means. Sodium and chloride are almost completely reabsorbed in the proximal and distal tubule, potassium and hydrogen ion are reabsorbed proximally then secreted in the distal tubule possibly by the same secretory mechanism. Water is reabsorbed in an obligatory fashion as the ions are reabsorbed and perhaps also directly in the loop of Henle and the collecting ducts. Most of these reabsorptive mechanisms are under hormonal control. For example, water reabsorption is influenced by antidiuretic hormone; Na^+, K^+ and H^+ secretion are influenced by aldosterone. Physical factors also play a role in regulating degree of ion and water reabsorption; decreasing the glomerular filtration rate increases the amount of sodium reabsorbed; increasing renal venous pressure also increases the amount of sodium reabsorption. For a more complete discussion of these mechanisms, see Pitts (1).

Most reabsorptive operations require the performance of metabolic work. Ions are "pumped" against electrochemical gradients throughout various protions of the kidney. The kidney is a vigorous metabolizing organ presumably utilizing the energy produced to reabsorb filtered materials.

Diuretic agents can affect tubular reabsorptions of ions and water in a variety of ways. Energy production or utilization mechanisms can be interfered with; the action of hormonal agents which enhance tubular reabsorption can be blocked; production of hydrogen ion in the proximal tubule which exchanges for Na^+ can be inhibited, and finally, membrane permeability to the passive movement of ions and other solutes can be decreased. Not all these potential mechanisms are represented by the mode of action of a current diuretic agent, nor has the mode of action of all diuretic agents been conclusively demonstrated. The purpose of this chapter is to summarize current knowledge of diuretics and to characterize their effects on urine electrolytes.

Water Diuretics. Water loading acts as a diuretic by inhibiting the production of anti-diuretic hormone. There is no clinical advantage because a net loss of water does not occur. Ethanol and chlorpromazine act directly to inhibit the supraoptico-neurohypophyseal system which controls the secretion of anti-diuretic hormone (2, 3). These drugs may be of use in selected clinical situations where "water intoxication" is a problem. They are not used widely for this purpose however. There is a relative increase in salt retention.

Osmotic Agents. Urea, glucose mannitol, isosorbide increase the solute load of the glomerular filtrate exerting an effective osmotic pressure in the renal tubule and in other body cells as well. Mannitol and isosorbide are not metabolized nor are they reabsorbable by the renal tubule, therefore their ability to exert an effective osmotic pressure exceeds that of glucose or urea. Since water reabsorption normally follows the osmotic gradient built up by the active reabsorption of Na^+ and Cl^-, during mannitol or isosorbide diuresis, the gradient is decreased and passive water transfer takes place to a lesser extent. In fact, there is an increase in salt excretion since the rate of active reabsorption of sodium is a function of its tubular concentration which under these circumstances would be reduced (4). The clinical usefulness of these agents is increasing and they may find an important place in the management of refractory edemas (5).

Acidifying Salts. Ammonium chloride, calcium chloride, lysine monohydrochloride result in an increased chloride load to the tubule by virtue of destruction or failure of absorption of the cation. Thus, a hyperchloremic acidosis is produced. The excess chloride in the urine claims a cation (Na^+, K^+ or NH_4^+). The response is only temporary since the kidney compensates by secreting more H^+ saving Na^+ (6). These agents are not widely used as primary diuretic agents.

Anti-aldosterone Agents. Spironolactone structurally resembles aldosterone and competitively blocks its action at the renal tubular level (7). In certain conditions, e.g., cirrhosis with ascites, the nephrotic syndrome, congestive heart failure, aldosterone secretion may be very high and contribute materially to the formation of edema. It is in these conditions that spironolactones work best to increase Na^+ excretion and decrease K^+ loss. Rarely are they the sole diuretic agent used, since their action is potentiated by combination with other agents discussed below.

Xanthines. Theophylline, caffeine and theobromine have purine-like structures and decrease the tubular reabsorption of

Cl$^-$ and Na$^+$. They are purported to inhibit the breakdown of cyclic AMP by phosphodiesterase and thus in some way enhance Na$^+$ and Cl$^-$ loss (8). They are not very powerful and side effects are common.

1, 3-Disulfonamides: Thiazides. These agents have revolutionized diuretic treatment in outpatients. The thiazides are well absorbed orally and relatively potent. There are many structural types but the action of any one of them resembles others in this class. Hydrochlorothiazide, the prototype, decreases distal tubular reabsorption of Cl$^-$ and Na$^+$ and some K$^+$ loss occurs. These drugs apparently work differently from others previously considered since effects are additive (6). As yet, no clue to their biochemical mode of action is known. They are weak acids, thus compete for uric acid secretion sites in the kidney resulting in mild elevation of serum urate (9). A diabetogenic action is partly due to excessive K$^+$ loss in the body as well as a direct effect on glucose metabolism (10). They are useful in hypertension through an effect most likely extra-renal (11).

Organomercurials. Mercaptomerin and mercuhydrin can only be used parenterally. They cause a loss of Na$^+$ and Cl$^-$. Potassium loss is not as much as that with the thiazides since the distal secretion of K$^+$ is inhibited by these agents. These drugs inhibit the transport ATP'ase in the kidney and perhaps this is their mode of action, however, some non-diuretic organomercurials have this property as well (12). They have the unique property of increasing free water clearance (13). Solute free water clearance (C_{H_2O}) is calculated by subtracting the osmolal clearance from the urine volume (V).

$$C_{H_2O} = V - \frac{U_{osm}}{P_{osm}} \times V$$

Organomercurials are thereby helpful in states of water intoxication or dilutional hyponatremic states where greater water than solute loss is desirable.

CARBONIC ANHYDRASE INHIBITORS

Acetazolamide, ethoxzolamide, methazolamide cause a bicarbonate diuresis and alkalinization of the urine. H$^+$ generation from CO_2 is inhibited, thus bicarbonate reabsorption is prevented. The excess proximal tubular bicarbonate claims Na$^+$. K$^-$ is excreted due to inhibition of distal H$^+$ production (14). Chronic administration results in a systemic acidosis which negates further bicarbonate loss. There is no progressive Na$^+$ or K$^+$ loss. These agents have limited usefulness as diuretics. Their chief use is in the treatment of glaucoma.

Ethacrynic Acid. A derivative of phenoxyacetic acid, it is the most potent of all diuretic agents. This agent has some features in common with organomercurials and thiazides but almost certainly acts on a different reabsorptive mechanism although still primarily distal. It also is a weak inhibitor of transport ATP'ase (12), a popular site for its mode of action in current literature. It binds to sulfhydryl groups of renal cellular proteins (15). Its major site of action is purported to be in the loop of Henle but this remains controversial. There is less K$^+$ loss for a given amount of sodium excreted than that seen with the thiazides, however, total body potassium loss is a problem.

Furosemide. Structurally unrelated to ethacrynic acid, it is as potent and behaves similarly. It appears to work along the entire nephron. Its effect is additive with hydrochlorothiazide suggesting a different site of action than these agents, however, there is no addition when combined with ethacrynic acid (16). Renal chloride excretion is greater than that of sodium. Furosemide shares the diabetogenic action and plasma urate elevating properties of the thiazides. It is well absorbed orally and has gained wide clinical acceptance.

Pteridines. Triamterene is the first agent of this new class of drugs that is remarkable for its effect on potassium excretion. It is only moderately effective as a natriuretic and chloruretic but actually causes *potassium retention* (17). When used in combination with other drugs, especially the thiazides, there is mutual potentiation, i.e., the effect of both is greater than the added effect of either.

Summary. The effect of the diuretics on the urinary electrolyte pattern is diverse. A summary of the effects of major representatives of the classes are given in section B of this chapter.

REFERENCES

1. Pitts, R. F.: Physiology of the Kidney and Body Fluids. Chicago, Year Book 1963, p.p. 52-115.
2. Gaunt, R., Chart, J. J., and Renzi, A. A.: Interaction of drugs with endocrines. A. Rev. Pharmac., *3:*109-128, 1963.
3. van Dyke, H. B., and Ames, Rose G.: Alcohol diuresis. Acta endocr. Copenh., *7:*110-121, 1951.
4. Walser, M., and Mudge, G. H.: Renal excretory mechanisms. Chapter 9 in Mineral Metabolism. (Comar, C. L., and Bronner, F. (ed.) New York, Academic Press, 1960.
5. Walker, W. Gordon, Cooke, C. Robert, Iber, Frank L., Lesch, Michael, and Caranosos, George: Topics in clinical medicine: A symposium on uses and complications of diuretic therapy. Johns Hopkins Med. J., *121:*194-216, 1967.
6. Pitts, R. F.: The Physiological Basis of Diuretic Therapy. Springfield, Thomas., 1959.
7. Kagawa, C. M., Sturtevant, F. M., and Van Arnam, C. G.: Pharmacology of a new steroid that blocks salt activity of aldosterone and desoxycorticosterone. J. Pharmacol., *126:*123-130, 1959.
8. Orloff, J., and Handler, J. S.: The cellular mode of action of antidiuretic hormone. Am. J. Med., *36:*686-697, 1964.
9. De Martini, F. E., Wheaton, E. A., Healey, L. A., Laragh, J. H.: Effect of chlorothiazide on the renal excretion of uric acid. Amer. J. Med., *32:*572-578, 1962.
10. Reutter, R., and Labhart, A.: Saluretica and Glukosetoleranz. Helv. med. Acta., *28:*487, 1961.
11. Wilson, I. M., and Freis, E. D.: Relationship between plasma and extracellular fluid volume depletion and the antiypertensive effect of chlorothiazide. Circulation, *20:*1028-1036, 1959.
12. Nechay, B. R., Palmer, R. F., Chinoy, D. A. and Posey, V. A.: The problem of Na^+ and K^+ ATP'ase as the receptor for diuretic action of mercurials and ethacrynic acid. J. Pharmacol. Exp. Therap., *157:*599-617, 1967.
13. Porush, J. G., Goldstein, M. H., Eisner, G. M., and Levitt, M. F.: Effect of Organomercurials on the renal concentrating operation in Hydropenic Man: Comments on site of action. J. Clin. Invest., *40:*1475-1485, 1961.
14. Berliner, R. W., Kennedy, T. J., Jr., and Orloff, J.: Relationship between acidification of the urine and potassium metabolium. Am. J. Med., *11:*274-282, 1951.
15. Beyer, K. H., Baer, J. K., Michaelson, Joan K., and Russo, H. F.: Renotropic characteristics of ethacrynic acid: a phenoxyacetic saluretic diuretic agent. J. Pharmacol. Exp. Therap., *147:*1-22, 1965.
16. Hook, J. B., and Williamson, H. E.: Addition of the Saluretic action of Furosemide to the Saluretic action of Certain Other Agents. J. Pharmacol. Exp. Therap, *148:*88-93, 1965.
17. Cohen, A. B.: Hyperkalemic Effects of Triamterene. Ann. Int. Med., *65:*521, 1966.

Tabulation of Diuretic Agents*

ROGER F. PALMER, M.D.

The following is a summary of major diuretic agents, their effects, and what is known of their mode of action. Examples were chosen to represent a class of agents with distinct actions.

1. "WATER DIURETICS"
    a) H_2O

Effect	Increases output of water by the kidney.
Mechanism	Reduces output of antidiuretic hormone by decreasing osmotic pressure of plasma.
Therapeutic Use	None. Electrolytes not affected, and no net loss of water.

    b) Ethanol; Chlorpromazine

Effect	Increases output of water by the kidney. Dehydrates.
Mechanism	Inhibition of supraoptico-neurohypophyseal system controlling secretion of antidiuretic hormone.
Therapeutic Use	None. Electrolytes not affected. Relative salt retention would be increased.

2. "OSMOTIC AGENTS" (Urea, Glucose, etc.)

Effect	Abstracts water from body, and in some cases Na^+ and Cl^-.
Mechanism	Increase in solute load of glomerular filtrate leads to obligatory water loss. Na^+ and Cl^- output due to tubule "flooding."

---

*This list was prepared by Dr. T. H. Maren and his associates of the Department of Pharmacology and Therapeutics, University of Florida.

Therapeutic Use	Limited, because of relative ineffectiveness; salt removal is negligible compared to other diuretics.

3. ACIDIFYING SALTS (NH_4Cl, $CaCl_2$, etc.)

Effect	Cation destroyed (NH_4Cl) or unabsorbed ($CaCl_2$), leaving excess Cl^- in plasma, and systemic acidosis. Excess Cl^- delivered to tubule, claiming Na^+. Na^+ and Cl^- excreted.
Mechanism	Cl^- partially replaces HCO_3^- in blood and glomerular filtrate. This is temporary, as the changes initiate a compensatory response, i.e., excretion of H^+, which carries off Cl^-, and saves Na^+.
Therapeutic Use	Limited to a few days, because of base saving mechanism. Used largely in connection with other drugs.

4. ANTIALDOSTERONE AGENTS

Effect	Loss of Na^+, Cl^-, and H_2O. Possible potassium retention.
Mechanism	Secretion of aldosterone inhibited (amphenones) or effect of aldosterone antagonized at tubular level (spirolactones).
Therapeutic Use	*Amphenones* experimental use only. *Spirolactones* used in edema secondary to liver disease and in some heart failure when aldosterone is elevated. Usually combined with thiazides.

Amphenone

H_2N—⟨benzene⟩—C(CH$_3$)(C=O, CH$_3$)—⟨benzene⟩—NH_2

5. XANTHINES (Theophylline, Caffeine, and Theobromine). (Note purine structure.)

Effect	Loss of Na^+, Cl^-, some K^+, and H_2O.
Mechanism	Decreases tubular reabsorption of Cl^- and Na^+.
Therapeutic Use	Well established, but these drugs are not very powerful; side effects, as emesis, are notable.

Theophylline

6. 1.—3-DISULFONAMIDES: THIAZIDES

Chlorothiazide, Hydrochlorothiazide, Dichlorphenamide, Benzthiazide, Trifluoromethylthiazide, Trichlormethiazide and late entries.

Hydrochlorothiazide

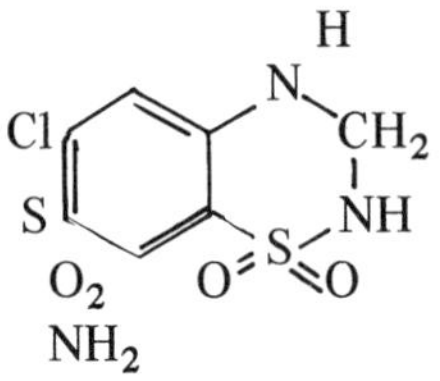

(Note chlorthalidone, an interesting structural variant with a carbon function replacing the second sulfamyl group.)

Effect

1) Loss of Na^+, Cl^-, and some K^+, and H_2O.
2) Depending on potency as a carbonic anhydrase inhibitor and dose, there may also be HCO_3^- in urine. *Hydrochlorothiazide* does not alkalinize the urine at any dose under 50 mg per kg, since it is an exceedingly weak C.A. inhibitor ($2 \times 10^{-5}M$). So it may be used as an example of this class, without the complication of renal HCO_3^- output.

Mechanism

On a biochemical or enzymatic basis unknown, decreases tubular reabsorption of Cl^- and Na^+, some K^+ is lost. Renal electrolyte pattern is the same as class 5 above, but biochemical mechanisms are different since effects of the two classes are additive. Action is probably chiefly on distal segment.

Therapeutic Use

Very great, in the treatment of cardiac edema. They have low systemic toxicity; however, there is some danger of K^+ loss. A few hypersensitive reactions have been reported. Also used in treatment of hypertension. Basis is probably salt and/or volume depletion with a possibility of a direct cardio-vascular effect. Also useful in both forms of diabetes insipidus. Decrease in urine volume possibly due to mild salt depletion.

7.   MERCURIALS (Mercuhydrin, Salyrgan, Mercaptomerin, etc.)

Effect   Loss of Na^+, Cl^-, and secondarily of H_2O. Erratically, K^+ loss.

Mechanism   Decreases tubular reabsorption of Na^+ and/or Cl^- by unknown mechanism (inhibition of Na^+ and K^+ dependent adenosinetriphosphatase?)

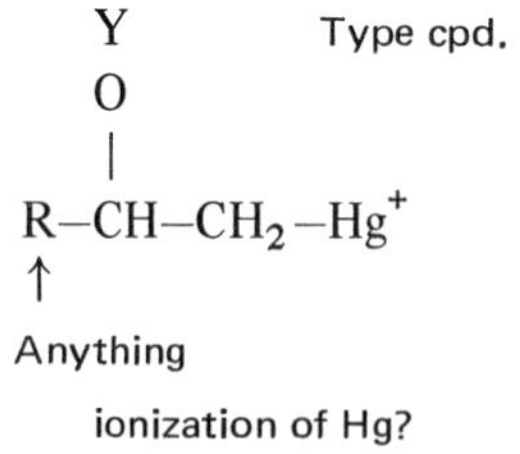

Y   Type cpd.

$$R\text{--}CH\text{--}CH_2\text{--}Hg^+$$

Anything

ionization of Hg?

Therapeutic Use   Very widespread, but not ideal due to toxicity, necessity for injection, and uneven course. Potentiated by acidosis due to NH_4Cl or acetazolamide. In contrast to thiazide increases free water clearance. If one wishes to treat edema complicated by dilutional hyponatremia, this is the drug of choice.

8. **CARBONIC ANHYDRASE INHIBITORS** (Acetazolamide, methazolamide, ethoxzolamide)

Effect

Increases output of HCO_3^-, Na^+, K^+, and secondarily of H_2O.

Mechanism

Slowing of the enzymatically controlled reaction $H_2O + CO_2 \xrightarrow[\text{Anhydrase}]{\text{Carbonic}} H_2CO_3$ in renal tubule. This in turn reduces the quantity of H^+ ions available for reaction with lumenal urine, leading to alkalinization of the final urine and loss of the ions noted above.

The promixal action leads to diuresis of Na^+ and HCO_3^-; the distal action to further repression of H^+ (and HN_4^+) output, and excretion of K^+.

Therapeutic Use

A. Acetazolamide is given orally and is well tolerated. Initial effect may be relatively small, but many ambulatory cardiacs are evenly maintained for many months or years at the low dose of 5 mg per kg per 24 or 48 hours. Not effective in severely ill cardiac patients, or in the presence of renal disease. Notably effective in cor pulmonale. Less active than the thiazides, but less toxic, since there is no danger of chronic K^+ loss.

B. After one or two days of administration at moderate dose (10 mg per kg 12 or 24 hours), the "stage is set" for the use of mercurial diuretics. Due to the metabolic acidosis, the effect of the mercurial is greater than if given alone.

9. **ETHACRYNIC ACID**

Effect

The most potent known inhibitor of Na^+ and/or Cl^-, and consequently water reabsorption by renal tubules. Na^+/K^+ ratios in urine considerably higher than after thiazides, but still danger of K^+ loss.

Mechanism

Probably inhibits utilization of ATP energy for Na^+ reabsorption. Binds to SH groups of renal cellular proteins.

Therapeutic Use

Because of its ability to overcome some homeostatic mechanisms causes death due to electrolyte imbalance after about one week of maximally effective dosing in dogs. However, the drug has received clinical acceptance, subject to judicial use, by virtue of being effective in some cases resistant to other diuretics.

10. FUROSEMIDE

Effect   Reduces tubular reabsorption of Na^+ and Cl^-. Some K^+ loss.

Mechanism   Unknown. Part of the effect is that of the thiazides. It is a "doubly acting drug", or a thiazide plus. Although it is a sulfonamide, carbonic anhydrase inhibition activity *in vivo* is negligible.

Therapeutic Use   Oral drug, gaining wide popularity. Although structurally related to thiazides, potency and electrolyte excretion is roughly similar to that of ethacrynic acid. Overdosage may result in electrolyte imbalance.

11. PTERIDINES (Triamterene)*
(Amiloride)

Effect   Increases urinary output of Na^+ and HCO_3^-. Causes retention of K^+ and *hyperkalemia*.

Mechanism   Unknown.

Therapeutic Use   Oral diuretic. Moderate effectiveness, less potent than thiazides. Used in edema due to cirrhosis of the liver. Like spirolactones, triamterene can sometimes be used in combination with thiazides to prevent hypokalemia. Needs more evaluation.

Not an aldosterone antagonist. Acts in the adrenalectomized animal.

---

*Dyrenium®

SUMMARY OF ACUTE RENAL ELECTROLYTE ACTIONS

Therapeutic Dose of:	Na^+	K^+	Cl^-	HCL_3^-	*Free Water Clearance $(T_c H_2 O)$*
Hydrochlorthiazide	+++	+	+++	0	↓
Acetazolamide	++	++	0	+++	↓ or 0
Meralluride	++++	+	++++	0	↑
Aminophylline	++	+	++	0	↑
Ethacrynic Acid	+++++	+	+++++	0	↑
Furosemide	++++	+	++++	0	↑ *
Triamterene	++		++	0	U

*May also decrease reabsorption during dilutional hyponatremia, thus, $T_c H_2 O$.

ACUTE EFFECTS OF SELECTED DIURETIC COMBINATIONS

Mercurials and acidifying salts	Potentiation
Mercurials and aminophylline	Additive on tubular level. May be more than additive due to improvement of renal circulation by aminophylline.
Mercurials and thiazides	Additive
Mercurials and carbonic anhydrase inhibitors, given simultaneously	Mercurial effect reduced. Note synergism under different circumstances of dosage, when acidosis is initially elicited by acetazolamide.
Thiazides and aminophylline	Additive
Thiazides and spirolactones	Reduces K^+ loss
Thiazides and triamterene	Reduces K^+ loss
Aminophylline and carbonic anhydrase inhibitors	Mutual potentiation
Thiazides, or ethacrynic acid, or furosemide; and carbonic anhydrase inhibitors.	Additive

EFFECT OF ALTERATIONS IN ACID–BASE BALANCE
ON REPRESENTATIVE RENAL DRUGS

	HCl	*K⁺ Depletion*	*Chronic Acetazolamide*	*NaNCO₃*
Hydrochlorothiazide	- - -	U	- - -	- - -
Aminophylline	↑	U	- - -	↓
Mercurials	↓	↓	↓	↑
Acetazolamide	↑	↑	↑	- - -
Ethacrynic Acid	- - -	U	U	- - -

- - - Effect as usual
↓ Increased effect
↑ Decreased effect
U Not known

REFERENCES

1. Earley, L. E., and Orloff, J.: Thiazide Diuretics. Amer. Rev. Med., *15*:149, 1964.
2. Kessler, R. H.: The clinical pharmacology of the mercurial diuretic compounds. Clin. Phar. & Therap., *1:*723, 1960.
3. Maren, T. H., *et al.*: Effect of diamox on electrolyte metabolism. Bull. Johns Hopk. Hosp., *95:*277, 1954.
4. Pitts, R. F.: Physiology of the kidney and body fluids. Chicago, Year Book 1963.
5. Pitts, R. F.: The physiological basis of diuretic therapy. Springfield, Thomas, 1959.
6. Symposium on the kidney. Amer. J. Med., May, 1964.

Chapter 8

Theoretical Considerations of Measurements of Renal Clearance

SIDNEY CASSIN, Ph.D., and BETTY VOGH, Ph.D.

About thirty-five years ago, the ability of normal and diseased kidneys of man to excrete urea was studied by Austin, Stillman and Van Slyke (2) in an effort to find a way to assess renal function. Unfortunately, the excretion rate of urea does not provide a particularly good measure of only renal excretory capacity, for the rate of excretion is influenced by endogenous production of urea. Another measure studied was plasma concentration of urea which is also a rather poor index of intrinsic renal excretory capacity, for it too is modified by the rate of production of urea as well as the state of body hydration (6, 13).

In a limited sense, the function of the kidneys is to "free" the blood of urea (1). A quantitative appraisal of this function is found in the expression first formulated by Mayrs and Watt (10) and later used by Moller, McIntosh and Van Slyke (12), i.e.,

$$\frac{\text{excretion rate of sulphate or urea.}}{\text{Blood conc. of sulphate or urea}}$$

"Moller, McIntosh and Van Slyke fully compensated in the direction of rationalism when they borrowed, perhaps from economic bankruptcy, the now familiar term *clearance* for the above ratio (21)."

"Like many good things, this term was born of necessity (21)." In 1926, Van Slyke was asked to discuss kidney function in Baltimore. When on the train from New York, he was suddenly taken with fear as he realized that he would have to discuss a mathematical equation with his audience. "He had learned what every lecturer must ultimately learn, that only experts can visualize and comprehend the true realities which the unreal symbols of a mathematical equation are intended to represent; the simplest equation has the fearsome power of completely dispelling the comprehension of an audience, at least in the fields of medicine (21)." As Van Slyke sat on the train seeking to resolve his dilemma, he suddenly realized that the ratio meant in effect that some constant volume of blood was being "freed" of urea each minute. Fortunately, Van Slyke preferred the term "clear" to "free" for the removal of urea from blood by the kidneys. Had he not shown this preference, we might be faced today with the concept of "freeance, a more horrible word than clearance (19)." Shortly after the introduction of Van Slyke's term "clearance broke loose from the excretion of urea, and taking conceptual wings, became a generalized notion applicable to all aspects of renal excretion (21)."

Since "clearance" is a rate of excretion divided by a concentration, it is not merely a numerical ratio, but has the dimensions of volume per unit time (ml/min.) . . . it is a rate. (It is not an excretion rate which would be expressed as mg/min.) Actually, the urea clearance described by Moller, McIntosh and Van Slyke (12) should have been calculated as a plasma rather than a blood clearance. Urea is excreted by filtration and reabsorption. The filtration of plasma water produces an insignificant change in the water content of the red cell (19). Thus, the urea in the erythrocyte undergoes no change during passage through the glomerular capillaries. In essence, the kidneys operate on plasma and treat erythrocytes as though they were inert floating bodies. In general, all kidney clearances refer to plasma or plasma water and must be considered as such for meaningful comparisons. By definition, "clearance" of any specified substance is the smallest virtual volume of plasma from which the kidneys can obtain in one minute an amount of that substance which they excrete in one minute. The volume is said to be "virtual," not to cause confusion, but because the clearance concept does not refer to a real value. In reality, the kidney does not free completely a small portion of the total renal plasma flow of any substance. In fact, the kidneys free a fraction of each ml of the total plasma flow through the kidney of any substance. Conceptually, it is *as if* a fractional volume of the total flow through the kidney is cleared completely of some substance. Figure 1 describes the two possibilities that may exist in nephrons of the kidney for the clearance of urea. It should be obvious from Figure 1 that situation B exists.

The clearance concept is simply an extension of the well known Fick Principle; it is not complicated and may be easily understood. Perhaps the fable described by A. Burton (5) to explain the Fick Principle would serve a useful purpose. In his rather comical presenta-

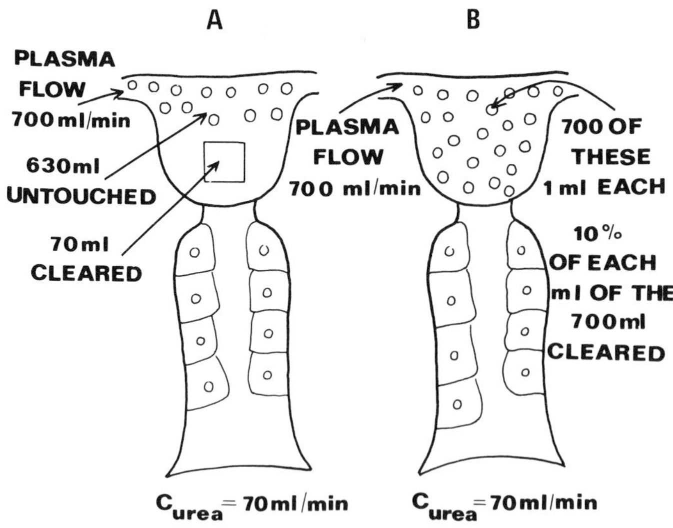

Fig. 1. Clearance concept. A. a small fraction of total flow completely extracted. B. a fraction of each ml of the total flow is extracted

tion of the Fick Principle, Dr. Burton describes the television broadcast of a recent world series game. For some reason, unexplained, the T. V. announcer deemed it of great importance to be able to announce the exact number of the paid attendance before the program was concluded. Unfortunately, the entrance gate counting machine broke down and the series officials were at a loss as to what to do. In desperation, a call was made over the loud speaker system for a "physiologist in the house." When the physiologist appeared, he explained that by using the Fick Principle it would be very simple to calculate the paid attendance. He noted that as he left the gate, he had \$5.00 less in his pockets than when he entered and he assumed that this was true for everyone at the game. Thus, he suggested counting the money at the gate and dividing by \$5.00 (the A-V difference) to obtain the number of persons entering.

The principle involved in the calculation is identical with that used by physiologists to measure blood flow through any region of the body (e.g., heart, lungs, kidneys). The following equations describe the flow in and out of the kidney:

1) Renal arterial plasma flow x plasma conc.$_x$ =
Renal venous plasma flow x plasma conc.$_x$ + Urine conc.$_x$ x Urine flow

2) $RPF_a \cdot Pa_x = RPF_v \cdot Pv_x + U_x \dot{V}$
where:

RPF = Renal plasma flow
P = Plasma concentration
U = Urinary concentration
$\dot{V}$ = Urine flow rate
x = Any material

3) Assume $RPF_a = RPF_v$; actually, they differ by a very small amount.

4) $RPF (Pa_x - Pv_x) = U_x \cdot \dot{V}$

5) $RPF = \dfrac{U_x \cdot \dot{V}}{Pa_x - Pv_x}$

6) Dividing numerator and denominator by Pa_x

$$RPF = \dfrac{\dfrac{U_x \circ \dot{V}}{Pa_x}}{\dfrac{Pa_x - Pv_x}{Pa_x}} = \dfrac{Clearance_x}{\dfrac{Pa_x - Pv_x}{Pa_x}}$$

where $\dfrac{Pa_x - Pv_x}{Pa_x}$ = Extraction Fraction or ratio = E

7) $RPF = \dfrac{Clearance_x}{Extraction\ Fraction_x} = \dfrac{C_x}{E_x}$

Utilizing the Fick Principle it may be seen that "clearance" is actually a product of the plasma flow to the kidney and the extraction fraction

$$\frac{\text{Volume}}{\text{Time}} \cdot E = \frac{\text{Volume}}{\text{Time}}$$

This product provides a number for the minimal volume of plasma which must be abstracted of material X in one minute in order to account for the amount of that material X which appears in the urine in one minute.

Thus, Van Slyke's urea clearance would in fact be equal to the product of the renal plasma flow and the extraction ratio for urea. For a renal plasma flow of about 700 ml/min. and an extraction ratio of 0.10, the urea clearance would be about 70 ml/min. Usually, in routine clinical or experimental investigations, one determines much more easily the concentration of X in the urine and plasma along with the urine flow rather than renal plasma flow and extraction fraction.

In normal adults with a moderately high urine flow rate (2 ml or more/min.) the urea clearance is about 75 ml/min. In a person on a high protein diet or in one who has ingested urea, the plasma urea increases. As the plasma urea increases, the rate of excretion of urea increases in direct proportion (6, 12). However, the ratio $\dfrac{U_{urea}}{P_{urea}} \cdot \dot{V}$, remains unchanged. In renal disease, the urea clearance is reduced, and the reduction within limits is useful as a measure of the degree of renal disease. There is no doubt that clearance was initially conceived as a way of assessing renal damage; however, as stated before, the number obtained for a clearance *per se* reveals nothing about how the kidney handles the material it clears.

In 1921, the first explicit attempt to measure glomerular filtration rate was made by Mayrs and Watt (10). Using a concentration ratio (U/P) for sulphate, they showed that the glomerular filtration rate should be equal to the product of the concentration ratio and urinary flow rate. However, the fact that a substance was needed which was neither reabsorbed nor secreted by the tubules was not fully appreciated. If this material could be found then one could establish an equivalence between the clearance for this material and glomerular filtration rate. In 1926, Rehberg (14) recommended exogenous creatinine for the purpose of measuring glomerular filtration rates on the grounds that this substance was concentrated in the urine to a greater extent than any other substance. Creatinine is generally used today by many investigators both in experimental work as well as in clinical evaluation. Work subsequent to Rehberg's (14) by Marshall and Grafflin (8, 9), Smith and Clarke (18) and Shannon (16) in the 1930's however, demonstrated that creatinine is secreted by aglomerular kidneys as well as by the kidneys of man, anthrapoid apes and other infra-human primates. (It is not secreted by canine kidneys.)

At about the same time, Shannon and Smith (17) and Richards, Westfall and Bott (15) proposed that inulin, a fructose polyaccharide derived from dahlia roots and Jerusalem artichokes, be used to measure glomerular filtration rate. Recently, a much more soluble substance polyfructose-S has been tried with success (11). In order to be used as a proper measure of glomerular filtration rate, Smith proposed the following specifications (19):

1. It must be filterable at the glomerulus and it must not combine with, or be absorbed by plasma proteins.
2. It must not be synthesized or destroyed by the tubules.
3. It must not be reabsorbed or secreted by the tubules.
4. It must be physiologically inert.

It is generally held that inulin fulfills all of these specifications. Its clearance when determined with suitable care is accepted as an accurate measure of the rate of glomerular filtration in all animals from fish to man.

On the average, about 700 ml plasma per minute perfuse the kidneys of man. About 125 ml per min. (Fig. 2) are filtered through the glomerulus. If each ml contains 1 mg of inulin and 125 ml are filtered, 125 mg per min will be presented to the tubules. If inulin is neither secreted nor reabsorbed, 125 mg per min. must be excreted. Since the bulk of the water is reabsorbed, 1 ml per min. appears as urine with 125 mg/min. inulin. It follows from Figure 2 that:

1. Filtered load = Excreted load
2. GFR $\times$ Plasma inulin conc. = Urine inulin conc. $\times$ urine flow rate
3. GFR = Urine conc. $\times \dfrac{\text{Urine flow rate}}{\text{Plasma inulin conc.}}$
4. GFR = Clearance of inulin = C_{in}

Creatinine may be given intramuscularly or in subcutanous pockets; however, since inulin is hydrolyzed to the sugar fructose in the gut and is poorly reabsorbed from subcutaneous pockets or muscle it must be administered intravenously. Generally, for the determination of a consecutive series of clearances, the inulin is administered in a priming dose to establish approximately the desired plasma level, and then at a constant rate by I.V. infusion to keep the plasma level constant. Since commercial preparations and material which has been recrystallized repeatedly from water and ethanol may contain quantities of dangerous pyrogen, it is necessary to use specially processed inulin. Fre-

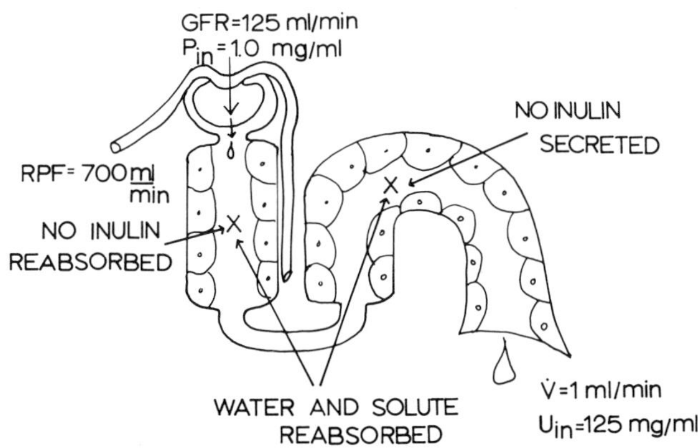

Fig. 2.   Equivalence of inulin clearance and glomerular filtration rate.

quent blood samples must be drawn (midpoint of 30 minute clearance periods). Urine collections must be accurate, preferably by a retention catheter in the bladder. The bladder must be emptied by application of suprapubic pressure if necessary and rinsed with measured volumes of sterile water or saline. Diuresis is generally induced by oral administration of water — up to 1 liter in man, 45 to 60 minutes prior to the first urine collection period. Finally, the chemical analysis of plasma and urine for inulin must be carried out with great care. This is certainly not the procedure for daily clinical evaluation.

Rather than inulin, urea and endogenous creatinine in man may provide on the spot useful information for assessing renal function clinically. However, in order to study secretion or reabsorption or abnormalities of these functions, measurement of inulin clearance is a necessity in man. As indicated previously, the clearance for creatinine is acceptable in dog for glomerular filtration rate (15), however in man creatinine clearances show discrepancies with G.F.R. measured by inulin. The clearance of endogenous creatinine in plasma is not a valid measure of glomerular filtration rate since not all of the plasma chromagen measured with standard Jaffe reagent is creatinine (19). The chromagen in urine (19) however is mostly creatinine. As a result, the clearance obtained with endogenous creatinine may be lower than the glomerular filtration rate. In contrast, exogenous creatinine clearances in man give values that are usually higher than glomerular filtration rate as creatinine is not only filtered, but it is also secreted by the tubules (19).

The glomerular filtration rate in normal young men is about 124 ± 25.8 ml/min. (20) per 1.73 sq. m. surface; in females it is about 109 ± 13.5 ml/min. per 1.73 sq. m. The G.F.R. varies not only with surface area but with age. In normal men, the glomerular filtration rate appears to be astonishingly constant on repeated measurements from day to day and month to month (19). The measurement of glomerular filtration rate in disease provides an extimate of renal impairment of one function — filtration.

Just as glomerular filtration rate can be measured as the clearance of a material, so can renal plasma flow be measured as a clearance. Clearly, a substance which is completely or almost completely eliminated by the kidneys in one pass would be ideal for this purpose. If the A-V difference is very large and the extraction almost 100% we may assume Pv_x is zero and drop the term in equation 5. An almost ideal substance is p-amino hippurate (PAH).

Going back to previously derived equations from the Fick Principle applied to the kidney, it may be seen from equation (5):

$$8)\ RPF = \frac{U_{PAH} \cdot \dot{V}}{Pa_{PAH} - Pv_{PAH}}$$

$$9)\ RPF = \frac{U_{PAH} \cdot \dot{V}}{\dfrac{Pa_{PAH}}{E_{PAH}}} = \frac{C_{PAH}}{E_{PAH}}$$

10) Since E is 0.92 (19) there is very little PAH in Pv_{PAH} and PAH may be assumed to be zero.

The actual value of renal clearance tells nothing about a particular operation by which it is excreted. However, the very fact that clearances are different for different substances must mean that these materials are handled differently by the kidneys. Excretion of a material may in fact occur as a result of net filtration, filtration + reabsorption or filtration + secretion. A substance may be filtered through the glomerulus — yet be reabsorbed completely, resulting in a zero clearance. If tubular reabsorption is steadily decreased, more and more of the filtered material will appear in the urine and the clearance will increase until it equals glomerular filtration rate. When clearance exceeds the glomerular filtration rate, it must do so by addition of substance by secretion (and the clearance can increase progressively while the extraction ratio increases). There is an obvious limit to the increase in clearance, for as the extraction ratio reaches a 100%, the upper limit of clearance is reached (Fig. 3). The kidneys cannot extract more than 100% and they cannot excrete more than is brought to them. The maximum amount of any substance brought to them is determined by the renal plasma flow. The average extraction fraction for PAH as indicated previously is about 92%. Since it is difficult if not impossible to determine E_{PAH} clinically, most investigators are content with C_{PAH} as an *estimate* of RPF fully aware that it is 8.0% too low. Thus, the clearance of PAH is referred to as effective renal plasma flow. The true renal plasma flow is $\dfrac{C_{PAH}}{E_{PAH}}$. One must realize that RPF may be measured with $\dfrac{C_x}{E_x}$ and not only $\dfrac{C_{PAH}}{E_{PAH}}$. However, as Wolf (22) has pointed out for substances with a low extraction ratio, the loss of urinary water from blood must not be ignored in the calculation. The equation for renal plasma flow then becomes:

$$\text{RPF} = \frac{\dot{V}(U_x - Pv_x)}{Pa_x - Pv_x} = \frac{U\dot{V}}{Pa_x - Pv_x} - \frac{\dot{V}P_x}{Pa_x - Pv_x}$$

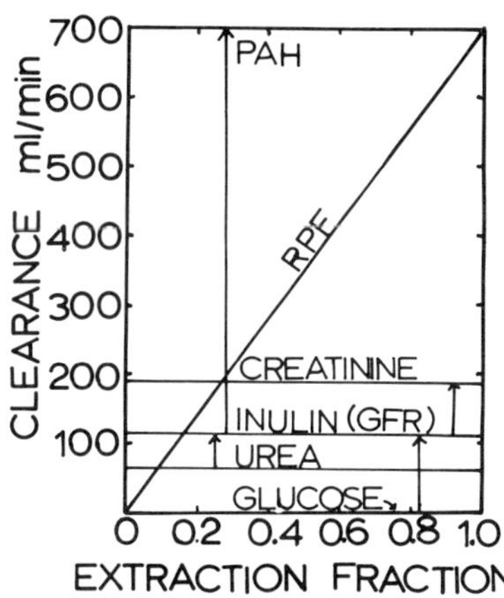

Fig. 3. Relationship between clearance, extraction fraction and renal plasma flow for substances reabsorbed, secreted or only filtered. The slope of the line labeled RPF is equal to the renal plasma flow.

For substances such as urea or inulin, neglect of the $\dfrac{\dot{V}P_v}{P_a - P_v}$ term as a correction factor, may result in an error of RPF of 4-14%. Balint, Fehete and Forgocs (3) and Bull and Metaxas (4) suggest additional correction factors for renal lymph drainage and renal storage. However, because the extraction fraction is so high for PAH, these correction factors may be omitted.

Having obtained the GFR and the RPF, one may estimate renal blood flow with knowledge of the hematocrit ratio:

$$\text{RBF} = \frac{\text{RPF}}{1\text{-Hct}}.$$ In addition, one may

calculate the *filtration fraction*, e.g., the fraction of plasma passing through the kidney which is filtered at the glomerulus, by dividing the clearance for inulin or creatinine by the clearance for PAH. The filtration fraction is normally about 20%. Alterations in renal plasma flow or glomerular filtration are thus reflected in changes in the filtration fraction.

In summary, an attempt has been made to define and describe the concept of renal clearance. Two clearances are of major importance in assessing renal function. The clearance of inulin (or creatinine with reservation) is a measure of glomerular filtration rate. The clearance of p-aminohippurate is a measure of effective renal plasma flow. Since creatinine determinations are much easier to make than inulin, endogenous creatinine clearances are usually done clinically. Actually, there is better agreement, in man, between endogenous creatinine and inulin, than between exogenous creatinine and inulin. This agreement probably results from the balance of two errors; (1) the apparent clearance of creatinine is lower than the true clearance because the apparant creatinine (chromagens) in plasma is higher than the true plasma creatinine; (2) the true clearance of creatinine is higher than the glomerular filtration rate because creatinine is secreted (13, 19).

The usefulness of the concept of clearance lies in the fact that it is possible to compare clearances of many substances in the same individual or one substance in many individuals. Thus, one may assess and compare the clearance of X with the clearance of inulin or creatinine. Since C_{inulin} or $C_{creatinine}$ may be equated with the glomerular filtration rate it can be established whether X is secreted or absorbed. As a test of complete renal function, no single clearance can be used. However, for practical purposes, the proper determination of creatinine, urea or inulin as tests of glomerular function and of p-aminohippurate for renal plasma flow are extremely useful.

REFERENCES

1. Addis, T.: The ratio between the urea content of urine and the blood after the administration of large quantities of urea. An approximate index of the quantity of actively functioning kidney tissue. J. Urol., *1*:263-287, 1917.
2. Austin J., Stillman, H. E., and Van Slyke, D. D.: Factors governing the excretion rate of urea. J. Biol. Chem., *46*:91-112, 1921.
3. Balint, P., Feheck A., and Forgocs, I.: Quantitative considerations on the storage of clearance substances in the kidney. Clin. Sci., *26*:345-350, 1964.
4. Bull, C. M., and Metaxas, P.: The theory and application of clearance methods for determining renal blood flow and lymph flow. Clin. Sci., *23*:515-523, 1962.
5. Burton, A. C.: Physiology and biophysics of the circulation. Chicago, Yearbook, 1965.
6. Dicker, S. E.: Standard renal clearances in mammals. *In*, Winton, F. R.: Modern Views on The Secretion of Urine. Boston, Little Brown, 1956, pp. 5-33.
7. Dunn, J. S., Kay, W. W., and Sheehan, H. L.: The elimination of urea by the mammalian kidney. J. Physiol. (Lond.), *73*:371-381, 1931.
8. Marshall, E. K., and Grafflin, A. L.: The structure and function of the kidney of Lophius Piscatorius. Bull. Hopkins Hosp., *43*:205-229, 1928.
9. Marshall, E. K., and Grafflin, A. L.: The function of the proximal convoluted segment of the renal tubule. J. Cell. Comp. Physiol., *1*:161-176, 1932.
10. Mayrs, E. B., and Watt, J. M.: Renal blood flow and glomerular filtration. J. Physiol. (Lond.), *56*:120-124, 1922.
11. Mertz, D. P.: Moderne Clearance Verfahren. Dtsch. Med. Wsche., *90*:1772-1775, 1965.
12. Moller, E., McIntosh, J. F., and Van Slyke, D. D.: Studies on urea excretion. II. Relation between urine volume and rate of urea excretion by normal adults. J. Clin. Invest., *6*:427-466, 1928.
13. Pitts, R. F.: Physiology of the kidney and body fluids. Chicago, Yearbook, 1963.
14. Rehberg, P. B.: Studies on kidney function. The rate of filtration and reabsorption in the human kidney. Biochem. J., *20*:447-460, 1926.
15. Richards, A. N., Westfall, B. B., and Bott, P. A.:

Renal excretion of inulin, creatinine, and xylose in normal dogs. Proc. Soc. Exper. Biol. & Med., *32*:73-75, 1934.

16. Shannon. J. A.: The renal excretion of creatinine in man. J. Clin. Invest., *14*:403-410, 1935.

17. Shannon, J. A., and Smith, H. W.: The excretion of inulin, xylose and urea by normal and phlorizinized man. J. Clin. Invest., *14*:393-402, 1935.

18. Smith, H. W., and Clarke, R. W.: The excretion of inulin and creatinine by the anthrapoid apes and the infrahuman primates. Amer. J. Physiol., *122*:132-139, 1933.

19. Smith, H. W.: The Kidney. Structure and Function in Health and Disease. New York, Oxford Univ. Press, 1955.

20. Smith, H. W.: Principles of Renal Physiology. New York, Oxford Univ. Press, 1956.

21. Smith, H. W.: Renal physiology between two wars. Reprinted from Lectures of the kidney., Welch Lectures, J. Mt. Sinal Hosp., *10*:59, 1943. In, Homer William Smith, his scientific and literary achievements. Ed., M. Chasis and W. Goldring. New York, N. Y. Univ. Press, 1965.

22. Wolf, A. V.: Total renal blood flow at any urine flow or extraction ratio. Amer. J. Physiol., *133*:496-497, 1941.

Renal Clearance Measurements in Man

WILLIAM J. FLANIGAN, M.D.

INTRODUCTION

The concept of renal clearance of a substance was introduced in 1917 by Thomas Addis (1). Subsequent pioneer work by Van Slyke (6), Rehberg (8) and Smith (5) proved this tool to be one of the most useful parameters for evaluating physiologic and clinical function of the kidneys. As defined by Van Slyke (6), the clearance value of any substance is that volume of plasma "cleared" of the substance per unit time (usually one minute). This volume is obviously a virtual rather than a real one since no single milliliter of plasma can be expected to have all of a substance removed during one passage through the kidney. Expressed in other terms, the clearance of any substance represents that volume of plasma necessary to furnish the amount of the substance which appears in the urine in one minute.

The renal clearance of any substance S is given by the formula:

$$C_S = \frac{U_S \cdot V}{P_S} \quad \text{where } U_S = \text{urinary concentration}$$

of substances S, P_S = the plasma concentration of S, and V = the urine volume in ml per minute. Inspection of the units will readily indicate that the numerator is actually the *amount* of substance S which appears in the urine in one minute.

Thus:

$$C_S = \frac{\text{mg/ml} \cdot \text{ml/min}}{\text{mg/ml}} = \frac{\text{mg/min}}{\text{mg/ml}} = \text{ml/min.}$$

Clear understanding of the units involved is essential in justifying certain "washout" procedures used in routine clearance measurements. Although any units of volume or time may be employed, it is customary to use ml per minute rather than liters per 24 hrs. or hogsheads per fortnight.

Glomerular Filtration Rate

Since all substances excreted by the kidney are filtered (and some, in addition, are secreted), measurement of glomerular filtration rate (GFR) is useful in assessing the mechanism by which certain substances are handled by the

86

kidney and, in pathologic states, the extent of functional renal impairment. In order to accurately determine the rate of glomerular filtration, it is necessary that one employ a substance which is: 1) non-toxic and physiologically inert; 2) freely filterable at the glomerulus (i.e., without significant protein binding and possessing a molecular radius small enough so that its passage from the glomerular capillary is not impeded), 3) neither secreted nor reabsorbed by the tubules, and 4) readily quantitated in both plasma and urine. Inulin, a fructose polysaccharide obtained from Jerusalem artichokes, is admirably suited for this purpose. Elegant micropuncture studies by Richards and co-workers (4) demonstrated that inulin is present in the glomerular filtrate in the same concentration as is present in the plasma. After intravenous injection, it can be recovered quantitatively in the urine indicating that it is physiologically inert and not metabolized under usual conditions. The chemical considerations in its laboratory determination are discussed on page 94.

Although other substances have been used to estimate glomerular filtration rate, the inulin clearance is generally accepted as the standard of reference. It would be ideal if there were an endogenous substance which would meet the above criteria. The clearance of creatinine in normal man offers a reasonable approximation of glomerular filtration; however, when renal function is reduced endogenous plasma creatinine increases, and tubular secretion of creatinine contributes significantly to the urinary excretion and thus overestimates glomerular filtration rate. This approximation of GFR is extremely useful in clinical medicine but is unsatisfactory for most physiologic studies.

Renal Plasma Flow

Identical clearance principles along with important supplementary requirements are utilized in determinations of renal plasma flow. Since the rate of glomerular filtration of any substance is dependent upon ultrafiltration of plasma water, it is obvious that no substance can be completely removed from blood during a single passage through the kidney. On the other hand, a substance secreted by the tubules may be completely extracted from the blood during its postglomerular contact with renal tubular cells providing its rate of excretion is below the maximal transport (secretory) capacity of the kidney.

The fractional removal of a substance during a single passage through the kidney is the extraction ratio and is determined by the formula:

$$E_s = \frac{(A_s - V_s)}{A_s}$$

where E_s = the extraction ratio of substance S, A_s = the arterial concentration of S, and V_s = the concentration of S in renal venous blood. Since tubular transport of S is not limited by the extent of protein binding, it is obvious that when the extraction ratio is high and the plasma concentration is *below* maximal tubular secretory capacity the clearance of substance S will reflect the effective renal plasma flow to that portion of the nephron capable of transporting substance S. Total renal plasma flow may then be obtained by the formula $TRPF = C_s \cdot 1/E_s$. The substance most commonly used in estimating renal plasma flow is para-aminohippuric acid (PAH). At low plasma concentrations, it is effectively excreted by the renal tubules, the extraction ratio averaging about 0.90 in man. The small fraction of PAH which escapes secretion presumably represents renal plasma flow to non-secretory portions of the kidney (perirenal fat, renal capsule, pelvis, etc.) and thus, the renal clearance of this substance accurately reflects the plasma flow to functioning kidney parenchyma. For this reason, PAH clearance is designated as *effective renal plasma flow* and can be determined by standard clearance techniques.

Glomerular filtration rate and renal plasma flow vary more or less directly with body size, and it is customary to correct inulin and PAH clearances to 1.73 m^2 body surface area. Nomograms relating height, weight and surface area are readily available. (See page 116.)

The chemical determinations of inulin (and to a lesser extent PAH) are rather tedious and time-consuming. For this reason, a number of investigators have adopted the use of isotopic derivatives of inulin and PAH in clearance determinations (2, 9). In particular, ^{131}I-ortho-iodohippurate for estimating RPF and ^{125}I-allyl inulin for determining GFR have been very satisfactory (10), yielding an extremely high correlation coefficient with the chemical determinations. Several reports have indicated that [57]Co $- B_{12}$ may be used to determine GFR (3, 7). Protein-binding in the plasma is saturated by injection of large quantities of "cold" B_{12} before administration of the radioactive material. In a limited number of simultaneous inulin and [57]Co $- B_{12}$ clearances, significant protein binding of the isotope has been found in spite of pre-injection of amounts of B_{12} calculated to raise the plasma level several thousand-fold. Correction for the protein-binding by determining dialyzable [57]Co $- B_{12}$ yielded good correlation with the inulin clearance. However, the necessity for determining protein-binding in each plasma sample seems to offset any advantage over the chemical determination of inulin.

CLEARANCE TECHNIQUES

Glomerular filtration rate and renal plasma flow are subject to spontaneous change induced by many environmental and subjective stimuli. Consequently, it is important that these studies be done with the subject at complete rest and under conditions approximating the basal state. Food and tobacco are withheld after midnight and complete bed rest is requested for hospitalized subjects. Outpatient subjects should arrive at the laboratory or hospital sufficiently early to permit at least two hours of quiet bed rest before the studies are begun. Clearance studies should be done in a pleasant, quiet, semi-dark room remote from the morning clamor and activity which usually characterize the busy hospital ward or laboratory. Traffic to and from the room should be minimal. Quiet conversation is permissible, and in many instances will allay the subject's anxiety or restlessness. Soft music from a radio or tape recorder will soothe both the patient and the investigator. Such ideal circumstances are difficult to achieve in practice but efforts along these lines will be rewarded by reproducible, stable results.

Preparation

Determinations of inulin and PAH clearances require much valuable time, both at the bedside and in the ensuing hours in the laboratory. Careful preparation and planning is the key to avoid wasting these precious hours. A roller cart containing all required syringes, needles, alcohol sponges, adhesive, catheterization set, constant infusion pump, intravenous solutions and appropriate collection beakers and graduated cylinders should be assembled on the day preceding the clearance. Acid-cleaned, heparinized specimen tubes for plasma and urine are labeled (P_0, U_0, P_1, U_1, etc.) for the anticipated number of clearance periods.

An important part of the preparation is concerned with estimation of the amounts of inulin and PAH which are to be administered during the clearance. The quantity required for the *priming dose* depends on the volume of distribution of the substance and the amount required to produce a readily measurable concentration in the plasma. The amount required for the *sustaining dose* will depend on the rate of excretion which must be estimated in order to achieve a constant plasma level.

The priming dose for both compounds will be considered first. Inulin is distributed throughout the extra-cellular fluid compartment of the body and its volume of distribution can be calculated as approximately 20% of the body weight. The volume of distribution of PAH is approximately twice that of inulin indicating some "leakage" into the cellular compartment. Inulin is supplied commercially as a 10% solution and PAH as a 20% solution. Optimum plasma concentration of these compounds for chemical determination are approximately 25 mg per 100 ml and 2 mg per 100 ml, respectively. Thus, in a 70 kg subject, the amounts required to achieve a readily measurable plasma concentration would be:

PRIMING DOSE

	Inulin	PAH
Vol. distribution	14 liter	28 liter
Conc. desired	250 mg/liter	20 mg/liter
Am't required	3.5 gm	0.560 gm
Vol. required	35 ml/10% sol.	2.8 ml/20% sol.

The amount of inulin and PAH required for the priming dose will obviously be independent of the level of renal function. In contrast, the amount of these substances required to achieve a constant plasma level in the sustaining dose will be dependent on their rate of excretion (i.e., level of renal function). The creatinine clearance or BUN will provide a framework for estimating these parameters. If renal function is estimated to be about 50% reduced, the following calculations would be made (based on a "normal" clearance of 120 ml per minute and 600 ml per minute for inulin and PAH, respectively):

SUSTAINING DOSE

	Inulin		PAH	
Desired plasma conc.	0.25	mg/ml	0.02	mg/ml
Est. clearance	60	ml/min	300	ml/min
Anticipated loss	15	mg/min	6	mg/min
Replacement	15	mg/min	6	mg/min

If the desired rate of constant infusion is 1 ml per minute, then it is obvious that each ml of the sustaining infusion must contain 15 mg of inulin and 6 mg of PAH. If one allows 60 min. for equilibration after injection of the priming dose and then plans for four 30-min. collection periods, the total time required will be four hours or 240 min. Allowing for an additional 60 min. "safety period," the total volume required will be 300 ml containing 4.5 gm inulin and 1.8 gm PAH. In this instance, the volume of sustaining fluid required could be made by adding 45 ml of 10% inulin and 9 ml of 20% PAH to 250 ml normal saline.

Calculation of the required priming and sustaining dose on the day preceding the clearance greatly facilitates the ease of the study the following morning.

Procedure

1. Priming and sustaining solutions are mixed on the morning of the study. The 10% solution of inulin is insoluble at room temperature and must be dissolved by heating the ampule in a boiling water bath for about 15 minutes. Approximately 30 minutes should be allowed for preparation of solutions and calibration of the infusion pump (if necessary).

2. The initial blood and urine sample (P_0, U_0) must be obtained *before* starting constant infusion. The priming dose of inulin and PAH are mixed in a 50 ml syringe and can be injected into the tubing from the infusion pump. An equilibration period of 30 to 60 minutes is then required for distribution of the priming dose in the various body compartments. This time can be utilized for inserting an in-dwelling needle in the opposite arm through which periodic blood samples may be obtained without the necessity for repeated venipunctures. Several types of plastic needles with stylets are available, but a 20 gauge, 1 inch spinal needle is satisfactory.

3. Accurate urine collections are essential and, except in unusual circumstances, should be obtained with an in-dwelling bladder catheter. A routine 14 to 16 Foley catheter is satisfactory, although some investigators prefer a multi-eyed plain French catheter. Needless to state that the insertion of the catheter should be done under strict, aseptic conditions. We have instituted the routine of obtaining a urine culture at the time the catheter is inserted. The urine is then permitted to drain freely into a beaker or narrow necked flask. Adequate urine flow introduces greatly reduced errors in volume, and in "routine" clearance measurements it is useful to establish a moderate water diuresis by oral ingestion of 10 to 20 ml

per Kg of tap water just prior to starting the intravenous infusions. Sustained diuresis can be achieved by periodically requesting the subject to drink a volume of water approximately equal to the amount of urine excreted during the preceding period.

4. The duration of clearance periods will vary with the urine flow, longer periods being required when flow is minimal. As a general rule, periods should be at least 15 minutes in duration and longer periods are usually desirable. Approximately 2 minutes before the period is completed the bladder should be emptied by gentle suprapubic pressure. Since the objective is to measure the amount of inulin and PAH excreted during a given period, it is permissible (and usually desirable) to use one or two bladder wash-outs with sterile saline at the end of the period. Our routine is to use two 50 ml saline washes, emptying the bladder between each injection by suprapubic pressure. The time is recorded to the nearest half-minute and the volume is measured and recorded. As a routine, it is wise to have duplicate volume readings by two people in order to avoid gross errors in measurement which are surprisingly common. Obviously, if additional studies are to be performed on the urine (e. g., sodium, potassium, osmolarity), it will be necessary to omit the saline bladder wash. In such circumstances, clearance periods should be somewhat longer and two air washes should be done.

5. Heparinized blood specimens are obtained at the mid-point of each clearance period and are immediately centrifuged. When plasma levels are constant, mid-point blood specimens are entirely satisfactory. If changing plasma levels are anticipated, blood specimens should be collected 4 to 6 minutes before the

mid-point in order to compensate for dead-space-lag between glomerulus and bladder.

6. Proper "bookkeeping" is essential and can conveniently be done by use of a work sheet similar to the one shown in Figure 1.

CLEARANCE RECORD

Name _________________________ Hospital No. _______________ Date _________

Wt. _____________ kg.   BP _________ P _________ Ht _________ Water Load ______

Catheter _______________ BSA _________ Estimated C_{IN} ____________ C_{PAH} __________

PRIME DOSE

Inulin 10% ___________ cc.   PAH 20% _______ cc.   Equilibration time __________ min.

SUSTAINING DOSE

Inulin 10% __________ cc/   PAH 20% __________ cc/   Infusion Rate __________ cc/min.

C_{IN} ________________ cc/min. C_{PAH} _____________ cc/min   f.f. _______

DIAGNOSIS:

No.	Period elapsed time	Sample No.	Time	Vol.	cc/min	U PAH	U In	P PAH	P In	C_{PAH}	C_{IN}	FF
		B_0										
		U_0											
1		B_1											
		U_1											
2		B_2											
		U_2											
3		B_3											
		U_3											
4		B_4											
		U_4											
5		B_5											
		U_5											
6		B_6											
		U_6											
7		B_7											
		U_7											
8		B_8											
		U_8											
9		B_9											
		U_9											

Fig. 1.

REFERENCES

1. Addis, T., Barnett, G. D., and Shevky, A. E.: The regulation of renal activity; regulation of urea excretion by the concentration of urea in the blood and in the urine. Am. J. Physiol., *46*:1-10, 1918.
2. Cotlove, E.: ^{14}C carboxyl-labeled inulin as a tracer for inulin. Fed. Proc., *14*:32, 1955.
3. Cutler, R. E., and Glatte, H.: Simultaneous measurement of glomerular filtration rate and effective renal Plasma flow with ^{37}Co-cyanocobalamin and ^{225}I-hippuran. J. Lab. Clin. Med., *65*:1041-1046, 1965.
4. Hendrix, J. P., Westfall, B. B., and Richards, A. N.: Quantitative studies of the composition of glomerular urine. XIV. The glomerular excretion of inulin in frogs and Necturi. J. Biol. Chem., *116*:735-747, 1936.
5. Jollife, N., and Smith, H. W.: The excretion of urine in the dog. 1. The urea and creatinine clearances on a mixed diet. Am. J. Physiol., *98*:572-577, 1931.
6. Moller, E., McIntosh, J. F., and Van Slyke, D. D.: Studies of urea excretion. II. Relationship between urine volume and the rate of urea excretion by normal adults. J. Clin. Invest., *6*:427-465, 1929.
7. Nelp, W. B., and Wagner, H. N.: Use of radioactive vitamin B_{12} to measure glomerular filtration rate (GFR). Clin. Res., *11*:93, 1963.
8. Rehberg, P. B.: Studies on kidney function. 1. The rate of filtration and reabsorption in the human kidney. Biochem. J., *20*:447-460, 1926.
9. Schlongbaum, W., and Billion, H.: Die Bestimung der effektivem Plasma—Nierendurchstromung mit radioaktieven mit ^{131}J markiertem perabrodil-M. Radioaktive Isotope in Klinik und Forschung, vol. 2. Munchen, Urban and Schwarzenberg, 1956, p. 145.
10. Summers, R. E., Concannon, J. P., Weil, C., and Cole, C.: Determination of simultaneous effective renal plasma flow and glomerular filtration rate with ^{131}I-ortho-iodohippurate and ^{125}I-allyl inulin. J. Lab. and Clin. Med., *69*:919-926, 1967.

The Measurement of Inulin, p-Aminohippuric Acid and Diodrast® in Biological Fluids

HOWARD QUITTNER, M.D., and PATRICK L. KNIGHT, M.D.

INTRODUCTION

A precise method for studying glomerular or tubular function requires the intravenous administration of an exogenous challenge substance. A stable blood level must be established through a priming dose and a sustaining infusion. These requirements and meticulous urine collection severely limit the use of the technique to research situations. Procedures have been described (10, 19) for determining renal clearances based upon the plasma disappearance curve of the administered substance. A timed series of plasma samples is taken after a single rapid injection. The mathematical computation is not simple, but clinical laboratories having access to computer facilities may find that their use converts exogenous clearance studies to practical procedures.

Inulin, a polyfructose, is the exogenous material chosen for measuring glomerular filtration. Although it has a molecular weight of 5,200 (4,457-7,777), the molecule is elongate and has the diffusion equivalence of a more spherical molecule of about 15,000 molecular weight. There is no difficulty for mo-lecules of this size to pass through the human glomerular filter. Other sugars which are not metabolized by the body have been used in a similar manner but offer no advantages over inulin. Polyethylene glycols and dextrans of varying weights can be synthesized, and the glomerular pore size in various animal species can be estimated with these materials (3). Problems relating to the stability of the glycols and their possible toxicity have restricted their use in human diagnostic studies, but dextran may prove to be clinically useful for studying pore size.

After acid hydrolysis of inulin to fructose, under carefully controlled conditions of temperature and acid concentration, advantage is taken of the fact that ketoses undergo dehydration to yield furfural derivatives more rapidly than do aldoses. Furfurals condense with any of a large number of phenols or aromatic amines to yield colored products. Modifications of the Selivanov resorcinol reaction (20) have been used by most workers (2, 18), but diphenylamine (1), anthrone (24), thiobarbituric acid (25), vanillin (14), skatole (16, 17), and indole-3-acetic acid (12) have been introduced as simpler and more sensitive reagents. Several of these methods have also been automated (7, 13, 23).

Although Diodrast® was the first substance widely employed to measure tubular secretion and renal plasma flow, the difficult chemical analysis led to its replacement by p-amino hippuric acid (PAH). This compound can be measured by the Bratton-Marshall reaction for sulfonamides (4, 8). The method of Brun (5) is also sensitive to sulfonamides, but it is simpler to perform and is described for this reason. A method for measuring Diodrast is included for its classical importance.

The extraction of PAH from the plasma is a function of renal tubular cell transport and is an active process in contrast to glomerular filtration which is a passive function of the kidney. Many albumin-bound organic acid anions share the same mechanism of movement into and through the renal tubule cell (22). The mechanism is the counterpart of a similar process involving bromosulfonphthalein in the liver cell (15).

A. INULIN IN BLOOD AND URINE (METHOD OF HEYROVSKY (12))

Principle

Inulin is treated with concentrated hydrochloric acid and indole-3-acetic acid at a controlled temperature. The acid and heat hydrolyze the inulin to fructose units which react to form a purple complex with the indole-3-acetic acid.

Reagents

1. *Indole-3-acetic acid.* Five hundred mg of indole-3-acetic acid (Calbiochem, Los Angeles, California) are dissolved in 100 ml of 95% ethanol, U. S. P. (Only pure white crystalline material should be used. If the preparation is colored, it must be recrystallized from hot dilute ethanol after charcoal treatment.) This reagent is stable in a brown bottle at room temperature for several months.

2. *Hydrochloric acid,* 37% (w/v), ACS.

3. *Inulin Standard Solution* (50 mg inulin per 100 ml). Fifty mg of inulin (Mann, New York) (dried overnight in a desiccator) are dissolved in 100 ml of distilled water. Since the color development follows the Lambert-Beer law, only a reagent blank and one standard are needed to construct a curve in the clinical range.

Procedure

The range of sensitivity of the procedure is between 0.01 and 0.1 mg inulin per ml. Protein-free filtrates of plasma (using 10 percent trichloroacetic acid, cadmium sulfate, or Somogyi reagents) are used at a 1:5 or 1:10 dilution of the original plasma. Urine diluted 1:100 may be used without deproteinization.

1. To 1.0 ml of reagent blank or specimen in a 19 mm Coleman cuvet are added 0.2 ml of indole-3-acetic acid solution and 8.0 ml of concentrated HCl.

2. The materials are mixed well, the tubes covered with parafilm, and placed in a 37°C water bath for exactly 60 minutes.

3. Upon removal from the water bath, the tubes are cooled to room temperature with running tap water, and the resulting purple color is read in a Coleman Jr. spectrophotometer at 530 mμ against the reagent blank.

4. $\dfrac{A_u}{A_s}$ x 5 x dilution = mg inulin per 100 ml original solution.

Discussion

The intensity of color formed depends upon the concentration of hydrochloric acid, the temperature, and the reaction time. If there is no urgency about the determination, the color may be developed at room temperature overnight. Temperatures above 37°C are not recommended even though color development is hastened because the color does not retain its intensity; there is rapid fading of the color and the reactivity of other sugars is increased. In an automated modification of the method where time is not a technical variable, Dawborn (7) has taken advantage of the temperature effect and runs the reaction at 60°C. When a large series of tests are run by hand at 37°C, standards should be interspersed through the group of readings to insure against errors owing to further increase in color.

Sources of Error

The method is not specific for inulin since inulin is hydrolyzed to fructose, and it is this sugar which participates in the reaction. Fructose and other ketoses (e.g., tagatose and sorbose) react equally. These sugars are easily excluded from the diet in the test period and, since they are rapidly metabolized, will not be encountered in the blood or urine. Other reducing substances and carbohydrate-like compounds do not produce significant color.

Dextran and glucose are minimally reactive at 37°C or room temperature but may produce significant errors if present in large amounts (Fig. 1). Glucose can be removed by yeasting (1), strong alkali (24), glucose oxidase (11), or gel filtration (6). If not removed, 120 mg glucose per 100 ml solution is equivalent to 0.5 mg inulin per 100 ml. Protein is removed in preparing the plasma to eliminate turbidity, a problem that is not encountered in using untreated urines.

The source of inulin must be as free of fructose and other inulinoid materials as possible, since these substances may be cleared from the blood stream by metabolism rather than by glomerular filtration.

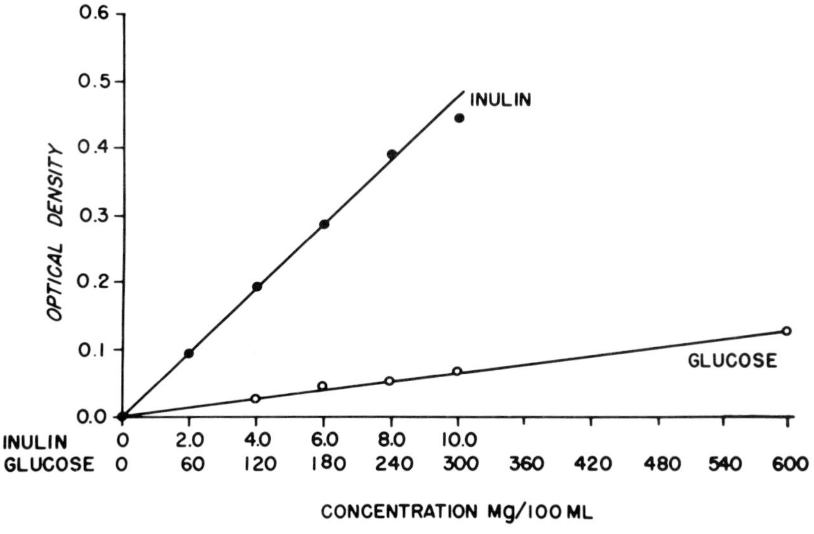

Fig. 1. Glucose and inulin equivalents with Heyrovsky's method.

B. DETERMINATION OF p-AMINOHIPPURIC ACID (PAH) IN PLASMA AND URINE (METHOD OF BRUN (5))

Principle

A yellow colored complex is formed by the reaction of p-amino compounds with p-dimethylaminobenzaldehyde (Ehrlich's reagent) at a low pH.

Reagents

1. *p-Dimethylaminobenzaldehyde Reagent.* Ten gm of p-dimethylaminobenzaldehyde (Eastman Chemical Company, Rochester, New York) are dissolved in 600 ml of 95% ethanol U.S.P. in a one-liter volumetric flask. Forty ml of 2N HCl (16.6 ml concentrated HCl, ACS, diluted to 100 ml with distilled H_2O) are added, followed by distilled H_2O to make 1 liter of reagent. Satisfactory reagent has a pale yellow color and gives a low blank reading. The reagent is stable for many months in a brown bottle at room temperature.

2. *PAH Standard Solutions* (100 mg per 100 ml p-aminohippuric acid solution). One hundred mg of p-aminohippuric acid (Sigma Chemical Company, St. Louis, Missouri) are dissolved in 100 ml of distilled water. For the direct method, water dilutions are made to prepare a curve representing 5, 10, 25, 50, and 100 mg per 100 ml. For the filtrate method, a 1:100 dilution of the stock standard is made with distilled water. Further dilutions are prepared from this: 0.5:10, 1:10, 2:10, 3:10, and 5:10. Three ml of each of these are used in the method to give values equivalent to 0.5, 1.0, 2.0, 3.0, and 5.0 mg per 100 ml.

Procedure

In plasma, when high concentrations (above 5.0 mg PAH per 100 ml plasma) are to be determined, one may perform the test directly without deproteinization. Urines are also analyzed directly. When very high concentrations of PAH are present in urine, it may be necessary to dilute the urine 1:25 with distilled H_2O prior to direct analysis. For low plasma levels, a 1:10 protein-free filtrate (10) percent trichloroacetic acid or Somogyi reagents) is used.

a) Direct Method

1. Plasma (0.05 ml) is pipetted into 10.0 ml of reagent in a 19 mm Coleman cuvet. Constant mixing is required during the addition to obtain a clear solution.

2. The resulting stable yellow color, which develops immediately, is read in a Coleman Jr. spectrophotometer at 465 $m\mu$ against undiluted reagent. The value is determined from a previously prepared calibration curve ranging from 5 to 60 mg PAH per 100 ml. This method should not be used outside of this range for accurate work.

b) Filtrate Method

1. Three ml of protein-free solution are added to 3 ml of reagent in a 19mm Coleman cuvet and mixed.

2. The yellow color, which develops immediately, is read against a similarly prepared reagent blank (3 ml of reagent and 3 ml of clear deproteinizing solution) at 465 $m\mu$. The value is determined from a previously prepared calibration curve ranging from 0.5 to 5.0 mg PAH per 100 ml.

Discussion

The advantage of the method is its simplicity and the stability of the reagent. The method is much less time-consuming than the more frequently used diazotization procedure of Bratton and Marshall. In the determination of concentrations above 5 mg per 100 ml, protein precipitation is unnecessary. The rapidity of color development and its stability at room temperature make this test much more practical than other methods. In an optically sensitive spectrophotometer (such as the Gilford 300), the curve may follow the Lambert-Beer law.

Sources of Error

As with the Bratton and Marshall method, sulfonamides and other p-amino compounds react with the reagent. In contrast to the Bratton and Marshall method, there is no interference produced by thiocyanates or traces of heavy metal. The pH of the reaction mixture must be below 2.0 for maximal color development.

C. DIODRAST® IN BLOOD AND URINE (METHOD OF FLOX, *et al.* (9))

Principle

Diodrast iodine is oxidized to iodate by heating with bromide. The excess bromine is removed with an alcoholic phenol solution and the iodate is measured colorimetrically as free iodine through its liberation by potassium iodide and the formation of a triiodide complex.

Reagents

1. *Bromine Reagent.* Ten gm of potassium bromate, ACS, and 80 gm of anhydrous soldium bromide (Analytical Reagent containing less than 0.01% iodide) are dissolved in 100 ml of distilled water in a brown glass-stoppered bottle. Forty ml of 85% phosphoric acid, ACS, are added with occasional shaking. The acid should be delivered from a buret under a hood. The reagent should stand for at least 24 hours before use, to insure complete reduction of the potassium bromate. The reagent keeps indefinitely.

2. *Phosphoric acid,* 17% H_3PO_4, (85%), is diluted 1:5 with distilled water.

3. *Phenol Reagent* (stable for only 3 days). Five gm of *fresh* reagent grade phenol are dissolved in 100 ml of 95% ethanol, U.S.P., in an Ehrlenmeyer flask. Ten ml of 17 percent phosphoric acid are added to complete the reagent.

4. *Potassium Iodide Reagent.* Fifty gm of potassium iodide are dissolved in 100 ml of approximately 0.01 N NaOH. This solution keeps indefinitely tightly sealed in a brown bottle.

5. *Standard Solutions.* An ampule of 35% Diodrast (Winthrop, New York) is diluted with deionized, iodine-free, distilled water to produce standards containing from 0.1 to 10.0 mcgm of iodine per ml. Five ml samples of the standards are treated in the same manner as the filtrates.

Procedure

1. To 5 ml of a protein-free filtrate (or appropriately diluted urine) in a 19 mm Coleman cuvet ($CdSO_4$ preferred; Somogyi or tungstic acid acceptable) is added 0.05 ml of bromine reagent.

2. The tube is agitated to distribute the bromide and is then placed uncovered in a boiling water bath which is deep enough for the solution in the tube to be below the water-line.

3. After exactly 3 minutes, the tube is removed from the bath and immediately brought to room temperature with cold water.

4. Five ml of phenol reagent are *slowly* added to the cuvet. If this is done carefully, the solution should become colorless before 3 ml of the phenol reagent has run into the solution. The last part of the delivery is used to rinse

the walls of the tube. The cuvet is shaken well to insure thorough mixing.

5. Exactly 0.05 ml of potassium iodide reagent is added to the cuvet and it is shaken immediately.

6. Exactly 10 minutes after the iodide addition, the cuvet is read at 400 mμ against distilled water in a Coleman Jr. spectrophotometer. The O.D. value of a reagent blank is subtracted from each specimen ($A_U - A_B$) and the new value is read from the calibration curve prepared from diodrast standards.

7. The value of a plasma blank prepared from a pre-injection specimen is subtracted from each post-injection value. If this is not available, zero time readings of the reagent blanks, specimens, and standards must be made in Step 6, and these optical densities must be subtracted from the final readings before deriving values from the curve. Urine blanks are not required.

Discussion

The color development increases with time. The time between the addition of the potassium iodide reagent and the spectrophotometer reading must be identical with all specimens. Greater sensitivity can be obtained at 365 mμ, if it is required.

It is possible to quantitate diodrast iodine with all of the standard methods used to determine protein—bound iodine. However, 1/100 or less of the amount of serum ordinarily called for in the procedure must be analyzed. The serum is delivered into the washed protein precipitating reagent or into the digestion mixture if a resin treatment method is used. When urine is used or if very great dilutions of serum are made, it is suggested that the final dilution be made into 3% glycine before addition to the reaction in order to minimize volatilization. Obviously, the range of iodine anticipated must be known in order to avoid contamination of the apparatus by volatilized iodine.

Source of Error

It is possible that other iodinated organic compounds may be oxidized to iodate in this method. Hippuran and skiodan are not affected. Iodeikon, Neoiopax, and inorganic iodides are oxidized. Diodrast clearances cannot be performed shortly after other tests using these iodine containing compounds and probably many others. The largest drawback to the diodrast test is that it is a major source of contamination for the PBI test.

Range of Values
(Studies of W. J. Flanigan):

	Mean Surface Area (M^2)	Mean Inulin Clearance (C_{IN})	Mean PAH Clearance (C_{PAH})
Males	1.92	(105)*116.3	(529)*587
Females	1.66	(103)* 98.9	(517)*496

*Values corrected to 1.73 m^2 body surface area are found in parentheses.

	Filtration** Fraction ($C_{IN/PAH}$)	Range of Values** C_{IN}	C_{PAH}
Males	19.9%	85-139	331–815
Females	19.9%	52-178	326-861

**All figures represent corrected values.

RÉSUMÉ OF CLINICAL INTERPRETATIONS

The information obtained may be used to estimate glomerular filtration (inulin), effective renal plasma flow (PAH, diodrast), and filtration fraction (inulin/PAH) (21). The maximal rate of tubular excretion (Tm_{PAH}) is an intricate study which has no practical diagnostic value. Diodrast clearance values are very similar to PAH clearance values.

REFERENCES

1. Alving, A. S., Rubin, J., and Miller, B. F.: A direct colorimetric method for the determination of inulin in blood and urine. J. Biol. Chem., *127:*609-616, 1939.
2. Bacon, J. S. D., and Bell, D. J.: Fructose and glucose in the blood of the foetal sheep. Biochem. J., *42:*397-405, 1948.
3. Berglund, F.: Renal clearances of inulin Polyfructosan-S and a polyethylene glycol (PEG 1,000) in the rat. Acta Physiol. Scand., *64:*238-244, 1965.
4. Bratton, A. C., and Marshall, E. K., Jr.: New coupling component for sulfanilamide determination. J. Biol. Chem., *128:*537-550, 1938.
5. Brun, C.: A rapid method for the determination of para-aminohippuric acid in kidney function tests. J. Lab. & Clin. Med., *37:*955-958, 1951.
6. Davidson, W. D., Sackner, M. A., and Davidson, M. H.: Use of gel filtration to remove chemically interfering glucose from blood and urine containing inulin. J. Lab. Clin. Med., *62:*501-505, 1962.
7. Dawborn, J. K.: Application of Heyrovsky's inulin method to automatic analysis. Clin. Chim. Acta, *12:*63-66, 1966.
8. Eckert, H. W.: Determination of p-aminobenzoic acid conjugated p-aminobenzoic acid and p-nitrobenzoic acid in blood. J. Biol. Chem., *148:*197-204, 1943.
9. Flox, J., Pitesky, I., and Alving, A. S.: A direct photoelectric colorimetric method for the determination of diodrast and iodides in blood and urine. J. Biol. Chem., *142:*147-157, 1942.
10. Fozzard, H. A.: Diodrast (I^{131}) whole blood clearance as an index of renal blood flow. Am. J. Physiol., *206:*309-312, 1964.
11. Froesch, E. R., Reardon, J. B., and Renold, A. E.: The determination of inulin in blood and urine using glucose oxidase for the removal of interfering glucose. J. Lab. Clin. Med., *50:*918-921, 1957.
12. Heyrovsky, A.: A new method for the determination of inulin in plasma and urine. Clin. Chim. Acta, *1:*470-474, 1956.
13. Krees, S. V., Baukal, A. J., and Wolff, F. W.: A semiautomated method for the simultaneous colorimetric determination of inulin and p-aminohippuric acid in blood and urine. Am. J. Clin. Path., *48:*95-99, 1967.
14. Levine, V. E., and Becker, W. W.: The determination of inulin in blood and in urine by means of vanillin in acid medium. Clin. Chem., *5:*142-148, 1959.
15. Quittner, H.: Excretion tests for measurements of liver function. In, Sunderman, F. W., and Sunderman, F. W., Jr. (eds.): Laboratory Diagnosis of Liver Diseases. St. Louis, Warren H. Green, Inc., 1968, pp. 237-243.
16. Ranney, H., and McCune, D. J.: A photometric micro-method for the determination of inulin in serum and urine. J. Biol. Chem., *150:*311-313, 1943.
17. Reinecke, R. M.: The application of the skatole color reaction to the determination of fructose in blood. J. Biol. Chem., *142:*487-490, 1942.
18. Roe, J. H.: A colorimetric method for the determination of fructose in blood and urine. J. Biol. Chem., *107:*15-22, 1934.
19. Sapirstein, L. A., Vidt, D. G., Mandel, M. J., and Hanusek, G: Volumes of distribution and clearances of intravenously injected creatinine in the dog. Am. J. Physiol., *181:*330-336, 1955.
20. Selivanov, F.: Notiz über eine Fruchtzuckerreaktion. Ber. dtsch. chem. Ges., *20:*181-182, 1887.
21. Smith, H. W., Goldring, W., and Chasis, H.: The measurement of the tubular excretory mass, effective blood flow and filtration rate in the normal human kidney. J. Clin. Invest., *17:*263-278, 1938.
22. Sperber, I.: Secretion of organic anions in the formation of urine and bile. Pharmacol. Rev., *11:*109-134, 1959.
23. Wright, H. K. and Gann, D. S.: An automatic anthrone method for the determination of inulin in plasma and urine. J. Lab. & Clin. Med., *67:*689-693, 1966.
24. Young, M. K., and Raisz, L. G.: An anthrone procedure for the determination of inulin in biological fluids. Proc. Soc. Exp. Biol. Med., *80:*771-774, 1952.
25. Zender, R., and Falbriard, A: Analyse colorimétrique des céto-hexoses et de l'inuline par la réaction à l'acide thiobarbiturique. Clin. Chim. Acta, *13:*246-250,1966.

Chapter 10

Measurements of Urea in Serum and Urine and the Estimation of Urea Clearance

J. DE LA HUERGA, M.D., PH.D., J. C. SHERRICK, M.D., and E. A. PETRUS, M.D.

INTRODUCTION

In 1773, Rouelle isolated urea from the solids of evaporated urine by alcohol extraction. Prevost and Dumas (1823) first found urea in the blood, and it was identified in other body fluids, including cerebrospinal fluid, by Rees in 1850. Urea was first synthesized in the laboratory by Wöhler, a student of Liebig, in 1828. Wöhler heated potassium cyanate and ammonium sulfate to produce ammonium cyanate. On further heating, the ammonium cyanate isomerized into urea. This simple experiment marked a new era in biological chemistry, because this was the first synthesis of a "vital" compound in the laboratory. About the time of Bright's classical description of nephritis, Christison found a large amount of urea in the blood serum of nephritic patients, and Bright, himself, found 1500 mg of urea per 100 ml of blood of a patient with uremia. Although the determination of urea in blood was proposed by Picard in 1856, the actual routine measurement of urea in the clinical laboratory was initiated in 1902 by Strauss, who employed more adequate methods than were previously available. Marshall, in 1913, proposed the use of urease for the determination, and this method is widely used to this day. This was the first use of an enzyme for a clinical laboratory determination. Urease was the first enzyme to be isolated in crystalline form, and this was done by Sumner in 1928.

Van Slyke and his co-workers pioneered in the quantitative evaluation of the mechanisms by which normal and diseased kidneys excrete urea (32). In this process, they developed the concept of "clearance" of urea from the plasma by the kidney. The principle of clearance, which was rapidly applied to other endogenous and exogenous substances, has proved to be fundamental in the understanding of renal function in health and disease, and is discussed in chapter 8.

The importance of the determination of urea in the clinical laboratory can be judged by the fact that it is one of the most commonly performed clinical chemistry tests, second only to the measurement of glucose. It is estimated that over 20 million determinations of the urea nitrogen were performed in the United States last year (56).

SITE OF UREA FORMATION

When it was observed that the concentration of urea in the blood of patients with nephritis was elevated, it became apparent that the kidneys were necessary for the excretion of urea but not for its synthesis. The experiments of Prevost and Dumas in 1823, who found urea in the blood of nephrectomized dogs, confirmed this theory. During the past century, various approaches were followed by investigators to identify the organs responsible for the synthesis of urea. Some workers compared urea concentrations in the arterial supply and venous drainage of various organs. The results were inconsistent, because the methods used were far from specific or reliable. Perfusion experiments performed by von Schroeder (1882) were more revealing. He perfused the livers of dogs with ammonium carbonate, and found that the hepatic vein contained a large concentration of urea. When other organs, including the kidneys were treated in a similar manner, this did not occur. In 1904, Kossel and Dakin discovered arginase, the enzyme that hydrolyzes arginine to urea and ornithine. They found arginase in large amounts in the liver but only in small amounts in the kidneys and lymph nodes. Some clinical observations by Stadie and Van Slyke (1920) were also in favor of the liver being the main site of urea formation, since in patients with "acute yellow atrophy" of the liver, the blood urea concentration became very low. Notwithstanding the extensive experiemental evidence, there were still investigators at the beginning of this century that denied that the liver was the main organ responsible for the synthesis of urea.

The elegant and extensive experiments of Bollman, Mann and Magath in 1924 finally proved that the liver is responsible for the synthesis of urea. These investigators were able to remove the livers of dogs in such a manner that the animals survived for relatively long periods and behaved fairly normally. They found that after hepatectomy, there was a progressive decline in the urea concentration in the blood and urine. When the kidneys were also removed, or if the animals became anuric, the level of urea in the blood remained constant. These experiments demonstrated that the main site of urea formation was the liver, and that urea is not utilized or excreted to any significant degree by organs other than the kidney.

Recent studies by Walser and Bodenlos with ^{15}N labelled urea show that even the urea secreted into the intestine can be hydrolyzed by the urea-splitting bacteria into ammonia, which is resynthesized to urea by the liver, thus confirming the studies of Bollman *et al.*

BIOSYNTHESIS OF UREA

The discovery of Kossel and Dakin of arginase explained the formation of only a minute amount of urea, since from 80 to 90% of the amino nitrogen catabolized is excreted as urea nitrogen. Consequently, if urea is formed from arginine, there must be a chain of events by which the arginine is regenerated. Krebs and Henseleit (1932) found that when ornithine, which is produced by hydrolysis of arginine, is incubated in liver slices in the presence of ammonium salts, large amount of urea were produced. They extended their studies and described what is now known as the ornithine cycle. The outstanding features of this cycle follow. For a detailed report of modern knowledge in this area, the papers of Cohen and Brown (1960) and Ratner (1954) may be consulted.

1. Ammonium and bicarbonate ions are activated by two molecules of adenosine triphosphate to form carbamyl phosphate. This reaction is due to carbamyl phosphate synthetase, which occurs in the liver of ureotelic vertebrates. Acyl glutamate acts as a co-factor in this reaction.

2. Carbamyl phosphate is incorporated into a molecule of ornithine by the enzyme ornithine transcarbamylase with the formation of another amino acid citrulline. This enzyme is present in the liver and intestine.

3. Citrulline is then combined to aspartic acid by argininosuccinate synthetase, which is also found in the liver. The condensation product is known as argininosuccinic acid. The energy for this synthesis is provided by a molecule of adenosine triphosphate.

4. Argininosuccinic acid is "cleaved" into arginine and fumaric acid by another enzyme.

5. Finally, arginine is hydrolyzed to urea and ornithine. The later becomes available to start the cycle again, beginning with 2.

During these enzymatic processes, carbon dioxide from the catabolism of carbohydrates, fats and proteins is combined with ammonia from the catabolism of amino acids with the formation of urea. Three molecules of adenosine triphosphate are necessary and five different amino acids actively enter into the reaction (acyl glutamic acid, ornithine, citrulline, aspartic acid and arginine).

PHYSICOCHEMICAL PROPERTIES OF UREA

Urea is assigned the following formula:

$$NH_2$$
$$|$$
$$C = O$$
$$|$$
$$NH_2$$

It may be considered as the amide of the hypothetical carbamic acid, which itself is a derivative of carbonic acid. Urea may also exist as the following tautomeric formula.

$$NH_2$$
$$|$$
$$C - OH$$
$$\|$$
$$NH$$

Urea has a molecular weight of 60, a molecular size of 3 Angstrom units, and is 47% nitrogen. Urea is extremely soluble in water and alcohol. The molecule, which is the same size as the molecule of water, can pass through almost all biological membranes, thus producing almost identical concentrations in the various body compartments, if the concentrations are calculated on a water content basis. It is very reactive, and many synthetic processes have been used in the preparation of industrial and medicinal compounds from urea.

BASIC CHEMICAL REACTIONS OF UREA

In the following, we will list some of the actions of urea which have found use in its determination in biological material.

I. Urea is easily hydrolyzed to ammonia and CO_2 by acids and alkalies at high temperatures.

$$H_2N - \overset{\overset{\textstyle O}{\textstyle \|}}{C} - NH_2 + 2\,H_2O \rightarrow 2\,NH_3 + H_2CO_3 \tag{I}$$

Similar reactions take place at physiological temperatures when urea is subject to hydrolysis by urease.

II. Alkaline hypobromite brings about the liberation of nitrogen from urea.

$$\underset{\textstyle NH_2}{\overset{\textstyle NH_2}{|\ \ C=O\ |}} + 3\,NaOBr + 2\,NaOH \rightarrow 3\,NaBr + Na_2CO_3 + 3\,H_2O + N_2 \uparrow \tag{II}$$

III. Alcohol or acetic acid solutions of xanthydrol in the presence of urea, produce an insoluble yellow precipitate of dixanthylurea.

$$\tag{III}$$

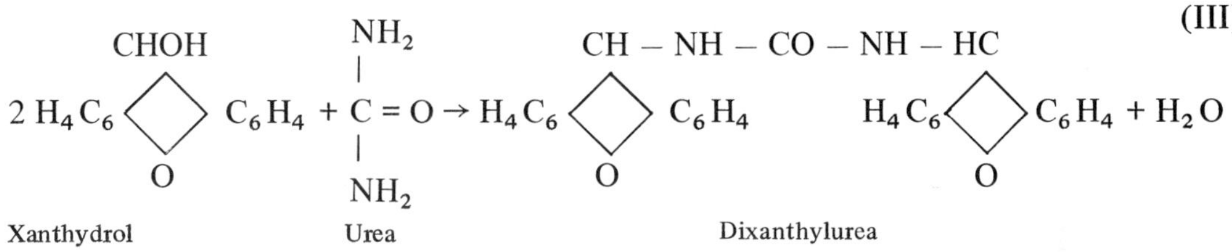

Xanthydrol + Urea → Dixanthylurea + H_2O

IV. Urea reacts with alpha ketones to produce a colored compound.

$$\tag{IV}$$

Substituted diketone + Urea → Colored complex + $2\,H_2O$

V. Miscellaneous reactions: Roijers and Tas have described a method based on the development of a yellowish-green color, when an alcoholic solution of p-dimethylaminobenzaldehyde (Ehrlich's reagent) reacts with urea in acid solutions. Sulfonamides and p-aminosalicylic acid interfere with this reaction.

METHODS FOR MEASUREMENT OF UREA IN BIOLOGICAL MATERIALS

Reaction I has been used extensively for the determination of urea. The ammonia which is formed may be measured in various ways. 1) It may be distilled isothermically using Conway units or aeration trains. In both instances, the ammonia neutralizes a stoichiometric amount of acid, which may later be titrated. 2) The ammonia formed may be measured colorimetrically by using Nessler's reagent, for which the following reaction has been suggested.

$$NH_4OH + 2\,(KI)_2\,HgI_2 + KOH \rightarrow NH_2\,Hg_2\,I_3 + 5\,KI + 2\,H_2O$$

The intensity of the yellow-orange color may be measured in the spectrophotometer. This is a sensitive reaction, but subject to turbidity under some conditions, which may interfere with the optical measurement. To avoid turbidity, various reagents have been utilized, such as gum ghatti, iodine, glucuronolactone, and potassium persulfate. The matter of turbidity has been studied by Boutwell.

3) If the ammonia formed is treated with an alkaline solution of sodium hypochlorite and phenol, an intense blue color is produced. This reaction, which was proposed over 100 years ago by Berthelot, has recently been revived for the measurement of urea in biological materials. The following explanation for the Berthelot reaction has been proposed (24).

$$NH_3 + O\,Cl^- + 2\;\langle\!\!\bigcirc\!\!\rangle\,OH \rightarrow O = \langle\!\!\bigcirc\!\!\rangle = N - \langle\!\!\bigcirc\!\!\rangle - O^-$$

This method is much more sensitive than the Nessler reaction, and may be used for ultramicromethods. Because of this sensitivity, various authors have suggested using it without deproteinizing serum. This may be satisfactory for measurement of urea in blood serum but not in urine, where interfering substances, such as ammonium salts, must be removed with permutit before the reaction is done.

If Reaction I is performed in a neutral or alkaline medium, sodium bicarbonate will be formed from the CO_2 released. If the solution is then acidified in a gasometric or manometric apparatus, the CO_2 collected may be measured, a somewhat tedious method.

Methods involving urease cannot be used on samples which contain fluoride, which inhibits the enzyme. Since a great many urea nitrogen and glucose determinations are performed together, this is a disadvantage. McNair has recently evaluated a proprietary paper strip test containing urease phosphate buffer and an indicator, and found that it differentiates between normal and abnormal levels of urea in heparinized plasma.

The reaction of alkaline hypobromites (Reaction II) was the method of choice during the last century, It is not specific for urea, because other substances, including ammonium salts, release nitrogen in a similar manner.

The xanthydrol methods (Reaction III) are quite specific for urea in biological materials, but to obtain quantitative precipitations takes several hours. This type of procedure is used extensively in radioisotope work. It is the basis of a screening test (50).

The alpha ketone reaction (Reaction IV) is one of the most widely used today (17). The determination may be performed in protein-free filtrates of plasma or whole blood treated with fluoride, so that glucose may be measured on the same specimen. Many diacetyl derivatives have been used. This type of reaction has been criticized because it takes a long time for complete color development, and because the color is not directly proportional to the urea concentration at all levels. The colored final product is sensitive to light, and the unpleasant odor of the color reagent is irritating to some persons.

Methods utilizing diacetyl monxime are commonly used in the automated techniques for the measurement of urea. According to a survey reported on in 1965, 47% of pathologists surveyed used a method of this type, while 30% employed urease and Nesslerization (52). In all probability, automated methods are even more commonly employed today.

Most of the automated procedures are based on the Fearon reaction (18) (Reaction IV). Skeggs (1957) and Marsh and associates (1957), after trying various reagents, recommended a ferric alum — sulfuric acid — phosphoric acid mixture for the acid reagent (61). In 1965 Moore and Sax presented an automated method based on the manual method of Coulombe and Favreau, which employs thiosemicarbazide as a sensitizing reagent. A somewhat similar method was reported by Marsh, Fingerhut and Miller in 1965, and this is used as the basis for other recently described methods (7, 62).

In our laboratories, the Fearon reaction and its modifications have been studied and a manual method has been devised which is simple, has good sensitivity at normal levels of urea, and has stable reagents. The use of a protein-free filtrate is not necessary.

Two methods have been selected for this chapter. The first is a modification of the Fearon reaction, and the second is a urease-Berthelot method. Both are accurate, reproducible, rapid and adaptable to automation.

Diacetyl Monoxime method
A. Serum or Plasma
Principle

The urea in serum reacts with diacetyl monoxime (2, 3-Butane-dione-2-oxime) in the presence of thiosemicarbazide in an arsenic sulfuric acid mixture to produce a red color with maximum absorbancy at 520 mμ.

Reagents

1. *Stock Diacetyl Monoxime Reagent.* About 500 ml of distilled water are added to a 1 liter volumetric flask, 10 gm of diacetyl monoxime and 0.3 gm of thiosemicarbazide are added, and mixed until dissolved. Distilled water is then added to the mark. This reagent should be prepared fresh every two months.

2. *Arsenic Acid Reagent.* Two hundred ml of distilled water are added to a 2 liter Erlenmeyer flask, and 200 ml of concentrated sulfuric acid are added slowly and carefully with mixing.. Twenty gm. of arsenic pentoxide are added, and the mixture is stirred on a hot plate, until solution is complete. It is cooled, and the volume made to 2 liters with distilled water. This reagent is stable indefinitely at room temperature.

3. *Standard Urea Nitrogen Solution* (20 mg per 100 ml). Reagent grade urea is dried over sulfuric acid in a desiccator

for at least 48 hours. Two hundred and fourteen mg of dried urea are transferred to a 500 ml volumetric flask, and dissolved by adding about 400 ml of distilled water and 0.2 ml of concentrated sulfuric acid. Distilled water is added to the mark. This solution is stable for at least 4 years at room temperature.

Procedure

Either serum of plasma may be used, and the plasma may be obtained from blood which has been treated with oxalate, fluoride, EDTA of heparin. This method *cannot* be used for whole blood, unless a protein-free filtrate is made.

1. *Color Reagent.* One volume of stock diacetyl monoxime reagent (Reagent 1) and five volumes of arsenic acid reagent (Reagent 2) are mixed immediately before performing the test. This reagent is stable for no more than 2 hours. Six ml of the reagent is necessary for each tube.

2. Six ml of color reagent are transferred to each of three 18x150mm test tubes, labelled "B," "S," and "X."

3. To "X" is added 10 μl of serum; to "S," 10 μl of urea nitrogen standard solution; and to "B," nothing is added.

4. The contents of the test tubes are well mixed, preferably in an oscillating type mixer, and placed in a boiling water bath for 12 minutes.

5. The tubes are cooled for 3 to 5 minutes in a covered container of cold water.

6. The contents of each tube are transferred to properly labelled 19 mm (3/4 inch) round cuvettes.

7. With the wave length of the spectrophotometer at 520 mμ, the galvanometer is adjusted to zero absorbancy with the tube labelled "B." Optical density readings of tubes "X" and "S" are made.

8. Calculations:

$$\frac{20 \times AX}{AS} = \text{milligrams of urea nitrogen per 100 ml}$$

AX = absorbancy of tube "X"
AS = absorbancy of tube "S"

If the absorbancy of "X" is between 0.9 and 1.5, the sample and blank are diluted with equal volumes of distilled water. The readings are repeated and the calculations are adjusted accordingly.

B. Urine

The principle, reagents and procedure are exactly the same as for the plasma method. In most cases, urine urea nitrogen is determined in the course of doing a urea clearance. The problem of determining the proper dilution of the urine, necessary because urine contains a great deal more urea nitrogen than plasma is considered in the section on urea clearance, where a nomogram for this purpose is presented. The nomogram furnishes the proper dilution whenever the urine flow in ml per min. is known. In case the urine flow rate cannot be ascertained readily, the specific gravity of the specimen may be utilized to assist in determining the proper dilution. In our laboratories, we have used the following simple formula:

$$\frac{20}{\text{Last two figures of specific gravity}} =$$

Volume of urine to be diluted to 25 ml

To be certain, 1 ml of the diluted urine specimen is added to 2 ml of distilled water, and the procedure is carried out on both dilutions. In the calculation, allowance is made for the dilutions.

Treatment to remove ammonia is not necessary.

The procedure is described for a Coleman instrument, or the Bausch and Lomb Spectronic 20, but may readily be adapted for other instruments by slight changes in dilution. For instance, for instruments using 12 mm. or similar round cuvettes, 10 μl of sample and 4 ml of color reagent will produce similar readings. For smaller cuvettes, 5 μl and 2 ml may be used. For those to whom a 20 μl volume is more convenient, 6 ml of water may be added after boiling is completed. Automatic pipetting devices are most helpful in this method. The usual quality controls should be applied.

Discussion

The procedure described here differs from other diacetyl monoxime methods in that it does not require the previous removal of proteins from the sample. This is possible because the sensitivity of the method allows for great dilution of the sample, about 1/600 in the method as described. An incidental benefit of this method is a significant decrease in the unpleasant odor under the conditions described.

EFFECT OF INTERFERING SUBSTANCES

Because simple dilution was the only treatment used for the plasma sample, the effect of interfering substances in the plasma was studied in some detail. Hemoglobin, obtained from washed red cells and treated with urease, produced no change in absorbancy with levels as high as 500 mg per 100 ml in the plasma sample, which represents marked hemolysis. Bilirubin in concentrations up to 100 mg per 100 ml produced no interference. Above 30 mg per 100 ml

the final mixture had a bluish-green hue, but the absorbancy at 520 mμ was the same as if bilirubin had not been added.

Turbidity due to the presence of protein was not observed, because of the dilution, and perhaps because the proteins were hydrolyzed by boiling in the strong acid solution.

The presence of gross lipemia in the serum specimens produced no interference.

In order to study the effect of interfering substances which might be present in random blood samples, 134 samples* (47 serum, 26 heparinized plasma and 61 EDTA plasma) from hospital patients were treated with urease for 3 hours at 37°C. When urea nitrogen was measured in these samples by the method described, values varied from 0 to 0.6 mg per 100 ml. These results compared favorably with those obtained from protein-free filtrates of the same samples, and are actually smaller than those obtained when the urea nitrogen of urease-treated plasma is measured by Nesslerization or the Berthelot reaction.

EFFECT OF VARIATION OF CONDITIONS

The method is based on that described by Coulombe and Favreau in 1963. When arsenic-sulfuric acid was substituted for the phosphoric acid which they recommend, the sensitivity was approximately doubled, and the blank readings were decreased.

When the diacetyl monoxime concentration in Reagent 1 was varied from 0.8 to 2%, no change in absorbancy was noted. However, the best compliance with Beer's law was found at a concen-

---

*Plasma samples treated with fluoride were not examined because fluoride inhibits urease.

tration of 1%, and this was selected for the method. At this concentration, the absorbancy of the blank was low, readings of 0.04 to 0.06 being obtained against distilled water.

When various thiosemicarbazide concentrations were tried, it was observed that concentrations above 50 mg per 100 ml in Reagent 1 produced higher blank readings, and that either 20 or 30 mg per 100 ml concentrations produced the same absorbancy. The latter concentration, which was that recommended by Coulombe and Favreau, was selected for the method.

Higher concentrations of the arsenic acid produced a yellow color in the blank without increasing the absorbancy. Concentrations down to 75% of that proposed produced the same absorbancy. The sulfuric acid concentration may be changed by 30% without affecting the absorbancy. In regard to the arsenic acid reagent, it may be convenient to prepare a stock solution which is five times more concentrated than Reagent 2. In this case, the color reagent is prepared by mixing one volume of diacetyl monoxime reagent, one volume of the concentrated Reagent 2, and four volumes of distilled water.

If the absorbancy of the final mixture is too great for accurate reading in the spectrophotometer, the final mixture may be diluted with an equal volume of water, and still comply with Beer's law, providing the blank is diluted correspondingly. This allows one to measure concentrations of urea nitrogen as high as 150 mg per 100 ml.

The time of boiling was studied under various conditions, and it was found that 8 minutes produced the maximum color for urea nitrogen concentrations up to 50 mg per 100 ml. For concentrations up to 150 mg per 100 ml, 10 minutes

was necessary. Therefore, a boiling time of 12 minutes was selected for the determination. The color remained the same when boiling time was increased up to 16 minutes, but when boiled for longer periods, the blank became discolored, and the color of the sample diminished, probaby due to destruction of the pigmented complex formed.

The effect of light on the color formed was studied under various light intensities. When the cuvettes were left in bright sunlight, the color faded 15% in 30 minutes. When kept in semi-darkness in a metal container without any direct light but without a cover, there was no color change in 30 minutes. In darkness, no color loss was noted. In actual practice, no special precautions were taken other than to turn off the light in the hood while the test tubes were boiling, to cover them while cooling, and to read them promptly. However, the color does fade in sunlight, and this must be considered in carrying out the procedure.

The absorbancy of the red color is maximum at 520 mμ, but sufficient absorbancy is present at 510 and 540 mμ, so that the procedure can be performed at these wave lengths without difficulty. At 520 mμ typical absorbancy readings for sample concentrations of 10 mg per 100 ml were 0.14 to 0.16; for 50 mg per 100 ml, 0.7 to 0.8.

This method is rapid, simple, and uses small volumes of serum or plasma. It can be performed on plasma treated with fluoride, and is not affected by ammonia in the atmosphere or the reagents. It can readily be adapted to automatic analysis, having the advantage that dialysis is not necessary because of the great dilution of the serum. Preliminary studies are now being carried out on automatic analysis, and at the present time the results seem most promising.

II. Urease-Berthelot Method

A. Serum of Plasma
Principle

The urea in serum is hydrolyzed by urease to ammonia and carbonic acid. Ammonia is measured colorimetrically by its reaction with sodium phenate and hypochlorite, in the presence of sodium nitroprusside, to form a stable blue color.

Reagents

1. *Stock Phenol Nitroprusside Reagent.* Fifty gm of phenol crystals and 250 mg of sodium nitroprusside (nitro-ferricyanide) are dissolved in distilled water to make a final volume of 1 liter. The phenol should not have a brown discoloration. When kept in a dark bottle in the refrigerator, this reagent is stable for at least 3 months.

2. *Working Phenol Nitroprusside Reagent.* One volume of stock phenol nitroprusside reagent (Reagent 1) is diluted with four volumes of distilled water. This reagent keeps for 1 month in a dark bottle in the refrigerator.

3. *Stock Alkaline Hypochlorite Reagent.* To a 1 liter volumetric flask is transferred 25 gm of sodium hydroxide pellets, which are dissolved in about 700 ml of distilled water. Forty ml of a solution of sodium hypochlorite, 3 to 6%, is added. Clorox, a bleaching compound, is satisfactory. Distilled water is added to the mark, and the reagent is mixed. When stored in a dark bottle in the refrigerator, this reagent is stable for at least 4 months.

4. *Working Alkaline Hypochlorite Reagent.* One volume of stock alkaline hypochlorite reagent (Reagent 3) is diluted with 4 volumes of distilled water. This reagent is stable for 1 month when kept in a dark bottle in the refrigerator.

5. *Stock Glycerol Urease Reagent.* Two gm of urease containing from 800 to 1000 Sumner units per gm is dissolved in 25 ml of distilled water, and 25 ml of glycerol is added slowly with mixing. Sigma II urease is satisfactory. This reagent keeps for at least a year in the refrigerator.

6. *EDTA Reagent.* Five gm of di-sodium ethylenediaminetetracetate is dissolved in about 400 ml of distilled water, and 1N sodium hydroxide is added to adjust the pH to 6.5. Distilled water is added to make a final volume of 500 ml. This reagent keeps well in the refrigerator.

7. *Working Urease Reagent.* One ml of the stock glycerol urease reagent (Reagent 5) is diluted to 100 ml with EDTA reagent (Reagent 6). In the refrigerator, this reagent keeps for 1 month.

8. *Urea Nitrogen Standard Solution, 20 ml per 100 ml.* Two hundred and fourteen mg of dried reagent grade urea is transferred to a 500 ml volumetric flask, and dissolved by adding about 400 ml of distilled water. Five hundred sodium azide is added and dissolved, and distilled water is added to the mark. This reagent keeps for at least 6 months in the refrigerator.

Procedure

Either serum or plasma may be used, and the plasma may be obtained from blood which has been treated by oxalate, EDTA or heparin. Plasma obtained with fluoride *cannot* be used. This method *cannot* be used with whole blood unless a protein-free filtrate is made.

1. One ml of working urease reagent (Reagent 7) is added to each of three 16x125mm. test tubes, labelled "X," "S," and "B."

2. To "X" is added 10 μl of serum, to "S" is added 10 μl of urea nitrogen

standard solution (Reagent 8), and to "B," nothing is added.

3. After mixing, the tubes are stoppered and placed in a 37° C water bath for at least 15 minutes.

4. Five ml of working phenol nitroprusside reagent (Reagent 2) are added to each tube, and the contents mixed. Five ml of working alkaline hypochlorite reagent (Reagent 4) is added to each tube, and the contents mixed well. The tubes are allowed to remain in the water bath for at least an additional 20 minutes.

5. The contents of each tube are transferred to properly labelled 19 mm (3/4 inch) round cuvets. With the spectrophotometer at a wave length of 600 mμ the galvanometer is adjusted to zero absorbancy with the cuvette labelled "B." Optical density readings of the standard and unknown are obtained.

6. Calculations:

$$\frac{20 \times AX}{AS} = \text{mg of urea nitrogen per 100 ml}$$

AX = absorbancy of tube "X"
AS = absorbancy of tube "S"

If the absorbancy of "X" is more than 0.8, the unknown and blank may be diluted with two volumes of distilled water, the readings repeated, and the calculations adjusted accordingly. The usual quality control methods should be applied.

B. Urine

The urine sample must first be treated to remove the preformed ammonia. This is accomplished by mixing 10 ml of urine with 2 gm of permutit and shaking intermittently for 10 minutes. The proper dilution of the urine sample is determined as described under the di-

acetyl monoxime method, and the procedure is then carried out exactly as described for plasma. In the calculation, allowance must be made for the dilution selected.

Discussion

The urease-Berthelot procedure follows in general one described by Kaplan (24), who has made a careful study of the method. Minor variations in the composition of the phenol nitroprusside and alkaline hypochlorite reagents will not produce changes in the final color. The method measures the ammonia nitrogen produced by the action of urease on urea. Because the sample is diluted 1.1100, the actual amounts of ammonia nitrogen present are on the order of 1 to 20 μg. Consequently, even minor contamination of reagents with ammonia must be avoided. During the incubation, the solution is slightly acid, an ideal condition for taking up ammonia from the atmosphere. This can be avoided by stoppering the tubes as recommended. As in any enzymatic procedure, contamination with heavy metals must be avoided, although the presence of EDTA in the urease reagent minimizes this danger to some extent.

The method is suitable for the use of automatic diluting devices. The method is described for the Coleman or Bausch and Lomb Spectronic 20 spectrophotometers, with the 19 mm (3/4 inch) covetts, but is readily adapted to other instruments. At the wave length recommended, absorbancies of about 0.15 will be obtained for samples containing urea nitrogen in concentrations of 10 mg per 100 ml. Without dilution, concentrations up to 60 mg per 100 ml can be measured. The final mixture may be diluted 1:3, so that sample concentrations up to

180 mg per 100 ml may be measured. However, at concentrations over 180 mg per 100 ml, it is best to repeat the determination, starting with a diluted sample. The wave length selected for our procedure is 600 mμ, but the blue color produced follows Beer's law above 520 mμ. To increase sensitivity, a wave length between 600 and 630 mμ may be used. To decrease sensitivity, a lower wave length may be selected. The maximum absorbancy is at 630 mμ.

As described, this determination takes about 40 minutes. The time may be shortened by carrying out the urease incubation at 50 to 55° C for 5 minutes, and the second incubation for 3 minutes, being sure that all reagents are at this temperature before starting. Fifty-five degrees C is optimum temperature for the urease reaction. This shortens the time to about 10 minutes.

The effect of bilirubin, hemoglobin and lipemia have been studied, and have been found to produce no interference.

STATISTICAL EVALUATION OF THE TWO METHODS

To study accuracy, urea nitrogen determinations were performed on 61 serum samples by the diacetyl monoxime and urease-Berthelot methods. The results were subjected to statistical evaluation by the method of paired samples (9, 23). The "t" value obtained was 0.813. Since t_{60}; 0.05 = 2.00, we can conclude that the results obtained gave no evidence of systematic differences between the two methods. The urease-Berthelot method is generally accepted as a standard reference method, and it may be concluded that the diacetyl monoxime method is equally accurate.

The precision of the methods was studied by performing 12 replicate analyses on each of three different serum samples by both methods. The following results were obtained:

	Sample I			Sample II			Sample III		
	AV.	S.D.	C.V.	AV.	S.D.	C.V.	A.V.	S.D.	C.V.
Urease-Berthelot	12.3	0.64	5.2	23.5	1.12	5.8	48.6	2.53	5.2
Diacetyl monoxime	12.7	0.75	5.9	24.3	0.78	3.2	49.9	2.89	6.0

AV. = Average, mg./100 ml.
S.D. = Standard deviation, ±
C.V. = Coefficient of variation, %

This table demonstrates good reproducibility (precision) for both methods.

The reproducibility of day-to-day analyses, often referred to as quality control, was studied by adding urea to a pooled serum sample to obtain a urea nitrogen concentration of about 20 mg per 100 ml, and distributing it in small test tubes that were kept frozen. One tube was taken daily for analysis by both methods. A total of 45 determinations were performed for each method with the following results:

	AV, mg %	S.D.	C.V., %
Urease-Berthelot	22.6	1.22	5.39
Diacetyl monoxime	21.7	1.43	5.49

These data demonstrate the high degree of precision of the methods.

Recovery experiements were performed as follows: 100 ml of pooled serum was dialyzed in the refrigerator against 2 liters of 0.85% sodium chloride solution for 72 hours, during which time the dialyzing solution was changed 5 times. The serum was then perevaporated until the serum protein concentration was 7.5 gm per 100 ml. The urea nitrogen content of the serum was practically zero by both methods. Urea was added to aliquots of this serum to obtain concentration of from 8 to 100 mg per 100 ml. The aliquots were analyzed in triplicate by both methods, and the average recovery was compared with the theoretical result. With the urease-Berthelot method, recovery varied from 95.1 to 106.3%, with the best recovery at the 30 mg per 100 ml. concentration. With the diacetyl monoxime method, recovery was from 94.5 to 104.6% of the theoretical result. Similar results were obtained when urea was added to native serum samples.

RANGE OF VALUES

In this country, concentration of urea in body fluids is usually expressed in terms of urea nitrogen, rather than urea. The value for urea nitrogen may be converted to the urea value by multiplying the former by 60/28 or 2.14.

The determination should be performed on plasma or serum, and these terms have been used interchangeably throughout this presentation. The reason for using plasma rather than whole blood is to obviate variations related to changes in the hematocrit. The red cells are usually considered to contain the same concentration of urea per unit of water as does the plasma (37, 38); but because the red cells contain only 71% water while the plasma is 93% water,* the whole blood urea nitrogen concentration of a given volume of red cells contains less urea than the same volume of plasma. In addition, recent studies appear to indicate that the water of the red cells actually binds more urea than the water content would lead one to expect, in a ratio to plasma of 1.19 to 1 (35, 43). The following table shows the ratio of whole blood urea to plasma urea at different hematocrit values, at cell/plasma urea binding ratios of both 1.0 and 1.19.

Hematocrit	*Whole Blood Urea / Plasma Urea at cell/plasma binding ratio of 1.0*	*Whole Blood Urea/Plasma Urea at cell/plasma binding ratio of 1.19*
20	1.05	0.99
45	1.12	1.04
60	1.16	1.05

According to this table, in a patient with a hematocrit of 45%, the plasma urea would be 1.12 times the whole blood urea, a difference of 12%. This might make a considerable difference in urea clearance calculations. It is true that if the cells bind 1.19 times as much urea as plasma, the differences due to hematocrit become somewhat less significant, 4% at a hematocrit of 45%.

---

*These figures are based on the careful work of Sunderman (58), and Williams and Sunderman (65).

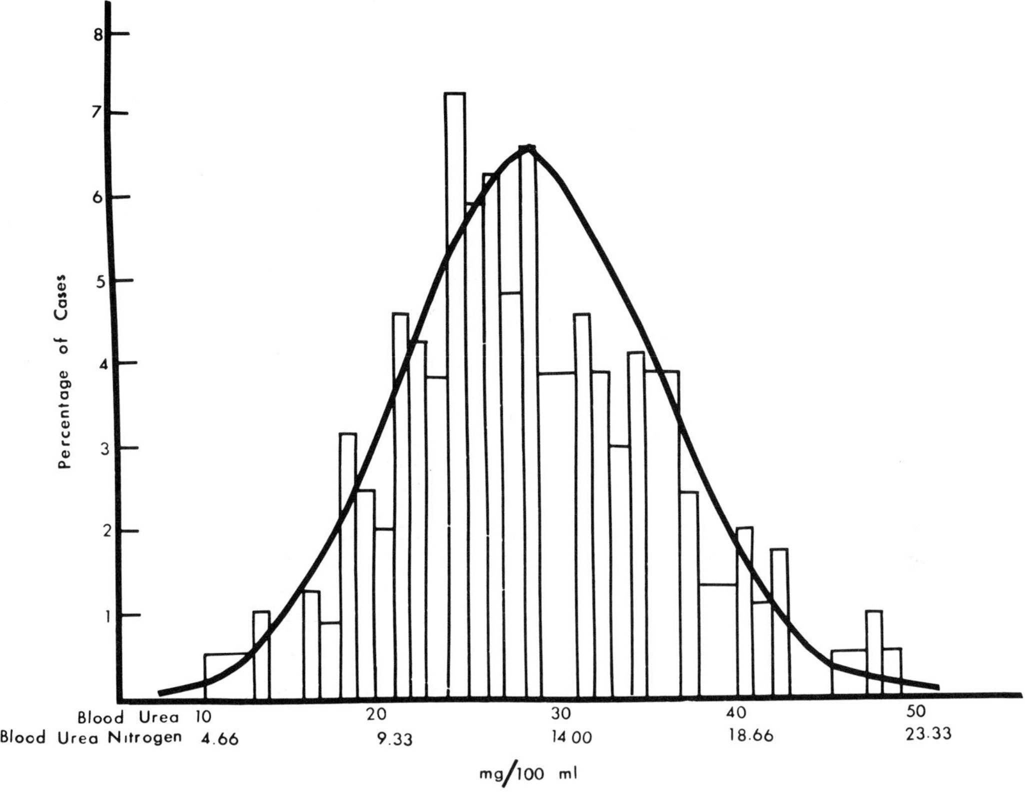

Fig. 1.   Normal values for blood urea nitrogen, from Mackay and Mackay.

Normal values for the blood urea were thoroughly studied by MacKay and MacKay in 1927. Their observations included 278 determinations, 58 on 47 female subjects, and 220 on 114 different male subjects, with an age range from 18 to 49. In Figure 1, Figure 3 from their article is redrawn. Blood urea nitrogen values are plotted along the abscissa. Using MacKay's data, the calculated normal distribution curve has been fitted onto their histogram, and it is obvious from simple inspection that the fit is good. To evaluate this statistically, the goodness of fit was tested by the chi square method (9). The compliance of chi square for 39 degrees of freedom was 18.37, which was lowered to 8.51, when using the Yates correc-tion. Both figures give a probability of over 99% compliance with the normal (Gaussian) distribution, meaning that distribution is normal, and not log-normal, as has been suggested (67).

In view of the normal distribution, the mean, ± two standard deviation, delin-eates the range of normal values. In MacKay's series, the mean was 13.7 mg./100 ml., and the range was from 7.2 to 20.2 mg per 100 ml, which would include 95% of cases. The male subjects had slightly higher values than the fe-males, but the fit of the curve is so excellent that this difference is not considered significant. Our own studies, and those of others, confirm this range of normal values.

RÉSUMÉ OF CLINICAL INTERPRETATIONS

The normal range for the plasma urea nitrogen is 7.2 to 20.2 mg per 100 ml. Concentrations above 18 mg per 100 ml. are more frequently found in abnormal than in normal individuals, so one should regard these patients with suspicion.

Abnormally high values are found in patients suffering from renal disease, cardiac decompensation, shock, gastro-intestinal hemorrhage, and similar conditions (33, 48).

Abnormally low values may be found in patients with severe liver disease, or in patients on a low protein diet with a high urinary output (19).

Part II: The Estimation of Urea Clearance

As methods for the accurate measurement of urea became available, investigators became interested in the evaluation of renal function by comparing the concentration of urea in the blood with that in the urine. Gréhant in 1904 was the first to investigate this subject by determinining the concentration of urea in urine and blood obtained at the same time. Later, Ambard carried this subject further by also taking into account the volume of urine excreted per unit of time. The pioneer investigations of Addis (1-4) elucidated this subject, and finally Van Slyke and his associates carefully evaluated the correlation between the concentrating power of the kidney and the rate of urea excretion. From these studies came the concept of clearance, as defined by Austin, Stillman and Van Slyke. The evaluation of renal function by renal clearance is a topic that is fully discussed in Chapter 8 and 9.

As established by Van Slyke and associates, urea clearance is the virtual volume of plasma cleared of urea per minute (32). It is calculated by the following formula, which is common to the calculation of the clearance of other substances from the plasma.

$$\text{Clearance} = \frac{\text{Urine concentration x ml. of urine excreted per minute}}{\text{Plasma concentration}}$$

However, it became apparent at once that the urea clearance of an individual was closely related to urine flow. In the same individual, urea clearance became constant when the rate of urine excretion was 2 ml per minute or more. This rate of urine flow was called the "augmentation limit," because little difference in the amount of plasma cleared was obtained when the urine volume rose from 2 ml per minute to higher volumes. On the other hand, if oliguria was produced by water restriction, the clearance as calculated by the above formula became much smaller. By actual experimentation in normal subjects,

Austin, Stillman and Van Slyke established empirically that another type of mathematical relationship prevailed when the urine flow was less than 2 ml per minute. In these cases, the urea clearance was related to the square root of the volume of urine per minute. The formula for the calculation of the urea clearance then became

$$\text{Clearance} = \frac{\text{Urine concentration} \times \sqrt{\text{vol./min.}}}{\text{Plasma concentration}}$$

The term, "standard clearance," was chosen for this relationship, the word, "standard," being used because 1 ml per minute is the average volume of urine excreted by a normal adult, that is, 1440 ml per day. It must be understood that "standard clearance" is not really clearance at all, but it does provide the clinician with an approximation about the excretory power of the kidney (41). In defense of the original investigators, it should be stated that they were interested in deriving a diagnostic procedure more than in establishing a physiological principle. They did not realize that for other substances the mathematical principles of maximum clearance would be the same at any urine flow rate. The effect of using $\sqrt{V}$ in the standard clearance formula is to correct the variable term $\frac{UV}{B}$ to that value which it would have if

$V = 1.0$, since $\sqrt{1} = 1$. The reason for this is that the square root of numbers between one and two is smaller than the original number; while the square root of numbers between zero and one is larger than the number itself. For example, the square root of 1.7 is 1.3; while the square root of 0.5 is 0.7. This allows a standard clearance of 54 ml per in. to be used as a normal value for all rates of urine flow below 2 ml per min., rather than having a separate normal value for each rate below 2 ml per min., as would be necessary if the square root of V were not used in the calculations.

The term, "maximum clearance," was then applied when the urine flow was more than 2 ml per minute, because flow rates higher than this do not change the urea clearance appreciably. As stated by the originators of the terms, "the standard clearance indicates the efficiency with which the kidneys excrete urea when the urine volume is at the average normal level of 1 ml per min. The maximum clearance indicates the maximum efficiency of urea excretion with high urine volume" (Möller *et al* ., 1928).

These investigators realized that the excretory function of the kidney was directly proportional to the surface area of the individual, and made allowances in the calculations based on the normal body surface of 1.73 square meters (60).

In contrast to other clearance studies, such as the creatinine clearance, the urea clearance must be performed over a relatively short period of urine collection. The reason for this is that the concentration of plasma urea varies with dietary intake, and has a significant diurnal variation. Because the plasma urea concentration is in the denominator of the fraction of the formula, small differences here may make significant differences in the final results. The procedure must, therefore, be done on a fasting patient, who is given a generous supply of water to produce an adequate urinary output. During the two-hour collection period, no appreciable variation of the blood urea is observed. The clearance is then calculated for each one-hour period, in order to confirm accurate urine collection. Complete emptying of the bladder is essential, and this has traditionally presented difficulties in hospital patients. Attempts at prolonging the collection period up to 24 hours, and utilizing an average of two blood urea nitrogen determinations, one obtained during fasting, and the other after the evening meal, have not been very successful. Some investigators have recommended a three-hour urine collection period in the morning (68).

In any case, urea is determined in the urine samples and in the plasma instead of blood, because it is the plasma that is cleared (41). The method for the determination of urea should be an accurate one, and because the concentration of urea in the urine is many times higher than in the plasma, the urine sample must be diluted so that the urea concentration is within the most accurate range of the method used. If the method chosen is one in which the amount of ammonia formed from the hydrolysis of urea is measured, the preformed ammonia in the urine must be determined and subtracted. Better yet, the preformed ammonia can be adsorbed by shaking the urine with permutit. The surface area of the patient must be

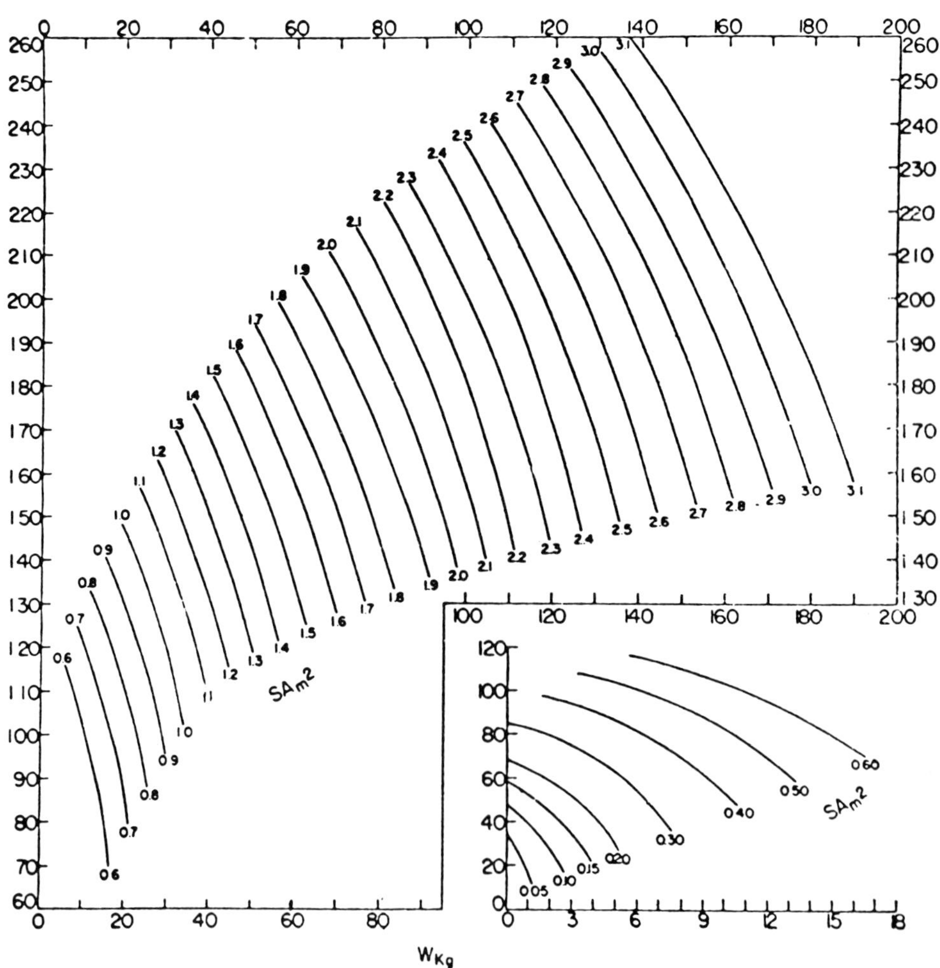

Fig. 2. Surface area nomogram, from Sendroy and Cecchini.

ascertained, for which the nomogram of Sendroy and Cecchini is convenient (51, 59) (Fig. 2).

The difficulty in obtaining a convenient dilution of the urine was appreciated by Van Slyke (37), who devised a nomogram to ascertain the proper dilution. His nomogram does not include the body surface area, the effect of which must be calculated separately. Van Slyke also devised nomograms for the calculation of the clearance itself. However, the ratio of urine urea and plasma urea must be calculated separately in his nomograms, and $\sqrt{V}$ must be obtained from a separate table. In the following, a simple set of nomograms is presented from which both urine dilution and urea clearance can be obtained without any calculations, and in which the body surface factor is automatically included. The mathematical basis for these nomograms is as follows:

The maximum clearance is calculated by the formula

$$C_M = \frac{UV}{P} \times \frac{1.73}{BS} = \frac{UV_C}{P}$$

where

U = urine urea nitrogen, mg/100 ml
V = urine volume, ml/min.
P = plasma urea nitrogen, mg/100 ml
BS = body surface, in sq. m
V_C = urine volume, ml/min.,

> corrected for body surface

Figure 3 is a nomogram which corrects the urine flow for the body surface, adjusting to a normal surface area of 1.73 sq. m. The urine flow is closely correlated with the urea nitrogen, and it has been found in actual practice that one may take an amount of urine equivalent to the corrected urine flow per minute, dilute it to 25 ml and obtain

urea nitrogen values which are similar to that in the plasma. This convenient relationship is utilized in the nomogram in Figure 3 to ascertain the urine dilution, and at the same time to correct it for body surface. Standard clearances are shown on the left side of the central oblique line, and maximum clearances on its right.

If one takes a volume of urine equal to V_C, dilutes it to 25 ml, performs a urea nitrogen determination on the specimen, and then expresses the results as mg per 100 ml of the diluted specimen (U_D), then

$$U = \frac{U_D \times 25}{V_C}$$

By substitution in the previous formula for maximum clearance, then

$$C_M = \frac{\dfrac{U_D \times 25}{V_C} \times V_C}{P} = \frac{U_D \times 25}{P}$$

A similar treatment may be applied to the standard clearance. Since 25 is a constant factor, it can be included in a modulus of a nomogram. Figure 4 is a nomogram derived from formula 2. By using this nomogram, one may obtain the urea clearance directly from the results obtained from the determination of urea nitrogen in the plasma sample and in the diluted urine sample. Both standard and maximum clearances may be obtained from this same nomogram. Since in the nomogram of Figure 3, the final results are expressed in terms of urea clearance for a normal body surface of 1.73 sq. m.

The results from the nomogram in Figure 4 are expressed as ml per min. Van Slyke and associates found that the

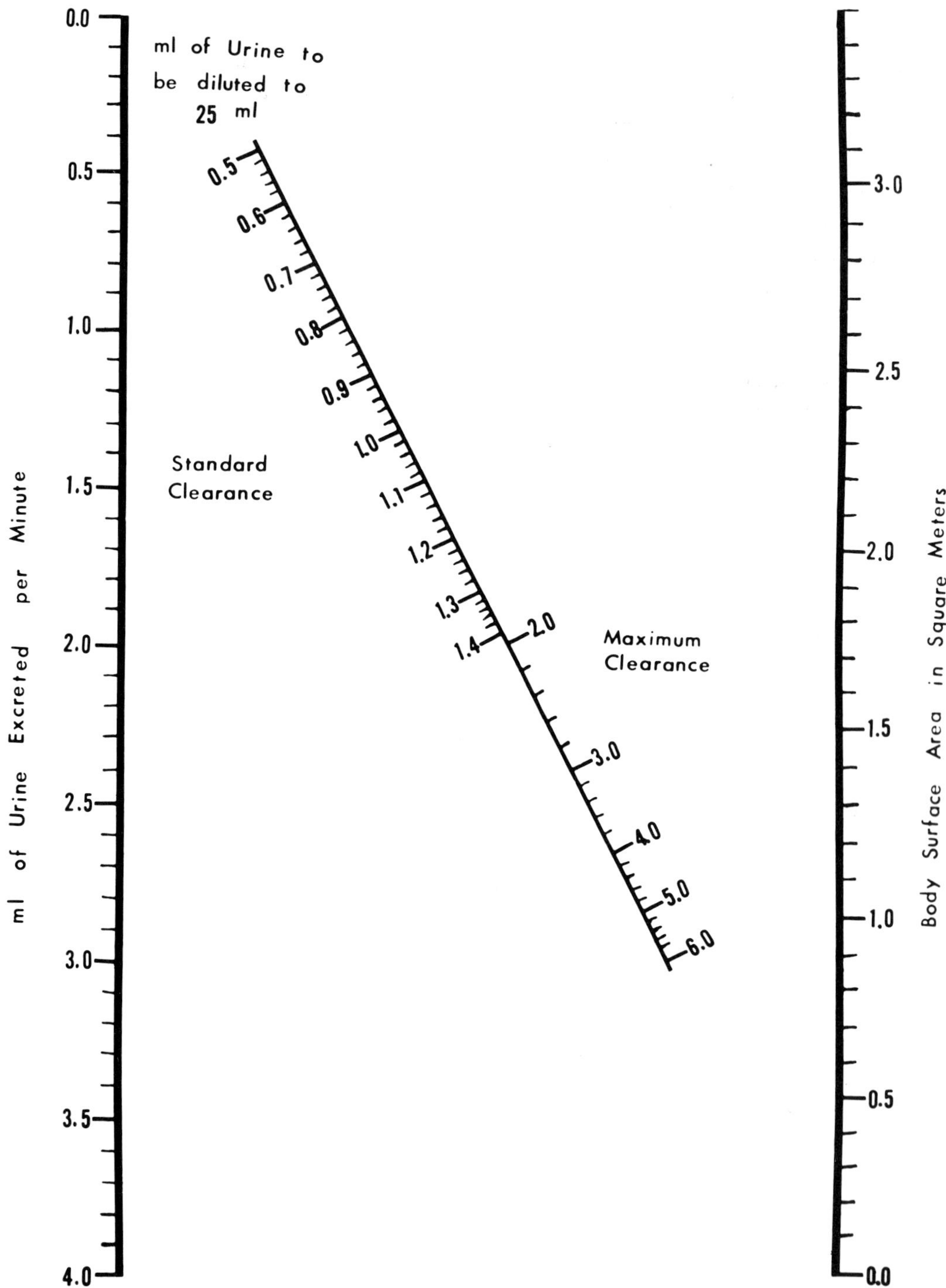

Fig. 3. Urine dilution nomogram. Note that both standard and maximum clearance can be obtained.

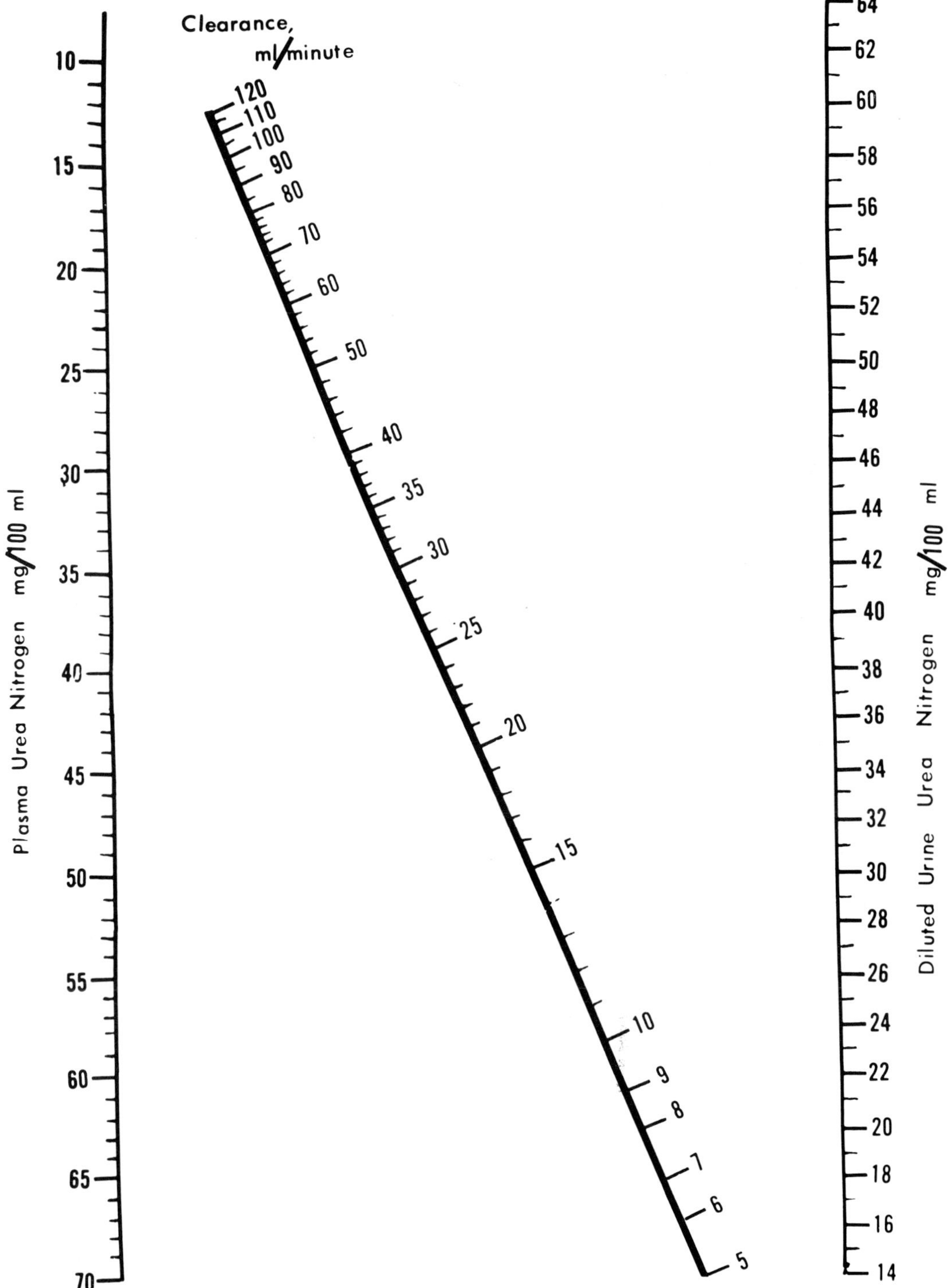

Fig. 4.   Urea clearance nomogram.

average value for C_M in the normal individual was 75 ml per min., with a range of 60 to 100 ml per min. The average for C_S was 54 ml per min., with a range of from 40 to 65 ml per min.

These results can be expressed in a different way, as a precentage of normal, as shown in the third nomogram, Figure 5. The calculation on which this percentage of normal is based is:

$$C_M \times \frac{100}{75} = C_M \times 1.33 = C_M, \text{ in } \% \text{ of normal}$$

$$C_S \times \frac{100}{54} = C_S \times 1.85 = C_S, \text{ in } \% \text{ of normal}$$

This rather old-fashioned means of expression eliminates the necessity of remembering normal values, but does not otherwise present any advantages.

As Pitts points out, crystalloids such as urea are dissolved in the water of the plasma, which makes up about 93% of plasma volume. Urea is filtered from this fraction of plasma through the glomerulus, because the proteins do not pass through; in other words, it is the plasma water that is actually being cleared of urea, not the whole plasma. One should keep this in mind at the same time as one realizes that urea clearance is reported in terms of whole plasma.

Method
A. Directions for Nurses

The urea clearance is performed in the morning on a fasting patient, who may have fruit juice for breakfast but not tea or coffee. To produce a good urine output, about a pint of water is given about 1/2 hour before the test is to begin. When the test begins, the patient is requested to empty the bladder completely, and discard this urine specimen. The time of voiding is recorded. Exactly 60 minutes later, the first hour sample is collected, and this sample should be labelled "first hour." At this time a blood sample is drawn, and another pint of water is given. One hour after the first

urine sample was collected, a second sample is collected and labelled "second hour."

It is imperative to know the exact time intervals of the urine sample collections, and it must be impressed on the nursing staff that a collection period of 50 minutes or 70 minutes is satisfactory, so long as it is known to the laboratory. All urine that is passed must be collected and brought to the laboratory. If urine collection is defective or incomplete, the test is useless.

The height and weight of the patient must be recorded on the requisition, accompanying the urine specimens.

B. Procedure

1. If all has gone well with sample collection, three specimens, properly labelled will be received; a first-hour urine specimen, a second-hour urine specimen, and a blood sample. The height and weight of the patient will be stated.

2. The volume of both urine specimens is accurately measured, and the volume per minute calculated for each specimen.

3. The surface area of the patient is obtained from Figure 2.

4. On Figure 3, the volume per minute and surface area are located, and when these are aligned with a straight-

edge, the ml. of urine to be diluted to 25 ml is obtained from the oblique line of the nomogram.

5. The volume of urine from Figure 3 is transferred to a 25 ml volumetric flask, which is then filled to the mark with distilled water.

6. Urea nitrogen determinations are performed on the two urine specimens and the plasma from the blood specimen. This procedure is suitable for any urea nitrogen method.

7. On Figure 4, the plasma urea nitrogen in mg per 100 ml (left-hand margin) and the diluted urine urea nitrogen in mg per 100 ml (right-hand margin) are located and aligned with a straight-edge. The clearance in ml per min. is obtained from the oblique line of the nomogram.

8. The percentage of normal is obtained from Figure 5, or calculated by other methods.

9. The urea clearance is reported for both one-hour periods, both in ml per min/1.73 sq.m, and as a percentage of normal.

Example

For example, a patient weights 70 kg, is 180 cm tall, and has a urine flow 2.5 ml per min.

1. The body surface area, obtained from Figure 2, is 1.85 sq.m.

2. The volume of urine to be diluted to 25 ml is obtained from Figure 3 by aligning 1.85 on the right margin with 2.5 on the left margin. It is 2.4 ml. Since the figure 2.4 is on the right side of the oblique line, the measurement is considered to be a maximum clearance.

3. The plasma urea nitrogen and the diluted urine urea nitrogen are measured. The former is 21 mg per 100 ml., and the latter 56 mg per 100 ml.

4. The urea clearance is obtained from Figure 4 by aligning 21 on the left margin with 56 on the right margin. It is 66 ml per min.

5. The percentage of normal is obtained from Figure 5. It is 88% of

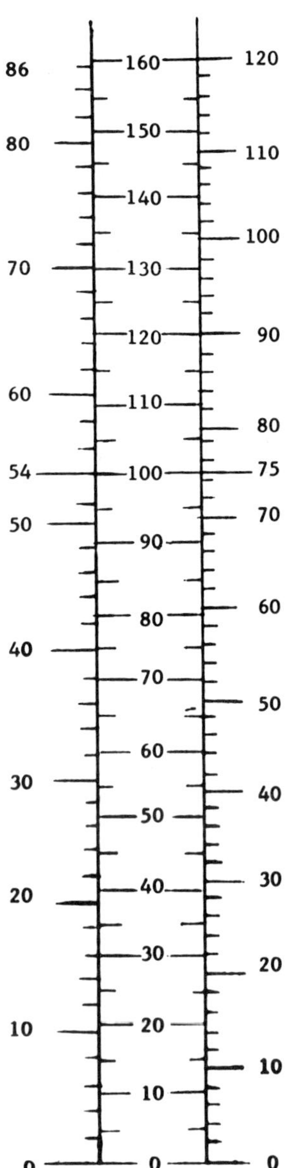

Fig. 5. Nomogram for obtaining urea clearance as % normal.

normal, already corrected to a normal body surface.

6. The procedure should be reported as follows:

Urea clearance:

$$C_M = 66 \text{ ml per min.}/1.73 \text{ sq.m}; \\ 88\% \text{ of normal}$$

7. An identical procedure is, of course, carried out stimultaneously for the other urine specimen.

Comments

1. If the plasma urea nitrogen is over 70 mg per 100 ml., one may divide the result by 2, find the clearance in ml per min. from Figure 4, and divide this value by 2 to obtain valid results. In general, the urea clearance does not provide reproducible or useful information in patients with this much nitrogen retention. It finds its greatest value in patients with nearly normal plasma urea nitrogen concentrations.

2. In very large patients, over 100 kg, with high protein intakes, the diluted urine urea nitrogen may be higher than 64 mg per 100 ml. In this case, the results of the diluted urine urea nitrogen may be divided by 2, and the results of the urea clearance may be multiplied by 2. This relationship applies because the two scales at the margins of Figure 4 are linear, with equal divisions, so that simple arithematic relations prevail. This is in contrast to nomograms devised by others.

Discussion

The urea clearance is most useful in evaluating the renal function of patients who have normal of slightly increased concentrations of plasma urea nitrogen. In evaluating the results of the plasma urea nitrogen, or the urea clearance, the effect of diet is often not appreciated. This effect was demonstrated by Addis (1948), who studied dogs after surgical reduction of the amount of functioning renal tissue. When this was reduced to 38% of normal, the serum urea concentration rose from 28 mg per 100 ml on a 5% lactalbumin diet to 183 mg per 100 ml when the diet was increased to 80% lactalbumin. These observations in animals were confirmed by studies in humans (21, 36).

The theoretical effect of diet may readily be seen from Table 6.

In this Table 6, line 1 shows a normal individual in nitrogen balance, eating a normal diet of 77 gm of protein daily, catabolizing 85% of the protein nitrogen as urea nitrogen, and having a normal urine flow of 1 ml per min. The combination of the effect of destruction of

TABLE 6—EFFECT OF DIET ON PLASMA UREA NITROGEN

Line	Daily Protein Intake gm	Urea Nitrogen Produced Per Day gm	Plasma Urea Nitrogen mg/100 ml	Urea Clearance ml/min	Urea Nitrogen Excreted Per Minute mg	Urea Nitrogen Excreted Per Day gm	Urea Nitrogen Retention Per Day gm
1	77	10.4	12.0	60	7.2	10.4	0
2	50	6.8	12.0	30	3.6	5.2	1.6
3	50	6.8	15.8	30	4.7	6.8	0
4	77	10.4	12.0	30	3.6	5.2	5.6
5	77	10.4	24.0	30	7.2	10.4	0
6	77	10.4	17.3	41.5	7.2	10.4	0

half his functioning renal tissue at the same time as his diet is reduced to 50 gm of protein daily without change in urine flow is shown in line 2. Parenthetically, it should be noted that many routine hospital diets contain no more than 50 gm of protein daily. On this diet, with a urea clearance of 30 ml per min., the patient retains 1.6 gm of urea nitrogen in one day. This causes the plasma urea nitrogen to become elevated to 15.8 mg per 100 ml, still a normal value. In line 3, one sees that at this level of plasma urea nitrogen, the patient is again in nitrogen balance. It is not until the diet is increased to 77 gm of protein daily, as shown in lines 4 and 5, that elevation of the plasma urea nitrogen above normal occurs.

The first five lines of this table assume a urine flow of 1 ml per min., which means that approximately 50% of the urea filtered through the glomeruli will be reabsorbed by the tubules. If urine flow rate is increased, tubular reabsorption decreases, more urea is cleared from the plasma, and the plasma urea nitrogen falls. An example is seem in line 6, which assumes the same conditions as line 5, except that the urine flow is increased to above 2 ml per min., a maximum clearance. The urea clearance increases to 41.5 ml per min (30 x 75/54). At this clearance level, the plasma urea nitrogen eventually falls from 24.0 to 17.3 mg per 100 ml, a normal value.

RÉSUMÉ OF CLINICAL INTERPRETATIONS

Although it is generally considered that the urea clearance measures glomerular filtration, it is evident that it does not measure this function alone, since 40 to 60% of the urea filtered through the glomeruli is reabsorbed by the tubules. The exact amount reabsorbed depends more on the rate of urine flow than on any other factor. In spite of this theoretical disadvantage, the urea clearance has been found to parallel the inulin clearance and the creatinine clearance, so that for practical purposes, it may be considered to be a general indication of the glomerular filtration rate.

Certain practical disadvantages are also inherent in the urea clearance. Among these are the difficulty of obtaining accurate collection of urine over the short period of time, the problem of securing satisfactory urine flow, and the wide variations that can be produced by diet. As Wrong points out, it is not uncommon to have 100% variation in the results of the two one-hour clearances. Because of these disadvantages, it is being replaced in many laboratories by the creatinine clearance.

However, the urea clearance is of great historical interest, and remains one of the traditional tests of renal function. It is still widely used clinically, and to quote one of the leading students of renal function, H. W. Smith, "Nevertheless, for ease and rapidity in the clinical assessment of renal function, the urea clearance is unsurpassed. More than any other single measurement, it has guided clinical investigation through many phases of disease."

REFERENCES

1. Addis, T.: The ratio between the urea content of the urine and of the blood after administration of large quantities of urea. An approximate index of the quantity of actively functioning kidney tissue. J. Urol., *1*:263-287, 1917.

2. Addis, T.: Glomerular Nephritis – Diagnosis and Treatment. New York, McMillan, 1948, p. 328.

3. Addis T., Barnett, G. D., and Shevky, A. E.: The regulation of renal activity. I. Regulation of urea excretion by the concentration of urea in the

blood and in the urine. Amer. J. Physiol., *46*:1-10, 1918.

4. Addis T., and Watanabe, C. K.: A method for the measurement of the urea excreting function of the kidneys. J. Biol. Chem., *28*:251-259, 1916.

5. Ambard, L.: Physiologie Normale et Pathologique des Reins. Paris, Masson et Cie., 1920, ed. 2.

6. Ambard, L., and Weill, A.: Les lois numériques de la secrétion rénale de l'urée et du chlorure de sodium. J. Physiol. Path. gén., *14*:753-765, 1912.

7. Annino, J. S.: An improved automated method for the determination of urea. Amer. J. Clin. Path., *37*:147-149, 1967.

8. Austin, J. H., Stillman, E., and Van Slyke, D. D.: Factors governing the excretion rate of urea. J. Biol. Chem., *46*:91-112, 1921.

9. Bennett, C. A., and Franklin, N. L.: Statistical Analysis in Chemistry and the Chemical Industry. New York, Wiley, 1954.

10. Berthelot, M. P. E.: Repert, Chim. Appl., *1*:282-284, 1859.

11. Bollman, J. L., Mann, F. C., and Magath, T. B.: Studies on the physiology of the liver. VIII. Effect of total removal of the liver on the formation of urea. Amer. J. Physiol., *69*:371-392, 1924.

12. Boutwell, J. H., Jr.: Direct nesslerization of blood and urine filtrates in the determination of urea (as ammonia). Clin. Clem., *3*:205-216, 1957.

13. Bright, R.: Cases and observations, illustrative of renal disease accompanied with the secretion of albuminous urine. Guy's Hosp. Reports, *1*:338-400, 1836.

14. Christison, R.: Observations on the variety of dropsy which depends on diseased kidney. Edinburgh Med. & Surg. J., *32*:262-290, 1829.

15. Cohen, P. P., and Brown, G. W., Jr.: Ammonia Metabolism and Urea Biosynthesis in Comparative Biochemistry (M. Florkin and H. S. Mason, eds.) Vol. II, Chap. 4. New York, Academic Press, 1960.

16. Coulombe, J. J., and Favreau, L.: A new simple semimicro method for colorimetric determination of urea. Clin. Chem., *9*:102-108, 1963.

17. Dickenman, R. C., Crafts, B., and Zak, B.: Use of alpha diketones for analysis of urea. Amer. J. Clin. Path., *24*:981-987, 1954.

18. Fearon, W. R.: The carbamide diacetyl reaction for citrulline. Biochem. J., *33*:902-905, 1939.

19. Gallagher, J. C., and Seligson, D.: Significance of abnormally low blood urea levels. New England J. Med., *266*:492-495, 1962.

20. Goldring, W., and Chasis, K.: Hypertension and Hypertensive Disease. New York, Commonwealth Fund, 1944, p. 253.

21. Goldring, W., Razinsky, L., Greenblatt, M., and Cohen, S.: The influence of protein intake on the urea clearance in normal man. J. Clin. Invest., *13*:743-748, 1934.

22. Gréhant, N.: Mesure de l'activitié physiologique des reins par le dosage de l'urée dans le sang et dans l'urine. J. Physiol. Path. gén., *6*:1-8, 1904.

23. Henry, R. J.: Improper statistics characterizing the normal range. Amer. J. Clin. Path., *34*:326-327, 1960.

24. Kaplan, A.: Urea nitrogen and Urinary ammonia. Standard Methods of Clinical Chemistry, Vol. 5, New York, Academic Press, 1965, pp. 245-256.

25. Kossel, A., and Dakin, H. D.: Über die Arginase. Z. f. Physiol. Chem., *41*:321-331, 1904.

26. Krebs, H. A., and Henseleit, K.: Untersuchungen über die Harnstoffbildung im Tierkörper. Z. f. Physiol. Chem., *210*:33-66, 1932.

27. MacKay, E. M., and MacKay, L. L.: The concentration of urea in the blood of normal individuals. J. Clin. Invest., *4*:295-305, 1927.

28. Marsh, W. H., Fingerhut, B., and Kirsch, E.: Determination of urea nitrogen with the diacetyl method and an automatic dialyzing apparatus. Amer. J. Clin. Path., *28*:681-688, 1957.

29. Marsh, W. H., Fingerhut, B., and Miller, H.: Automated and manual direct methods for the determination of blood urea. Clin. Chem., *11*:624-627, 1965.

30. Marshall, E. K., Jr.: A rapid clinical method for the estimation of urea in urine. J. Biol. Chem., *14*:283-290, 1913.

31. McNair, R. D.: Use of a screening procedure for blood urea nitrogen. Clin. Chem., *11*:74-76, 1965.

32. Möller, E., McIntosh, J. F., and Van Slyke, D. D.: Studies of urea excretion. II. Relationship between urine volume and the rate of urea excretion by normal adults. J. Clin. Invest., *6*:427-465, 1928.

33. Möller, E., McIntosh, J. F., and Van Slyke, D. D.: IV. Relationship between urine volume and the rate of urea excretion by patients with Bright's disease. J. Clin. Invest. *6*:485-504, 1928.

34. Moore, J. J., and Sax, S. M.: A revised automated procedure for urea nitrogen. Clin. Chim. Acta, *11*:475-477, 1965.

35. Murdaugh, H. V., Jr. and Doyle, E. M.: Effect of hemoglobin on erythrocytic urea concentration. J. Lab. Clin. Med., *57*:759-762, 1961.

36. Nielsen, A. L., and Bang, H. O.: The influence of diet on the renal function of healthy persons. Acta Med. Scandinav., *130*:382-388, 1948.

37. Peters, J. P., and Van Slyke, D. D.: "Quantitative Clinical Chemistry. Methods," Vol. II. Baltimore, Williams and Wilkins, 1932.

38. Peters, J. P., and Van Slyke, D. D.: "Quantitative Clinical Chemistry. Interpretations," Vol. I, Baltimore, Williams and Wilkins, 1946, pp. 835-872.

39. Picard (1856): As quoted by Bollman, Mann and Magath, 1924.

40. Picard (1881): As quoted by Bollman, Mann and Magath, 1924.

41. Pitts, R. F.: Physiology of the Kidney and Body Fluids. Chicago, Year Book, 1963, p. 87.
42. Prevost, J. L., and Dumas, J. A.: Examen du sang et de son action dans les divers phenomenes de la vie. Ann. de Chim. et de Phys., 2 me serie, *23:*90, 1823.
43. Ralls, J. O.: Urea is not equally distributed between the water of the blood cells and that of the plasma. J. Biol. Chem., *151:*529-541, 1943.
44. Ratner, S.: Urea synthesis and metabolism of arginine and citrullin. Advances in Enzymology, *15:*319-387, 1954.
45. Rees, G. U. On the Nature and Treatment of Diseases of the Kidney with Albuminous Urine (Morbus Brightis). London, Longman, Brown, Green and Longmans, 1850, p. 134.
46. Roijers, A. F. M., and Tas, M. M.: The determination of urea with p-dimethylaminobenzaldehyde. Clin. Chim. Acta, *9:*197-202, 1964.
47. Rouelle, H. M.: Observations sur l'urine humaine, E. fur alles de vache e de cheval comparees ensemble. J. de Med., *40:*451-468, 1773.
48. Schreiner, G. F., and Maher, J. C.: Uremia: Biochemistry, Pathogenesis and Treatment. Springfield, Thomas, 1961.
49. Schroeder, W. von: Über die Bildungstätte des Harnstoffs. Arch. exp. Path. Pharmakol., *15:*364-402, 1882.
50. Searcy, R. L., Korotzer, J. L., Douglas, G. L., and Bergquist, L. M.: Quantitation of serum urea as a microcapillary column of dixanthylurea. Clin. Chem., *10:*128-135, 1964.
51. Sendroy, J., Jr. and Cecchini, C. P.: Determination of human body surface area from height and weight. J. Appl. Physiol., *7:*1-12, 1954.
52. Shively, J. A.: Evaluation of methodology in clinical chemistry. Amer. J. Clin. Path., *43:*505-516, 1965.
53. Skeggs, L. T., Jr.: An automatic method for colorimetric analysis. Amer. J. Clin. Path., *28:*311-322, 1957.
54. Smith, H. W.: Principles of Renal Physiology. New York, Oxford, 1956.
55. Stadie, W. C., and Van Slyke, D. D.: The effect of acute yellow atrophy on metabolism and on the composition of the liver. Arch. Int. Med., *25:*693-704, 1920.
56. Stevenson, G. F.: Personal communication.
57. Strauss, H.: Die chronischen Nierenentzündungen in ihrer Einwirkung auf die Blutflüssigkeit under deren Behandlung. Berlin, A. Hirschwald, 1902.
58. Sunderman, F. W.: Studies in serum electrolytes. X. The water of serum and factors for the calculation of the molality of a solute in serum from the measurement of the specific gravity. J. Biol. Chem., *113:*111-115, 1936.
59. Szakacs, J. E., and Borowsky, M.: Clearance and tubular function tests. In: Fuller, J. B. (ed.): Workshop on Urinalysis and Renal Function Studies, Technique Mamual. Commission on Continuing Education, Council on Clinical Chemistry, American Society of Clinical Pathologists, 1962, p. 21.
60. Taylor, F. B., Drury, D. R., and Addis, T.: The regulation of renal activity. VIII. The relation between the rate of urea excretion and the size of the kidneys. Amer. J. Physiol., *65:*55-61, 1923.
61. Technicon Autoanalyzer Method File N-la, Technicon Instruments Corporation, Chauncey, New York, 1963.
62. Technicon Autoanalyzer Method File N-1c, Technicon Corporation, Ardsley, New York, 1967.
63. Van Slyke, D. D., and Hiller, A.: Determination of ammonia in blood. J. Biol. Chem. *102:*499-504, 1933.
64. Walsler, M., and Bodenlos, L. J.: Urea metabolism in man. J. Clin. Invest., *38:*1617-1626, 1959.
65. Williams, E. S., and Sunderman, F. W.: The distribution of sugar and chloride in the blood of diabetic individuals. Amer. J. Med. Sci., *187:*462-469, 1934.
66. Wöhler, F.: Über Künstliche Bildung des Harnstoffs. Ann. Phys. Chem., *12:*253-256, 1828.
67. Wootton, I. D. P., King, E. J., and Smith, J. M.: The quantitative approach to hospital biochemistry. Brit. Med. Bull., *7:*307-311, 1951.
68. Wrong, O. M.: Test of renal functions. In Renal Disease, Black, D.A.K. (ed): Philadelphia, F. H. Davis, 1962.

The Measurement of Creatinine Clearance

IRENE E. ROECKEL, M.D.

Assessment of glomerular filtration is important in evaluating renal function. Inulin clearance is the most precise method of measuring glomerular filtration rate (23), but it involves the intravenous infusion of an accurate dose of inulin. Also, the subsequent measurement of inulin in blood and urine (21) is cumbersome. These problems with the inulin clearance test have prompted reconsideration of the clinically and technically less intricate endogenous creatinine clearance test. Moreover, with the present knowledge of factors influencing the endogenous creatinine clearance in health and disease, there is no need to consider it a measurement of the "poor man's polysaccharide" (2, 7, 14).

FACTORS INFLUENCING CREATININE CLEARANCE

1. *Chemical Creatinine Measurement.* Though many authors speak of "true creatinine" determinations, a critical evaluation reveals that we are today without a genuine method for creatinine measurement in biologic fluids (1-5, 10, 11, 14-20, 25-28). Of all the methods proposed (15, 27, 24), the modified reaction with alkaline picrate described by Jaffe (13) in 1886 is still the method of choice. A detailed description of the laboratory procedure is given in section B of this chapter. With the proper performance of the alkaline picrate method, serum and urine creatinine determinations reflect, as nearly as possible, the true creatinine levels in these biologic fluids.

2. *Tubular Secretion.* Creatinine clearance has been compared with inulin clearance data (6, 7, 23). In normal man, the ratio of endogenous creatinine clearance to inulin clearance (C_{cr}:C_{in}) is 1.11. In renal insufficiency, the ratio increases up to 1.50, and this increased ratio has been attributed to tubular secretion of part of the creatinine appearing in the urine. Recent studies by Goldman (9) and his associates have thoroughly investigated this relationship. By performing exogenous creatinine clearance studies in normal subjects and uremic patients, they showed there is not a simple "rate limited" secretory mechanism responsible for the rate of tubular creatinine transport. As the serum creatinine level in normal subjects is raised, the ratio of the exogenous creatinine clearance to inulin clearance

reaches a high of $\approx$ 1.73, then gradually falls to an endogenous clearance ratio as seen in patients with uremia, $\approx$ 1.40. Since creatinine infusion in uremic patients fails to give this steep rise in ratio seen in the normal subject, it must be attributed to tubular excretion being at its maximum and therefore the difference in the observed creatinine inulin clearance ratio in renal failure is due to tubular creatinine excretion (3, 9).

3. *Dependence on Lean Body Mass.* Doolan (7) and co-workers examined their endogenous creatinine clearance data for correlation with lean body weight and for estimated body surface area. In their study of 30 subjects with accurate antropometric measurements, the correlation analysis of creatinine excretion with lean body weight revealed a correlation coefficient of 0.878 and 0.887 for surface correction area respectively. These data are better than the ones previously reported since they more closely approximate the straight line coefficient of correlation of one.

It appears that endogenous creatinine clearance data applied to normal subjects and uremic patients are highly reproducible in the individual subject but without correction for either surface area or lean body mass show a great deal more variation in a group of subjects. Most clinical situations are concerned with the improvement or deterioration of a patient, and dependable data will be obtained without correction, provided there is no extensive muscular wasting.

4. *Diurnal Variation.* Dodge (6) and his co-workers have recently considered the possibility of a significant variation in plasma and urinary creatinine content during a 24-hour period. Their patient material consisted of children only. If a 24-hour urine collection is employed it would obviously compensate for any variation in excretion. Unfortunately, complete collection of urine for 24 hours poses a very difficult problem even for hospitalized patients. Doolan (7) and his group studied adults during morning and afternoon periods and compared these data with data obtained from 24 hour collections in the same subjects. They were unable to demonstrate any difference in clearance data, although plasma creatinine concentration was significantly higher in the afternoon. Also, they established that a one-hour clearance study will be significantly 7 to 11% higher for women and recommend a longer urine collection period.

5. *Sex and Age Differences.* Durbach (8) and co-workers attempted to answer the question of variation in serum creatinine due to age and sex by studying 1107 men and 1151 women varying from 15 to 69 years of age. The subjects studied were volunteers in the Swiss watch industry and were not selected by normal physical examination. Without correcting their values for lean body mass, they found a mean serum creatinine for men to be 1.19 ± 0.33 mg per 100 ml and for women 0.96 ± 0.28 mg per 100 ml. The authors point out that young males between 15 to 19 years of age are demonstrating a significantly lower value than the remainder of the adult male and female population.

By re-evaluating published reports, newborn infants have adult serum creatinine values. These levels fall during the first week of life and slowly rise again to reach adult levels by age 20 (8). The data in the literature are not large enough to calculate authoritative normals for each age group.

This leaves the problem of normal urinary creatinine excretion unanswered on a scale comparable to the studies of serum creatinine levels. Doolan (7) and co-workers data show that 24-hour clearance values for healthy males corrected for a standard surface area of 1.73 sq. M are 123 ml per min ± 19.3 and for women 114 ml per min ± 16.0. The uncorrected values are 140 ml per min ± 27.2 and 112 ml per min ± 20.3 respectively. If lean body weight data are available for correction, Doolan (7) and co-workers demonstrated that the sex difference is completely removed. It seems reasonable to conclude that body surface corrections are not contributing to the accurate evaluation of creatinine clearance data and should be abolished, leaving a significant difference between adult male and female subjects (7, 12).

SUMMARY

It has been shown that creatinine clearance measurements can be used effectively in following the progress of a patient's renal status. The measurement can be carried out even in the presence of renal disease as long as the interpretation is done with the realization that with increasing serum creatinine content the measurement does in part reflect tubular secretion. Abnormal values obtained in one patient cannot readily be matched with values in other patients since lean body mass measurements are needed to correct the data for comparison.

REFERENCES

1. Biggs, H. G., and Cooper, J. M.: Modified Folin methods for the measurement of urinary creatine and creatinine. Clin. Chem., *7:*655-664, 1961.
2. Blondeel, N. J., Goodman, S., Simon, N. M., and Greco, F. del: Production of urea nitrogen and creatinine in chronic azotemia and effect of hemodialysis. Proc. Soc. Exp. Biol. Med., *122:*156-160, 1966.
3. Bonsnes, R. W., and Taussky, H. H.: On the colorimetric determination of creatinine by the Jaffe reaction. J. Biol. Chem., *158:*581-591, 1945.
4. Brod, J., and Sirota, J. H.: The renal clearance of endogenous "creatinine" in man. J. Clin. Invest., *27:*645-654, 1948.
5. Cooper, J. M., and Biggs, H. G.: An evaluation of four methods of measuring urinary creatinine. Clin. Chem., *7:*665-673, 1961.
6. Dodge, W. F., Travis, L. B., and Daeschner, C. W.: Comparison of endogenous creatinine clearance with inulin clearance. Amer. J. Dis. Child., *113:*683-692, 1967.
7. Doolan, P. D., Alpen, E. L., and Theil, G. B.: A clinical appraisal of the plasma concentration and endogenous clearance of creatinine. Am. J. Med., *32:*65-79, 1962.
8. Dubach, U. C., Metz, I., und Schmid, P.: Serum-Kreatininwerte bei 2258 arbeitstatigen Personen verschiedenen Alters und Geschlechts. Klin. Wschr., *45:*621-629, 1967.
9. Goldman, R., Yadley, R. A., and Nourok, D. S.: Comparison of endogenous and exogenous creatinine clearances in man. Proc. Soc. Exp. Biol. Med., *125:*205-210, 1967.
10. Hare, R. S.: Endogenous creatinine in serum and urine. Proc. Soc. Exp. Biol. Med., *74:*148-151, 1950.
11. Haugen, H. N., and Blegen, E. M.: Plasma creatinine concentration and creatinine clearance in clinical work. Ann. Int. Med., *43:*731-739, 1955.
12. Harvey, A. M., Malvin, R. L., and Vander, A. J.: Comparison of creatinine secretion in men and women. Nephron, *3:*201-205, 1966.
13. Jaffe, M.: Ueber den Niederschlag, welchen Pikrinsaeure in normalen Harn erzeugt und ueber eine neue Reaction des Kreatinins. Z. Physiol. Chem., *10:*391-400, 1886.
14. Josephson, B.: The clinical value of the "apparent" serum creatinine concentration. Scand. J. Clin. Lab. Invest., *69:*121-129, 1963.
15. Langley, W. D., and Evans, M.: The determination of creatinine with sodium 3, 5-dinitrobenzoate. J. Biol. Chem., *115:*333-341, 1936.
16. Lauson, H. D.: Sources of error in plasma creatinine determination. J. Applied Physiol., *4:*227-244, 1951.
17. Mandel, E. E., and Jones, F. L.: Studies in nonprotein nitrogen. III evaluation of methods measuring creatinine. J. Lab. & Clin. Med., *41:*323-334, 1953.
18. Mattar, G., Barnett, H. L., McNamara, H., and Lauson, H. D.: Measurement of glomerular filtration rate in children with kidney disease. J. Clin. Invest., *31:*938-946, 1952.
19. Owen, J. L., Iggo, B., Scandrett, F. J., and Stewart, C. P.,: The determination of creatinine in plasma or serum, and in urine; A critical examination. Biochem. J., *58:*426-437, 1954.

20. Polar, E., and Metcoff, J.: "True" creatinine chromogen determination in serum and urine by semi-automated analysis. Clin. Chem., *11:*763-770, 1965.
21. Schreiner, G. E.: Determination of inulin by means of resorcinol. Proc. Soc. Exp. Biol. Med., *74:*117-120, 1950.
22. Sirota, J. H., Baldwin, D. S., and Villarreal, H.: Diurnal variations of renal function in man. J. Clin. Invest., *29:*187-192, 1950.
23. Smith, H. W.: The Kidney. New York, Oxford University Press, 1951.
24. Sullivan, M. X., and Irreverre, F.: A highly specific test for creatinine. J. Biol. Chem., *233:*530-533, 1958.
25. Taussky, H. H.: A procedure increasing the specificity of the Jaffe reaction for the determination of creatine and creatinine in urine and plasma. Clin. Chim. Acta, *1:*210-224, 1956.
26. Tobias, G. J., McLaughlin, R.F., and Hopper, Jr. J.: Endogenous creatinine clearance: A valuable clinical test of glomerular filtration and a prognostic guide in chronic renal disease. New Eng. J. Med., *255:*317-323, 1962.
27. Van Pilsum, J. F., Martin, R. P., Kito, E., and Hess, J.: Determination of creatine, creatinine, arginine, guanidinoacetic acid, guanidine, and methylguanidine in biological fluids. J. Biol. Chem.,*222:*225-236, 1956.
28. Van Pilsum, J. F., and Bovis, M.: Effect of various protein precipitants on recoveries of creatinine added to plasma. Clin. Chem., *3:*90-94, 1957.
29. Zender, R., et Falbriard, A.: Analyse Automatique de la Creatinine Dans Le Serum et Dans L'Urine, Valeurs "Normales" Chez L'Homme de la Creatininemie et de la Clearance. Clinica Chim. Acta, *12:*192-190, 1965.

Measurements of Creatinine in Serum and Urine and the Estimation of Creatinine Clearance

IRENE E. ROECKEL, M.D.

Introduction

The need for a simple and dependable measure of glomerular filtration rate has focused the interest on the measurement of serum and urine creatinine (1, 2). In spite of the problems encountered in measuring creatinine, and the fact that there is a small amount of tubular secretion of creatinine, endogenous creatinine clearance studies in normal and uremic patients (3) are useful in assessing renal function.

Principle

Creatinine in an acid protein free filtrate of serum and in diluted urine reacts with alkaline picrate to form a red color. This color follows Beer's law in a linear relationship of optical density to concentration at 520 mμ up to a sample concentration of 6 mg per 100 ml. The construction of a calibration curve permits accurate determinations up to 12 mg per 100 ml (4). To avoid chromogens in serum adding to the creatinine alkaline picrate complex, strict adherence to the procedure is required. Automatic equipment utilizing dialysis and accurate timing of the reaction make this method most suitable for the laboratory which processes a large number of specimens.

Reagents

1. *Tricholoracetic Acid, 1 N.* Exactly 16.3 gm of reagent grade CCl_3COOH are weighed and 100 ml of distilled water added.

2. *Picric Acid, 0.04 N.* A saturated picric acid solution is prepared from reagent grade picric acid by dissolving 16 gm of picric acid in one liter of distilled water. The solution is heated to 80°C. and cooled to room temperature. About 690 ml of this saturated solution are diluted to one liter. The concentration is adjusted between 0.0395 N and 0.0405 N by titrating with 0.1 N NaOH with phenolphthalein as indicator.

3. *Sodium Hydroxide, 2.5 N.*

4. *Alkaline Picrate Working Reagent.* Ten volumes of 0.04 N picric acid solution are mixed with 2 volumes of 2.5 N NaOH just before use since this reagent is not stable.

Standard Solutions

1. *Stock Creatinine Standard.* Exactly 0.201 gm of creatinine zinc chloride are

weighed and dissolved in 0.1 N hydrochloric acid and diluted to 100 ml in a volumetric flask. This solution is stable in refrigerator for one month.

2. *Working Creatinine Standard S_1.* Two ml of the stock standard are diluted to 100 ml with 0.1 hydrochloric acid.

3. *Working Creatinine Standard S_2.* Twelve ml of stock standard are diluted to 100 ml with 0.1 N hydrochloric acid.

Procedure
A. Serum

A protein-free filtrate is prepared by mixing 2 ml of serum, 4 ml of distilled water, and 4 ml of 1 N trichloroacetic acid. The mixture is shaken well and allowed to stand for 10 minutes before centrifugation and filtration. Two ml of the working standard S_1 creatinine solution and 4 ml of distilled water and 4 ml of 1 N trichloracetic acid are processed instead of serum in identical fashion. Five ml of the serum filtrate, working standard, and a blank are placed in a 15-ml capacity colorimeter tube and 10 ml of the freshly prepared alkaline pricric acid reagent added to each tube and mixed. Exactly 16 minutes after the addition of the alkaline picrate reagent, the color is read at 520 mμ. The reading of the standard should be checked with a previously obtained calibration curve.

Calibration Curve

Eight 15-ml cuvets are prepared and labeled as listed in Table I. To each tube are added 10 ml of the freshly prepared alkaline picrate reagent. After mixing, the color is read at exactly 16 minutes. The calibration curve is prepared by plotting the concentrations of the creatinine standard as abscissa against the blank corrected meter readings as coordinate.

TABLE I

Tube Numbers	Standard	H_2O	Creatinine (mg per 100 ml)
Blank	0	5 ml	0.0
1	1 ml S_1	4 ml	0.5
2	2 ml S_1	3 ml	1.0
3	4 ml S_1	1 ml	2.0
4	1 ml S_2	4 ml	3.0
5	2 ml S_2	3 ml	6.0
6	3 ml S_2	2 ml	9.0
7	4 ml S_2	1 ml	12.0

B. Urine:

The same method should be used as for serum excepting for two modifications: a) the urine should be diluted approximately 1:50 resulting in a concentration comparable to serum, and b) if the urine is protein-free, the deproteinizing step can be omitted.

To a 250-ml volumetric flask 1 ml of urine and 100 ml of 20% trichloroacetic acid are added and diluted to volume with distilled water. Five ml of this diluted urine are mixed with 10 ml of the freshly prepared alkaline picrate reagent. Exactly 16 minutes later the developed color is read at 520 mμ.

Calculations

$$\frac{\text{serum creatinine}}{\text{(mg per 100 ml)}} = \frac{\text{O.D. unknown}}{\text{O.D. Standard } S_1} \times 5$$

$$\frac{\text{urine cretinine}}{\text{(mg per 100 ml)}} = \frac{\text{O.D. unknown}}{\text{O.D. Standard } S_1} \times 250$$

Creatinine Clearance

The patient must be well hydrated to establish maximal flow of urine, drinking at least 3 glasses of water. (Coffee and tea should be avoided.) The patient empties the bladder completely, and the time of voiding is recorded as the beginning of the test period. Exactly 5 hours later, the patient empties the bladder completely, and the entire specimen is collected and measure accurately. At the same time, a blood sample is drawn for the determination of serum creatinine.

Calculations

$$\text{Creatinine clearance} = \frac{\text{urine creatinine} \times \text{urine flow}}{\text{serum creatinine}} \frac{\text{(mg per 100 ml)} \quad \text{(ml per min)}}{\text{(mg per 100 ml)}}$$

Discussion

The modified picric acid determination of serum and urine creatinine (4-6) compares favorably with more specific but cumbersome procedures. It is suitable to the study of normal subjects as well as patients with various stages of renal disease (3, 7). The results can be improved by correcting clearance data for body surface.

Sources of Error

1. Poor quality of picric acid.

2. Reading the picric acid creatinine color complex after more than 16 minutes time has elapsed. This is most important for serum samples since the chromogens in serum form a color complex on standing.

3. Incomplete collection of urine owing to inability of the patient to empty the bladder for the collection of urine. If the patient is unable to empty the bladder, catherization is necessary.

4. Inadequate hydration of the patient.

Range of Values

A. Serum Creatinine
    Men: 1.19 ± 0.33 mg per 100 ml
    Women: 0.96 ± 0.28 mg per 100 ml

B. Endogenous Creatinine Clearance
    Men: 140 ± 27.2 ml per minute
    Women: 112 ± 20.3 ml per minute

Resume of Clinical Interpretations

In renal failure, the serum creatinine level is elevated and the endogenous creatinine clearance decreases. Creatinine determinations and serial clearance studies permit an appraisal of the patient's clinical course.

REFERENCES

1. Rehberg, P. B.: Studies on kidney function. The rate of filtration and reabsorption in the human kidney. Biochem. J., *20*:447-460, 1926.

2. Holten, C., and Rehberg, P. B.: Studies on the pathologic function of the kidney in renal disease, especially Bright's disease. Acta Med. Scandinav., *74*:479-518, 1931.

3. Goldman, R., Yadley, R. A., and Novrok, D. S.: Comparison of endogenous and exogenous creatinine clearance in man. Proc. Soc. Exp. Biol. Med., *125*:205-210, 1967.

4. Owen, J. A., Iggo, B., Scandrett, F. J., and Stewart, C. P.: The determination of creatinine in plasma and serum, and in urine; a critical examination. Biochem. J., *58*:426-437, 1954.

5. Biggs, H. G., and Cooper, J. M.: Modified folin methods for the measurement of urinary creatine and creatinine. Clin. Chem., *7*:655-664, 1961.

6. Cooper, J. M., and Biggs, H. G.: An evaluation of four methods of measuring urinary creatinine. Clin. Chem., *7*:665-673, 1961.

7. Doolan, P. D., Alpen, E. L., and Theil, G. B.: A clinical appraisal of the plasma concentration and endogenous clearance of creatinine. Am. J. Med., *32*:65-79, 1962.

8. Dubach, V. C., Metz, I., and Schmid, P.: Serum creatinine values of 2258 working persos with age and sex differences. Klin. Wschr., *45*:621-629, 1967.

Nomograms for Creatinine Clearance

J. DE LA HUERGA, M.D., PH.D., and J. C. SHERRICK, M.D.

The creatinine clearance can readily be related to the body surface by employing a set of nomograms in the same manner as for the urea clearance (chapter 10). Because the excretion of creatinine is much more constant than that of urea, the problem of determining the proper urine dilution is less acute, but it still exists. The following nomograms have been devised for creatinine measurements done with the Auto-Analyzer, although they can be used for manual methods with certain modifications.

It is first necessary to ascertain the body surface, which can conveniently be done from a nomogram such as that of Sendroy and Cecchini (chapter 10). Then, in Figure 1, urine flow in ml per minute and the surface area in square meters are located and aligned with a straightedge. The ml of urine to be diluted to 100 ml is obtained from the oblique line of the nomogram. The proper volume of urine is transferred to a 100 ml volumetric flask, which is filled to the mark with distilled water. Creatinine determinations are performed on the samples of plasma and diluted urine with the AutoAnalyzer. In Figure 2, the plasma creatinine in mg per 100 ml is aligned with the urine creatinine in mg per 100 ml of diluted sample, and the creatinine clearance in ml per minute is obtained from the oblique line the nomogram.

These nomograms will apply to the majority of creatinine clearances. Should the plasma creatinine be higher than 5.0 mg per 100 ml, it may be divided by 2, the clearance obtained from Figure 2, and the result divided by 2 to obtain valid results. This is true because the two vertical scales at the margin of figure 2 are linear, with equal divisions, so that simple arithmetic relations prevail.

ML OF URINE TO BE DILUTED TO 100 ML FOR CREATININE CLEARANCE
URINE FLOW
ml. per min.
BODY SURFACE
square meters
0
0.5
1.0
1.5
2.0
2.5
3.0
3.5
4.0
2.3
2.2
2.1
2.0
1.9
1.8
1.7
1.6
1.5
1.4
1.3
1.2
1.1
1.0
0.9
1.2
1.6
2.0
2.4
2.8
3.2
3.6
4.0
4.4
4.8
5.2
5.6
6.0
6.4
6.8
7.2
7.6
8.0
8.4
8.8
9.2
9.6
10.0
10.4
10.8
11.2
11.6
12.0
12.4
12.8
13.2
13.6
14.0
14.4
14.8
15.2
16.0
16.8
17.6
18.4
19.2
20.0
20.8
21.6
22.4
23.2
24.0
24.8
25.6
26.4
27.2
28.0
28.8
29.6
30.2

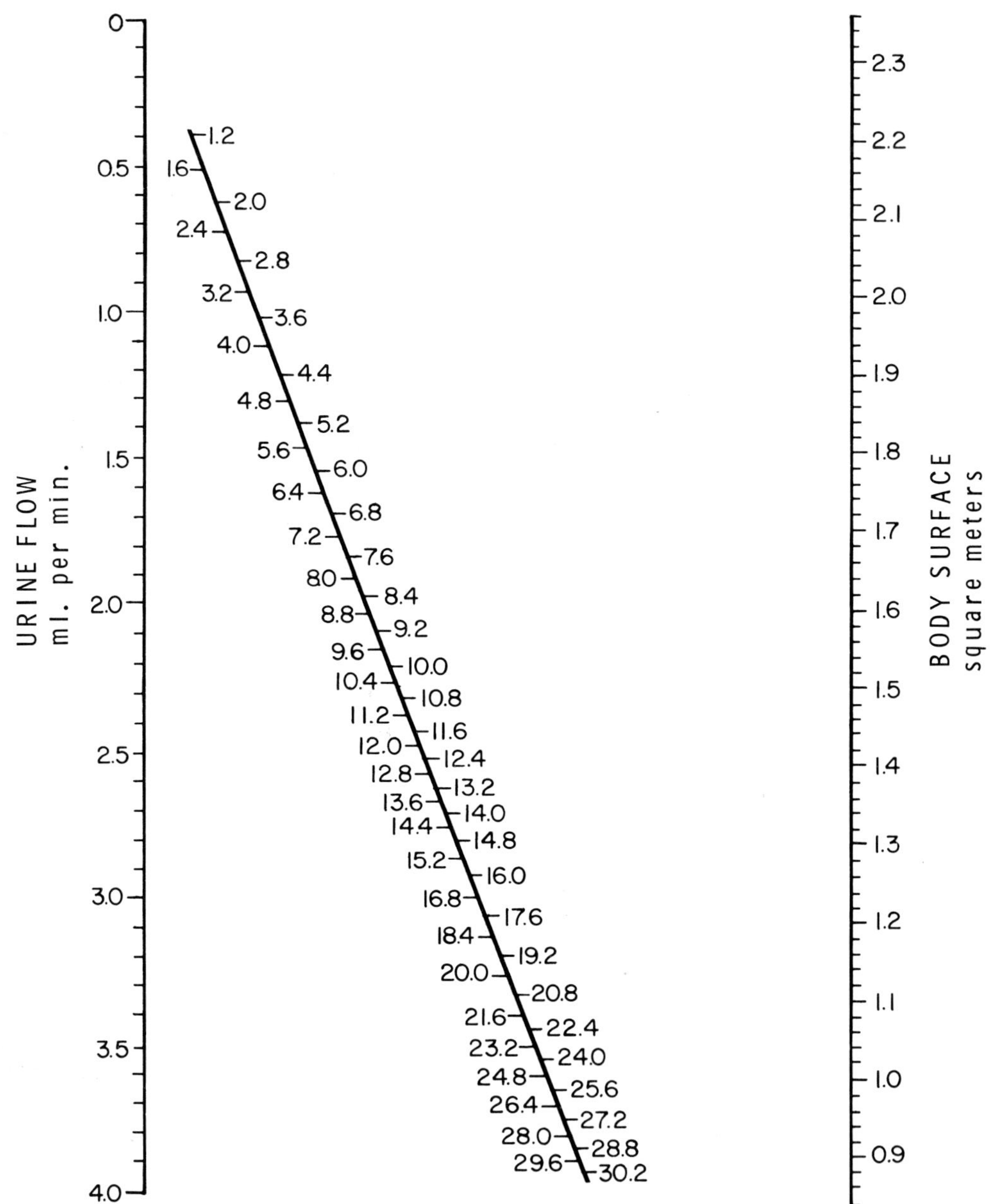

Fig. 1.

CREATININE CLEARANCE
ml. per min.
PLASMA CREATININE
mg. per 100 ml.
DILUTED URINE CREATININE
mg. per 100 ml.
0.8
1.0
1.5
2.0
2.5
3.0
3.5
4.0
4.5
5.0
160
140
120
100
80
70
60
50
40
35
30
25
20
15
12
6.0
5.5
5.0
4.5
4.0
3.5
3.0
2.5

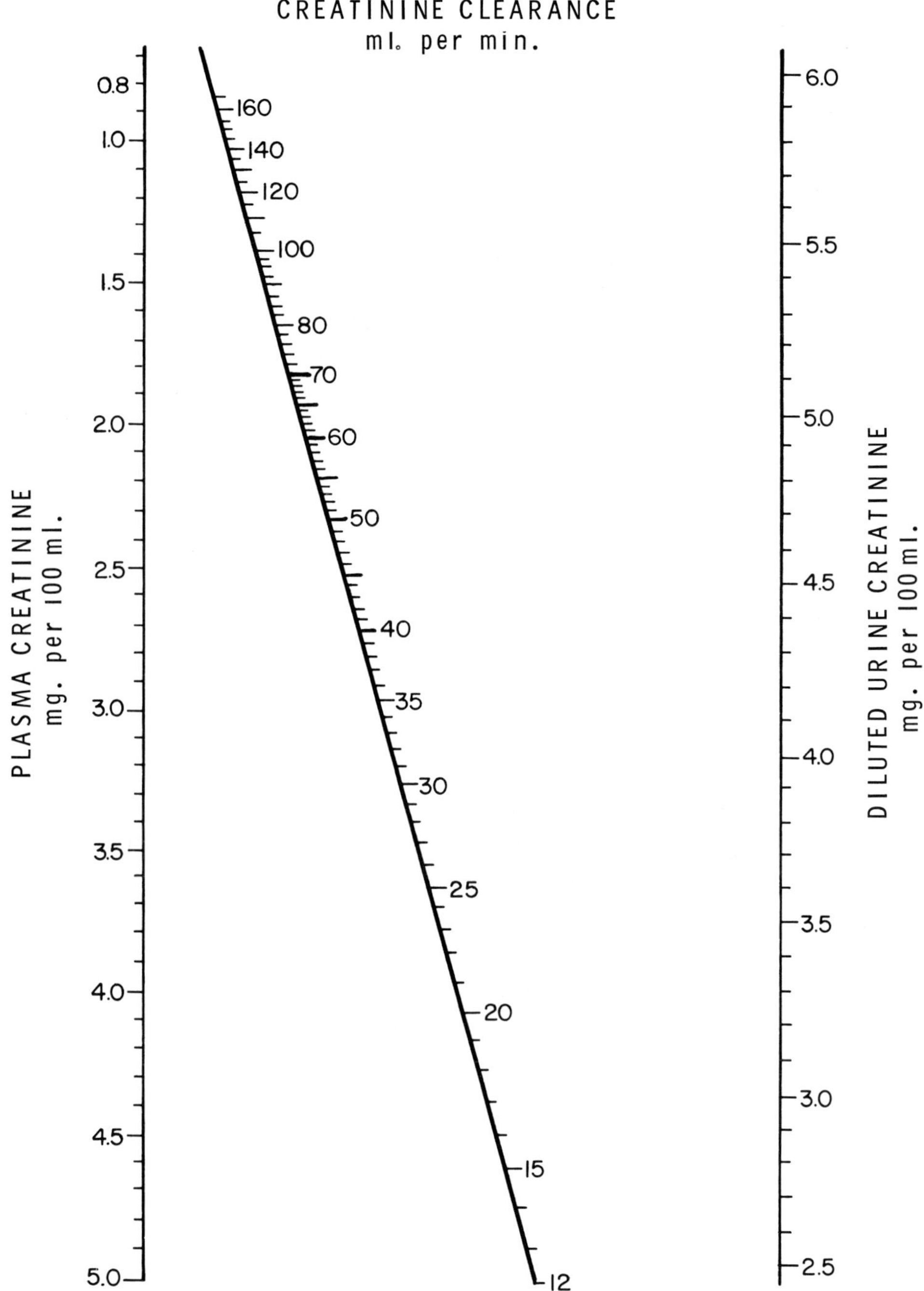

Fig. 2.

Chapter 12

Phenolsulphonphthalein Excretion and Concentration-Dilution Tests in the Evaluation of Renal Function

FREDERICK VOLINI, M.D., J. DE LA HUERGA, M.D., PH.D., and FRANK MADERA-ORSINI, PH.D.

INTRODUCTION

The excretion of phenolsulphonphthalein (PSP) and the concentration-dilution tests are commonly used clinical procedures which can provide an estimate of functional capacity of the kidney. While these tests do not indicate a particular species of renal disease, they do indicate when functional capacity is reduced, whether due to intrinsic renal abnormality or extra-renal factors. In cases where kidney disease is established, the severity of the condition can be reflected by these function tests and also the progress of the renal abnormality can be followed.

While PSP excretion is a rather specific function of the proximal renal tubules and concentration a proper function of the distal portion of the nephron these tests are not highly specific the way they are usually employed in clinical medicine. Owing to their less specific character, they are best viewed as screening procedures. They are also easier to perform analytically than the more specific tests such as inulin clearance and para-aminohippuric acid (PAH) clearance and this accounts for their more widespread use in clinical medicine.

I. Phenolsulphonphthalein Excretion

The administration of colored substances for the evaluation of kidney function has the advantage of easy identification and quantitation in urine within short periods of time after injection. Heidenhain, in 1874 (21), injected indigocarmine into rabbits and found this dye in the tubular cells. He concluded that the tubules were involved in the excretion of urine. Bouchard (7), in 1877, proposed the use of fuchsin but no further investigation of this dye was undertaken. Achard and Castaigne (2), in 1897, devised the first clinical trial using methylene blue. Fifteen minutes after injection, they could detect its presence in urine. Lepine (29), in the following year, proposed the use of rosaniline in the same manner. Voelker and Joseph (49) revived the use of indigocarmine in 1903. All these dyes had the disadvantage of being painful when injected and were partially metabolized and thus not available for excretion in the same form.

In 1909, Abel and Rowntree (1) studied various phthaleins with the intention of proposing one for subcutaneous use as a purgative. They found that phenolsulphonphthalein (PSP) was non-toxic, not irritating when injected and appeared in the urine shortly after administration.

The use of PSP as a test of renal function was pursued by Rowntree and Geraghty during 1910 (39) and 1912 (40) in two extensive and well-documented publications. From their observations, they concluded that the injection of 6 mg of PSP was followed by the excretion of dye in the urine in less than 10 minutes and that about 85% of the injected amount was excreted in the urine within 2 hours after administration. They also found some excretion in bile, but the dye was rapidly reabsorbed from the intestine. An interesting finding was that the frog *Rana Catesbiana* eliminated the dye by tubular secretion when the independent blood supply to the glomeruli was circumvented and glomerular filtration thus excluded. However, the mechanism of its renal excretion had to await the elucidation of the basic physiologic events underlying glomerular filtration, tubular secretion and renal blood flow. Even so, the results of the studies of Rowntree and Geraghty were immediately useful in evaluating various medical and surgical diseases of the kidney and their test has enjoyed wide usage since its introduction.

PSP is a phthalein derivative frequently used in the laboratory as a pH indicator. It was prepared by Remsen in 1844 by treating the anhydride of ortho-sulfonbenzoic acid with phenol.

The dye (Fig. 1, formula A), is an orange-red powder which when dissolved in water acquires a negative charge at the benzenesulfonic group and a positive charge at the carbon linking the two phenols with the benzenesulfonic group. At the same time, one of the phenols also ionizes, thus providing a hybrid ion containing two negative and one positive charges and giving a yellow solution (formula B). If alkali is added, the other phenol group ionizes, giving a more ionized form containing three negative and one positive ions, in which state it has an intense red color (formula C). Finally, if a strong acid is added, the ionized phenol group of form (B) gains back a hydrogen ion and the molecule becomes less ionized containing a positive and a negative charge and the solution takes on a weak pink color (D). These changes are reversible. The useful pH range extends from the yellow color at a pH of 6.8 to pH 8.4 when it develops the highest intensity red color with an absorption maximum at 558 (6) to 562 (22) millimicrons. In alkaline solutions, fading of the red color is noted, but this takes place only after long periods of standing.

BIOLOGICAL PROPERTIES OF PSP

The experiments of Rowntree and Geraght demonstrated the excretion of PSP by the renal tubules of *Rana Catesbiana*. However, due to the influence of the Cushny School (13) the tubules were denied any secretory function. Between 1923 and 1931, Marshall (32, 33) and his group noted that a large proportion of the PSP present in the plasma was in a form

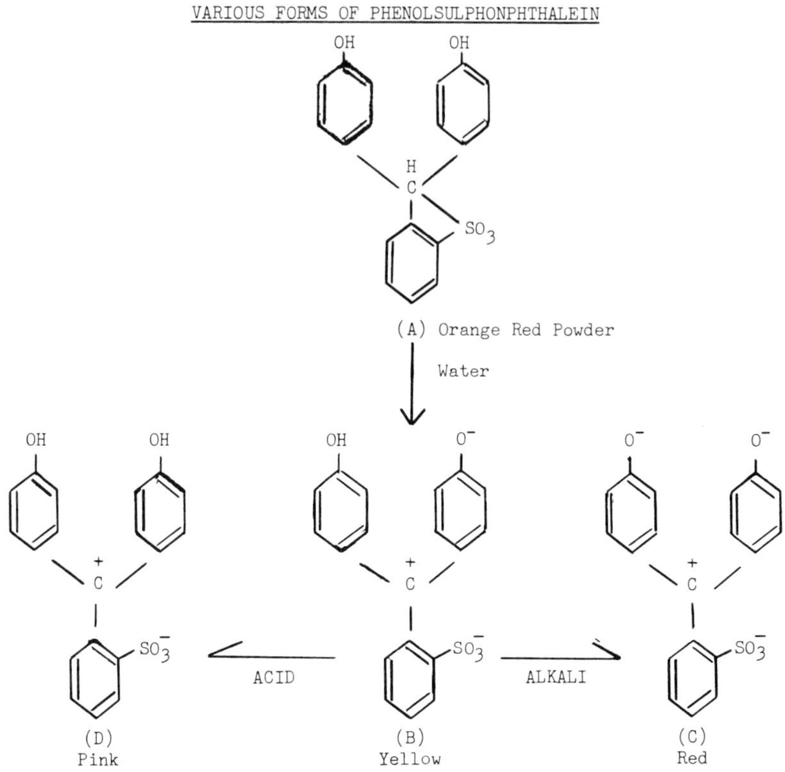

Fig. 1

bound to protein. Allowing for the small concentration of the filterable, free dye in the plasma, an enormous volume of filtrate would have to be formed to explain the excretion of PSP. Moreover, when the dye was injected in increasingly larger amounts, the rate of excretion also increased progressively up to a point beyond which the excretion diminished in relation to the concentration of dye in the plasma. This finding militated against glomerular filtration as the only means by which PSP could be excreted in the urine. Finally, it was found (33) that the clearance of PSP was higher than the clearance for creatinine in dogs in which animal the latter is a measure of glomerular filtration. While the secretory property of the tubules had up to this time been vehemently denied, these

basic studies of Marshall and Vickers using PSP, provided incontrovertible proof of secretion by the mammalian renal tubules.

A more direct approach was used by Chambers and his co-workers (10) who discovered an ingenious method of studying tubular secretion. They noted that when placing chick mesonephros in a culture medium, the ends of the tubules closed up and became little cysts. When adding PSP to the medium, they found that the cysts contained more than 20 times the concentration of PSP than was present in the surrounding medium.

Similar studies were later performed by Forster and his group (17, 18, 24) using teased tubules from the flounder kidney. They could observe also the excretion of PSP in the closed tubules and carried out investigations to elucidate its excretion. In the presence of dinitrophenol, the tubules did not excrete PSP and so it was concluded that the excretion of dye was an energy-dependent reaction requiring the activity of oxidative enzymes. Other inhibitors of respiration, like the heavy metals, cyanide and azide also inhibited the excretion of PSP. Two different steps were clearly identified. The first was the uptake of dye by the tubular cells from the surrounding media for which energy is needed together with potassium ions, and second, the actual excretion of the dye from the cells into the lumen, for which calcium ion was required (37).

These studies performed in cold-blooded animals were later applied to mammals by Forster and Copenhaver (18) using slices from the cortex of rabbit kidneys. They were able to observe the uptake of PSP from the surrounding medium by the tubular cells, but there was no transfer of dye into the lumen of tubules. The latter step was thought to be unnecessary in mammals on account of the profuse flow of glomerular filtrate which of itself would supposedly cause a leaching out of dye from tubular cells.

The excretion of PSP from animals and humans was further elucidated by comparing its excretion to that of inulin and the iodine-containing organic acids as well as para-aminohippuric acid (PAH). Studies with inulin which is excreted entirely by glomerular filtration, established that a normal adult human has a glomerular filtration rate of approximately 120 ml per minute. Data from the study of PAHA clearance at low plasma levels indicated that practically all of the plasma is cleared of PAHA during a single passage through the kidneys by combined glomerular filtration and tubular secretion. This latter finding became the basis for determination of effective renal plasma flow and whole blood flow through the kidneys.

With the usual clinical test dose of PSP (6 mg), a plasma concentration of approximately 0.2 mg per 100 ml is obtained. At this low concentration, and with a normal albumin content of 4 gm per 100 ml, only 20% of the dye is in the free form and capable of being filtered by the glomerulus. Given a glomerular filtration rate of 120 ml per minute, there will be 0.048 mg appearing in the glomerular filtrate each minute (120 x 0.04/100). With a plasma flow rate of 650 ml per minute, 1.3 mg of PSP will enter the kidneys each minute (650 x 0.2/100). At the plasma level of 0.2 mg per 100 ml the extraction of PSP is only 66% complete, so the amount of PSP excreted will be 0.86 mg per minute (66 x 1.3/100). Of this amount 0.048 mg is due to glomerular filtration as shown above and the remainder, 0.812, is due to tubular excretion. Thus, the amount of PSP eliminated by glomerular filtration is only about 6% (100 x 0.048/0.868) of the total excreted. This clearly indicates that other conditions being normal, destruction of the glomeruli will influence the PSP excretion negligibly.

When much larger doses of PSP are administered, the amount of PSP excreted per minute at the glomerular level will be proportionately higher; but when a very high plasma level is reached, the tubules become saturated and no greater amount of PSP is excreted per unit of time by the tubules. This situation is reached when the tubules excrete about 40 mg of PSP per minute and has been referred to as the Tm for PSP (42).

Returning to the example under study, it is evident that the tubular maximum capacity for excretion of PSP is about 50 times greater (40/0.812) than that required for excretion of the PSP injected in the usual clinical dose. If the plasma flow per unit of time remains normal, there would have to be an extensive destruction of tubules to bring about a diminished excretion of dye when using the regular 6 mg test dose. The only possible deduction is that when PSP excretion is abnormally low, it is due mainly to a deficiency of effective blood flow to the kidneys, whether due to intrinsic renal disease or extra-renal factors affecting renal blood flow. Much of the physiological studies regarding PSP excretion were carried out by Homer Smith and colleagues (43, 44, 12).

Reagents and Equipment
1. NaOH, 10% aqueous solution
2. Glacial acetic acid
3. Na_2CO_3, 10% aqueous solution
4. Spectrophotometer with 19 mm (3/4" cuvette)
5. Centrifuge
6. Filter paper, Whatman #2 paper or any other retentive filter paper.

Procedure
1. It is desirable to withhold medication for at least 24 hours, since various drugs such as aspirin, butazolidine, penicillin, etc., compete with the renal tubular transport of PSP (15). If there is reason to suspect urinary retention or inability to void completely, catheterization of the urinary bladder should be considered.

2. One-half hour before the test is begun, approximately 500 ml of water is given by mouth.

3. Exactly 1 ml of sterile PSP dye is withdrawn from a vial with an insulin syringe and rapidly injected intravenously, noting the time precisely.

4. Urine is collected 15 minutes after the injection, and also at 30 minutes, 1 and 2 hours into separate labeled containers.

5. Each urine specimen is then transferred to separate 500 ml volumetric flasks, followed by addition of 5 ml of 10% sodium hydroxide and finally water to the mark. The contents of each flask are well mixed, then filtered using retentive filter paper.

6. A 7 ml aliquot from each flask is then added to each of a pair of 19 mm cuvettes. To one of the pairs is added one drop of glacial acetic acid. The red color should disappear; if not, add another drop.

7. The spectrophotometer is set to 560 millimicrons and with the cuvette containing acidified urine, the galvanometer is set to read 100% T. If the sample reads less than 15% T, 7 ml of water is added to both cuvettes. The same procedure is carried out for all samples.

8. The per cent dye excretion is read from a graph (see standardization below).

Standardization
It has been found (22) that variations between different manufacturers and dirrerent lots of dye may be as great as 17%. In our own evaluation, nine different lots from five manufacturers showed a variation from 96 to 104% of the average obtained for all lots examined.

For preparation of a standard solution of PSP, about 400 ml of water is transferred to a 500 ml volumetric flask and 500 microliters of PSP dye is added from an ampule having the same lot number as that used for injection. Five ml of 10% sodium hydroxide is then added, followed by water to the mark. To a series of seven pairs of 19 mm (3/4") cuvettes, the following amounts of dye are transferred: 7, 6, 5, 4, 3, 2, 1 ml and water is added to a total volume of 10 ml. To one pair of the seven cuvettes is added one drop of glacial acetic acid. Using the cuvettes with acidified dye the glavanometer is set to 100% T at 560 millimicrons and the per cent transmittance of the other cuvettes is obtained. With the spectrophotometer (Coleman Junior) used in our laboratory, the solution containing the equivalent of 50% dye excretion gave a reading of 26% transmission. Using semilogarithmic graph paper, these readings are plotted against equivalent dye excretion. Beer's Law is followed in this range. *The PSP standards given here are equivalent to the range 70 to 10% dye excretion when the urine sample has been diluted to 1 liter.* Since most of the samples will be read at the 500 ml dilution, the above standards then will be equivalent to 35 to 5% dye excretion.

Interferences

The two main interfering substances are hemoglobin and bilirubin. If the urine sample contains blood, centrifugation is performed after measuring the total volume. Following centrifugation, 1/5 of the total volume is transferred to a 100 ml volumetric flask, followed by 2 ml of 10% sodium hydroxide and water to the mark. Filtration is then carried out and calculations used as noted above. If centrifugation does not clear the urine of blood, as in cases with hemoglobinuria, 4 ml of 10% anhydrous Na_2CO_3 is added instead of NaOH to avoid the formation of alkaline hemochromogen. Also, for the blank setting, a smaller amount of glacial acetic acid (0.06 to 0.10 ml) is used to avoid the

production of acid hematin. Bilirubin at levels of 10 mg per 100 ml will produce a positive error not greater than 5% because its absorption at 560 millimicrons is very low and the difference between the acid and alkaline solution is practically nil. Bromosulphthalein dye used in liver function studies may appear in urine and cause interference with readings of PSP. For this reason, it is best not to perform both of these tests on the same day. Since the most important sample is the 15-minute collection of urine, and it is difficult to be exact unless catheterization is used, Pierce (36) has recommended that a deduction of 1.25% dye excretion be made for each minute in excess of the 15-minute standard collection.

Normal Values

Normal values for the intravenous method as given by Chapman and Halstead (11) are as follows:

	Percent Dye Excretion	
Specimen	*Range*	*Average*
15 minutes	28 – 51	35
30 minutes	13 – 24	17
60 minutes	9 – 17	12
120 minutes	3 – 10	6
Total 2 hours	63 – 84	70

Interpretation

The PSP test as originally proposed by Rowntree and Geraghty (40) involved the measurement of only the 2-hour excretion of dye. Performed in this manner the test was found to be insensitive to mild degrees of renal functional impairment. However, the original authors of the procedure noted that the curve of elimination of PSP dye was different in normal subjects and in those with nephritis. In disease states, a maximum excretion was reached more slowly. This formed the basis for the Fractional PSP Test developed by Shaw (41) and by Chapman and Halstead (11). The latter employed the fractional test in the study of a large number of patients with chronic renal disease and found the test more sensitive than urea clearance as an index of renal dysfunction. In routine practice, the 15-minute sample alone is sufficient for it is this specimen which provides maximum sensitivity in detection of impaired renal function. Excretion of less than 25% of the administered dye during the first 15 minutes provides significant evidence of impaired renal function. If the urinary bladder cannot be emptied in 15 minutes, the 30-minute sample can be used and normally is found to contain more than 40% of the administered dye.

The PSP test has also been done using intramuscular injection followed by urine collection at 1 and 2 hours. By this method, 40 to 60% of the dye is found in the first hourly specimen and an additional 20 to 25% in the second hourly specimen. Although the intramuscular route was recommended in the original work of Rowntree and Geraghty in 1912, it is considered generally less satisfactory and would be impractical to use for the 15-minute excretion. Higher than normal PSP excretion has been noted in some cases of liver disease presumably because the liver cannot excrete the usual small fraction of dye normally found in bile. However, the 15-minute excretion is not affected by the presence of liver disease. Usually, the PSP excretion is decreased before there is a significant decrease in glomerular filtration rate. The concentration tests, however, are generally regarded as more sensitive indicators of early renal impair-

ment, however, in some patients these are contraindicated. When azotemia supervenes, PSP excretion is decreased quite uniformly. In the presence of obvious azotemia, however, the test is not recommended because of the potentially harmful effects of hydration used in this test. While normally the quantity of dye eliminated is relatively independent of urine volume, in states of moderate renal impairment, the output of PSP varies more or less directly with the urine volume. As mentioned previously, PSP elimination is more a test of renal plasma flow than a test of tubular integrity. This is true because in the usual clinical procedure, the tubules are not challenged with sufficient dye to test a reduced tubular capacity for excretion. The finding that PSP excretion is reduced early in such a wide variety of renal diseases (11) attests to the fact that decreased renal plasma flow is a frequent concomitant of many renal diseases.

Lapides and Bobbitt (27) compared the results of the 15-minute PSP excretion to the endogenous creatinine and urea clearance in 350 patients with such diseases as acute and chronic pyelonephritis, tuberculous pyelonephritis, nephrosclerosis, acute and chronic glomerulonephritis and polycystic disease. They found that the values for urea or creatinine clearance were often normal in the presence of established renal disease while the PSP excretion was usually abnormal. In some patients, the clearance values and PSP excretion were equally reduced but in no patient was the PSP excretion significantly closer to normal than the urea or creatinine clearance. Patients with 60% of normal values for PSP excretion had associated urea or creatinine clearance which were 62 to 100% of normal. Also, patients with a 15-minute PSP dye excretion of zero had urea or creatinine clearances which ranged from 5 to 82% of normal. A combination of various renal function tests including the PSP have been used by some authors. Raisz *et al* (38) combined a water load with endogenous creatinine clearance and after collection of blood and urine for creatinine, administered PSP dye. The procedure was also used to measure the function of each kidney separately during cystoscopy. Healy, Edwards and Whyte (20) performed creatinine clearance, PSP excretion and concentration tests with vasopressin sequentially and found considerable value in the latter two tests in predicting the glomerular filtration rate.

From the foregoing discussion, it is evident that the usual clinical tests including PSP do not predict specific functional capacities of the kidney. However, by using tests such as inulin clearance, PAH clearance and transfer maxima, more specific patterns of renal dysfunction have been found in various diseases. Bradley and co-workers (8), were able to characterize various renal diseases in terms of glomerular filtration, effective renal plasma flow, filtration fraction, extraction percentage of PAHA and tubular maximum excretion of PAHA and Diodrast. In acute glomerulonephritis, the glomerular filtration rate was reduced to a greater degree than plasma flow apparently in relation to the swelling of capillary endothelium. In nephrosclerosis, the renal plasma flow was disproportionately reduced while in pyelonephritis the most characteristic finding was reduction of tubular maxima for Diodrast and PAH. Despite the demonstration of more characteristic findings with these specific tests, such studies are seldom performed. In the initial evaluation of patients for renal dysfunction, the less specific procedures such as the concentration test, 15-minute PSP excretion and urea or creatinine clearance still prevail in routine clinical practice.

II. Concentration and Dilution Tests

The importance of the concentration of solutes in urine and their estimation by specific gravity was appreciated in the writings of Richard Bright (9) as early as 1827. He found that the specific gravity of urine was diminished in cases of chronic renal disease. The studies of Albarran (5) in 1905 laid the foundation for the use of specific gravity in distinguishing normal and abnormal kidney function. In his studies, a simple type of dilution test was employed. Vaquez and Cottet (48) in 1912 contributed to the study of specific gravity of urine as affected by water loading and alterations induced by diet, posture and diurnal variation. The estimation of urinary solutes by specific gravity did not become widely used, however, until popularized by Volhard (50) in the early part of this century. He developed a technique for evaluating renal function with a concentration and dilution test and appreciated the alterations occurring in renal disease. A modification of this test was introduced in this country by Mosenthal (35) and became widely used. The work of Addis (3, 4) and later

Fishberg (16) firmly established the concentration test as a valuable procedure in clinical studies of renal function.

The concentration and dilution tests depend on the ability of the kidney to excrete a urine of high or low solute content according to the stress imposed by restriction or excess of water intake. A brief review of the physiological mechanisms underlying the concentration and dilution tests is presented here so that these tests may be used and interpreted to best advantage.

The glomeruli which are heavily perfused with blood produce an average of 180 liters of filtrate per day in the normal adult. This filtrate has about the same composition of crystalloids as the plasma and consequently the same osmolality (approximately 290 milliosmoles). This filtrate is first modified in the proximal tubules in such a fashion that upon its entrance into the Henle tubules, it has the same osmolality as when originally formed although some of the solutes have been reabsorbed. Glucose is the most typical example of a substance which is completely reabsorbed in the proximal tubules. About 85% of the water and the same proportion of sodium have also been reabsorbed, yet the osmolality remains the same as that found initially in the glomerular filtrate. During its passage through the Henle's tubules, there is a concentrating process in the descending limb and a diluting process during its passage through the ascending limb, so that at the beginning of the distal tubules, the modified filtrate is actually less concentrated than the original glomerular filtrate. The volume of fluid passing to this point each day is about 30 liters. Finally, at the end of the collecting tubules, the urine will have a volume of about 1.5 liters with a total

excretion of 1000 milliosmoles of solute per day, the net difference of 28.5 liters of water and about 6000 milliosmoles of solute having been reabsorbed in the distal segments. The reabsorption of water and electrolytes, and some organic components of the filtrate is accomplished in the proximal tubules under the influence of exclusively renal factors. In contrast, the reabsorptive activities of the distal segment are under hormonal influence. In the final analysis, the latter determines the osmolality and volume of the urine voided, in other words, the production of a concentrated or diluted urine.

During water deprivation and following water loss through the urine and the insensible loss from skin and the respiratory tract, the water content of the body diminishes (hydropenia). This in turn stimulates the hypophysis to release anti-diuretic hormone (ADH) into the circulation. This hormone acts upon the distal segments of the nephron to increase the permeability for water, thus, increasing the water reabsorbed and decreasing water excretion, the final product being a concentrated urine. On the other hand, during water loading, the mechanism is inverted and the kidneys excrete a copious but diluted urine.

Of the 9000 milliosmoles of solute that reach the distal segment, most is in the form of sodium salts. Normally, about 95% of these salts must be reabsorbed (parenthetically the over-all reabsorption of sodium is greater than 99% but at the proximal tubules about 85% had already been reabsorbed). Obviously, if more sodium is reabsorbed while the other solute and water excretion remains constant, a less concentrated urine will be excreted. The reabsorption of sodium in the distal segment is under the influence of aldosterone.

A third important factor in urine concentration is the amount of urea excreted. Urea contributes significantly to the urine specific gravity and osmolality and is in fact second only to the electrolytes in this respect. A diet rich in protein will produce a urine of higher specific gravity and this factor is of importance in evaluating the concentration test.

The fourth important factor is the functional integrity of the renal tubules. In disease states, the renal tubules may fail to reabsorb water normally, resulting in a decreased urine osmolality so that it may approach the same osmolality as that of plasma. An exception to this would be the condition of diabetes insipidus where the tubules are intact and yet due to the deficiency of ADH a voluminous urine of low specific gravity is excreted.

When voided urine has the same osmolality as that of plasma (isosthenuria), no osmotic work has been performed. The excreted urine contains the same proportion of water as the plasma indicating that the distal segments are neither excreting nor reabsorbing any relative excess of water (table 1, example 1). If the final urine has a higher osmolality than the plasma (hypersthenuria) more water than solids have been reabsorbed and this excess of water reabsorption is referred to as $T^c_{H_2O}$ (Table 1, example 2). On the other hand, if the urine has a lower osmolality than the plasma (hyposthenuria), then water has been excreted and this portion of the solute-free water is measured as the clearance of free water, C_{H_2O} (Table 1, example 3). These parameters are easily determined by measuring the volume of urine excreted per minute, its osmolality and the osmolality of plasma. The osmotic clearance can then be calculated as in any other clearance study: Cosm = Urine osm x ml urine per minute/plasma osm.

TABLE 1

CONCENTRATION AND DILUTION OF URINE IN A NORMAL INDIVIDUAL
HAVING A PLASMA OSMOLALITY OF 290 MOSM/ L AND EXCRETING 1040 MOSM/24 HRS

Example	Urine Volume ml/min.	Urine Osmolality mosm/L	Cosm ml/min.	Water Reabsorbed or Excreted ml/min.
1	2.5	290	$\frac{290 \times 2.5}{290} = 2.5$ $2.5 - 2.5 = 0$	$\begin{vmatrix}2.5\\ \downarrow \\ 2.5\end{vmatrix}$
2	1.0	725	$\frac{725 \times 1}{290} = 2.5$ $2.5 - 1.0 = 1.5\ T^c_{H_2O}$	$\begin{vmatrix}2.5\\ \downarrow \\ 1.0\end{vmatrix} \rightarrow 1.5\ T^c_{H_2O}$
3	3.6	200	$\frac{200 \times 3.6}{290} = 2.5$ $3.6 - 2.5 = 1.1\ CH_2O$	$\begin{vmatrix}2.5\\ \downarrow \\ 3.6\end{vmatrix} \leftarrow 1.1\ CH_2O$

METHODS FOR DETERMINING THE CONCENTRATION OF URINE

Water is the most abundant single component of the urine as it is for all fluids and most tissues. Under the severest conditions of dehydration, the most concentrated urine that can be excreted is at least 85% water and the remainder solids. The presence of the latter bring about physical changes in the urine which are proportional to the amount of solids present. Since the solids as such weigh more than the water and also because of the lowering of the volume which takes place when solids are dissolved, the density of the urine is always higher than that of water, and is increased in proportion to the amount of dissolved solids per unit volume of urine. This can be measured by various simple densitometers or specifically urinometers which have been used in the clinical laboratory for many years. The main disadvantages are the inaccuracy occurring especially with dilute urines, and also the fact that rather large volumes of urine are required. A more accurate method for measuring density is that employing the pycnometer but its use is very tedious. The Westfal balance is also an accurate instrument but is not used in clinical laboratories.

The results obtained with all these instruments are dependent upon the temperature at which test measurements are taken. To complicate matters further, various temperatures have been taken as reference standard. In this respect, it must be mentioned that the true density of the urine refers to the weight of a known volume in comparison to that of water at 4°C (at which temperature it is heavier). The specific gravity as commonly used in the clinical laboratory refers to the density of the urine in relation to that of water when both have been measured at the same temperature or adequate corrections made when performed at different temperatures. As already mentioned, the specific gravity of the urine is an index of the solids content, and various factors have been proposed to calculate the total solids of the urine based on specific gravity. More recently, the total solids of the urine have been measured by refractometric methods which are simple, accurate, precise and require only one drop of urine. A convenient and reliable instrument is the Goldberg type refractometer which can be obtained from most laboratory supply companies. With refractometers, there is a better correlation between the total solids and specific gravity. The latter can be obtained by direct reading from special scales relating the two and no temperature correction is necessary.

However simple or accurate any of the methods described may be, in reality they do not measure very exactly the concentrating or diluting function of the kidney. Any particle regardless of size, whether it be organic or inorganic, polymolecular or monomolecular, positive or negative in charge, will produce the same osmotic pressure when dissolved in the same weight of water. The same osmotic work will be performed by the distal tubules in diluting or concentrating a luminal fluid if it has the same number of particles. This physiological function can only be measured by determining the osmolality of urine. The best method currently available employs the cryoscopic technique which depends on lowering of the freezing point of an aqueous solution such as urine which in turn is proportional to the osmolality. That this latter approach is different from the densitometric methods is emphasized in the following example. If the same weight of urea or sodium chloride is dissolved separately in one kilogram of water, the specific gravity will be almost the same, while the osmolality will be twice as much for the sodium chloride solution as for the urea solution. It is apparent that osmolality is a more adequate way of measuring the concentrating and diluting power of the distal tubules.

Until recently, the instruments available for measuring osmolality were very cumbersome. Today, various manufacturers have marketed simple and accurate instruments. However, they are not yet in wide use in clinical laboratories. For the measurement of urinary solids in the concentration and dilution tests, the densitometric methods seem to be adequate, judging from the work of Miles *et al* (34), Jacobson *et al* (26), and Holmes (23) amongst others. They have shown sufficient correlation between osmolality and specific gravity so that serious errors do not occur when using specific gravity alone. The various parameters of urine concentration such as specific gravity, refractive index, osmolality and total solids are well illustrated in the following abridged table from the article by A. V. Wolf (51).

Most of the concentration tests which have been used successfully involve a period of dehydration varying from 12 to 36 hours. While tests using short periods of dehydration are employed by some, a minimum of 24 hours is recommended in view of the demonstration by Miles *et al.* (34) that a period of 22 hours is required for most individuals to reach 90% of their maximum urine concentration. The earliest procedures called for rigorous control of solid intake as in the special diet of Lashmet and Newburg (28). Experience with these tests has shown that in subjects previously on a normal diet and fasting during the dehydration period, it is unnecessary to more rigidly control the intake of solids prior to the test proce-

TABLE 2—VALUES FOR URINARY CONCENTRATION TESTS IN MAN

	Specific Gravity $(D_{20^o}^{20^o})$	Refraction $(\Delta n \times 10^4)$	Osmolality $(m\ Osm/kg)$	Total Solids $(g/100\ g\ urine)$
Normal	1.022–1.035 Eugravuria	85–134 Eurefracturia	800–1300 Eusthenuria	5.4–8.5 Eusteruria
Below Normal	(Moderate) 1.011–1.017 Hypogravuria	44–66 Hyporefracturia	400–600 Hyposthenuria	2.8–4.2 Hyposteruria
	(Severe) $<$1.011 Isogravuria	$<$44 Isorefracturia	$<$400 Isosthenuria	$<$2.8 Isosteruria
Above Normal	1.035–1.040 Hypergravuria	134–159 Hyperrefracturia	1300–1450 Hypersthenuria	8.5–10.0 Hypersteruria

dure. Of some importance, however, is the contribution of urea in reaching adequate urinary solid levels and for this reason, sufficient protein intake must be assured.

Concentration Test Procedure

The procedure recommended here is that given by Fishber (16)

1. The patient is allowed to have the usual breakfast but thereafter no more fluids are allowed until the test is completed twenty-four hours later. The patient is instructed to have a dry lunch and an evening meal containing protein, potatoes and vegetables but no fluid.

2. All urine passed during the day is discarded and before retiring the patient is instructed to void and discard the urine.

3. On awakening the following morning, the patient is instructed to void and save the urine and if possible to void one and two hours later into separate containers.

4. The specific gravity of each specimen is measured using an accurately calibrated hydrometer or refractometer.

Normally, the specific gravity of at least one of the three specimens will exceed 1.022, however, in many patients much higher values are noted. In conditions of impaired renal function, lower specific gravities are found. Some workers (30) have reported a diminished ability to concentrate with advancing age. In estimating the specific gravity in the concentration test, a correction must be made for heavy glucosuria and proteinuria, otherwise a false idea of excretion of urinary solids is obtained. For each 1 gm protein per 100 ml, one must subtract 0.003 units and for each 1 gm glucose per 100 ml, subtract 0.004 from the observed specific gravity.

Because of the fact that prolonged fluid deprivation is unpleasant for many patients and occasionally dangerous if a severe negative fluid balance develops, various modifications of the basic test have developed. One of these is the Pitressin Test suggested by Sodeman and Engelhardt in 1941 (45).

Procedure

1. The subject without prior special diet is instructed to void and save the urine specimen.

2. Thereafter, 10 units of posterior pituitary extract is given subcutaneously (1 ml of obstetrical or 0.5 ml of surgical pituitrin).

3. Food and fluids are withheld until the test is completed.

4. Urine specimens are obtained at the end of the first and second hour.

5. The specific gravity of the three urine specimens is determined with the usual corrections for temperature, proteinuria and glucosuria.

The authors regard a specific gravity of 1.023 or higher in either of the two post-injection specimens as indicating normal concentrating ability.

The procedure of Sodeman and Engelhardt was modified by lengthening the period of urine collection for 9 hours and giving pituitrin as the tannate in oil by intramuscular injection. Three urine specimens were obtained at 3, 6 and 9 hours post-injection (20). Normal values were similar to those obtained with the shorter urine collection period. The osmolality exceeded 900 milliosmoles per kg in all cases. Patients with renal disease generally did not exceed a specific gravity of 1.020 or 650 milliosmoles per kg. Administration of pituitrin may have some undesirable side effects (19) including elevation of blood pressure and aggravation of symptoms in angina pectoris. Its use is contraindicated in pregnancy, epilepsy, infancy and severe arteriosclerotic heart disease.

Dilution Test Procedure

1. The test should be performed independently of the concentration test. After an overnight fast, the patient is instructed to void and discard all urine.

2. The patient is given 1200 ml of water within one-half hour.

3. For the next four hours, urine is collected at hourly intervals into separate containers. The specific gravity is determined using an accurately calibrated hydrometer or refractometer.

With normal renal function, most of the 1200 ml of ingested fluid will be eliminated within the four-hour test period. The specific gravity of one of the specimens normally will fall to 1.003 or below. In states of impaired renal function, smaller amounts of urine are eliminated and the specific gravity is higher than 1.003 and in some patients values of 1.010 may be seen. The clinical value of the dilution test is questionable because impaired diluting ability is most often seen in advanced renal failure and the latter is usually evident form less drastic procedures. In such patients, a large water load may precipitate water intoxication or marked sodium diuresis with danger of circulatory collapse. While the regulation of excess water excretion is primarily dependent upon distal tubule function and secretion of ADH, other factors may alter the amount and specific gravity of urine. In states of diminished glomerular filtration, as for example, in acute glomerulonephritis, tubular function may not be severely affected and yet the decreased amount of filtrate results in smaller urine volume and high specific gravity.

REFERENCES

1. Abel, J. J., and Rowntree, L. G.: On the pharmacological action of some phthaleins and their derivatives with special reference to their behavior as purgatives. J. Pharmacol. & Exp. Therapeutics, *1:*231-264, 1909-1910.
2. Achard and Castaigne: Bull, et mem. soc. med. d. hop. de Par., p. 637, April 1897. Gaz, hebd. de med., Para., no. 37, p. 433, 1897.
3. Addis, T., and Foster, M. G.: The specific gravity of the urine. Arch. Int. Med., *30:*555-558, 1922.
4. Addis, T., and Shevky, M. C.: A test of the capacity of the kidney to produce a urine of high specific gravity. Arch. Int. Med., *30:*559-562, 1922.
5. Albarran: Exploration des fonctions renales, Paris, 1905.
6. Bates, R. G.: Determination of pH, Theory and Practice. New York, London, Sydney, John Wiley & Sons, Inc., 1954.
7. Bouchard: Quoted by Rowntree, L. G., and Geraghty, J. T.: Arch. Int. Med., *9:*284-338, 1912.
8. Bradley, S. E., Bradley, G. P., Tyson, C. J., Curry, J. J., and Blake, W. D.: Renal function in renal diseases. Amer. J. Med., *9:*766-798, 1950.
9. Bright, R.: Reports of Medical Cases. Longmans, Rees, Orme, Brown and Green, London, 1827.
10. Chamber, R., and Kempton, R. T.: Indications of function of the chick mesonephros in tissue culture with phenol red. J. Cell. & Comp. Physiol., *3:*131-160, 1933.
11. Chapman, E. M., and Halstead, J. A.: The fractional phenolsulphonephthalein test in Bright's disease. Amer. J. Med. Sc., *186:*223-232, 1933.
12. Chasis, H., Redish, J., Goldring, W., Ranges, H., and Smith, H. W.: The use of sodium p-aminohippurate for the functional evaluation of the human kidney. J. Clin. Invest., *24:*583-588, 1945.
13. Cushny, A. R.: The Secretion of the Urine. Longsman, Green, 1917.
14. de Wardener, H. E.: The Kidney. London, J & A Churchill Ltd., p. 38, 1958.
15. Edwards, K. D. G.: Renal tubular activities. Austral. Ann. Med., *11:*59-70, 1962.
16. Fishberg, A. M.: Hypertension and Nephritis, Fifth Ed. Philadelphia, Lea and Febiger, 1954.
17. Forster, R. P., and Taggart, J. V.: Use of isolated renal tubules for the examination of metabolic processes associated with active cellular transport. J. Cell. & Comp. Physiol., *36:*251-270, 1950.
18. Forster, R. P., and Copenhaver, J. H., Jr.: Intracellular accumulation as an active process in a mammalian renal transport system *in vitro.* Am J. Physiol., *186:*167-171, 1956.
19. Goodman and Gilman: Pharmacological Basis of Therapeutics, 2nd Ed. New York, MacMillan Co., 1955.

20. Healy, J. K., Edwards, K. D. G., and Whyte, H. M.: Simple tests of renal function using creatinine, phenolsulphonphthalein, and pitressin. J. Clin. Path., *17:*557-563, 1964.

21. Heidenhain, R.: Versuche uber den vorgang der harnabsonderung. Arch. gest Physiol., *9:*1-27, 1874.

22. Henry, R. J.: Clinical Chemistry: Principles and Techniques. Hoeber Medical Division, Harper & Row, 1964.

23. Holmes, J. H.: Measurement of Osmolality in Serum, Urine and other Biological Fluids by the Freezing Point Determination. Booklet published by Advanced Instruments. Newton Highlands, Mass.

24. Hong, Suk Ki, and Forster, R. P.: Run-out of Chlorphenol red following luminal accumulation by isolated renal tubules of the flounder *in vitro.* J. Cell. & Comp. Physiol., *51:*241-247, 1958.

25. Jacobson, M. H., Levy, S. E., Kaufman, R. M., Gallinek, W. E., and Donnelly, O. W.: Urine osmolality. Arch. Int. Med., *110:*83-89, 1962.

26. Jacobson, M. H., Levy, S. E., Kaufman, R. M., Gallinek, W. E., and Donnelly, O. W.: Urine osmolality. Arch. Int. Med., *110:*121-127, 1962.

27. Lapides, J., and Bobbitt, J. M.: Preoperative estimation of renal function J.A.M.A., *166:*866-869, 1958.

28. Lashmet, F. H., and Newburgh, L. A.: An improved concentration test of renal function J.A.M.A., *99:*1396-1398, 1956.

29. Lepine: Lyon Medical, 1898.

30. Lewis, W. H., Jr., and Alving, A. S.: Changes with age in the renal function in adult men. Am. J. Physiol., *123:*500, 1938.

31. Lewis, W. H., Jr., and Alving, A. S.: Changes with age in the renal function in adult men. Am. J. Physiol., *123:*500-507, 1938.

32. Marshall, E. K., Jr., and Vickers, J. L.: The mechanism of the elimination of phenolsulphonphthalein by the kidney; a proof of secretion by the convoluted tubules. Bull. John Hopkins Hosp., *34:*1-6, 1923.

33. Marshall, E. K., Jr.: The secretion of phenol red by the mammalian kidney. Am. J. Physiol., *99:*77-86, 1931.

34. Miles, B. E., Paton, A., and de Wardener, H. E.: Maximum urine concentration. Brit. Med., J., *2:*901, 1954.

35. Mosenthal, H. O.: Renal function as measured by the elimination of fluids, salt and nitrogen and the specific gravity of the urine. Arch. Int. Med., *16:*733-774, 1915.

36. Pierce, J. M., Ruzamna, R., and Segar, R.: Standardization of the phenolsulphonphthalein excretion test in clinical practice. J. A. M. A., *175:*711-713, 1961.

37. Puck, T. T., Wasserman, K., and Fishman, A. P.: Some effects of inorganic ions on the active transport of phenol red by the isolated tubules of the flounder. J. Cell. & Comp. Physiol., *40:*73, 1952.

38. Raisz, L. G., Rosenbaum, J. D., Prout, T. E., and Russell, W. H.: Procedure for clinical evaluation of renal function. J. A. M. A., *162:*266-268, Sept., 1956.

39. Rowntree, L. G., and Geraghty, J. T.: An experimental and clinical study of the functional activity of the kidneys by means of phenolsulphonphthalein. J. Pharmacol. & Exp. Therap., *1:*579-661, 1909-1910.

40. Rowntree, L. G., and Geraghty, J. T.: The phthalein test. An experimental and clinical study of phenolsulphonphthalein in relation to renal function in health and disease. Arch. Int. Med., *9:*284-338, 1912.

41. Shaw, E. C.: A study of the curve of elimination of phenolsulphonphthalein by the normal and diseased kidneys. J. Urol., *13:*575-592, 1925.

42. Smith, H. W.: The Physiology of the Kidney. New York, Oxford University Press, 1937.

43. Smith, H. W., Goldring, W., and Chasis, H.: The measurement of the tubular excretory mass effective blood flow and filtration rate in the normal human kidney. J. Clin. Invest., *17:*263-278, 1938.

44. Smith, H. S.: Principles of Renal Physiology. New York, Oxford University Press, 1956.

45. Sodeman, W. A., and Engelhardt, H. T.: Renal concentration test employing use of pituitary extracts. Response of normal subjects. Proc. Soc. Exp. Biol. Med., *46:*688-691, 1941.

46. Taggart, J. V., and Forster, R. P.: Renal tubular transport: Effect of 2, 4-dinitrophenol and related compounds on phenol red transport by the isolated tubules of the flounder. Am. J. Physiol., *161:*167-172, 1950.

47. Van Slyke, D. D.: Renal function tests. N. Y. State J. Med., 825-833, 1941.

48. Vaquez and Cottet: Eprevue de la Diurese provoquee. Presse Med., *20:*993-995, 1912.

49. Voelker, F., Joseph, F.: Funktionelle nierendiagnostik ohne ureterenkatheter. Munch. med. wschr., *50:*2081-2089, 1903.

50. Volhard, F.: Uber die funktionelle unterscheidung der schrumpfnieren. Verhandl. deutsch. Kong inn. med., *27:*735, 1910.

51. Wolf, A. V.: Urinary concentrative properties. Amer. J. Med., *32:*329-331, 1962.

Chapter 13

Physical and Physicochemical Techniques of Urine Examination

MICHAEL LUBRAN, M.D., Ph.D.

The physical properties of urine are determined by all its constituents. Measurement of these properties gives, as a rule, information about groups of substances rather than a single constituent, although it is sometimes possible to modify the technique to measure mainly one substance. Thus, the refractive index of urine depends on all its dissolved constituents; by suitable modifications, refractive index may be used to determine urinary protein.

Although very many physical properties of urine can be measured, and many have been investigated by physical and physicochemical methods, only a few of these properties have been related to disease, perhaps because simple, usually imprecise, methods of measurement have been employed. The availability of easily used, more sophisticated, apparatus capable of good precision, may awaken renewed interest in the clinical application of some of these properties, currently considered to be unhelpful.

The most widely used physical property of urine is its specific gravity; more recently, measurement of this property has been supplemented (or, in some laboratories replaced) by measurement of refractive index and osmolality. Surface tension, viscosity and optical activity of urine have also been measured, but much less frequently. The methods of measurement of these six properties, and the interpretation of their values. will be discussed. Other properties, such as pH, and other physical techniques such as polarography, spectroscopy, absorptiometry and chromatography will not be discussed, as they are used, essentially, to measure individual constituents of urine.

SPECIFIC GRAVITY AND DENSITY

The absolute density of a solution at a given temperature is defined as mass (in grams) of unit volume (in cc): in symbols,

$$d^t = m/v \qquad g/cc$$

The relative density is defined as the mass (in grams) of unit volume (in ml). As the liter is defined in terms of water at its maximum density (this occurs at 3.98° C; for convenience, 4° C is usually used) and is, in fact, very slightly larger than the cc, the relative density $d_4^t = m/v$ g/ml is very slightly smaller than the absolute density. Neither of these measurements is of great practical value when precision is required, because of the difficulty of precise measurement of volume of liquids. Instead, specific gravity is used. This is a ratio of densities and is a pure number (i.e., without units). It is defined as the ratio of the weight of the solution to the weight of an equal volume of water, both volumes being measured at the same temperature. Provided the solution and water are weighed in the same place, the ratio of the weights is the same as the ratio of the masses. Specific gravity can be written as d_t^t.

As water expands slightly when heated above 4° C, while its weight remains constant, the density of water decreases with an increase in temperature. However, as urine and water have nearly equal coefficients of expansion, specific gravity of urine is not greatly altered by change in temperature. When relative density d_4^t is measured (this is what is usually meant by 'specific gravity') the temperature of measurement, t, should be given.

Measurement of Specific Gravity and Density

1. *The Pycnometer.* This is a glass container, usually of 10 to 30 ml capacity, which can be completely filled with liquid and kept at constant temperature. By filling it in turn with urine and water, and weighing the contents, the specific gravity can be determined with 0.1% precision, at a known temperature. Various pycnometers and the method of their use are described by Bauer and Lewin (1). Although accurate and precise, the technique is tedious. The pycnometer is not suitable for routine use: it can be used for measurement of the specific gravities of reference solutions.

2. *The Urinometer.* This is a form of hydrometer widely used for measuring the specific gravity of urine, consisting of a bulb to which is sealed a graduated cylindrical stem. The scale on the stem is calibrated in terms of specific gravity. It is therefore necessary for the urinometer to be used at the temperature of calibration of the scale or the reading corrected for temperature. The scale reading at the position of the meniscus gives the specific gravity. The precision of the instrument is not great. Galambos *et al.* (6) reported that when 71 observers, composed of doctors and laboratory staff, read the specific gravity of two allegedly different (in reality, the same) urines, differences as great as 0.005 were reported. The mean value of the specific gravity was 1.0244, standard deviation 0.0019. Many urinometers are incorrectly calibrated. The scale should be checked using solutions of known specific gravity. Convenient solutions are 65.07 g $CuSO_4 \cdot 5H_2O$/liter and 17.39 g $CuSO_4 \cdot 5H_2O$/liter; the respective specific gravities (at 20°/4°C) are 1.040 and 1.010.

3. *Westphal Balance (Fisher Scientific Company).* This balance employs the principle of Archimedes. A sinker, adjusted to have a definite displacement, is hung from one arm of the balance and suspended in about 50 ml of the urine contained in a cylinder. Riders, graduated in terms of density, are moved along the beam until a balance is obtained. The values of the weights and the position of the riders give the density. The temperature should be noted. The method is rapid, precise and convenient. Its disadvantage for clinical use is that it requires a large volume of urine. An analytical balance can be adapted to this technique, to provide a method suitable for small volumes.

Interpretation of Specific Gravity

The purpose of measuring the specific gravity of urine is to provide information about its solute content, as a guide to renal function and water metabolism. How useful is specific gravity for this purpose? Wolf (27) points out that opinions, not scientific evidence, govern the points of view of adherents of and opponents to the clinical use of specific gravity. It is possible, however, without adjudicating on this issue, to determine the relationship between specific gravity and total urinary solute concentration.

A solute can be considered to occupy a definite volume of the solution; in a molar solution this volume is its partial molar volume. For most substances, the partial molar volume is not constant, but varies with concentration. Partial molar volumes are additive, provided the substances do not interact. In a solution containing several components, the volume of the solution will be the sum of the products of partial molar volume and molar concentration of all the components, including water. As the density of the solution depends upon weight and volume, it can be seen that both the molar concentration of the substance (*not* its concentration in g/100 ml) and partial molar volume determine the density. Galambos *et al.* (6) have shown that the specific gravity of urine increases by 0.001 when the following weights of substance are added to a liter: 1.47g of sodium chloride, 3.8g of sodium dihydrogen phosphate, 3.6g of urea, 2.7g of albumin.

Rules of thumb for converting specific gravity to solute concentration, such as Long's rule (14) (which uses the factor 2.6 to multiply the last two digits of the specific gravity to give g of solute/liter) can at the best give only rough approximations to total solute concentration.

Protein and glucose in the urine cause considerable error in the calculation. It can be concluded that specific gravity does not provide a good measure of urinary total solute concentration.

REFRACTIVE INDEX

The refractive index of a solution (relative to air) is the ratio of the velocity of light in air to the velocity of light in the solution. The refractive index of pure water at 20°C is 1.3330 (using sodium light at 5893 Å). It falls with rising temperature, by about 0.0001 per °C at room temperature but at a greater rate at higher temperatures. The refractive index of water decreases with increasing wavelength, over the visible spectrum. However, if an aqueous solution contains substances which absorb light of particular wavelengths, abrupt changes of refractive index occur when those wavelengths are used for its measurement.

The refractive index can be described by Snell's law: $n = \sin i / \sin r$ where i and r are the angles of incidence and refraction of light entering the solution at an angle. Geometrical considerations show that if light passes from a substance of higher refractive index to one of lower, there is a certain value of i (the critical angle) which must not be exceeded if light is to pass out of the more refractive medium. Thus, a fish-eye view of the world outside its habitat is restricted to a cone of vision of angle about 97° ($2 \sin^{-1} 0.75$). Many refractometers depend upon the critical angle for their function.

Measurement of Refractive Index

Many types of instruments exist for measuring the refractive index of liquids, but in practice either a refractometer or an interferometer is used. The interferometer is the more precise instrument, capable of measuring the difference in refractive index of urine and water with a precision of 0.00001 (e.g., Laborinterferometer LI 3, Carl Zeiss). However, the instruments are expensive and require a highly skilled operator. Refractometers are more convenient though less accurate. The classical instrument is the Abbé refractometer, a critical angle instrument. It requires accurate control of temperature, and monochromatic light. A convenient critical angle refractometer, which is temperature compensated and suitable for use with daylight or artifical light, is now available. This instrument, the Goldberg refractometer (American Optical Co., Buffalo, N. Y.) is a small, hand, instrument requiring only a drop of urine, It is extremely simple to use and gives the refractive index to the fourth decimal place. The scale of the instrument is calibrated in terms of refractive index, or in terms of total solid. The latter scale is based on certain assumptions, discussed below. A scale is also available calibrated in terms of specific gravity, based on similar assumptions. Within limitations, the refractometer can be used to measure the specific gravity of urine.

Interpretation of Refractive Index

The refractive index of urine is measured in order to provide information about the total solids of urine. By measuring the refractive index before and after heat-coagulation of proteins with acetic acid, urinary protein can be measured, if its concentration exceeds 300 mg/100 ml (26). The relationship between refractive index, specific gravity and total solids of urine has been investigated by Rubini and Wolf (19), who have extended the work of Blohm (3). Studies of 190 urines, free from detectable protein or glucose, revealed a high correlation between refractive index and total solids, and between refractive index and specific gravity. In both cases, the curves connecting these quantities were slightly curved. However, by fitting the best straight line, the following formulae were calculated

$$U_s = 639.52 \, (n - 1.33320)$$
$$U_v = 212.6 \, (D - 1.0000)$$

where U_s is the weight of urinary solids in grams per 100 g of water, U_v is the weight in grams of urinary solids in 100 ml of urine, D is the specific gravity of urine at 15°C and n is the refractive index of urine at 17.5°C using the sodium D line. The respective standard errors of the estimate were 0.062 g per 100 g and 0.419 per 100 ml. These figures show that the reliability of the total solid concentration derived from refractive index is good, from specific gravity measurements poor.

It is not certain that the formulae would have been so successful if grossly abnormal urine had been included, or urine containing glucose or protein. The relationship between refractive index and solute concentration is complex. While, in general terms, refractive index is a colligative property of solutions (i.e., dependent on the number, not the chemical nature, of the particles in solution), this generalization has so many exceptions that it is necessary in every case to determine empirically the relationship between refractive index and concentration of the solute. Essentially, the refractivity of a substance depends on the interaction of light with the valency electrons of the atoms; the type and number of bonds may modify the interaction. As refractive index is a colligative property, the molecular weight of the compound dissolved, not the weight per unit volume, is the determinant. As urine contains salts of differing molecular weights, it is surprising that there is such a close relationship between concentration (in g per 100g) and refractive index. However, so far as ions are concerned, anions make a much larger contribution towards refractive index than cations (15); organic solutes are more refractive than inorganic solutes, on a molar basis. The refractive increment for inorganic salts is roughly constant at about 0.0020, for protein about 0.0019. It appears, therefore, that in normal urine the inequalities of refractivity due to the differences among the salts have cancelled out. Considerable glucosuria or proteinuria will produce anomalous results. Wolf (27) has suggested that refraction (i.e., the difference in refractive index of the urine and water, multiplied by 10,000 to get rid of decimals) should be employed as an independent measurement, without an attempt to translate it into solute concentration. He defines the "normal range" as 85-134. Now that refractometry is widely practised, it should be possible to obtain extensive data concerning the diagnostic value of refractive index of urine.

OSMOLALITY

Osmolality, a colligative property of solutions, is an index of osmotic concentration. Osmotic pressure is the pressure which must be applied to a solution to prevent the passage into it of solvent when the two liquids are separated by a semipermeable membrane (i.e., one permeable only to the solvent). In an 'ideal' solution, osmotic pressure and concentration are related by the equation $P = RTC$, where P is the osmotic pressure measured in atmospheres, R is the gas constant, T the absolute temperature and C is the molarity of the solution. This relationship (van t'Hoff's law) is, in fact, obeyed only in very dilute aqueous solutions of non-electrolytes. The osmotic pressure of ionic solutions is made up of contributions from each ionic species; these contributions are, on the whole, additive. The osmotic pressure of a molar solution of sodium chloride is about twice that of a molar solution of glucose.

Thermodynamic considerations show that osmotic pressure is related to the activity of the solute, not its concentration. A factor, ϕ (the osmotic coefficient) is therefore used to convert concentration into osmotic activity. The osmotic coefficient is not a constant, but varies with temperature and concentration of solute. Stokes (22) has measured the osmotic coefficient of urea. At low urea concentrations, urea solutions are almost 'ideal,' but at concentrations greater than 0.5 molal, the osmotic coefficient falls rapidly as the concentration rises. At these higher concentrations, the osmotic coefficient decreases as the temperature falls. Osmotic coefficients of electrolytes can be calculated from formulae given by Leskovsek (13), or may be measured directly. For 0.06M NaCl, ϕ is 0.974, for 0.1M NaCl, ϕ is 0.932; the corresponding figures for KCl are 0.974 and 0.927. Temperature variation of electrolyte osmotic coefficients is small.

The osmotic pressure of a solution can be defined in terms of osmolality: osmolality = $\phi\, n\, c$, where ϕ is the osmotic coefficient, n is the number of ionic species derived from the solute (e.g., two for sodium chloride) and c is the molal concentration (moles per 1000 g of water). Osmolality is a concentration: it is the number of osmols of a solute per

1000 g of water. Solutions of the same osmolality have the same osmotic pressure.

Measurement of Osmolality

Although osmotic pressure is described in terms of semi-permeable membranes, it is usually measured indirectly by making use of another colligative property of solutions. Membranes permitting the passage of water only and not of electrolytes do not currently exist. Two types of instrument are available for measurement of the osmotic pressure of urine: one type measures the freezing point of the urine, the other its vapor pressure.

Freezing Point Osmometer

The freezing point of a solution is lower than that of the solvent; the difference, i.e., the depression of the freezing point, is proportional to the molality of the solution. The depression of freezing point of a molal solution of an 'ideal' aqueous solution is 1.858°C. Osmolality, therefore, equals the observed depression of freezing point divided by 1.858. The problem, then, is to measure the freezing point of urine, with adequate accuracy.

An aqueous solution is at its freezing point when it is in equilibrium with ice, i.e., when the temperature of the equilibrium mixture is constant in the presence of small changes in external temperature. In principle, it is necessary only to cool the solution slowly, keeping it stirred to prevent supercooling, until ice appears and the temperature of the solution remains constant: this temperature is the freezing point. Very accurate thermometers, capable of recording temperature differences of 0.001°C are required. A thermistor is suitable. In practice, it is difficult to measure the freezing point of urine by the method described, because as the solution freezes and ice separates, the solution becomes more concentrated, its freezing point is lowered and its temperature continues to fall. If a solution of a single substance were being examined, it would be relatively simple to remove a sample of the solution in equilibrium with ice at a particular temperature and determine the composition by an appropriate procedure. In this way, the depression of freezing point of a solution of particular composition would be determined. The problem with urine, however, is to determine the freezing point of an actual solution, and thus deduce its osmolality. A convenient method of measuring the depression of freezing point is through the use of supercooling. The Cryoscopic Osmometer (Advanced Instruments, Inc., Newton Highlands, Mass.) or Osmette (Fisher Scientific Co) may be used. The instruments, calibrated in terms of temperature and osmolality, are convenient for routine use. One determination takes about three minutes and requires about three ml of urine. The measurement can be repeated as often as required on the same sample.

Sunderman (23) has discussed the measurement of osmolality with particular reference to serum. Stadie and Sunderman (21) have described a technique for measuring osmolality which avoids supercooling. However, the procedure is time-consuming for routine work.

In the supercooling method, urine is cooled rapidly to below freezing point. Ice does not separate until the solution is stirred, when there is a rapid release of the heat of fusion of ice and the temperature rises. By means of suitably adjusted conditions, the heat of fusion balances the cooling effect, to give a temperature plateau lasting about a minute. This temperature is not the true freezing point of the solution, but the apparent freezing point. The difference between these two values is directly proportional to the degree of supercooling. The true freezing point can be determined by measuring the apparent freezing point with different degrees of supercooling and extrapolating to zero supercooling. However, it is more convenient to have a fixed cooling bath temperature, to follow carefully a definite procedure and to calibrate the instrument using solutions of precisely known osmolality. Precisely measured sodium chloride and potassium chloride solutions are available for use as standards. Other salt standards also are available. Provided the procedure is correctly carried through, very reproducible results are obtained. It must be stressed that the supercooling technique described here does not measure the true freezing point of urine: it measures an apparent freezing point, which, by an empirical calibration procedure, can be related to the osmolality of the urine. If the protein concentration is high, a small error may be introduced.

The osmolalities determined by cryoscopic methods are those at the freezing temperature measured. The osmolalities at room temperature will be slighly higher, because of the variation of osmotic coefficient with temperature. The difference is unimportant in clinical work.

Vapor Pressure Osmometers

Osmotic pressure can, in theory, be measured indirectly by measuring the elevation of boiling point, depression of freezing point or vapor pressure depression of the solution. Boiling point measurements are impracticable for urine; depression of freezing-point is widely used, but the method is empirical and suffers from the theoretical disadvantage of not measuring the true freezing-point. The vapor pressure method depends on the physicochemical fact that the vapor pressure of a solution is lower than that of the solvent. The depression of vapor pressure is proportional to the osmotic pressure of the solution, and is affected by similar factors, such as activity, departure from 'ideal' behavior and temperature.

Until recently, vapor pressure osmometry was difficult and imprecise, and hardly suited to routine work. However, an instrument has recently become available, which measures vapor pressure differences thermoelectrically. This instrument (Model 302 VPO, Hewlett Packard, F & M Scientific Division, Avondale, Pa.) is simple to use and very sensitive. The VPO works in the following way. A drop of solvent is placed on a thermistor bead and a drop of urine on another, in a vapor-filled temperature-controlled box. Solvent condenses on the solution drop, releasing the heat of vaporisation, which warms up the drop. This process is progressive, but in about 4 minutes (for urine) a steady state develops. The difference in temperature between the drops is measured as a difference in resistance, ΔR, by appropriate bridge circuitry. Calibration with known NaCl, KCl or other solutions gives a factor for converting ΔR to osmolality. Ehrmantraut (5) describes the principle and operation of an earlier type of VPO. Unlike cryoscopy, vapor pressure differences can be measured at any convenient temperature. In particular, osmolality can be measured at 37°C.

Interpretation

The 'normal range' for osmolality is

800 to 1300 milliosmols per kg (27). More information about renal function, however, is obtained by considering the ratio of plasma to urine osmolalities. This ratio measures the concentrating ability of the kidney. Jacobson *et al.* (10) found urine osmolality in 26 healthy subjects to vary between 855 and 1335 mOsm per kg, and the plasma/urine ratio to lie within the range 3.0 to 4.7. Polacek *et al.* (16) give the values of urine osmolality and renal concentrating power in infants and children.

Osmolality is a better guide to renal function than specific gravity or refractive index. The two latter measurements are greatly affected by protein; osmotic pressure is hardly affected by the protein concentration of most pathological urines. The osmotic effect of glucose is about one sixth that of the same concentration of sodium chloride. Osmotic pressure, therefore, is essentially related to electrolyte and urea osmolalities, except when glycosuria is marked. Osmolality should be used as a measurement in its own right, not as a means of determining solute concentration, with which its correspondence is very approximate.

SURFACE TENSION

Surface tension was one of the earliest physical properties of urine to be related to disease. Hay's test for bile salts, in which flowers of sulphur sprinkled onto the surface of urine fall to the bottom of the container if excess of bile salts is present, depends upon the ability of bile salts to lower surface tension. Quantitative measurements on urine had been made sporadically, but a systematic study of surface tension was stimulated by the work of Butt *et al.* (4) who emphasized the role of protective

urinary colloids in the treatment and prevention of renal lithiasis. To facilitate clinical studies of surface tension in urinary lithiasis, a simple apparatus was devised (Revici urotensiometer). Most of the small number of authors who have published on urinary surface tension have employed this apparatus (7, 12, 17, 18). Hauser and le Beau (9) employed the pendant drop method. No work appears to have been published using modern, reliable, instruments, such as are described below.

Surface tension is a phenomenon common to all surfaces separating two phases. Usually, air is one phase. A surface possesses free energy (in the thermodynamic sense), measured by the work required to increase the area by 1 sq. cm. Surfaces assume a shape which results in a minimum value for the free energy. The effect is equivalent to the surface being under tension. If a cut were made in a solid surface under tension, it would gape and a force would be required to close the cut, proportional to its length. Similarly, surface tension can be described as a force acting along the surface of a liquid at right angles to any line 1 cm in length. The force is measured in dynes per cm. Although the force of surface tension appears to be linear, it is exactly equivalent to surface energy, which is measured in ergs per sq. cm. As an erg is a dyne x a cm, it can be seen that the two methods of measurement are identical. It is purely a convention to use the unit of dyne per cm.

The surface tension of most aqueous solutions of inorganic salts is not very different from that of water (72 dynes per cm at 25°C). However, there are some substances that lower the surface tension considerably. These substances are surface active, and are concentrated in the surface of the solution. When a new surface is formed, surface active substances pass from the bulk of the solution to the surface. This process may not be instantaneous; in fact, it may take many minutes for equilibrium to be established when new surfaces are created in protein solutions. Methods of measuring surface tension may be static (the surface is stable) or dynamic (the surface is being created). Dynamic methods are not suitable for surfaces which reach equilibrium slowly. As most biological fluids show this feature, dynamic methods of measurement of surface tension will not be considered.

Measurement of Surface Tension

1. *Capillary Height Method* If a narrow-bore glass capillary tube open at both ends is placed vertically in urine, the liquid rises in the tube. The difference in height between the liquid surface in the tube and the liquid surface outside the tube is related to the surface tension. It is also necessary to know the diameter of the tube, the density of the urine and the temperature of measurement. In practice, the bore must be about 0.5 mm, and the interior of the glass must be completely wetted (i.e., the contact angle must be zero). Because of the difficulty of measuring the diameter of the tube with precision, the apparatus should be calibrated with water at a known temperature. As long as dilute aqueous solutions, not differing greatly from water in surface tension, are measured, the method gives reliable results. However, when much surface active material is present, the method becomes erroneous, unless corrections are introduced, because the contact angle becomes significantly different from zero. Erroneously high results are produced.

2. *Revici Urotensiometer (18).* This is a capillary tube (thermometer tubing) about 15 cm long, with a bore of 0.5 mm. It is graduated in dynes/cm. To use it, a column of urine is sucked into the tube to the top mark, the tube is held vertically and the fall of the column observed. After a few seconds, the flow stops or is markedly slowed. The reading at this point gives the surface tension. The flow speeds up again, then slows down and stops leaving a residual column of urine. The apparatus is calibrated on the assumption that the specific gravity of the urine is 1.015; suitable density corrections must be made. The temperature should be noted. Surface tension decreases by about 0.16 dynes per cm for each degree centigrade rise in temperature. The value obtained with this instrument is also affected by the viscosity of the urine, which is altered by protein.

3. *Pendant Drop.* This method has been applied to urine by Hauser and le Beau (9) and is described in detail by Hauser (8). Essentially, if a drop of liquid is allowed to form at the end of a capillary tube and hang there without falling, it will assume a particular shape related to its surface tension. It is necessary to photograph the drop. Many measurements are required and a complex formula has to be used. There is divided opinion about the accuracy of the method. It is certainly unsuitable for routine use, whatever its merits.

4. *Forced Bubble Method.* The pressure required to form and burst a bubble of inert gas in a liquid is related to its surface tension. The gas is introduced through a capillary tube of known bore, into a liquid kept at constant temperature. The method is simple, rapid and accurate (provided the capillary is calibrated by use in water). No systematic

study of the surface tension of urine using this method has been reported.

5. *The du Nouy Balance.* This apparatus measures the force required to detach a platinum-iridium ring from the surface of a liquid. A torsion balance or more accurate analytical balance can be used. The force required is very simply related to the surface tension of the solution, which can be maintained at any desired temperature. Many of the problems associated with the use of this instrument (non-verticality of the stirrup, tilting of the ring, dipping the ring too far into the solution, recognising the moment of detachment) have been overcome by the introduction of an automated apparatus, the Tensiomat (Fisher).

Other methods of measuring surface tension, such as drop weight, drop volume, hanging drop and sessile drop methods will not be described.

Interpretation

The surface tension of pure water is 72.0 dynes per cm at 25°C and 72.8 dynes per cm at 20°C. In general, electrolytes produce a very small rise in surface tension, although ammonium salts cause a lowering. Surface tension is also reduced with increasing acidity. Organic substances produce different effects; glucose produces a very small increase, organic acids a well-marked decrease, amino acids may increase or decrease the surface tension. Proteins form films in the surface, reducing the surface tension in a manner varying with pH and salt concentration. Bile salts decrease surface tension markedly; glucuronides also decrease surface tension.

It is apparent that there are considerable difficulties in interpreting the surface tension values of urine. From the data of Harlin and Wiesel (7) on 1200 urines obtained from 100 healthy, non-pregnant subjects, the mean urinary surface tension can be calculated to be 67.2 dynes per cm, standard deviation 0.96 dynes per cm. A small number of urines had values as high as 73 dynes per cm. Ravich and Ravich (17) reported a similar mean value. They also showed there was a diurnal variation of about 6 dynes per cm in surface tension, the minimum being at about 5 p.m., the maximum about 5 a.m. Pregnancy and jaundice are associated with low tensions (about 55 dynes per cm). Infections may give rise to an increase or decrease in surface tension. Stress and steroid therapy are associated with raised surface tensions, Addison's disease with a low surface tension. In the face of all these known variables, and many unknown ones, it is difficult to know how to interpret the slightly elevated tensions (about 70 dynes per cm) occasionally found in patients with renal lithiasis. It is very probable that there is no connection between surface tension of urine and stone formation. Smiddy (20) was unable to confirm any relationship. He found, using the Revici instrument, that surface tension of urine was correlated with specific gravity. Von Berlepsch (24) reinvestigated the factors affecting the surface tension of urine and concluded that there was no basis for relating 'protective colloids' to stone formation. It would appear that, with the possible exception of measurement of bile acids, there are no clinical conditions for which the measurement of urinary surface tension is indicated.

VISCOSITY

The viscosity of a fluid is defined as the tangential force per unit area (i.e., shearing force) on either of two horizontal planes at unit distance apart in the fluid, one fixed, the other moving at unit velocity. If the viscosity is constant when different shearing forces are applied, the fluid is called Newtonian. Normal urine is a Newtonian fluid. The unit of viscosity is the poise (after Poiseuille), defined as the viscosity of a material which requires a shearing force of 1 dyne per sq. cm to maintain a velocity gradient of 1 cm/sec. between two planes 1 cm apart. The viscosity of water at 20°C is 1.005 centipoises.

Measurement of Viscosity

Viscosity is conveniently measured in terms of water. The relative viscosity is the ratio of the viscosity of the solution to that of water measured at the same temperature. Flow must be streamlined (i.e., non-turbulent) and slow. Most measurements on aqueous solutions are carried out by timing the rate of flow through a capillary tube. A typical instrument is the Ostwald viscometer, in which liquid flows through a narrow vertical capillary from a reservoir. The rate of flow is measured and compared with that of water run under identical conditions. The ratio of the rates is the relative viscosity, allowance being made for the difference in densities of the liquids. If the densities are markedly different, corrections have to be made for the differences in kinetic energy. However, no corrections for kinetic energy are necessary with urine. Many varieties of the Ostwald viscometer exist, designed to improve accuracy and reproducibility. A useful type for work with urine is the Ostwald-Cannon-Fenske capillary viscometer, with flow times of more than 200 seconds, and the Ubbelöhde viscometer. Temperature must be accurately controlled, as vis-

cosity falls by about 2.5% per °C rise. In the capillary viscometer, surface tension effects may be important; corrections may have to be applied. An automated viscometer is available (Auto-viscometer 5901 B, Hewlett Packard, Avondale, Pa.) in which the sample is automatically introduced into the capillary and the efflux time measured very precisely.

Interpretation

There is little reliable data in the literature on urine viscosity. The relative viscosity is about unity. Gergentz *et al.* (2) found values of 0.9 to 2.3 centipoises (mean 1.15) in 12 dehydrated patients with normal renal function; these values correspond to a mean relative viscosity of 1.10. The viscosiy of a 2% solution of urea at 25° is 1.013 (11); aminoacids have small effects on viscosity (24). The inorganic salts and other constituents of urine account for the small excess of the relative viscosity over unity. Proteins have a larger effect, difficult to quantitate with precision, as capillary flow methods are unsuitable for measuring the viscosity of protein solutions. However, a 3% solution of albumin has a relative viscosity of 1.22 at 25°C. It would appear, therefore, that proteinuria would affect the viscosity of urine; other pathological constituents would have minor effects only. Measurement of viscosity of urine does not appear to be of value in the clinical laboratory.

POLARIMETRY

Optically active substances rotate the plane of polarisation of light passing through them. The rotation depends upon the wavelength of the light, the temperature, the density of the solution and its concentration. In some cases, the solvent, although optically inert, may have an effect on rotation. The specific rotation is defined as the rotation in degrees of 1g of the substance in 1 ml of solution, in a tube with path length of 10 cm. The direction of rotation of a substance is not always constant and may change from right to left (i.e., positive to negative) with concentration and solvent. However, for the substances found commonly in urine, the direction of rotation of the plane is either right or left.

Measurement of the plane of polarisation

Many types of polarimeter are available. The solution to be examined is placed in a narrow tube 10 cm long. Monochromatic light must be used, usually a sodium lamp. In a common type of instrument, both halves of an optical field are evenly illuminated; if the plane of polarisation is rotated, one half of the field becomes dark. By suitable adjustment of a compensating device, the original brightness is restored. The degree of rotation of the plane can then be deduced. Temperature must be kept constant. If the urine is deeply colored, it should be decolorised by treatment with a solution of basic lead acetate.

Interpretation

The optical rotation of urine is caused by its optically active organic constituents. The major contributors to the optical activity of urine are the amino-acids and glucuronides; to a lesser degree, urinary steroids make a contribution. In pathological urines, protein and glucose rotate the plane of polarisation. Glucose and glucuronic acid are dextrorotatory in aqueous solution. Aminoacids, although configurationally L-isomers, rotate the plane either to the right or left, depending on pH. Rotation becomes more positive in acid solutions, although it may still be to the left. The net result, in normal urine, may be a small degree of optical rotation in either direction.

In pathological urines, protein always gives negative rotations, the exact value depending on pH. The specific rotation of serum albumin is about -50°, over the pH range 4 to 11. Glucose gives a positive rotation, the specific rotation being +52.5°. This value has to be slightly increased in concentrated solutions. Polarimetry can be used to give an approximate value for glucose concentration, provided there is no proteinura. However, the ketoacids often present in diabetic urine are levorotatory. Cystine has a very large specific rotation (-214° at pH 1); polarimetry can be helpful in the examination of cystinuric urine. On the whole, polarimetry has little place in the routine examination of urine. Better methods exist for measuring glucose and protein. However, it has an occasional use. Bergentz *et al.* (2) used polarimetry to measure the dextran concentration of urine of patients receiving dextran infusions. The specific rotation of the material used was +199°, making this method of analysis both precise and practical.

REFERENCES

1. Bauer, N., and Lewin, S. Z.: In Weissberger, A. (ed.): Technique of Organic Chemistry, Vol. 1. New York, Interscience, 1959, Part 1, pp. 148-175.
2. Bergentz, S. E., Falkheden, T., and Olson, S.: Diuresis and urinary viscosity in dehydrated patients. Ann. Surg., *162*:582-586, 1965.
3. Blohm, G. J.: On the determination of the content of solid constituents in the urine. Upsala lakf. forh., *23*:283-304, 1918.
4. Butt, A. J., and Hauser, E. A.: The importance of protective urinary colloids in the prevention and

treatment of kidney stones. Science, *115*:308-310, 1952.

5. Ehrmantraut, H. C.,: The Measurement of Serum Osmolality by Vapor Pressure Osmometry. Clinical Pathology of the Serum Electrolytes. Springfield, Thomas, 1966, pp. 181-188.

6. Galambos, J. T., Herndon, E. G., and Reynolds, G. H.: Specific-gravity determination. Fact or fancy?. New Eng. J. Med., *270*:506-508, 1964.

7. Harlin H. C., and Wiesel, L.: Modification of urinary surface tension by oral glucuronolactone: its application in prophylaxis of urinary calculi. J. Urol., *72*:1046-1049, 1954.

8. Hauser, E. A.: In Glasser, O. (ed.): Medical Physics, Vol. 1., Chicago, Year Book Publishers Inc., 1944, pp. 1494-1497.

9. Hauser, E. A., and le Beau, D. S.: Urinary calculi. Kolloid Zeitschr., *132*:78-84, 1953.

10. Jacobson, M. H., Levy, S. E., Kaufman, R. M., Gallinek, W. E., and Donnelly, O. W.: Urine Osmolality. Arch. Int. Med., *110*:83-89, 1962.

11. Kawahara, K., and Tanford, C.: Viscosity and density of aqueous solutions of urea and guanidine hydrochloride. J. Biol. Chem., *241*:3228-3232, 1966.

12. Kocar, von J.: The surface active substances in urine. Zeitsch. f. die gesamte Innere Medizin, *19*:491-495, 1964.

13. Leskovsek, D.: One-parameter equations for activity and osmotic coefficients for 1, 1 valent electrolytes, Zeitschr. f. phys. Chem. (Neue Folge), *46*:251-253, 1965.

14. Long, J. H.: On the relation of the specific gravity of the urine to the solids present. J. Amer. Chem. Soc., *25*:257-262, 1903.

15. Moelwyn-Hughes, E. A.: Physical Chemistry. New York, Pergamon, 1961, pp. 370-400.

16. Polacek, E., Vocel, J., Neugebauerova, L., Sebkova, M., and Vechetova: The osmotic con-centrating ability in healthy infants and children. Arch. Dis. Child., *40*:291-295, 1965.

17. Ravich, R. A., and Ravich, A.: Study of the urinary surface tension and protective colloids in urolithiasis; use of the Revici urotensiometer. J. Urol., *72*:1050-1056, 1954.

18. Ravich, R. A.: Relationship of colloids to the surface tension of urine. Science, *117*:561-563, 1953.

19. Rubini, M. E., and Wolf, A. V.: Refractometric determination of total solids and water of serum and urine. J. Biol. Chem., *225*:869-876, 1957.

20. Smiddy, F. G.: Estimations of the surface tension of human urine and the effect of hyaluronidase. Brit. J. Urol., *26*:270-273, 1954.

21. Stadie, W. C., and Sunderman, F. W.: A method for the determination of the freezing-point depression of aqueous solutions, particularly those containing protein. J. Biol. Chem., *41*:127-226, 1931.

22. Stokes, R. H.: Osmotic coefficients of concentrated aqueous urea solutions from freezing-point measurements. J. Phys. Chem., *70*:1199-1203, 1966.

23. Sunderman, F. W.: Clinical Pathology of the Serum Electrolytes. Springfield, Thomas, 1966, pp. 176-181.

24. Tsangaris, J. M., and Martin, R. B.: Viscosities of aqueous solutions of dipolar ions. Arch. Biochem. Biophys., , *112*:267-272, 1965.

25. von Berlepsch, K.: Surface tension and protective colloids of the urine and their questionable relation to the formation of kidney stones. Urol. Int., *5*:149-173, 1957.

26. Wolf, A. V., Fuller, J. B., Goldman, E. J., and Mahony, T. D.: New refractometric methods for the determination of total proteins in serum and urine. Clin. Chem., *8*:158-165, 1962.

27. Wolf, A. V.: Urinary concentrative properties. Amer. J. Med., *32*:329-332, 1962.

Chapter 14

Screening Tests for Chemical Components of Urine

ALFRED H. FREE, PH.D., and HELEN M. FREE, B.S.

INTRODUCTION

One of the first instances of a test being applied to urine for the recognition of a chemical component was the study of Richard Bright (3) at Guy's Hospital in London in the early part of the 19th century. Bright's test would not correspond to our present-day classification of screening but he was able to clearly demonstrate that the urine from patients with a specific type of kidney disease showed coagulation when boiled in a pewter spoon held over a candle. Bright's work was so clear-cut and outstanding that even today the disorder which he studied bears his name.

During the ensuing one and one-half centuries, a number of screening tests for chemical components of urine have evolved which provide identification of renal disorders. This presentation describes and discusses screening tests commonly used to identify chemical components of the urine which are suggestive of renal disease.

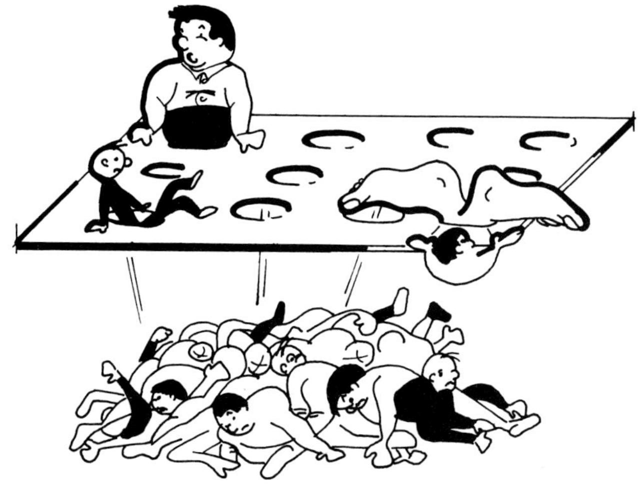

Fig. 1.   Screening.

SCREENING

Screening tests are continuing to show an increasingly great popularity as they have in recent years. Figure 1 is a cartoon depicting the concept of screening. In essence, one might envision separation of a group of individuals into those who would pass through the screen and those who would not — much as one might separate the large stones from the gravel on a screen. In screening for disease, the atypical individual who does not pass through the screen is not necessarily regarded as having the disease. He is simply separated for further study which is designed to determine the presence or absence of the disease considered.

Specific tests which may be regarded as screening procedures for renal disease are incorporated into many examinations such as those conducted by a physician in an office examination or those test procedures which are involved with hospital admissions. There is at present a very minimal amount of screening of healthy population groups for renal disease in a manner comparable to screening for diabetes.

SCREENING TESTS
FOR PROTEINURIA

The examination of urine for protein is such a common procedure and is so much a part of most routine examinations that it is sometimes taken for granted. The utility of the information obtained from this test, although it is integrated into the patient's profile, is not always recognized.

Until the last few years, practically all tests for protein were based on procedures which caused a precipitate or turbidity. Tests of this type have certain aspects of inconvenience. One is that many urine specimens from patients are already turbid at the time they are tested. Turbidity can be removed from most samples by filtering or centrifuging, but this is inconvenient. Older tests for proteinuria often require heating or involve the use of a strong caustic acid. The turbidity tests for proteinuria are non-specific and may give precipitates with any type of acid-precipitable material — notably metabolites of tolbutamide and certain x-ray contrast media. The recently-introduced colorimetric tests for protein are based on the protein error of certain pH indicators, as first described by Sorenson (25). Using tetrabromphenol blue as an example, Figure 2 illustrates the principle involved in these tests. Tetrabromphenol blue shows a color change from yellow to blue as the pH increases from 3 to 4. The top row of beakers indicates that normally the indicator is yellow at pH 2 and 3 but blue at pH 4. The indicator exhibits the protein error since, in the presence of protein, the pH of color change is altered as shown by the lower row of beakers. In the presence of protein at pH 2, the indicator is yellow, but at pH 3 and 4, the mixture is blue. The colorimetric test for protein involves buffering the indicator at a pH of 3. This composition is impregnated into cellulose attached to a plastic strip. The testing procedure simply involves dipping into the urine and matching to a color chart. In the absence of protein, the color will be yellow and in the presence of protein, the color will be green or blue (8).

Colorimetric tests for protein in urine present advantages but are also subject to certain sources of error. Urines which are very alkaline, particularly if highly buffered, have sufficient buffering capacity to overcome the buffer of the

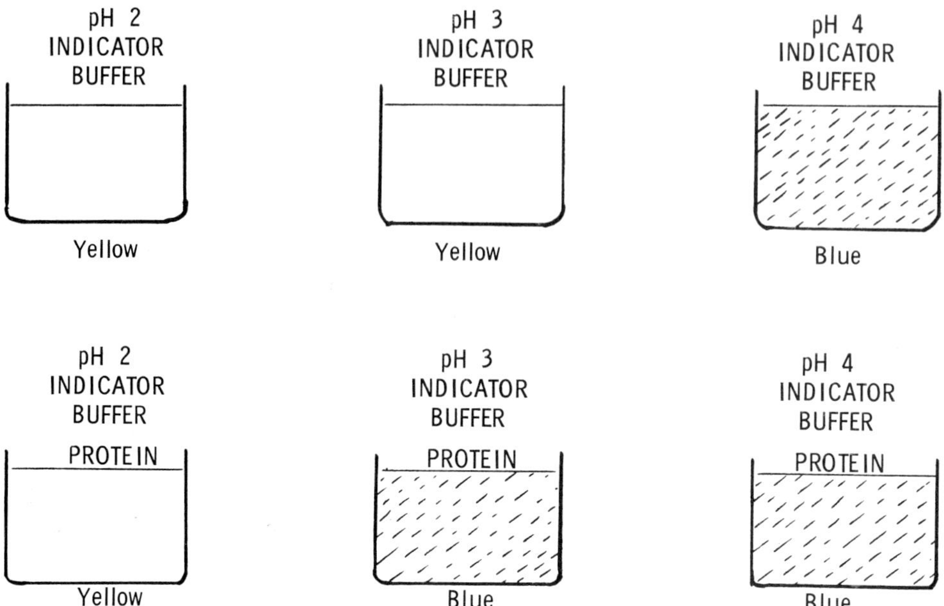

Fig. 2. The protein error of indicators.

impregnated reagent. Accordingly, such urines may give false positive results. Certain quaternary compounds which may be added to urine as an antiseptic will also give false positive reactions (12).

Table I presents a list of disorders of the kidney in which proteinuria may occur. This table was prepared simply by listing the kidney disorders which might have proteinuria as they are discussed in current textbooks of medicine, surgery, pediatrics, obstetrics and gynecology, and renal disease (2, 14, 5, 22, 24, 27, 26). The list is impressive in that most renal diseases may show proteinuria. It should be pointed out, however, that proteinuria is not a constant finding in all of these disorders. It is also important to recognize that proteinuria may occur in non-renal disorders.

SCREENING TEST FOR OCCULT BLOOD IN URINE

Screening tests for blood in urine have only recently come into widespread usage. This, in part, relates to the fact that reliance has been placed on the microsopic examination of urine sediment for red cells. This procedure is of value but it does not recognize all cases of blood in urine. Until quite recently, the chemical tests for blood in urine were quite unsatisfactory. Older chemical tests involved the addition of reagents directly to urine. The inadequacy of such a procedure is identified by Hoffman (15) who states "The benzidine test for blood in urine should not be applied directly to the urine specimen. Something in the urine decomposes the blue color as fast as it is formed, even in the presence of much blood."

Recognition of the presence of blood

in urine can reliably be established by the use of a colorimetric "dip-and-read" procedure which utilizes the peroxidase-like property of hemoglobin (1). The reagent area of the system is impregnated with cumene hydroperoxide, o-tolidine, and a buffer. The procedure for the test involves dipping the reagent into the urine and comparing with a color chart at 30 seconds. Hemoglobin, if present, will catalyze the oxidation of o-tolidine by the hydroperoxide. If there is no catalysis by hemoglobin or myoglobin, the oxidation will not occur under the conditions of the test. Oxidation gives rise to a blue color, an oxidized derivative of o-tolidine.

The microscopic identification of red cells in urine sediment as a test for occult blood in urine is satisfactory only when hemolysis has not occurred and when performed in a standard manner by qualified personnel. Fetter and Free (6), in discussing the difficulty of distinguishing red cells from other components of the urine sediment state "The usual procedure is to examine the unstained sediment and the usual person to make the identification is the laboratory person least qualified to do it." With the establishment of good chemical procedures for recognizing occult blood in urine, it has become evident that with a very appreciable proportion of excreted blood, the erythrocytes are hemolyzed. Leonards (20) indicated that 95% of urines containing occult blood contain some portion of it as free hemoglobin. Figure 3 presents a summary of data from random urines from hospital patients containing occult blood (1). In this figure, the approximate amount of hemolysis is shown. In this series, all but 10% of the urines contained free hemoglobin.

A dip-and-read test for occult blood provides for rapid screening for occult blood in urine since it reacts with free hemoglobin as well as intact red cells. Sources of error with the procedure may arise from improper mixing of the urine sample prior to testing so that cells which have settled to the bottom are not made available to the reagent system. Very large quantities of ascorbic acid in the urine will inhibit or interfere with

TABLE I—RENAL DISEASE IN WHICH PROTEINURIA AND HEMATURIA MAY OCCUR

Acute Glomerulonephritis	Malignant Nephrosclerosis
Acute Pyelonephritis	Multiple Myeloma
Acute Renal Failure	Nephrolithiasis
Amyloid Kidney	Nephrosis
Angioseratoma Corporus Diffusum	Obstructive Uropathy
Chronic Glomerulonephritis	Papillary Necrosis
Chronic Pyelonephritis	Periarteritis
Chronic Renal Failure	Polycystic Kidney
Chyluria	Preeclampsia
Eclampsia	Radiation Nephritis
Fanconi Syndrome	Renal Arterial Occlusion
Grawitz's Tumor	Renal Vein Thrombosis
Hereditary Nephritis	Scleroderma of the Kidney
Hypercalcemia Nephropathy	Sickle Cell Nephropathy
Intercapillary Glomerulosclerosis	Systemic Lupus Erythematosis
Kimmelsteil-Wilson Disease	The Kidney of Gout
Lipoid Nephrosis	Wilms's Tumor

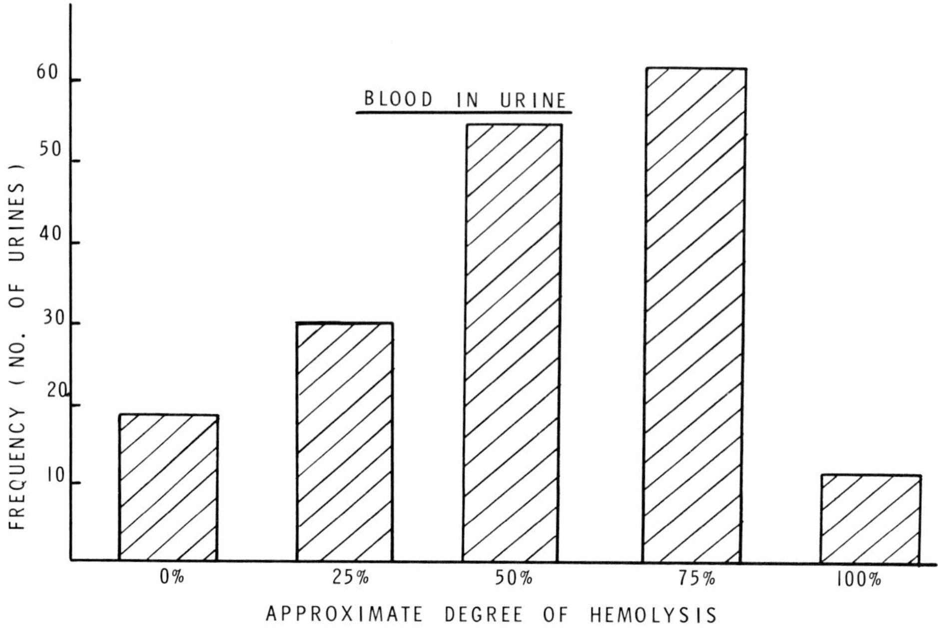

Fig. 3. Extent of hemolysis in urines giving positive chemical test for occult blood.

proper reactivity. Normally, there is not occult blood present in the urine. Positive reactions will occur when quantities of blood of the order of 1 part in 50,000 to 1 part to 100,000 are present. Equivalent amounts of myoglobin have the same reactivity to the test system as hemoglobin. Since erythrocytes may be hemolyzed and since hemoglobin or myoglobin may be excreted directly from the plasma into the urine, it is not practical to precisely relate the sensitivity of an occult blood test to the number of cells per high power field. Ordinarily, any urine in which there are 10 or more red cells per high power field will give a positive reaction with the dip-and-read test for occult blood in urine. In some instances where hemolysis has occurred or where hemoglobin or myoblogin has been excreted, the reactivity will occur with fewer cells or no cells in the sediment.

Table I also presents a compilation of information on the occurrence of occult blood in urine in disorders of the kidney. The information on occult blood was derived in the same manner that was used for proteinuria (2, 14, 5, 22, 24, 27, 26). It is quite striking that practically all disorders of the kidney may result in the excretion of occult blood in the urine. This does not mean that every case of these diseases will show urinary occult blood and it must be remembered that blood may occur in the urine in diseases other than those of renal origin.

SCREENING TESTS
FOR URINARY pH

The kidney has a remarkable ability to excrete urine which is much more acid than the blood from which it is formed or, alternatively, much more alkaline than the blood. By this mechanism, the kidney plays an important role in maintaining the acid-base balance of the blood.

Colorimetric tests for pH are popular and most are satisfactory. However, some are not made specifically for use with urine and, consequently, may have some deficiency in this area. The pH area of Labstix is specifically designed for use with urine. It utilizes two separate indicators — methyl red and bromthymol blue — to provide a wide color span throughout the urinary pH range of 5 to 9. Color changes from orange through green to blue allow easy differentiation of each pH unit. Nitrazine paper is frequently used to measure urinary pH but the directions call for a correction factor when the test is used with urine. Urinary pH can be measured electrometrically with a pH meter but this is inconvenient as a screening method.

Sources of error in urinary pH measurement may arise from bacterial decomposition of the urine after voiding. Bacterial decomposition may make the pH more acid or more alkaline but most commonly the change is to a more alkaline pH. Certain materials (such as acids) used as urine preservatives modify the pH of the urine.

There is a wide "normal" range for pH, from approximately pH 5 to a pH slightly over 8. pH values which are potentially useful in providing screening information fall into approximately the same pH range. However, identification of certain urine pH values tends to indicate possible renal disorders.

In renal tubular acidosis, the kidney is unable to excrete an acid urine with a pH of as low as 5 (16, 23). Accordingly, if urine pH is part of a screening program, the possible correlation of urine pH with suspected renal tubular acidosis is provided. In many urinary tract infections, an alkaline urine may be excreted

TABLE II

URINE PH IN SCREENING FOR RENAL DISEASE

Renal Tubular Acidosis
Urinary Tract Infection
Drug Therapy Monitor
Prophylaxis of Renal Calculi
Renal Tubular Alkalosis
Fanconi Syndrome

as a result of the influence of bacteria in causing breakdown of urea to alkaline decomposition products. The excretion or retention of certain drugs is markedly influenced by urinary pH and in such instances information on urine pH is important. Renal calculi are formed from a number of materials. Acid urine tends to favor the formation of certain types of stones and the solution of other types. Correspondingly, alkaline urine has an influence in favoring stone formation from phosphate but minimizing the formation of stones from cystine and uric acid. In renal tubular alkalosis (26), the kidney is unable to excrete an alkaline urine and in such instances the urine pH never falls in the upper pH range. In Fanconi's syndrome a tubular defect in reabsorption occurs and in this condition, and acid urine is never excreted (26).

SCREENING FOR URINARY GLUCOSE

Usually, the major objective in screening for glucose in urine is the detection of diabetes. Detection of renal disease per se is a minor objective, although severe untreated diabetics may have already developed nephropathy. The principle on which screening tests for glucose are based involves the use of enzyme glucose oxidase to catalyze the oxidation of glucose to form gluconic acid and hydrogen peroxide. In turn, a second enzyme peroxidase catalyzes the reaction of hydrogen peroxide with o-tolidine to form a blue color. Reagents for this screening procedure are the "dip-and-read" type and consist of cellulose areas impregnated with the components required for this reaction. The composition is dipped into the urine specimen and if glucose is present, the color changes from red to purple in 10 seconds.

A possible source of error in urinary glucose tests is the presence of very large amounts of ascorbic acid in the urine which may inhibit or delay color development with the enzymatic tests. Ascorbic acid is a powerful reducing agent and affects the oxidation system in the test reagent. It must be present in very large amounts such as those excreted by patients receiving intravenous feedings or other types of therapeutic doses including the large amounts added as antioxidants to various parenteral preparations. Another minor source of error is contamination of the urine specimen by collection in a container not previously rinsed free of strong oxidizing agents (such as bleaching compounds, either chlorine type or hydrogen peroxide). Another possible source of error in glucose testing is the destruction of glucose by bacteria if the samples are not tested soon enough after collection.

Normally the urine does not contain glucose in sufficient quantities to be detected by the usual sensitive screening procedures. In renal glycosuria, the range is variable but tends to be more in the range of lower levels excreted by untreated diabetics.

Screening for glucose for detection of renal glycosuria is of clinical importance. For example, with present methods it is much easier to apply a test for urine glucose than it is to apply a test for amino acids to detect the Fanconi syndrome, which can then be confirmed by amino acid analysis (26). A screening test for blood glucose is often of value in separating those patients with renal glycosuria from those with glycosuria due to diabetes mellitus.

SCREENING FOR CYSTINURIA

W. E. Knox (19) defines cystinuria as a hereditary anomaly of renal function in which there is impaired renal tubular reabsorption of cystine, lysine, arginine and ornithine. Cystinuria was one of the first four "inborn errors of metabolism" described by Garrod (10) in 1908. There are two types of cystinuria which seem to be related to two separate autosomal recessive genes. Around 1930, Lewis (21) used a simple screening test on 10,000 students at the University of Michigan and from these data estimated the incidence of cystinuria to be 1 in 600 in a typical American population. Some of the positive reactions may include heterozygotes of Type II cystinuria who excrete cystine in abnormal quantities but do not form stones.

Lewis used a screening test involving nitroprusside and cyanide solutions added to urine to give a purple color. Fischl *et al.* (7) simplified testing by mixing sodium nitroprusside, sodium cyanide, sodium carbonate and ammonium sulfate as a powder. A few drops of urine added to a little of the powder produced a purple color with abnormal amounts of cystine. A convenient screening test was reported by Cheuk *et al.* in 1963. (4) This procedure uses a 10% solution of sodium cyanide in 1N NaOH along with a stable tablet (Acetest) as the source of nitroprusside and buffer. The method for this screening test is:

Place an Acetest tablet in the depression of a spot plate. Add one drop of 10% sodium cyanide in 1N NaOH to the tablet and immediately add one drop of urine. Use droppers which will deliver drops sufficiently large so that two drops make enough solution around the tablet to observe for color. Observe the solution around the tablet for a cherry-red color at one minute which indicates the presence of cystine in concentrations of 25 mg. or more per 100 ml. The intensity of cherry-red color is roughly proportional to the amount of cystine.

The convenience of the test is obvious. A large series of urine specimens can be screened in a few minutes. This is in contrast to the test-tube screening test which requires a longer period for color development. Hambraeus (13) in Sweden has reported false negative reactions on urines containing cystine but his technic differed from that of the authors. He examined the surface of the tablet for color formation whereas the method states that the *solution in the spot plate around the tablet* gives the cherry-red color change. In this regard, it is important to use drops big enough to allow two drops to flow off the surface of the tablet. Cyanide is a dangerous chemical. Employment in an alkaline solution minimizes volatilization. If proper precautions are taken, it can be used safely in spite of its poisonous nature.

The powder test produces a purple color with urine containing ketone bodies. However, the tablet test, though it was designed as a test for ketonuria, will not give a color with even large amounts of acetone or acetoacetic acid using the cystine detection procedure just described. This is because the addition of the cyanide solution to the tablet prevents its reaction with ketones. The incidence of ketonuria is much greater than that of cystinuria. In a recent screening program, 9 of 1,702 urines from healthy subjects gave positive reactions for ketones. It is, therefore, important to prevent color formation with ketones in a screening program for cystinuria.

The basis of the color reaction of cystine is the reduction of cystine to cysteine which then forms the cherry-red color with nitroprusside. Cysteine is not found in urine in concentrations great enough to give a positive reaction. Homocystine is the only other substance occurring in urine which is known to give the cherry-red color typical of cystinuria. However, it is also of extreme importance to detect homocystine in urine, since it, too, signifies a genetic defect with even more serious consequences than cystinuria since there is a threat of mental deficiency with homocystine (11).

The normal excretion of cystine is reported to be 40 to 80 mg per day whereas the amount excreted by cystinurics ranges from 700 to 1,500 mg per day. The recognition of cystinuria is of importance to the clinician because after a positive screening test is confirmed with follow-up studies, dietary treatment can be instituted to prevent the formation of cystine stones in the kidney.

NITRITE IN URINE AS A SCREENING TEST FOR BACTERIURIA

Over the course of a half century, consideration has been given to the use of a test for nitrite in urine as an indicator of bacteriuria. Normally, there is approximately one-half gram of nitrate excreted in the urine each day. There is no significant amount of the reduced nitrite in urine but this material appears if urine in the urinary tract is subject to the reducing activity of certain bacteria.

Nitrite can be demonstrated in urine by the use of a diazotizing reaction in which the nitrite in urine provides the basis for the formation of a diazonium compound from a precursor such as sulfanilic acid. This diazonium compound then couples with a suitable compound to form a colored complex. A positive reaction for nitrite is evidenced by the appearance of a pink color when the reagents are added to urine. Recently, two commercial test systems for nitrite in urine have appeared (Stat-test; Nitur-test). Each of these is based on the employment of the diazonium reaction. Each provides a convenient approach to a test for urinary nitrite which is readily adapted to screening.

Nitrite in urine can be accurately and confidently recognized by a chemical test. The principal problem or "source of error" is that in a very considerable proportion of cases of bacteriuria, there is not any nitrite in the urine. This may be due to low dietary nitrate intake with consequent inadequate nitrate in the urine to serve as a precursor for nitrite. Certain organisms involved in renal infections do not effect a reduction of nitrate. Finally, there may be an inadequate time exposure of the urine to allow for nitrite formation. Ordinarily, there is no nitrite in urine and bacteriuria is the only significant factor giving rise to nitrite formation so, consequently, nitrite tests for bacteriuria do not show many false positive reactions.

Bacteriuria is regarded as an important medical problem. Kass (17) suggests that approximately 3,000,000 females and 300,000 males in the United States have infections of the urinary tract at any given moment. Current day studies of the nitrite test as a means of identifying bacteriuria have given definition of the correlation between positive nitrite tests and bacteriuria identified by a conventional bacteriological procedure. Kincaid-Smith and associates (18) found 35% of established cases of bacteriuria showing nitrite in the urine. Fuchs and Gutensohn (9) in a similar study observed a positive nitrite in 10% of urines containing 100,000 to 1,000,000 gram negative organisms per ml, 46% positive nitrite when the count was 1,000,000 to 10,000,000 and 78% positive with cases where the count exceeded 10,000,000 per ml.

During the fifty years that tests for nitrite have been available, such tests have not achieved any significant popularity or usage. This is attested to by the fact that most compilations of laboratory procedures in either clinical pathology or clinical chemistry make no reference to the testing for nitrite. With interest in screening becoming widespread, it will be interesting to observe the degree of popularity achieved by a test procedure which recognizes approximately one-half of the cases of what is generally agreed to be an important medical problem.

SUMMARY

A number of screening procedures are available for recognizing chemical components of urine which may be associated with renal disease. Positive screening tests provide the basis for further study. Extension of the usage of these screening tests should contribute to the earlier and more accurate diagnosis of renal disease.

REFERENCES

1. Adams, E. C., Jr., Fetter, M. C., Free, H. M., and Free, A. H.: Hemolysis in hematuria. J. Urology, *88*:427-430, 1962.
2. Beeson, P. B., and McDermott, W.: Cecil-Loeb Textbook of Medicine, 12th ed. Philadelphia, W. B. Saunders, 1967.
3. Bright, R.: Reports of Medical Cases Selected with a View of Illustrating the Symptoms and Cure of Disease by a Reference to Morbid Anatomy. London, Longman, Rees, Orme, Brown and Green, 1827.
4. Cheuk, Y. H., Free, H. M., and Free, A. H.: A simple test for cystinuria. Proceedings of Division of Biological Chemistry. Abstracts of 143rd Meeting of American Chemical Society, Cincinnati, Ohio, 1963. p 43A.
5. Davis, L.: Christopher's Textbook of Surgery, 8th ed. Philadelphia, W. B. Saunders, 1964.
6. Fetter, M. C., and Free, A. H.: The inadequacy of microscopic exaimations of urine for occult blood. Amer. J. Med. Tech., *28*:135-140, 1962.
7. Fischl, J., Sason, I., and Segal, S.: A rapid spot test for the determination of cystinuria and aminoaciduria. Clin. Chem., *7*:674-677, 1961.
8. Free, A. H., Rupe, C. O., and Metzler, I.: Studies with a new colorimetric test for proteinuria. Clin. Chem. *3*716-727, 1957.
9. Fuchs, T., and Gutensohn, G.: Wert and Grenzen des Nitrit-Tests bei der Diagnostik einer Pyelonephritis. Dtsch. Med. J., *18*:343-347, 1967.
10. Garrod, A. E.: Inborn errors of metabolism. Lancet, *2*:1, 1908.
11. Gerritsen, T., and Waisman, H. A.: Homcystinuria, an error in the metabolism of methionine. Pediatrics, *33*:413-420, 1964.
12. Hall, R.: Albustix: False-positive reactions. Brit. Med. J., *2*:1566, 1961.
13. Hambraeus, L.: Comparative studies of the value of two cyanide-nitroprusside methods in the diagnosis of cystinuria. Cystinuria in Sweden. Part IX. Scandinav. J. Clin. and Lab. Invest., *15*:657-659, 1963.
14. Harrison, T. R., *et al.*: Principles of Internal Medicine, 5th ed. New York, McGraw-Hill, 1966.
15. Hoffman, W. S.: The Biochemistry of Clinical Medicine, 3rd ed. Chicago, Year Book Medical Publishers, 1964.
16. Huth, E. J.: Renal tubular syndromes and immunologic disorders. Bull. Path., *8*:294-295, 1967.
17. Kass, E. H.: Geographic pathology of bacteriuria. In Mostofi, F. K., and Smith, D. E. (eds): The Kidney. Baltimore, Williams and Wilkins Co., 1966, pp 469-475.
18. Kincaid-Smith, P., Bullen, M., Mills, J., Fussell, U., and Huston, N.: The reliability of screening tests for bacteriuria in pregnancy. Lancet, *2*:61-62, 1964.
19. Knox, W. E.: Cystinuria. In, Stanbury, J. B., Wyngaarden, J. B., and Fredrickson, D. S. (eds): Metabolic Basis of Inherited Disease. New York, McGraw-Hill, 1966 pp 1262-1282.
20. Leonards, J. R.: Simple test for hematuria compared with established tests. J. A. M. A., *179*:807-808, 1962.
21. Lewis, H. B.: The occurence of cystinuria in healthy young men and women. Ann. Int. Med., *6*:183-192, 1932.
22. Nelson, W. E.: Textbook of Pediatrics, 8th ed. Philadelphia, W. B. Saunders, 1964.
23. Relman, A. S.: Renal acidosis and renal excretion of acid in health and disease. Advances in Int. Med., *12*:295-347, 1964.
24. Schaffer, A. J.: Diseases of the Newborn, 2nd ed. Philadelphia, W. B. Saunders, 1965.
25. Sorenson, S. P. L.: Enzymstudien. II. Uber die Messung and die Bedeutung der Wasserstoffenkonzentration bei enzymatischen Prozessen. Biochem. Z., *21*:131, 1909. O26.
26. Strauss, M. B., and Welt, L. C.: Diseases of the Kidney. Boston, Little, Brown and Company, 1963.
27. Willson, J. R., Beecham, C. T., and Carrington, E. R.: Obstetrics and Gynecology, 2nd ed. St. Louis, C. V. Mosby Co., 1963.

Chapter 15

Qualitative Identification of Urinary Pigments

EARL B. WERT, M.D.

INTRODUCTION

The metabolites of certain drugs and metabolic substances coloring the urine defy chemical identification, while others (homogentisic acid, porphyrins) can be identified simply and with relative assurance. No satisfactory scheme is available for rapid identification of all urinary chromogens, many of which are complex and of uncertain and often inconsistent chemical structure. The pigments appearing in the urine will be considered under the headings of: a) drugs, foods, and dyes; b) bile pigments; c) porphyrins; d) melanogens-melanins; e) hemoglobin and derivatives; f) myoglobin; g) inborn errors of metabolism; and h) miscellaneous conditions.

In recent years, the demonstration in the urine of increasing numbers of chemical compounds has provided exacting technics for the diagnosis of inborn errors of metabolism, porphyria, etc. On the other hand, less attention is now paid to other time-honored substances; for example, the demonstration of urinary bile pigments in differential diagnosis. Some of these substances are merely of academic or historic interest, for example, "biliverdin," since the chemical nature of certain compounds has become more dubious rather than established, and the products shown to be those of reversible oxidation reduction reactions of a spurious nature, not consistently related to specific biochemical processes.

The pigmentation of normal urine is due to "urochrome," apparently a compound of urobilin and peptide, and its concentration is proportional to the metabolic rate, as in fever, and to the specific gravity of the specimen. In spite of complexities, most pigmentary substances can be identified by the following simple schema:

1. Consider the possibility of more than one substance coloring urine.

2. Eliminate formed elements as a cause of the abnormal appearance by centrifugation (phosphate crystals, erythrocytes).

3. Check the patient's drug and diet intake. See list of drugs, foods, and dyes which follows.

4. Eliminate common pigments by simple tests for:

    a. Bile pigments ("Ictotest"–Ames Co.)

b. Hemoglobin derivatives (Hema-test"–Ames Co.) (Spectral Absorption)

5. Note effect of mild oxidizing agents, especially on standing in light, and with $FeCl_3$.

6. Note fluorescence under Wood's light.

7. Special screening procedures:
   a. Watson-Schwartz test for porphobilinogen.
   b. Coproporphyrin screening test.

8. Spectral absorption curves in ultraviolet region.

Ferric chloride has been used commonly for qualitative identification of a variety of urinary chromogens. The components in urine that react with ferric chloride have been listed in Table I. The color produced by ferric chloride results from oxidation of the compound in question, often with chelation of the Fe ion into the complex. The long list of substances reacting attests to the non-specificity of the reactions, and the colors are often difficult to distinguish. Nevertheless, no reaction serves to rule-out suspected conditions, and the test remains a valuable adjunct to screening methods. Ferric chloride is available also as the reagent in an impregnated paper (marketed by Ames Co. as "Phenistix") designed originally to detect phenylpyruvic acid in a semi-quantitative fashion. Magnesium is included to minimize interference, and an acid buffer facilitates maximal color.

Consistency in color nomenclature should be sought. To this end, Circular 553 and color-name chart supplement prepared by the U. S. Department of Commerce, Nationa Bureau of Standards, is recommended (1). Kelley and co-workers present in the circular a "universal color language," some thirty years in development. Using the charts and text, a color can be coded. Thus, a shade of yellow can be designated "#67 Brill. OY" (color number 67 on the color charts, named "brilliant orange yellow"). Thus, the light rose of porphobilinogen may properly be designated "#2 s. pk." (color number 2, strong pink). "Mauve" and "mauvette" have found their way into no less than 38 color names identifying hues from light pink to dark green!

In Table II are listed procedures for the qualitative identification of miscellaneous substances that may color the urine.

A) DRUGS, FOODS, AND DYES

Introduction

"Mysterious" substances coloring the urine transiently are numerous, and usually are the metabolic products or the dye contained in drugs, foods, and dyes.

Riboflavin (Vitamin B_2) may cause the urine to be green, green-yellow, or brightly yellow. Identification may be effected microbiologically using Lactobacillus casei (2) correcting for the inhibitory effect of urea (3), especially at low riboflavin levels. Photometric (4) and fluorometric (5, 6) methods are available for urine identification and quantitation. In 1935, Koschara (7) isolated a crystalline flavin which he termed uroflavin, a pigment almost identical to riboflavin and apparently an excretion product. The method for identification is fluorometric. The urinary output of riboflavin varies with dosage immediately before the test and gives no indication of body stores of this vitamin (8). The output varies greatly from 50 to 7,500 μg per 24 hours.

TABLE I—URINARY CHROMOGENS: REACTANTS IN FERRIC CHLORIDE TESTS
(From: Henry, R. J.: Clinical Chemistry, Principles and Technics. Hoeber and Row, Pub., 1964 (15))

Substance	Color Produced With	
	Ferric Chloride Solution	*Phenistix*
Phenylpyruvic acid	Green or blue-green eventually fading to yellow	Gray-green or blue-green, max. 1 min., fade slowly
p-Hydroxyphenyl pyruvic acid	Green, fades in seconds	Green, fades in seconds
o-Hydroxyphenyl pyruvic acid	Initial red-brown turning green or blue then fading to mauve	Green, max., at 1 min.
o-Hydroxyphenyl acetic acid	Mauve	Very pale Mauve
Acetoacetic acid	Red or red-brown	Nil
Pyruvic acid	Deep gold yellow or green (?)	Gold yellow
Homogentisic acid	Blue or green, fades quickly	Nil, brown with stronger solution
3-Hydroxyanthranilic acid	Immediate deep brown	Yellow, turns green at 1 min., later brown
Salicylates	Stable purple	Stable purple
p-Aminosalicylic acid	Red-brown	Pink to purple
Phenol derivs.	Violet	Nil
Vanillic acid	Red-manve, turns deep brown	Brown
Xanthurenic acid	Deep green, later brown	Nil
α-Ketobutyric acid	Purple, fades to red-brown in 1 to 2 min.	Faint brown-purple
Maple syrup disease urine	Gray with green tinge	Nil
Cyanates	Red	?
Phenothiazine derivs. (Compazine, Thorazine)	Purple	?
Bilirubin	Blue-green	?
Melanin	Gray ppt., turning black	?
Antipyrines & aceto-phenetidines	Red	?
Imidazolepyruvic acid	Green or blue-green	Gray green or blue-green

TABLE II—IDENTIFICATION OF MISCELLANEOUS SUBSTANCES

Substance	Acid (HCl)	Alkaline (NaOH)	Remarks
Anthracine derivatives yielding emodin and chrysophanic acid (aloe, cascara, rhubarb, and senna)	yellow-brown	red-violet	negative tests for bilirubin
Phenolphthalein	colorless	red	absorption band 556 mμ
Phenolsulphonphthalein	colorless	red	absorption band 556 mμ
Bromsulfalein	colorless	red	
Eosin	clear	pink	green fluorescence, absorption band 520 mμ
Phenol, cresol	clear	olive to black	
Pyridium	red	colorless	clear at either extreme of the pH scale
Santonin	yellow	pink-scarlet	
Thymol	colorless	olive on oxidation	
Anthocyanin (blackberries, beat root)	red	yellow	

Spectral Absorption Curves

The accurate determination of absorption spectra in acid, neutral, and alkaline media is indispensable for identification of certain urinary substances, especially drugs. A recording spectrophotometer, preferably of the double-beam type with ultraviolet capabilities, is required. The urine sample (1.0 ml) is diluted with 50 to 100 ml of absolute ethanol until the absorbance is less than 0.5 O.D. units. Neutrality of the specimen is thus produced and a blank composed of normal urine similarly treated is prepared. The spectral absorption curve is run between 325 and 200 mμ in the ultra-violet range. (The greatest degree of specificity for compounds is achieved in this ultraviolet region. The visible portion of the spectrum may be used but is limited by the lack of specific absorption pattern.) The sample and blank are then acidified with 0.5 N H_2SO_4, and the absorption pattern again recorded. If necessary, the sample may be further diluted with the acid until the optical density remains below 0.5 units, in the interest of accuracy of the readings. The same acidified sample and blank (or a second sample from the alcohol treated urine specimen and freshly prepared blank) are alkalinized with 0.5 N NaOH similarly maintaining the optical density at less than 0.5 units. The absorption curve of the alkalinized specimen is read. The curves of absorption obtained in acid, neutral, and alkaline solution are now compared. The amount of shift due to change in pH is noted. The absorption maxima and minima and the change are characteristic for the compound. For example, the change of maximal absorption from 255 mμ

in alkaline media to 240 mμ in acid media is characteristic for secobarbital. Reference volumes (9-11) provide comparison data for provisional identification of compounds. While compounds are generally identified in tables by both maximal and minimal points of absorbance, only maximal points (usually 2, rarely 1 or more than 4) are referred to in other descriptive literature of the essay type. It is important, however, to verify the values by running the absorption curves on the same instrument as the unknown, using the known solution of the suspected drug.

In the interest of compiling a complete reference list of material capable of coloring the urine, questionnaires were submitted to 25 leading drug manufacturers. Their answers tabulated together with similar lists previously published. Metabolites are included for reference purposes.

REFERENCE LIST OF MATERIALS WHICH MAY COLOR URINE

Urine Color	Associated Drug, Food, Dye, or Metabolite
Blue	acid copper sulfate (Diagnix:Squibb) methylene blue pseudomonas ingestion Certified color in water and propylene glycol.
Blue Fluorescence	triamterene (Dyrenium: Smith, Kline, French)
Blue-Green	amitriptyline (Elavil:Merck, Sharpe, Dohme) tetralin tolonium (Blutene Chloride:Abbott) Doan's liver pills
Green-to Dark Green	anthraquinone arbutin bile pigments copper sulfate, acid solution (Diagnix:Squibb) creosote eosins methocarbamol (Robaxin:Robins) phenyl salicylate resorcinol (resorcin) tetrahydronaphthalene thymol Certified color in water and propylene glycol.
Green or Yellow	carotene-containing foods methylene blue riboflavin Vitamin B complex yeast concentrate
Yellow	benefin (Balan:Elanco) phenacetin picric acid quinacrine (Atabrine:Winthrop) riboflavin santorin trifluralin (Treflan:Elanco) Certified color in water and propylene glycol.

URINE COLOR	ASSOCIATED DRUG, FOOD, DYE, OR METABOLITE
Orange to Yellow-Brown in alkaline urine	salicylazosulfapyridine (Azulfidine:Pharmacia)
Yellow or Pink (acid urine)	aloe, cascara

Orange	furazolidine (Furoxone:Eaton)
	Inandione derivatives in alkaline urine, e.g.,
	    anisindione (Miradon:Schering)
	    diphenadione (Dipoxin)
	    phenindione (Danilone, Eridione, Hedulin)
	phenazopyridine HCI (Azotrix:Bristol; Urobiotic:Pfizer)
	rhubarb
	senna
	azo gantrisin

Orange to Orange Red	ethoxanzene (Serenium:Squibb) phenylazopyridine (Pyridium:Warner-Chilcott; Azo-Mandelamine: Warner-Chilcott; Dolonil: Warner-Chilcott)
Orange or Purplish Red	chlorzoxazone (Paraflex:McNeil)
Orange to Red Brown	phenylazopyridine (Pyridium:Warner-Chilcott) santonin
Orange or Brown	furaxolidone (Furoxone:Eaton)
Rust Yellow or Brownish	chlorzoxazone (Paraflex:McNeil) danthron (Dionone:Dorbane, Istizin) (acid urine) heavy metals (bismuth, mercury) liver poisons: jaundice (alcohol, arsenicals, carbon tetrachloride, chloral hydrate, chlorinated hydro-carbons, chlorobutanol, chloroform, cincophen) naphthalene neocinchophen nitrofurantoins (Furoxone, Furacin, Furadantin:Eaton) pamaquine (Aminoquin, Beprochine, Gamegar, Plasmoquine, Pracquine, Quipenyl) pamaquine naphthoate (Plasmochin:Winthrop) primaquine chloroquine (Aralen:Winthrop) Sulfonamides tribromomethanol with amylene hydrate (Avertin)
Browish Red	metronidazole (Flagyl:Searle)
Pink and Red to Red Brown	aloin aniline dyes (in sweets) aminopyrine, dipyrone anthraquinone and its dyes antipyrine (Pyrazoline) pyridium (amido pyrine) beet root (red dye) benyene carbontetrachloride chrysarobin (alkaline urine) cinchophen danthron (Dorbane) (pink to violet–alkaline urine) diphenylhydantoin (Dilantin:Parke-Davis) emodin (alkaline urine) eosins (red with green fluorescence) hematuria producers (mercuric salts, irritants, etc.)

URINE COLOR   ASSOCIATED DRUG, FOOD, DYE, OR METABOLITE

                           hemolysis producers
                           indanedione derivatives; anisodione (Miradon:Schering);
                               phenindione (Hedulin:Walker, Danilone)
                           trional
                           phenolic metabolites (glucuronides)
                           phenolphthalein (alkaline urine)
                           phenothiazines
                           phensuximide (Milontin:Parke-Davis)
                           picoic acid
                           porphyrins
                           Povan (for pinworms)
                           prochlorperazine (Compazine)
                           santonin (alkaline urine)
                           sulfonal
                           thiazolsulfone (Promizole)
                           urates (especially newborn infants and during tumor lysis)
                           Certified color in water and propylene glycol.

Brown   funazolidone (Furoxone:Eaton)
                           nitrofurantoin (Furadantin:Eaton)
                           nitrofurazone (Furacin:Eaton)

Brown to Black   aniline dyes
                           cascara
                           chlorinated hydrocarbons
                           hydroxyquinone
                           melanin
                           methocarbomol (Robaxin:Robins)
                           naphthalene
                           naphthol
                           nitrites
                           nitrofurans: furazolidone (Furoxone:Eaton); nitrofurazone (Furacin:Eaton)
                           phenol
                           phenyl salicylate (salol)
                           pyrogallol
                           quinine and its derivatives
                           resorcinol (resorcin)
                           rhubarb
                           santonin
                           senna
                           thymol

Black   iron-sorbitol-citric acid complex (Jectofer:Astra)

Magenta to   fuchsin
Purple   phenolphthalein (in alkaline urine)

Darkening on   cascara
standing   chlorpromazine (Thorazine:Smith, Kline, French)
                           methocarbamol (Robaxin:Robins)
                           methyldopa (Aldomet:Merch, Sharpe, Dohme)
                           methronidazole (Flagyl:Searle)

Discoloration   naphthol

non-specific   nitrogenzene
                           p-aminosalicylic acid and its derivatives
                           phenals
                           salol

B) BILE PIGMENTS

DETERMINATION OF BILIRUBIN IN THE URINE

Introduction

Bile pigments, some colored and some colorless, find their way into the urine. Their (straight chain) molecules are made of 4 pyrrole rings joined by methene ($-CH_2$) or methyne ($-CH=$) groups. While much of the chemistry of bile pigments is obscure, the following provides a working concept for clinical purposes. Bilirubin (free, unmodified, indirect) is formed in the reticulo-endothelial system by breakdown of hemoglobin and is transported in plasma as protein (albumin)-bound complex. The liver and perhaps other extrahepatic sites conjugate the (free, albumin bound) bilirubin with acids (glucuronic, sulfuric, etc.) and excrete the (modified, direct conjugated) bilirubin into the bile-ducts. Thus, jaundice is of two chemical types due to either free bilirubin (hemolytic jaundice) or conjugated bilirubin (obstructive jaundice).

Billing (12) points out that conjugated bilirubin is easily converted to free bilirubin by alkalinization and suggests a linkage of the ester type,—the propionic side chain of the bilirubin linking with the hydroxyl of the aldehyde group of glucuronic acid. Direct proof of this has been provided by Schachter (13) and by Yamaoka (14). The insolubility of free bilirubin in water at neutrality and its attachment to albumin may explain its absence in the urine. On the other hand, the albumin-free conjugated bilirubin, including conjugates with bile salts (e.g., glycocholate), enters the urine freely.

Tests for bilirubin in the urine fall into 4 groups:

1. Observation of yellow color or brown color (foam test)

2. Addition of dye until bile color is obscured (methylene blue)

3. Oxidation of bilirubin to characteristic color (iodine ring, HNO_3)

4. Diazotinization ("Ictotest" of Free) These tests have been summarized by Henry (15). The method of Free ("Ictotest" — Ames Co.) approaches the ideal as a qualitative test for bilirubin and is the procedure of choice.

Principle

Bilirubin is detected by diazotinization, employing a tablet containing p-nitrobenzenediazonium p-toluenesulfonate, sodium bicarbonate, sulfosalicylic acid, and boric acid.

Reagents

Test mats and "Ictotest" reagent tablets (kit form — Ames Co.)

Procedure

Five drops of urine are placed on one square of special test mat. An "Icotest" reagent tablet is placed in the center of the moistened area, and two drops of water are allowed to flow onto the tablet. If the mat around the tablet turns blue or purple within 30 seconds, the test is positive. Any color after 30 seconds and slight pink or red colors are ignored. The amount of bilirubin is proportional to the speed and intensity of the color developed.

Discussion

A rough quantitation may be made by serial dilution of the urine, — the highest dilution giving a positive color reaction will contain 0.1 mg per 100 ml, the sensitivity of the test.

Sources of Error

Bilirubin is unstable, and tests may become negative in one hour if in sunlight or elevated temperatures. The oxidation products include "biliverdin", which can be detected by oxidation tests (e.g., Harrison's spot test employing $FeCl_3$ in trichloracetic acid on urine concentrated on $BaCl_2$). The non–specificity of the oxidation tests for bilirubin limits their value.

Ascorbic acid (100 mg per 100 ml) will preserve bilirubin in urine even if allowed to stand at room temperature for 24 hours in alkaline media. Ascorbic acid interferes with the diazo tests, however, while oxidative tests remain positive.

The diazo test ("Ictotest") has a very high degree of specificity, and many studies have failed to show a single false positive. Care must be taken to recognize the effect of urobilin or indican (red color) and salicylates (orange-yellow to red-purple).

UROBILINOIDS
(UROBILINOGEN AND UROBILIN)

Introduction

As secreted from the liver, bilirubin is conjugated, water soluble, and accounts for the yellow color of "bile." On entering the intestine, bacterial action reduces conjugated bilirubin to a variety of colorless chromogens (most of which enter the portal vein to be returned to the liver). A small amount appears in the urine as the colorless chromogenic precursors of the colored urobilin. Together, they (the colorless precursors or chromogens, collectively referred to as "urobilinogen," and their colored oxidation products, collectively referred to as the "urobilin pigments") are known as "urobilinoids."

Urobilinoids are identified by two methods: *Method 1* — All urobilins are reduced to chromogens and determined by benzaldehyde reaction. *Method 2* — All chromogens are oxidized to urobilins and determined by zinc fluorescent reaction. Method 2 is simpler and is recommended as a screening test to exclude urobilinoids. The former method of Watson (16) modified by Henry (15) is preferred.

Method 1. Semi-quantitative Determination of Urobilinogen in Urine

Principle

Urobilins are reduced to urobilinogens by $Fe(OH)_3$ and read photometrically with Ehrlich's aldehyde reaction. Reduction is effected with ascorbic acid, and the color of the complex is intensified with sodium acetate. Alkaline phenolsulfonephthalein (PSP dye) is used as an artificial standard, and results expressed as "Ehrlich units" (1 unit = 1 mg urobilinogen) indicate semi-quantitative and non-specificity of the reaction.

Reagents and Standard Solutions

1. *Ehrlich's Reagent.* Seven-tenths gm of p-dimethylaminobenzaldehyde is dissolved in 150 ml conc. HCl (A.R. grade). One-hundred ml distilled water are added and mixed. Purity of the HCl is important. The reagent is stable.

2. *Sodium Acetate (Saturated).* Anhydrous or triple hydrate acetate (A.R. grade) may be used, leaving some undissolved salt to insure saturation.

3. *Ferrous Sulfate*, 20% solution is kept in a refrigerator and is stable only 24 hours.

4. *Sodium Hydroxide, 2.5 N.*

5. *PSP Dye Standard.* Twenty mg of the acid form of the dye (Eastman Kodak, LaMotte, Mann) are dissolved in 100 ml of 0.05% NaOH, and diluted to one liter with 0.05% NaOH. Thus, 0.20 mg per 100 ml of the dye will give same

absorptivity as 0.346 mg urobilinogen. Unfortunately, not all batches of dye are similar, and the working standard should have an absorbance of 0.384 at 562 mμ. The dye as obtained for intravenous injection is unsuitable.

Procedure

Although any urine may be used, an afternoon specimen is preferred. The bladder is first emptied at 2:00 pm. Then, at 4:00 pm, the specimen is obtained and analyzed promptly without exposure to bright daylight.

1. The volume of the specimen is measured.

2. The urine is tested for bilirubin. If more than a faint trace of bilirubin is present, 2.0 ml of 10% $BaCl_2$ are mixed with 8.0 ml of urine and filtered. The final result must be multiplied by 1.25 to correct the 4:5 dilution.

3. One-hundred mg of ascorbic acid are dissolved in 10 ml of clear urine (centrifuged if turbid), and 1.5 ml aliquots are placed in each of two test tubes or cuvets labeled "X" (unknown) and "B" (blank).

4. To "B" — 4.5 ml freshly prepared mixture of one vol. Ehrlich's reagent and two vol. saturated sodium acetate are added and mixed.

5. To "X" — 1.5 ml Ehrlich's reagent are added and mixed well; then 3.0 ml saturated sodium acetate are *immediately* added to inhibit the development of other Ehrlich reacting substances.

6. The absorbance of "X" and "B" are read at 562 mμ (a filter at 540 mμ is satisfactory) against water, and the PSP standard is read against water at the same wavelength.

7. Calculations are made as follows:

$$\text{Ehrlich units per 100 ml urine} = \frac{A_x - A_b}{A_s} \times 0.346 \times \frac{6.0}{1.5}$$

$$= \frac{A_x - A_b}{A_s} \times 1.38$$

$$\text{Ehrlich units per 2 hours} = \frac{A_x - A_b}{A_s} \times 0.0138 \times \text{volume in ml}$$

Discussion

The method is non-specific and includes other Ehrlich reactors. Fortunately, its clinical use is not usually impaired since these substances increase proportionately with urobilinogen. However, false negative results may approach 15% of cases, and recovery of added urobilinogen is only 40 to 68% depending on the urine, suggesting a variety of inhibiting substances.

Normal Values

0 — 1.1 Ehrlich units per 2 hours. Daily and hourly variation is marked, related to food intake; noctural values are quite low.

Method 2 – Demonstration of Urobilin in Urine by the Zinc Fluorescence Reation

Principle

Urobilinogen is oxidized to urobilin by iodine. Alcoholic zinc acetate produces a zinc-urobilin complex which fluoresces green. The reaction is sensitive, detecting 0.005 mg of urobilin per 100 ml.

Reagents

1. *Alcoholic Suspension of Zinc Acetate.* About 10 gm of zinc acetate are suspended in 100 ml ethanol.

2. *Lugol's Solution.* About 5 gm iodine and 10 gm KI are dissolved in 100 ml water.

Procedure

1. Ten ml of fresh urine are mixed with 10 ml of well-shaken alcoholic zinc-acetate suspension and filtered. Two test tubes (10 mm diam.) are used to collect the filtrate equally.

2. One drop of conc. HCl is added to one tube. Two drops of Lugol's solution are added to *each* tube, and the tubes are mixed by inversion.

3. Fluorescence is observed using a Wood's light. Only a green-yellow fluorescence appearing in the *unacidified tube alone* constitutes a positive test. (HCl is known to destroy urobilin.)

Discussion

Substances which give fluorescence in this test are:

Substance	Color of Fluorescence
biliviolins, bilipurpurins, porphyrins	red
phylloerythrinogen (from chlorophyll found in patients on high vegetable diet)	red
riboflavin, acriflavin, fluorescein	yellow-green
eosin, mercurochrome, erythrosin	mauve (dull)

Bilirubin in the urine does not react.

BILIVERDIN

In the present state of our knowledge, the true nature and significance of biliverdin seem uncertain. It seems reasonable that the oxidation of heme produces verdohemochrome or iron-biliverdin, a green pigment; loss of iron and the addition of two hydrogen atoms produce biliverdin, a green pigment not detectable in normal serum. In obstructive jaundice, high concentrations (up to 2 mg per 100 ml) of a green pigment are found in the serum which can be read at 660 mμ. However, this compound adds little in the differential diagnosis at present and perhaps should be considered merely of historic interest. In recent studies, the chemical nature of biliverdin has become more dubious rather than better established and seems to represent a mixture of substances with spurious oxidation-reduction in the tissues. The demonstration of the compound "biliverdin" in the urine probably depends on secondary processes in the bladder rather than on metabolic alterations secondary to an identifiable disease.

In fact, the chief interest in biliverdin may lie in the recognition that in poorly

TABLE III–CLASSIFICATION OF PORPHYRIA AND RESULTS OF
WATSON–SCHWARTZ TEST FROM SERIES OF 275 CASES (18)

Variety	Number of Cases	Percent of Total Cases	Watson-Schwartz Test Results
Porphyria erythropoietica	7	3	Negative
Porphyria hepatica			
Acute, intermittent, hereditary	161	60	Positive
Cutaneous, hereditary	*	*	Negative
Mixed or varigate, hereditary	14	5	Positive or Negative**
Latent, hereditary	38	15	Positive or Negative**
Constitutional or idiosyncratic (cutanea tarda)	55	20	Negative
Acquired***	- - -	- - -	- - -
Chemical toxicity			
Hepatoma			

*   Percentage included under constitutional or idiosyncratic.

**   Usually positive in patients with abdominal symptoms.

*** Information not available.

preserved urine specimens (in sunlight or at room temperature for periods even less than one hour), bilirubin will have been oxidized to a mixture of substances (chiefly biliverdin) and will give negative tests with diazo procedures for bilirubin ("Icototest" – Ames Co.). The oxidative tests (Harrison's spot test) may remain positive for bilirubin.

C) PORPHYRINS

Introduction

Although the subject of porphyrins and their precursors is complex, two screening tests are available which solve most clinical problems. These tests are the Watson-Schwartz test for porphobilinogen (PBG) in the urine (indicated when any dark or red color is present in the urine, or when urine shows these changes on standing) and the Screening Test for porphyrins which demostrates increased porphyrins, especially coproporphyrins, as encountered in lead poisoning. For a concise review of this subject, the reader is referred to the paper by Patterson and co-workers (17) which appeared in the "Manual on the Porphyrins and the Porphyrias."

PORPHOBILINOGEN

In the most common type of porphyria (acute intermittent porphyria) (A.I.P.), porphobilinogen (PBG) can be demonstrated by the Watson-Schwartz test. Table III, taken from Watson's paper (18), indicates the classification of the porphyrias and the value of the test. Townsend, in testing 1000 routine urine samples with the Watson-Schwartz technic, found no false-positive results

(19). Rarely, due to high concentrations of inhibitor substances, porphobilinogen (PBG) cannot be demonstrated by this method, and one must employ column chromatography by the method of Mauzerall and Granick (20).

QUALITATIVE DETERMINATION OF PORPHOBILINOGEN (PGB)
(METHOD OF WATSON AND SCHWARTZ)

Introduction

The test can be performed on random or 24-hour specimen, but the 24-hour specimen should be collected in a brown bottle containing 5 gm of sodium carbonate (pH below 6.0 is not reliable) to prevent destruction of porphyrins and inhibit conversion of PBG to porphobilin (which is negative with Ehrlich's aldehyde and negative in Wood's light).

Principle

PBG is a precursor of other porphyrins which reacts with Ehrlich's aldehyde reagent (para-di-methyl-aminobenzaldehyde) to form a red color.

Procedure

Urine (2.5 ml) cooled to room temperature and Ehrlich's reagent (2.5 ml) are well-mixed in a test tube. The solution is observed for a pink-red color developing at this stage if PBG is present.

Saturated sodium acetate (5.0 ml) is added. It is important to mix well at this point to insure color enhancement. The solution is tested with Congo red paper, and the color of the paper should remain red. (While the PBG pigment may deepen at this point, deepening may also be due to the presence of urobilinogen.) In any event, if no pink-red color has developed, PBG is absent and no further testing is necessary. If pink-red color is present, urobilinogen and other non-specific Ehrlich-reacting substances may be extracted as follows:

Chloroform (5.0 ml) is added and the solution is shaken and allowed to settle. The chloroform will go to the bottom carrying with it urobilinogen and other interfering substances. The aqueous phase is now at the top, — if colorless, the test is negative. If the pink or red color remains in the top (aqueous) layer it is aspirated and placed in another test tube. Then 5.0 ml butyl alcohol are added to this tube, the tube is shaken well, and the solution is allowed to settle. However, if the butanol (upper) layer is definitely colored pink, the aqueous (lower) layer is again extracted with butyl alcohol to insure that all of the butyl-alcohol soluble color has been removed from the aqueous phase, thus avoiding a false positive reaction.

In the event that pink color remains in the aqueous phase after two thorough extractions with butyl alcohol, additional technics are available, any or all of which should be used to verify the presence of PBG in the aqueous phase.

These are as follows:

1. The Watson-Schwartz test as described previously is repeated employing 22% HCl in place of Ehrlich's reagent. This procedure is followed especially if marked deepening of color has occurred on adding the sodium acetate in the Watson-Schwartz test. If the color deepens or turns a peculiar hue with the HCl reagent, one can suspect interfering drugs (tranquilizers, methyl red, pyridium, etc.) as the cause of the color change.

2. A mixture of equal parts of freshly voided urine and Ehrlich's reagent is examined spectroscopically. PBG will show absorption bands at 560 to 570 mμ and at 515 to 530 mμ (the latter

somewhat weaker). (CAUTION: These bands fade rapidly; examine immediately.)

Note: Additional confirmatory tests have been described, requiring quantitation of uroporphyrin (16).

URINE SCREENING TEST FOR PORPHYRINS (Designed especially to detect coproporphyrins of lead intoxication.)

Procedure

To about 5 ml of freshly voided urine in a test tube are added the following reagents:

0.1 ml of 1% alcoholic iodine solution
1.0 ml of glacial acetic acid
5.0 ml of ether
3 drops of hydrogen peroxide

The reagents are mixed by inversion 8 to 10 times to insure extraction. The solution is then allowed to stand for 15 minutes and is examined in a dark room with Wood's light, noting fluorescence of the ether layer. A pale blue ether layer is a negative reading indicating absence of porphyrins, while violet to pink is 1+, pink to light rose is 2+, light rose to medium rose is 3+, and deep red rose is 4+.

Clinical Interpretation

A repeatedly negative test practically rules out lead poisoning. In the author's laboratory, no false negative results have been found in 100 consecutive urine specimens suspected of lead poisoning. Positive specimens are found in industrial groups proportional to the degree of exposure. Mild exposures produce strongly positive urines, and positive urines can be demonstrated before stippling is seen in the erythrocytes. The excretion of porphyrin continues for considerable periods after exposure to lead.

The urine of patients in sickle-cell crises deserves special attention. Urines thus voided show a characteristic dark-brown color, independent of volume or specific gravity, and the depth of this color darkens on standing or on exposure to sunlight. The sediment of such urine shows magenta fluorescence under Wood's light. Coproporphyrins, uroporphrins, and total porphyrins are quite regularly increased and occasionally the porphyrin precursors porphobilinogen and delta-aminolevulinic acid.

D) MELANOGENS – MELANIN

Introduction

The finding of these tyrosine derivatives in the urine of patients suspected of having disseminated malignant melanoma is of value. The sequential oxidation of tyrosine through indole derivatives may produce melanogens (colorless chromogens) in the urine.

Principle

The urine is oxidized by standing in light and observed for the formation of the melanogen-melanin-protein complex, or oxidized by ferric chloride, or treated with Ehrlich's reagent. More recently, an approach employing spectrophotometry and paper chromatography has added in the identification of these compounds.

Methods

1. *Ferric Chloride Test* (von Jaksch-Pollak Test)

To 5 ml of urine in a test tube, several drops of 10% (w/v) ferric chloride aqueous solution are added until a good precipitate has formed. The tube is centrifuged at 2000 rpm for 5 minutes, and the supernatant and precipitate are examined.

2. *Thormahlen Test*

To 5 ml of urine in a test tube, 0.3 ml of freshly prepared 40% (w/v) aqueous solution of sodium nitroprusside is added and mixed. Five-tenths ml of sodium hydroxide (10%, w/v) is added and mixed. The solution is acidified with the addition of 0.5 ml of glacial acetic acid. The color of the solution is then observed.

3. *Ehrlich Test*

To 2 ml of urine in a test tube are added 2 ml of Ehrlich's aldehyde reagent (0.7 gm para-dimethylaminobenzaldehyde and 150 ml of concentrated hydrochloric acid plus 100 ml of distilled water). Four ml of 70% (w/v) aqueous solution of sodium acetate ($NaC_2H_3O_2 3H_2O$) are added. The color of solution is observed. If solution is red, 5 ml of chloroform are added. The color of the chloroform and aqueous layers is observed.

Discussion

The exact chemical composition of the melanin complex has not been established with certainty due in part to the insolubility of melanin, and attempts to analyse the complex into identifiable fragments have failed. The procedures listed have been critically evaluated and found to be insufficiently sensitive, liable to misinterpretation, and not much more useful than the simple observation of the urine darkening on standing. One should rule out other cause for darkening of the urine by the Watson-Schwartz test for porphobilinogen.

Sources of Error

Salicylates give a red-brown or purple suspension making interpretation difficult. Further, a brown precipitate may form in control specimens which are difficult to distinguish from melanin-containing urines. It is important that only truly gray-black precipitates be regarded as positive. Helman (21), Spencer (22), and Ham (23) modifications of the ferric chloride test do not render it more useful.

Resumé of Clinical Interpretation

About 20% of patients with dissemination of malignant melanoma have melanogenuria. Following resection of sites of dissemination or chemotherapy, the chromogens may diminish or disappear. Duchon and Pechan (24) have reviewed the problems in interpretation of the literature on this subject.

E) HEMOGLOBIN (Occult Blood)

Introduction

Since *some* hemoglobin is always present in urine, it is thus the *excessive* amount of occult blood which concerns the clinician, and the demonstration of hemoglobin (or erythrocytes) in the urine, therefore, must be essentially *quantitative*. Urine normally contains about 0.5 million rbc per liter, and one is unable microscopically to distinguish between a normal urine and one containing 5.0 million rbc per liter. Actually, studies indicate a much more severe limitation in the microscopic determination of abnormal hematuria, suggesting one cannot be certain of an abnormal content of rbc until the urine contains 50 million rbc per liter, or 100 times the normal concentration. Certainly, other factors are operative — hemolysis increases as the pH increases and as the specific gravity falls; sediment obscures the erythrocytes; and yeast cells, oil droplets, and crystals have confused even experienced microscopists.

Principle

The method for the detection of occult blood is based on the peroxidase activity of hemoglobin and its derivatives. The peroxidase activity acts as a catalyst to oxidize the substrate o-tolidine (and the less sensitive substances benzidine, phenolphthalein, and guaiac in that order) in the presence of H_2O_2, resulting in a color change.

Procedure

Free, in 1956, produced a tablet now available as Occultest (Ames Company). One drop of uncentrifuged urine is placed on a piece of filter paper provided, and the tablet placed in the center of the moist area. Two drops of water are placed on the tablet. A diffuse blue color appearing on the filter paper around the tablet within 2 minutes is a positive reaction. The amount of blood present is proportional to the intensity of the blue color, to its area on the filter paper and to its speed of color development.

Discussion

The tablet contains sodium bicarbonate and tartaric acid to provide effervescence which facilitates solution of the ingredients. A red dye present is intended to mask confusion which might result from the discoloration of the tablet. The tartaric acid and the calcium acetate present react with strontium peroxide to form H_2O_2. The peroxidase activity of hemoglobin produces the blue color change in the o-tolidine.

Sources of Error

Pus, iodides, and bromides may give false positive tests. Boiling diminishes reaction with hemoglobin, but a positive reaction persists if due to helogens. Ascorbic acid, which can be avoided by acidification of urine, many have some inhibitory effect. The test appears to be quite specific otherwise for hemoglobin and its derivatives. Iron salts and chlorophyll do not produce false positive results, and porphyrins do not react. All hemoglobins and myoglobins and their derivatives are detected in acid or alkaline solution. The sensitivity of the test is reported to be in the order of 0.00015 to 0.0015 mg per ml (25) which is at least 200 times the sensitivity required.

F) MYOGLOBIN

Introduction

Myoglobin, a muscle pigment serving to store oxygen in the muscles, differs from hemoglobin in that it contains only one Fe atom and one heme atom (in contrast to the four of hemoglobin) and is incompletely bound in the plasma. It thus has a low renal threshold and a high urinary excretion rate. A simple schema for distinguishing between hemoglobin and myoglobin in the urine is as follows:

Appearance of Urine	Tests on Urine	Appearance of Plasma	Interpretation
Red to red-brown or chocolate color	Benzidine pos.	Normal	Myoglobin
	Hematuria neg. (No r.b.c. on microscopic)	Pink	*Hemoglobin

Note: *Hemoglobin will be found in the urine only after its concentration exceeds the plasma binding capacity, about 125 mgm per 100 ml of plasma.

**Absence of fluorescence will distinguish these pigments from porphyrins.

The *chemical* distinction between hemoglobin and myoglobin in the urine is not a simple matter and is discussed elsewhere in this manual. The methods commonly in use may be summarized here as follows:

1. *Spectrophotometric Identification*

Absorbance peaks of the two compounds are too close for accuracy; interfering substances are commonly present; and myoglobin may be largely in "met" form.

2. *Ultracentrifugal Identification*

Although the constants are adequately separated, other urinary proteins have similar constants making the technique unreliable.

3. *Salt Precipitation*

Based on the solubility of myoglobin in 75 to 80% $(NH_4)_2 SO_4$ following precipitation of protein with sulfosalicylic acid, Blondheim (26) reported an ingenious and simple procedure. Others have reported false negative results (27) with this technique.

4. *Electrophoresis*

Whisnant (28) has reported effective separation by paper electrophoresis with pH 8.6 barbital buffer in which myoglobin migrates half the distance of hemoglobin.

5. *Differentiation Based on Molecular Size*

A collodion membrane or Millipore (pore 9) filter permits myoglobin but not hemoglobin to pass.

6. *Immunologic Identification*

The sensitivity of this method is 20 times that of the spectrophotometric method.

G) INBORN ERRORS OF METABOLISM

ALKAPTONURIA (OCHRONOSIS)

Introduction

Of the major disturbances in the aromatic amino acid metabolism (namely phenylketonuria, tyrosinosis, and alkaptonuria), only the latter produces a pigmentary disturbance in the urine. This darkening is due to homogentisic acid. However, contrary to many previous reports, the urine of the alkaptonuric may be clear when passed and does not darken for many hours if it remains at an acid pH. When allowed to stand exposed to air or made alkaline, the urine gradually darkens after 24 to 48 hours to dark brown or black, beginning at the surface and spreading inward. Darkening of the urine on standing, alkalinization, or oxygenation is, of course, non-specific and may indicate gentisic acid (a metabolite of salicylates), melanogen, indican, urobilinogen, porphyrins, phenols, unidentified metabolites of salicylates, etc.

Homogentisic acid accumulates in the blood and is excreted in the urine. Apart from the homogentisic acid itself, no other abnormal substances are excreted in the urine as a result of the metabolic block. The homogentisic acid is, in part, responsible for the deposition of pigment and ochronosis in the tissues.

The demonstration of homogentisic acid by paper chromatography is definitive. Using a system of n-butanol saturated with water and a few drops of formic acid, stained with ammoniacal silver nitrate bath for about 5 minutes, and cleared with 1 M sodium thiosulfate until the background is white, the presence of homogentisic acid is indicated by black spots on a white background.

Homogentisic acid may be quantitated by the reduction of phosphomolydbic acid to molybdenum blue according to the methods of Biggs (29) and LaDu and Zannoni (30). Recently, a simple qualitative method (31) of demonstrating homogentisic acid has been devised.

Hyperuricuria

The red to red-brown urine sometimes seen in patients excreting uric acid has received little attention. Uric acid in pure form is a white crystalline substance. Apparently forming a complex with urochrome under certain conditions, the crystals impart a red color to the urine, and the sediment is red to red-brown. These crystals are negative for hemoglobin, but give weakly positive tests for bilirubin. Such discoloration does not occur in all patients having heavy urate or uric acid concentrations in the urine, for reasons not yet clear.

Oxalosis

A whitish cloud is seen in oxalosis, or primary hyperoxaluria, a rare disease with increased oxalic acid synthesis and oxalate crystals throughout the body, including the urine and urinary tract (32, 33). Up to 10 times the normal oxalate excretion is seen in this condition, with deposits of calcium oxalate stones throughout the urinary tract. Diagnosis is made by showing excessive oxalic acid and glycolic acid in the urine.

The "Blue Diaper" Syndrome

The "blue diaper" syndrome (34) may represent a further entity in the spectrum of defects of infancy accompanying hypercalcemia of an idiopathic nature. In this rare defect, probably caused by a defect in tryptophan absorption, indigo blue appears in the urine. This pigment is insoluble in water, absolute ethanol, and in ether, but is readily soluble in acetone, chloroform, and benzene. Spectrophotometric studies in chloroform reveal peaks of absorption at 246, 285, and 610 mu and a shoulder at 340 mu, identical values to those given for indigot (indigo blue). The conditions which produce increased urinary excretion of indometabolites (indicans, etc.) include phenylketonuria, Hartnup disease, maple syrup urine disease, pellagra, schizophrenia, and intestinal malabsorption owing to a variety of causes. Why the process goes on to coupling of 2 molecules in indican outside the body to form the insoluble dye indigo blue in the syndrome, accompanied by hypercalcemia and nephrocalcinosis, is not understood.

H) MISCELLANEOUS CONDITIONS

Cream-colored Urine (Chyluria)

A cream-colored urine suggests chyle. Often a red zone of stratified erythrocytes may be seen on standing, which appears at the bottom beneath the chyle.

Discussion

Lipuria and pyuria may be confused with chyluria although, in the former, the fat is present in droplet form, rarely emulsified. Microscopy will identify pyuria. The fat in chyluria is molecular but coagulants are present due to abundant fibrin. Specific gravity is low; the reaction is acid, and abundant albumin is present. Microscopic study shows fat globules, some erythrocytes, and hematoidin plates. A test meal employing 2 glasses of equal parts milk and cream should cause chyle to appear in a catheterized specimen after 1 hour, but may not appear for 4 hours. The patient should be in recumbent position to enhance appearance of chyle in the urine.

Blue or Green Urine

Blue or green urine may be due to pseudomonas infection although analysis of 2000 consecutive urine cultures in the author's laboratory (3% of which yielded pseudomonas in significant colony counts — over 10,000 per ml) failed to detect a single instance of discoloration of the urine by a blue or blue-green color. As a cause of discoloration of urine, pseudomonas infection must be quite rare possibly because the deep-blue pigment "pyocyanin" and phenazin dye are not water soluble and require chloroform extraction for demonstration. This pigment is formed only by pseudomonas. The second pigment is less well defined, is yellow-green in color, fluorescent, water soluble but not soluble in chloroform, and is a product of organisms other than psuedomonas.

The term "green urine syndrome" has been applied to severely burned patients showing verdoglobinuria as a result of pseudomonas aeruginosa septicemia. All such cases have proved fatal. The green coloring matter has been detected by fluorescence several days to a week before the urine becomes visually discolored.

REFERENCES

1. Kelley, K. L., and Judd, D. B.: The ISCC-NBS method of designating colors and a dictionary of color names. U. S. Dept. of Commerce, National Bureau of Standards, Circular 53 and color chart supplement. U. S. Gov't. Printing Office, Washington, D. C. 20025, price $2.00.
2. Snell, E. E., and Strong, F. M.: Lactobacillus casei in the identification of Riboflavin. Anal. Chem., *11*:346, 1939.
3. Isbell, H., Wooley, J. G., and Frazer, H. F.: Inhibiting effect of urea on microbiological assay of riboflavin. U. S. Public Health Report, *56:*282, 1941.
4. Emmerie, A.: Determination and excretion of flavins in normal human urine. Nature, *138:*164, 1936.
5. Ferrebee, J. W.: Urinary excretion of riboflavin; fluorometric methods for its estimation. J. Clin. Invest., *19:*251, 1940.
6. Najjar, V. A.: Fluorometric determination of riboflavin in urine and other biological fluids. J. Biol. Chem., *141:*355, 1941.
7. Koschara, W.: Uber Harnlyochrome, Hoppe-Seylers Z. Physiol. Chem., *232:*101, 1935.
8. Najjar, V. A., and Holt, L. E., Jr.: Excretion of riboflavin related to body stores. Bull. Johns Hopkins Hosp., *204:*476, 1941.
9. Ungnade, H. E. (ed.): Organic Electronic Spectral Data, Vol. 2. Interscience Publishers, Inc., N.Y. 1960.
10. Sunshine, I., and Gerber, S. R.: Spectrophotometric Analysis of Drugs Including Atlas of Spectra. Springfield, Thomas, 1963.
11. Hayden, A. L., Sammul, O. R., Selzer, G. B., and Carol, J.: Infrared, ultraviolet, and visible absorption spectra of some USP and NF reference standards and their derivatives. Assoc. Official Agric. Chem., *45:*797, 1962.
12. Billing, B. H., Cole, P. G., and Lathe, G. H.: Excretion of bilirubin as a diglucuronide giving the direct Vandenberg reaction. Biochem. J., *65:*714, 1957.
13. Schacter, D.: Natural glucuronide in direct-reacting bilirubin. Science, *126:*507, 1957.
14. Yamaoka, K., *et al.:* Ester type linkage in the conjugation of bilirubin. Proc. Japan Acad., *27:*715, 1951.
15. Henry, R. J.: Clinical Chemistry, Principles and Technics. Hoeber Medical Division, Harper and Row, Publishers, 1964.
16. Watson, C. J., Bossenmaier, I., and Cardinal, R.: Acute intermittent porphyria. J. A. M. A., *175:*1087, 1961.
17. Patterson, J. N., Catanzaro, C., and Dede, D. M.; Manual on the porphyrins and the porphyrias. Commission on Continuing Education, Council of Clinical Chemistry, 1966.
18. Watson, C. J.: The problem of porphyria-some facts and questions. New Eng. J. Med., *263:*1205-1215, 1960.
19. Townsend, J. D.: An evaluation of a recent modification of the Watson-Schwartz Test for porphobilinogen. Ann. Int. Med., *60:*306-307, 1964.
20. Mauzerall, D., and Granick. S.: Occurrence and determination of delta-aminolevulinic acid and porphobilinogen in urine. J. Biol. Chem., *219:*435, 1956.
21. Helman: In, Cecil, R. L., McDermott, W., and Wolff, H. (ed.): Textbook of Medicine. *7:*1011, 1947.
22. Spencer, R. P.: Medical progress: Malignant melanoma. New Eng. J. Med., *253:*18-23, 1955.
23. Ham, T. H. (ed.): Syllabus of Laboratory Examinations in Clinical Diagnosis, Cambridge, Havard University Press, 1950.
24. Duchon, J., and Pechan, Z.: The biochemical and clinical significance of melanogenuria. Ann. N. Y. Acad. Sci., *100:*1048, 1963.
25. Cook, M. H., *et al.:* The detection of blood in urine. Amer. J. Med. Tech., *22:*218, 1956.

26. Blondheim, Solomon, Margoliash, E., and Shafir, E.: A simple test for myohemoglobinuria (myoglobinuria). J. A. M. A., *167:*453, 1958.
27. Dumas, R. J., Trigg, J. W., and Hammack, W. J.: Primary myoglobinuria, A case report emphasizing recent diagnostic techniques. Ann. Int. Med., *56:*97, 1962.
28. Whisnant, C. L., *et al.:* Primary idiopathic myoglobinuria in a Negro female; its implications and a new method of laboratory diagnosis. Ann. Int. Med., *51:*140, 1959.
29. Briggs, A. P.: A colormetric method for the determination of hemogentisic acid in urine. J. Biol. Chem., *51:*453-454, 1922.
30. LaDu, B. N., and Zannoni, V. G.: The tyrosine oxidation system of liver, II. Oxidation of p-hydroxyphenylpyruic acid to homogentisic acid. J. Biol. Chem., *217:*777-787, 1955.
31. Valmikinathan, K., and Verghese, N.: Simple color reaction for alkaptonuria. J. Clin. Path., *19:*200, 1966.
32. Hsia, D. Y.: In, Inborn Errors of Metabolism, Part 1, Clinical Aspects, 2nd Ed. Year Book Medical Publishers, Inc. 1966.
33. Hsia, D. Y., Inouye, T.: In, Inborn Errors of Metabolism, Part 2, Laboratory Methods, 2nd Ed. Year Book Medical Publishers, 1966.
34. Drummond, K. N., Michael, A. F., Ulstrom, R. A., and Good, R. A.: The blue diaper syndrome: Familial hypercalcemia with nephrocalcinosis and indicanuria. A new familial disease with definition of the metabolic abnormality. Amer. J. Med., *37:*928-948, 1964.

Chapter 16

Differentiation of Hemoglobinuria and Myoglobinuria in Renal Diseases

ERNEST C. ADAMS, Jr., Ph.D., and MARGARET J. ROZMAN, B.S.

INTRODUCTION

Myoglobinuria — the presence of the oxygen carrying pigment of muscle in urine — is associated with damage to muscle which causes the release of the pigment into the plasma and its subsequent excretion into the urine. Hemoglobinuria — the presence of the oxygen carrying pigment of the erythrocytes in urine — is associated with hemolysis of erythrocytes which releases the pigment into the plasma and its subsequent excretion into the urine. Myoglobinuria and hemoglobinuria thus may be symptoms of a variety of clinical conditions and occasionally even occur together. In Table 1 are listed some of the conditions reported to result in myoglobinuria and hemoglobinuria. Some of the conditions such as the crush syndrome may result in both myoglobinuria and hemoglobinuria. In all the described cases of myoglobinuria and most of those of hemoglobinuria there are large quantities of the pigment. There has been little attention paid to smaller amounts that can be detected by one of the more sensitive methods. Further, many reported cases of hemoglobinuria may really have been myoglobinuria. A particular example of this may be some of the reported cases of march hemoglobinuria.

Myoglobin and hemoglobin are similar in structure but have some distinctly diffferent physical, chemical, and immunochemical properties. Some of these properties are listed in Table 2. These properties may be used to differentiate one of the proteins from the other. With the exception of the immunochemical methods, such differentiation requires the presence of relatively large quantities of myoglobin and hemoglobin.

Usually, the diagnosis of myoglobinuria, if made at all, is a presumptive one based on the clinical symptoms and the color of the urine and plasma. The presumptive diagnosis then may be confirmed by methods based on spectral properties, molecular size, electrophoretic behavior, ion exchange, solubility in 80% saturated ammonium sulfate, etc.

Some (17, 20, 21, 31) suggest the diagnosis of myoglobinuria from the clinical symptoms of muscle weakness and pain, when there is a peroxidase positive pigment in the urine and no observable pigment in the plasma. When there is sufficient pigment in the urine to be clearly visible, comparison of the color of the urine with the color of the plasma leads to the differentiation of myoglobinuria from hemoglobinuria. Failure of the urine to fluoresce under ultra-violet

TABLE I—CONDITIONS ASSOCIATED WITH MYOGLOBINURIA OR HEMOGLOBINURIA

A. MYOGLOBINURIA (31)

I. Hereditary myoglobinuria
  a. Phosphorylase deficiency
  b. Unknown metabolic defects
    1. Some associated with muscular dystrophy
II. Sporadic myoglobinuria
  a. Exertional myoglobinuria in untrained individuals
    1. Squat-jump syndrome
    2. Anterior tibial syndrome
    3. March hemoglobinuria (some cases)
    4. Other forms of exertion
  b. Crush Syndrome
  c. Ischemic myoglobinuria
    1. Arterial occlusion
    2. Myocardial infarction (35)
  d. Metabolic myoglobinuria
    1. Haff disease
    2. Alcoholism
    3. Sea-snake bite poisoning
    4. Carbon monoxide intoxication
    5. Diabetic acidosis
    6. Hypokalmia
    7. Systemic infection and fever
    8. Barbiturate poisoning
    9. Others
  e. Myoglobinuria with progressive muscle disease
  f. Electrical shock
  g. Seizures such as in epileptic convulsions
  h. Myoglobinuria due to unknown cause

B. HEMOGLOBINURIA (22)

CONDITION	MECHANISM OR PRESUMPTIVE CAUSE OF HEMOGLOBINURIA
Hematuria with hemolysis of cells in the urine	1. Red cells in the urine (hematuria) may be hemolyzed osmotically in the urinary tract in urine of low specific gravity.
Infarction of the kidney	2. Hemoglobinuria and some hematuria may occur.
Intravascular hemolysis of exercise	3. Strenuous running by trained athletes may produce hemoglobinemia and hemoglobinuria.
	4. March hemoglobinuria may occur in some individuals after brief run or walk.
Intravascular hemolysis resulting from hypotonicity of plasma	5. Intravenous injection of distilled water will produce hemoglobinemia and hemoglobinuria.
	6. In transurethral resection of the prostate and irrigation of the bladder with distilled water, the water may gain access to the blood plasma through ruptured vessels and make the plasma hypotonic.
Paroxysmal cold hemoglobinuria	7. An autohemolysin is attached to the red cells when chilled in the presence of serum complement. Hemolysis occurs on warming to room or body temperature with serum complement. This occurs *in vitro* and after chilling *in vivo*.
Hemolytic transfusion reactions	8. Isoagglutinins without isohemolysins such as anti-A, anti-B, anti-D may produce hemolysis *in vivo*.
	9. Isohemolysins with isoagglutinins are a major cause for hemolytic reactions.
Autohemolysins in acquired hemolytic anemia	10. Hemolysins occur which may be active at body temperature, acid pH or in the cold in the hemolysis of the patient's cells and normal cells.
Autoagglutinins and incomplete antibodies in acquired hemolytic anemia	11. Hemoglobinuria occasionally occurs in the absence of demonstrable hemolysins but in the presence of cold agglutinins, warm agglutinins and incomplete antibodies.
Paroxysmal nocturnal hemoglobinuria	12. Patient's abnormal red cells are hemolyzed *in vitro* in the patient's serum and compatible normal serum containing complement, properdin, Mg^{++}, and an acid pH.

TABLE I (CONT'D) CONDITIONS ASSOCIATED WITH MYOGLOBINURIA OR HEMOGLOBINURIA

CONDITION	MECHANISM OR PRESUMPTIVE CAUSE OF HEMOGLOBINURIA
Thermal injury to red cells	13. In thermal burns the red cells which are injured by heat become spheroidal and increased in susceptibility to osmotic and mechanical fragility.
Chemical agents acting directly on red cells.	14. Certain chemical agents such as arsine, sulfonamides, phenylhydrazine, naphthaline, quinine, and certain oxidant compounds produce acute hemolytic anemia with spheroidicity, fragmentation and increased osmotic fragility of red cells.
Chemical agent acting with an agglutinin	15. In fuadin hemolytic anemia an antibody for red cells in the serum combines with red cells only in the presence of fuadin.
Infestation of red cells	16. In severe malaria, marked infestation of the red cells by the plasmodium may be associated with hemoglobinuria.
	17. In oroya fever, the red cells are infested with the Bartonella bacilliformia; fatal hemoglobinuria may result.
Favism	18. Sensitivity to the fava bean may result in severe hemolytic anemia.
Toxemia of Pregnancy	19. Hemoglobinuria, thrombocytopenia and clotting defects of unknown origin have been observed in toxemia of pregnancy.

light rules out porphyria as a cause of the pigmentation. The urine is tested with Hemastix® or some other "peroxidase-like " test system. A positive test indicates that hemoglobin, myoglobin, or intact erythrocytes are present and the pigment is not the result of alimentary ingestion or is a drug metabolite. A blood sample is collected (heparin or oxalate), care being taken to avoid hemolysis. The cells are centrifuged down and the plasma inspected. A definite pink color indicates that the pigment is hemoglobin while a straw color indicates that the pigment in the urine is myoglobin (28). Hemoglobin when released into the plasma is immediately bound to the serum protein haptoglobin; the complex is too large to be excreted into the urine and thus plasma hemoglobin must exceed 100 to 150 mg per 100 ml before appearing in the urine.

This hemoglobin level is 2 to 4 times that needed to color plasma (9, 37). Myoglobin is only 1/4 the size of hemoglobin and is not bound to haptoglobin. Accordingly, it appears in the urine once a level of 15 – 20 mg per 100 ml plasma is exceeded, this is only 1/2 of the level needed to give a visible color to the plasma.

This presumptive evidence, of course, depends on the plasma and urine representing approximately the same time sequence. Also, the pigment in the urine could be a result of hemolysis of erythrocytes after excretion of the urine.

A somewhat more complicated clinical method is to assay for serum haptoglobin since a hemoglobinemia at a level of 100 to 150 mg per 100 ml will deplete the serum of haptoglobin. Of course, this depletion may be the result of earlier hemolytic episodes.

TABLE II (17)—COMPARISON OF HEMOGLOBIN AND MYOGLOBIN

	Hemoglobin	*Myoglobin*
Molecular Weight	68000	17000
Prosthetic Group	Ferroprotoporphyrin	Ferroprotoporphyrin
%Fe^{++}	0.34	0.34
Fe^{++}/Molecule	4	1
Dissociation Curve	S-Shaped 90% saturated with oxygen at 55 mm Hg	Hyperbolic 90% saturated with oxygen at 30 mm Hg
Occurrence	15 g/100 ml blood	1-3 g/100 g muscle
Electrophoretic Mobility	Myoglobin one-half that of hemoglobin	
Sedimentation Constant (S 20 Saline)	4.5	4.5
Solubility in 80% Ammonium Sulfate	Precipitated	Soluble
"Renal Threshold"	100-140 mg/100 ml plasma	20 mg/100 ml plasma
Renal Clearance	Myoglobin clearance 25 times that of hemoglobin	
Serum Binding	Bound to haptoglobin to 100-135 ml/100 ml serum	Not appreciably bound to Hpt.
Isoelectric Point	pH 6.99	pH 6.78

Spectra	*oxy-*	*carboxy-*	*met-*	*oxy-*	*carboxy-*	*met-*
max.	577	570	630	582	579	630
	560	560	600	564	560	595
	540	539	500	542	540	500
	500	492	460	500	500	465

A. IMMUNOCHEMICAL DIFFERENTIATION OF HEMOGLOBINURIA AND MYOGLOBINURIA

Principle

The most definitive differentiation of hemoglobinuria and myglobinuria can be acheived by using relatively simple immunochemical methods. These methods, which include immunodiffusion, hemagglutination inhibition, and immunoelectrophoresis, are dependent upon the fact that specific antisera will react only with its homlogous antigen (1, 32, 33). Moreover, the methods quantitate the hemoglobin or myoglobin present in the urine.

Reagents

1. *Ammonium Sulfate.*

2. *Tris-EDTA-Borate Buffer*, pH 9.2

   200   gm Tris (Hydroxymethyl) aminomethane
   20   gm Disodium ethylenediaminetetra-
      acetate
   7.6 gm Boric acid
   20   liters distilled water

3. *Acrylamide Gel,* 7.5%. Fifteen gm Cyanogum® are dissolved in 200 ml Tris-EDTA-Borate Buffer.

Four-tenths ml N,N,N',N'-Tetramethylethylenediamine is added and the solution is filtered through coarse filter paper. Four-hundred mg ammonium persulfate are dissolved in approximately 1 ml tris buffer. This solution is added to the cyanogum solution and mixed thoroughly. It is immediately poured into the electrophoresis apparatus. The gel will begin to from in 5 to 10 minutes.

4. *Phosphate-Saline Buffer,* pH 7.4.

   6.8 gm Disodium hydrogen phosphate
   0.64 gm Potassium dihydrogen phosphate
   0.2 gm Sodium azide
        diluted to 1 liter with isotonic saline (0.85%)

5. *Agar, 0.6%.*

   0.6 gm Difco Bacto Agar in 100 ml phosphate –
        saline buffer, pH 7.4

6. *Phosphate Buffer,* 0.15 M.

   107.45 gm $Na_2HPO_4 \cdot 12H_2O$
          diluted to 2000 ml with distilled water
   40.83 gm KH_2PO_4
          diluted to 2000 ml with distilled water
   80.8   ml of the sodium phosphate solution is
          mixed with 19.2 ml of the potassium
          phosphate solution.

7. *Phosphate Buffer,* pH 7.

   22.7 ml 0.5 M Na_2HPO_4
   1.6 ml 4.0 M NaH_2PO_4
        diluted to 2000 ml with isotonic saline

8. *Sodium Acetate Buffer.*

   20   ml 2.0 M sodium acetate
   33.7 ml 3.5 M acetic acid
        diluted to 2000 ml with isotonic saline
        and pH adjusted to 3 to 4 with glacial acetic
        acid

9. *Barbital Buffer.* For stability at room temperature, a buffer solution 5 X concentrated is prepared.

   2.88 gm barbital are dissolved in 250 ml hot
        distilled water
   42.5 gm Na Cl and
   1.88 gm barbital sodium are dissolved in approx.
        700 ml distilled water.

The two solutions are combined, cooled to room temperature, and diluted to 1000 ml with distilled water. To use, the 5 X concentrated barbital buffer is diluted with 4 volumes of distilled water.

10. *Bis-diazobenzene Solution (BDB).* A 5-ml aliquot of cold $NaNO_2$ solution (0.68 gm sodium nitrite in 10 ml distilled water) is added dropwise to a cold benzidine solution [0.64 gm benzidine • 2HCl in 100 ml dilute HCl (1.5 ml of 37% HCl diluted to 100 ml with distilled water)] over a period of 10 minutes with magnetic stirring (1 drop every 4 to 6 seconds). The solution is allowed to stir an additional 20 minutes. (It should give only a trace reaction with starch iodide test paper.) The BDB is ready for immediate use. If it is not to be used immediately, it will remain stable if frozen immediately and kept at -60°C. To store frozen, one dram screw cap vials are set upright in crushed dry ice and 3 ml BDB is pipetted into each vial. These vials are placed in a -60°C freezer.

11. *Formalinized Sheep Cells*

Fresh sheep blood mixed with an equal volume of Alsever's solution (usually 100 ml total volume) is obtained from Cappel Laboratories and refrigerated until formalinization 7 days after shipment. The blood is centrifuged and the supernatant siphoned from the cells (usually 20 ml). The cells are washed 3 times with saline.

To 20 ml fresh, packed sheep cells are added 230 ml saline and 250 ml 3% formalin solution, pH 7.3. This is thoroughly mixed and placed in a stoppered Erlenmeyer flask in the 37°C. incubator for 18 to 20 hours with magnetic stirring.

The formalinized cells are washed 5 times with distilled water and stored as a 10% suspension of cells in distilled water in the refrigerator. The formalinized cells can be used for 1 month for conjugate preparation. At the end of 1 month, any remaining cells can be lyophilized for storage in dry form and used for adsorption of antisera.

Special Apparatus
High Voltage Electrophoresis Apparatus
Convection Elution Apparatus
Repp Lyophilizer

Procedure
Antigen Preparation
Myoglobin is isolated according to the selective precipitation method of Luginbuhl (24). Muscle proteins, including hemoglobin, are precipitated from prepared muscle extracts at pH 8 with 80 percent ammonium sulfate saturation. Under these conditions, myoglobin remains in solution. It is precipitated at pH 7 with 100% ammonium sulfate saturation and collected on 0.45 micron Millipore filters. The myoglobin is further purified by electrophoresis on acrylamide gel which removes albumin, a potent antigen contaminant (33). A 7.5% acrylamide gel is prepared with Tris buffer for use in the EC Apparatus high voltage electrophoresis cell. The crude myoglobin is dissolved in the buffer (80 to 120 mg per run), and several crystals of sucrose and bromphenol blue to mark the albumin migration are added. After 3 hours at 300 V, the electrophoresis is stopped. The albumin has migrated to the end of the gel and can be cut away. The portion of the gel containing the myoglobin is placed in the convection elution apparatus (EC Apparatus Corp.) and myoglobin in eluted from the gel in 3 hours at 300 milliamps. The myoglobin is then lyophilized.

The hemoglobin antigen is prepared from freshly drawn oxalated whole blood. A hemoglobin determination is performed. The blood is centrifuged at 2000 rpm for 30 minutes and the plasma is carefully removed. The cells are washed several times with an equal volume of saline. The cells are then lysed with 8 to 10 volumes of distilled water. The hemoglobin solution is centrifuged 2 times at 16000 rpm for 30 minutes to remove cell stroma. Hemoglobin must be purified by electrophoresis also.

Immunization
Young white rabbits of either sex are used for immunization. The antigen solution of 0.4 ml, equivalent to 1 mg per rabbit in equal volumes of Freund's complete adjuvant, is given initially in each foot pad. Inoculum for intravenous injections consists of 0.5 ml antigen solution (diluted with saline and equivalent to 1 mg antigen per rabbit) and is injected into the left external marginal ear vein.

Bleedings are made from the right external marginal ear vein after carefully shaving the ear. A lengthwise (1/8 to 1/4 inch) slit in the vein is made with a sharp razor blade. Xylene wiped on the ear will cause vasodilation, but care should be taken to avoid getting any xylene in the wound. Approximately 50 ml blood can

IMMUNIZATION SCHEDULE	
Day 0	Foot Pad
21	1st IV
23	1st Booster IV
33-35	1st Full Bleeding
54	2nd IV
56	2nd Booster IV
66-68	2nd Full Bleeding
87	3rd IV
98	3rd Booster IV
99-101	Final Bleeding

be collected within 30 minutes. A piece of cotton, held in place by a paper clip will stop the bleeding.

Antiserum Preparation

The rabbit blood is allowed to stand at room temperature for 1 to 2 hours to clot. The clot is loosened from the sides of the tube and the tube is refrigerated overnight. The clot is centrifuged at 2000 rpm for 15 minutes. The serum is poured off and centrifuged again. Complement is destroyed by heating the serum in water bath at 56°C for 30 minutes. Heterophile antibody is removed by absorption with lyophilized formalinized sheep red cells (10 mg per ml sera). The serum is stored undiluted at -60°C.

Methods for Detecting Antigen-antibody Reaction

1. *Immunodiffusion.* This method was originally described by Ouchterlony (27). Agar is pipetted into 9 cm Petri dishes to a depth of 3 mm. After standing for 2 hours, the agar is cut with a Feinberg agar gel cutter.

The antiserum is placed in the center well and the suspect urines in the outer wells. A moistened filter-paper disc is placed in the cover of the Petri dish. Positive precipitin lines can be read in 16 to 48 hours. Relative quantitation can be achieved by diluting the urine until either the hemoglobin or myoglobin antiserum fails to give a positive test.

2. *Immunoelectrophoresis.* Modifications of the Scheidegger microimmunoelectrophetic technique as reviewed by Crowle (18) are employed. Microscope slides are coated with 1% Noble Agar in barbital buffer (0.025 μ, pH 8.6). Merthiolate (0.01 percent) is added as a preservative. Electropheretic migration is carried out for 2 hours at 47 volts across the slides. The electrophoresed urines are diffused against the specific antisera for 16 to 48 hours. The slides are stained with amidoschwartz 10B.

3. *Hemagglutination Inhibition. Myoglobin Conjugate Preparation*

A modification of the Howard and Wild (23) technique is used for coupling myoglobin to the red cell. This procedure is especially applicable to myoglobin because the first step reacts the protein with pyrrole-2-carboxylic acid azide at pH 9 to 10. Myoglobin, extracted by Luginbuhl's method, is least insoluble at this pH. Next, formalinized sheep red cells are diazotized with bis--diazobenzidine at pH 3 to 4. Finally, the two solutions are reacted at pH 7.

Step 1.

Crude myoglobin (24 mg) is homogenized in 10 ml phosphate buffer, 0.15 M, with 100 mg sodium bicarbonate. The pH is adjusted to 9 to 10. One hundred mg of pyrrole-2-carboxylic acid azide (29) is dissolved in 2 ml dioxane and 2 ml distilled water. The pyrrole is added dropwise to the buffered myoglobin solution. The pH is maintained at pH 9 to 10. The myoglobin-pyrrole solution is dialyzed for 3 days against cold phosphate buffer (pH 7).

Step 2.

Seven ml of 10% formalinized sheep red cells are centrifuged and resuspended in 8 ml of sodium acetate buffer, pH 3.5. The bisdiazobenzidine solution is added dropwise to the red cells with shaking and the pH is adjusted to 3 to 4. The solutions are rotated for 30 minutes at room temperature. After this reaction time, the cells are washed 3 times with sodium acetate buffer and suspended in 8 ml saline.

Step 3.

The myoglobin-pyrrole is added dropwise, with mixing, to the cells. The pH rises gradually and is finally adjusted to 6 to 7. The conjugates are rotated at room temperature for 4 hours and refrigerated overnight. The conjugates are washed 4 times with saline and finally suspended in 40 ml of saline.

Hemoglobin Conjugate Preparation

Acrylamide gel electrophoresed hemoglobin is coupled to formalinized sheep red cells through bis-diazobenzidine according to the Arquilla method (4). Three ml of 10% formalinized sheep red cells are centrifuged and resuspended in 17 ml of phosphate buffer, 0.15 M. To this is added 10.5 mg acrylamide gel electrophoresed hemoglobin in 1 ml phosphate buffer, 0.15 M (or 1.5 mg crude hemoglobin antigen in 1 ml phosphate buffer, 0.15 M).

Two ml of bis-diazobenzidine are diluted with 8 ml phosphate buffer, 0.15 M. Six ml of distilled bis-diazobenzidine are added immediately to the red cell hemoglobin mixture. It is rotated for 20 minutes at room temperature. After reaction time, the conjugate is washed 4 times with saline and resuspended in 17 ml saline.

Hemagglutination inhibition is carried out in wet system in Cooke "U" plates or lyophilized in the reaction capsule (patent pending).

Wet System

Specific myoglobin and hemoglobin sera are serially diluted 1:75, 1:150, 1:300, 1:600, 1:1200, 1:2400, and 1:4800 in 1 X barbital buffer or 1:225-1:14400 in the test. The myoglobin conjugate is suspended in saline. The hemoglobin conjugate is suspended in 1 percent bovine serum albumin in 1 X barbital buffer solution. The red cell concentration is approximately 1.25%. One drop of antiserum dilution is placed in each vertical column. The eighth vertical column is a control of 1 X barbital buffer solution. One drop of inhibitor or suspect urine is placed in the horizontal

Work Sheet for Hemagglutination Inhibition Test

	Myoglobin antiserum in 1 x Barbital buffer solution.							
	1:225	1:450	1:900	1:1800	1:3600	1:7200	1:14400	Buffer Control
Titer								
Inhibitor								
Urine #1								
Urine #2								
Urine #3								
Urine #4								
Myoglobin Control								

	Hemoglobin antiserum in 1 x Barbital buffer solution.							
	1:225	1:450	1:900	1:1800	1:3600	1:7200	1:14400	Buffer Control
Titer								
Inhibitor								
Urine #1								
Urine #2								
Urine #3								
Urine #4								
Hemoglobin Control								

rows. The first horizontal row has 1 drop 1 X barbital buffer solution in each well in place of the inhibitor to determine the titer. Then one drop of conjugate is placed in every well in the plate that contains antiserum and inhibitor. The plate is swirled carefully to mix the contents thoroughly. Wood applicator sticks can be used to stir each well if a clean stick or piece of a stick is used in each well.

Cooke Plate

The Cooke plate is placed on a level surface, free of vibration, for one hour. A positive test for myoglobinuria or hemoglobinuria is indicated by an inhibited pattern or ring of cells at the bottom of the well. A negative test or hemagglutination is seen as a smooth mat of cells.

Lyophilized System

The specific antiserum is serially diluted in 2% peptone in 1 X barbital buffer solution. The conjugate is suspended in 1% bovine serum albumin in barbital buffer solution. The purpose of the peptone is to protect the gamma globulin during lyophilization and reconstitution. One drop of conjugate is dropped into the cap of the opened reaction capsule and one drop of antiserum is dropped into the base of the reaction capsule. Lyophilization is allowed to proceed according to manufacturer's instructions. The lyophilization reaction capsules are then closed and stored in bottles with desiccant packets. To use the capsules, they are opened and one drop distilled water is added to each. To differentiate myoglobinuria from hemoglobinuria, one drop of the suspect urine is added to a hemoglobin reaction capsule and one drop to a myoglobin reaction capsule. The capsules are closed

and shaken vigorously and allowed to stand undisturbed for one hour. The presence of myoglobin in the urine is indicated by a ring of cells in the bottom of the myoglobin reactive capsule. As in the wet system, a negative test is shown by a smooth mat of cells at the bottom of the capsule. It is preferable to use the immunochemical method on fresh urine. If the urine has become alkaline, it should be neutralized before testing.

B. SPECTRA

It has been suggested by a number of investigators (9, 31, 37) that myoglobinuria can be differentiated from hemoglobinuria by a spectral examination of the urine. Others (10, 19, 20, 25) apparently believe that this method is of little use or extremely difficult. The absorption bands of oxyhemoglobin and oxymyoglobin are very close together, 578 and 581 mμ for the α and 540 and 542 mμ for the β. The separation of the α bands can be increased by converting both pigments to the carbomonoxy derivatives. The method of Berenbaum (6) is used. The urine is buffered to pH 8 and filtered. The filtrate is placed in a spectrophotometer cuvette. Carbon monoxide is bubbled into the liquid for 3 to 4 minutes and a pinch of sodium hydrosulfite added. The surface of the solution is covered with liquid paraffin and carbon monoxide is bubbled into the solution for another 3 to 4 minutes. The cuvette is covered with a lid and placed in a spectrophotometer with a wavelength drive and scanned. The absorption band for the carbomonoxyhemoglobin in 568 millimicrons and that for the carbomonoxymyoglobin is 578 millimicrons.

This method has the disadvantages of requiring the use of toxic gas and the presence of clearly visible quantities of myoglobin or hemoglobin. Denaturation of the proteins which occur in urine may alter the spectral characteristics.

In our experience, the hand spectroscope is of no use in differentiation of myoglobin from hemoglobin.

C. ELECTROPHORESIS

Principle

Positive differentiation of myoglobin from hemoglobin is made by electrophoreisis on paper, cellulose acetate, starch, or acrylamide gel. In all methods, hemoglobin A migrates twice as fast as myoglobin.

Reagents
1. *1.5 M acetate buffer pH 4.7*
   1.46 gm sodium acetate
   0.52 ml glacial acetic acid
   distilled water to a volume of 500 ml
2. *o-Dianisidine solution*
   1.43 gm o-dianisidine
   95% ethanol to a volume of 1000 ml
3. *3 percent H_2O_2* – Prepared fresh
   10 ml 30% H_2O_2
   diluted to 100 ml with distilled H_2O
4. *Barbital buffer, pH 8.6, 0.05 μ*
5. *Dianisidine Stain – Prepared Fresh*
   70 ml alcoholic o-dianisidine solution
   10 ml acetate buffer
   18 ml distilled H_2O
   2 ml 3 percent H_2O_2

Special Apparatus
   Electrophoresis apparatus

Procedure
1. *Cellulose Acetate.* (12) Cellulose acetate strips are premoistened and prepared for electrophoresis. Seven microliters of suspect urine and control are applied on separate strips. Electrophoresis is carried out for 90 to 120 minutes at 150 to 200 V (not to exceed 0.2 ma per 2.5 cm strip width). After electrophoresis, the strips are dried and stained by floating on o-dianisidine solution for a period of 3 to 5 minutes. The strips are rinsed with distilled water and dried.

2. *Paper (38).* Whatman #3 filter paper is cut to fit the apparatus. Electrophoresis is carried out at 200 V for 22 hours in pH 8.6 barbital buffer, 0.05 u. The suspect urine specimen is prepared by diluting it 1:2 with human serum. The purpose of the addition of serum is to prevent the myoglobin or hemoglobin from adsorbing to the filter paper. After electrophoresis, the filter paper is dried and fixed in oven at 125°C for 10 minutes. A fine caliber glass hand spray is used to apply the o-dianisdine stain.

Discussion

A control hemoglobin hemolysate should be included in each electrophoresis run.

With midline application, hemoglobin and myoglobin migrate toward the cathode. Hemoglobin will be closest to the point of application. Hemoglobin C and E can not be differentiated from myoglobin under these conditions of electrophoresis.

D. AMMONIUM SULFATE PRECIPITATION TEST

Principle

At 80% saturation with ammonium sulfate, hemoglobin, along with denatured myoglobin, is completely precipitated from solution with only minor amounts of underatured myoglobin also precipitated. At 100% saturation, myoglobin is completely precipitated (8).

Reagents
  Ammonium Sulfate
  Hemastix®
  Sodium Hydroxide 5N

Procedure
The filtered urine is brought to 80% saturation by dissolving 2.8 gm ammonium sulfate in 5 ml urine. The mixture is warmed under the hot water tap to hasten solution. The pH is adjusted to 8 by adding 1 to 2 drops of 5N sodium hydroxide. The urine is centrifuged and the supernate tested with Hemastix® (11) (Dip the stick into the supernate, wait 10 seconds and wash the stick with a stream of water, read after another 30 seconds; the washing is necessary to remove the ammonium sulfate which inhibits the reaction).

If a negative Hemastix® test is obtained on the supernatant from the 80% saturation, the precipitated protein is hemoglobin. If the Hemastix® test is positive, and the protein precipitated by 100% ammonium sulfate saturation, the protein is probably myoglobin.

E. ULTRAFILTRATION STUDIES

Principle
Since hemoglobin has a molecular weight of 68000 and myoglobin a molecular weight of 16500, theoretically, it should be possible to separate them by ultrafiltration through a membrane that discriminates between molecules with molecular weights below 20000 and those with molecular weights above 20000; myoglobin passes through and hemoglobin tends to be retained. Several filters have been suggested in the literature — VF Millipore filter (20) with pore size of 10 millimicrons or 9 millimicrons (Gradacol Elford) collodion filter (36).

Our experience has been with the Amicon Diaflo® XM 50 ultrafilter.

Special Apparatus and Reagents
  Diaflo® ultrafiltration cell model
  50 Amicon Corporation
  Diaflo® ultrafilter XM 50
  Nitrogen tank plus necessary fittings
  Hemastix®

Procedure
The urine is centrifuged. The supernate is tested with Hemastix®. The supernate is placed in the assembled filter cell and forced through with 50 pounds nitrogen pressure. The ultrafiltrate is tested with Hemastix®. If the reaction with the filtrate is markedly less than with the original supernate, the urine probably contains hemoglobin.

F. ULTRACENTRIFUGE STUDIES

Special Apparatus
Spinco Model E Analytical Ultracentrifuge

Photographs are made at 8 minute intervals after a speed of 59,780 rpm is attained. The urine is studied undiluted (20).

Discussion
The procedure is long, requires expensive equipment and is not readily adaptable to the routine laboratory.

These results furnish substantiating evidence.

G. COLUMN CHROMATOGRAPHY

1. DEAE Cellulose
Principle
This method uses a cellulose ion

exchange column for separation of hemoglobin and myoglobin with Tris buffer, pH 8.2 to 8.6, and concentrations of 0.005 to 0.05 M (13).

With 0.05 M buffer, myoglobin is eluted near the hold-up volume and is increasingly retained as the molarity of the buffer is decreased. Under these conditions, hemoglobin is retained at the top of the column. Hemoglobin may be removed from the column by increasing the ionic strength or decreasing the pH of the buffer.

Reagents
1. DEAE-Cellulose
2. Trishydroxymethylaminomethane

Procedure
The DEAE is washed several times with water and repeatedly with buffer until pH equilibration is achieved. The 0.5 x 7 cm column is packed by gravity. Myoglobin is eluted starting with the same buffer with which the column is equilibrated. (Tris, pH 8.2 to 8.6, 0.005 to 0.05 M); hemoglobin and other soluble proteins are eluted by a change to buffers of lower pH or higher ionic strength (usually 0.02 to 0.2 M NaCl). The change in buffers on the column is made directly. The concentration of proteins in the effluent is assayed by measurement of the Soret absorption peak of ultraviolet absorption in the 280 mμ region in a spectrophotometer.

Discussion
This procedure is also suitable for quantitative determinations of myoglobin in extracts and isolation of myoglobin from muscle.

2. Dextran Gel
Principle
Gel filtration utilizes the differing rates of diffusion of molecules within the interstices of a cross linked gel to fractionate molecular size and shape. Several investigators (5, 7, 15,) report the separation of hemoglobin and myoglobin by molecular sieve filtration.

Reagents
1. Sephadex G-50 or G-75, fine grain
2. 0.1 M KCl
3. 0.1 M Phosphate Buffer, pH 7.3
4. 0.25 M NaNO$_2$
5. 25% Sucrose Solution

Procedure
Approximately 3 gm of dry Sephadex powder is suspended in 0.1 M KCl and decanted several times to remove the fines. This preconditioned Sephadex is poured as a slurry into a glass chromatographic column (1 cm diameter) to give a settled column height of 30 cm. The column is equilibrated with 0.1 M phosphate buffer, pH 7.3.

Two tenths ml of 0.25 M NaNO$_2$ is added to 2.0 ml of suspect urine. The urine is then dialyzed overnight at 4°C against 0.1 M phosphate buffer, pH 7.3 and filtered. One ml of the filtrate is mixed with 1 ml of 25% sucrose solution and an aliquot of this mixture (0.1 ml to 1 ml) is carefully added to the top of the column.

The fractions are collected and analyzed spectrophotometrically or with a peroxidase activity method.

Discussion
Hemoglobin (MW 68,000) is eluted first from the column followed closely by myoglobin (MW 16,500).The fractionation can be followed easily as both proteins are highly colored. The separation can be increased by adding haptoglobin to the urine.

The pH of 7.3 and ionic strength are

not critical. In view of the possibility investigated by Rossi-Fanelli (30) of dissociation of hemoglobin into smaller subunits at higher net concentrations, buffers of ionic strength higher than 0.2 M should not be used.

There is slight overlap which would allow only rough quantitation of the heme proteins.

H. IN VIVO RENAL CLEARANCE

The difference in renal clearance of hemoglobin and myoglobin can be used in an *in vivo* animal test (2). The suspect urine is injected intravenously (saphenous) into a rat. After 10 to 30 minutes, the urine of the rat is tested with Hemastix.® A positive test indicates that myoglobin is in the urine. The suspect urine may be injected intraperitoneally, but then it requires about an hour before myoglobin appears in the rat urine. In the cited experiments it required 0.2 ml of 1% myoglobin solution to give a positive test.

I. QUANTITATIVE DETERMINATION OF HEMOGLOBIN AND MYOBLOBIN

The method is based on the "peroxidase-like" activity of hemoglobin and myoglobin — the ability to catalyze the oxidation by hydrogen peroxide of an indicator such as o-tolidine. Hemoglobin and myoglobin act the same in this system. Because there are potent inhibitors of this oxidation in urine, the "peroxidase-like" methods lack accuracy unless there is sufficient hemoglobin present for the inhibitors to be diluted out or the inhibitors can be removed. The described method is adapted from that of Mattenheimer and Adams (26).

Reagents

1. *0.1 M tartrate, pH 4.2*
77.3 ml 0.1 M sodium tartrate, 17.7 ml 0.1 M tartaric acid
2. *o-tolidine.*
50 mg o-tolidine dihydrochloride in 100 ml tartrate buffer
3. *Hydrogen Peroxide, 15%*
4. *Sephadex Column.*
Either Sephadex G 25 or G 50 is equilibrated with isotonic saline and a 1 x 20 cm column prepared.

Standards

The cells are centrifuged from fresh whole blood, washed several times with saline and laked with 10 volumes of water. After centrifuging off the cell debris, the hemoglobin solutions is frozen and stored. The hemoglobin of the original blood is determined with a cyanide method. Standards containing 1 to 10 micrograms hemoglobin per ml are prepared by diluting the hemolysate.

Method

One ml of standard or sample is added to 2 ml of o-tolidine reagent. After mixing, 0.25 ml of the hydrogen peroxide is added and mixed. The color development is measured against distilled water at 635 milimicrons in a spectrophotomer. The maximum optical density is recorded. A standard curve of maximum optical density is plotted for the standards.

The urine is diluted 1/500 with saline before assaying. If the optical density is at least 0.1 when 1 ml of the dilution is used, the hemoglobin level of the urine can be calculated directly. If the optical density is less than 0.1, it will be necessary to remove the inhibitors from the original urine by passing it through the Sephadex column. Two ml of urine are placed on the column and washed through with saline. When the effluent from the column becomes positive to Hemastix® the effluent is collected until it is no longer positive. The volume of the collected effluent is measured and then one ml of the effluent or a suitable dilution is used in the described assay. The hemoglobin or myoglobin in the original urine is calculated by multiplying the value from the standard curve by the dilution factor and the volume of the effluent divided by 2.

Ammonium Sulfate Precipitation Method

For each 5 ml of urine, 3.5 gm of ammonium sulfate is added and the pH is adjusted to 8 with a sodium hydroxide solution. After being mixed well, the mixture is placed in the refrigerator overnight. The precipitate is collected on 0.45 micron Millipore filters. The precipitate is removed from the filter with a pH 9.2 buffer. The resulting solution is dialyzed against saline and one ml of the dialysate or suitable dilution used in the described assay procedure.

Sensitivity of Methods

The most sensitive method is that of hemagglutination inhibition. Using a urine that contained only myoglobin and not hemoglobin, it was shown that the hemagglutination inhibition method will detect as little as 0.3 micrograms per milliliter. Likewise, the hemagglutionation inhibition method will detect as little as 0.3 micrograms hemoglobin per milliliter. Since there is no cross reaction between the two, the presence of a minute amount of one can be detected in the presence of large amounts of the other.

The sensitivity of the immunodiffusion method as defined in our earlier papers (1, 32, 33) is about 10 micrograms per milliliter.

The sensitvity of the "peroxidase-like" methods depend on a variety of conditions. The more sensitive ones such as Hemastix® will detect as little as 1 to 2 micrograms of hemoglobin or myoglobin per milliliter. Of course, this is without differentiation of the two. Concentration of the pigment by ammonium sulfate precipitation, dialysis, column chromatography, evaporation, etc. combined with Hemastix® May enable the differentiation of 2 to 10 micrograms per milliliter if the urine is fresh.

Normal Levels

The normal levels of hemoglobin or myoglobin in urine have never been clearly defined. From our experience with the hemagglutination inhibition methods, and the stick test, it appears that the normal level of the pigments is less than 0.3 micrograms per milliliter. With vigorous muscular activity myoglobin in the urine sometimes increase to detectable levels.

Difficulties and Possible Sources of Error

A number of the methods for differentiation of myoglobinuria from hemoglobiuria require that large, clearly visible quantities of the pigment be present. These methods include the clinical interpretation involving comparison of serum and urine, the *in vivo* renal clearance, the spectral comparisons, and possibly the chromatographic separations.

The methods depending on molecular size such as ultrafiltration and molecular sieving are subject to errors caused by dissociation of the hemoglobin tetramer to the dimer and possibly the monomers. This dissociation of hemoglobin in dilute solutions which has been described in the literature (3, 16, 30, 34) would result in reactive material passing through the filter or being retarded on the Sephadex column. Separation on Sephadex may also lead to destruction of the peroxidase-like activity of hemoglobin and myoglobin as reported by Mattenheimer (26). Addition of haptoglobin will prevent the destruction of hemoglobin but not myoglobin. Use of haptoglobin will also nullify the effect of hemoglobin dissociation.

Denatured myoglobin has an electrophoretic mobility about the same as hemoglobin.

In addition to needing large quantities of pigment, the spectral method requires the use of the highly toxic carbon monoxide.

The ultracentrifuge is useful for the most part for confirming the other tests. The instrument is expensive and requires skill in operating and in interpreting the results. Since the sedimentation in the ultracentrifuge is related to the molecular weight, the dissociation of the hemoglobin tetramer may confuse the results. Finally, there may be other proteins in the urine with the same sedimentation constants as hemoglobin and myoglobin (38).

The major disadvantage of the immunochemical methods is that at present the antisera, the conjugates, and the unitized tests are not commerically available. It is desirable to use fresh urines if at all possible, although the immunochemical methods appear to perform better with old urines than do the other methods. If the urine is alkaline, the pH must be adjusted to neutral before applying an immunochemical method. The immunodiffusion method requires a waiting time of at least 16 hours for the precipitin line to develop.

SUMMARY

Means of differentiating myoglobinuria from hemoglobinuria are described. The sensitivities, the utility, precautions, and possible errors of the various methods are given. The most sensitive and reliable method appears to be an immunochemical one based on hemagglutination inhibition. Ultrafiltration, ammonium sulfate precipitation, and the clinical picture can be useful in the differentiation. The other methods serve mainly for confirmation.

REFERENCES

1. Adams, E. C., Rozman, M. J., and Free, A. H.: Immunochemical recognition of hemoglobin and myoglobin. In, Sunderman, F. W., and Sunderman, F. W., Jr. (eds.): Hemoglobin: Its Precursors and Metabolites. Philadelphia, J. B. Lippincott Co., pp. 81-89, 1964.
2. Adams, E. C., and Peterson, J. A.: Unpublished, 1962.
3. Antonini, E: Interrelationship between structure and function in hemoglobin and myoglobin. Physiol. Rev., 45:123-170, 1965.
4. Arquilla, E. R.: Pregnancy Test with an Immunological Indicator. No. 3, 236, 732, U. S. Government Printing Office, Washinton, D. C., February 22, 1966.
5. Awad, E., Cameron, B., and Kotite, L.: Chromatographic separation of hemoglobin and myoglobin on "Sephadex" gel. Nature, 198: 1200-1201, 1963.
6. Berenbaum, M. C., and Birch, C. A.: Paroxysmal myoglobinuria. Lancet, 1:892-896, 1955.
7. Berman, M. C., and Kench, J. E.: Separation of myoglobin and hemoglobin on a column of dextran gel. J. Clin. Path., 16:385, 1963.
8. Blondheim, S. H., Margoliash, E., and Shafrir, E.: A simple test for myohemglobinuria (myoglobinuria). J. A. M. A., 167:453-454, 1958.
9. Boroian, T. V., and Attwood, C. R.: Myoglobinuria. J. Pediat., 67:69-75, 1965.
10. Bowden, D. H., Fraser, D., Jackson, S. H. and Walker, N. F.: Acute recurrent rhabdomyolysis (paroxysmal myohaemoglobinuria). Medicine, 35:335-353, 1956.
11. Brodine, C. E., and Vertrees, K. M.: Differentiation of myoglobinuria from hemoglobinuria, A. Procedure based upon differential solubility. In, Sunderman, F. W., Jr. (eds.): Hemoglobin: Its

precursors and Metabolites. J. B. Lippincott Co., pp. 90-91, 1964.

12. Brodine, C. E., and Vertrees, K. M.: Differentiation of myoglobinuria from hemoglobinuria, B. Electrophoretic procedure. In, Sunderman, F. W., and Sunderman, F. W., Jr. (eds): Hemoglobin: Its Precursors and Metabolites. Philadelphia, J. B. Lippincott Co., pp. 91-93, 1964.

13. Brown, W. Duane: Chromatography of myoglobin on diethylaminoethyl cellulose columns. J. Biol. Chem., 236:2238-2240, 1961.

14. Bywaters, E. G. L., Delory, G. E., Remington, C., and Smiles, T.: Myohaemoglobin in urine of air raid casualties with crushing injury. Biochem. J., 35:1164-1168, 1941.

15. Cameron, B. F., Azzam, S. A., Kotite, L., and Awad, E. S.: Determination of myoglobin and hemoglobin. J. Lab. Clin. Med., 65:883-890, 1965.

16. Chiancone, E., and Gilbert, G. A.: Dissociation of hemoglobin into subunits. I. Oxyhemoglobin: effect of acetic acid. J. Biol. Chem., 240:3866-3867, 1965.

17. Comings, D. E., and Rosenfeld, H.: Idiopathic paroxysmal myglobinuria. Ann. Int. Med., 55:647-661, 1961.

18. Crowle, A. J.: Immunodiffusion. New York, Academic Press, 1961, p 231.

19. Duma, R. J., Trigg, J. W., and Hammack, W. J.: Primary myoglobinuria . . . a case report emphasizing recent diagnostic techniques. Ann. Int. Med., 56:97-104, 1962.

20. Farmer, T. A., Hammack, W. J., and Frommeyer, W. B.: Idiopathic recurrent rhabomyolysis associated with myoglobinuria. New. Eng. J. Med., 264:60-66, 1961.

21. Gillett, R. L.: Primary myoglobinuria. New Eng. J. Med., 260:1156-1160, 1959.

22. Ham, T. H.: Hemoglobinuria. Am. J. Med., 18:990-1006, 1955.

23. Howard, A. N., and Wild, F.: A two-stage method of crosslinking proteins suitable for use in serological techniques. Brit. J. Exptl. Pathol., 38:640-643, 1957.

24. Luginbuhl, W. H.: Immunologic investigation of preparations of human myoglobin. Am. J. Clin. Path., 38:487-493, 1962.

25. Mengel, C. E., and Scarpelli, D. G.: A clinicopathological conference. Ohio Med. J.,

62:466-471, 1966.

26. Mattenheimer, H., and Adams, E. C.: Quantitative determination of hemoglobin in urine. 1. The inhibitory effect of urine on the peroxidase-like activity of hemoglobin and on horseradish peroxidase. Z. klin. Chem. u. klin. Biochem., 5:48-54, 1967.

27. Ouchterlony, O.: Diffusion-in-gel methods of immunological analysis. Prog. Allergy, 1-78, 1958.

28. Pearson, C. M., Beck, W. S., and Blahd, W. H.: Idiopathic paroxysmal myoglobinuria. A. M. A. Archives of Int. Med., 99:376-389, 1957.

29. Piccinini, A., and Salmonini, L.: Idrazidi degli acidi α-pirrolo ed α-indolmonocarbonici e loro transformazioni: Gazz. Chin. Ital., 32:246-253, 1902.

30. Rossi-Fanelli, A., Antonini, E., and Caputo, A.: Hemoglobin and myoglobin. Adv. Prot. Chem., 19:73-222, 1964.

31. Rowland, L. P., Fahn, S., Hirschberg, E., and Harter, D. H.: Myoglobinuria. Arch. Neurol., 10:537-562, 1964.

32. Rozman, M. J., Peterson, J. A., and Adams, E. C.: Differentiation of hemoglobin and myoglobin by immunochemical methods. Invest. Urol., 1:518-525, 1964.

33. Rozman, M. J., and Adams, E. C.: Specific antisera to myoglobin. Invest. Urol., 4:436-438, 1967.

34. Schachman, H. K., and Edelstein, S. J.: Ultracentrifuge studies with absorption optics. IV. Molecular weight determinations at the microgram level. Biochemistry, 5:2681-2705, 1966.

35. Strausser, H. R., Rothfeld, E. L., and Bucsi, R. A.: Isolation and preservation of human myoglobin for use in immunologic detection of myoglobinuria. P. S. E. B. M., 122:621-624, 1966.

36. Sunderman, F. W., MacFate, R. P., MacFadyen, D. A., Stevenson, G. F., and Copeland, B. E.: Symposium on clinical hemoglobinometry. Am. J. Clin. Path., 23:519-598, 1953.

37. Wheby, M. S., and Miller, H. S.: Idiopathic paroxysmal myoglobinuria. Am. J. Med., 29:599-610, 1960.

38. Whisnant, C. L., Owings, R. H., Cantrell, C. G., and Cooper, G. R.: Primary idiopathic myoglobinuria in a negro female: Its implications and a new method of laboratory diagnosis. Ann. Int. Med., 51:140-150, 1959.

Chapter 17

Estimation of Urinary Reducing Substances

MANFORD D. MORRIS, Ph.D., and HOWARD QUITTNER, M.D.

Along with the examination of urine for protein, the semiquantitative test for urinary reducing substances is one of the oldest routine diagnostic chemical tests in medical practice (5). The test of Benedict (1) in its original form, or a close modification, is widely used as a standard screening procedure.

The non-specific nature of the reducing substance test allows for its use in a dual manner. It can be employed as an important diagnostic agent for the detection of glycosuria, the most frequent of the melliturias, and at the same time be employed as a general screening method for the large array of other urinary compounds that have reducing activity. With the availability of a specific qualitative enzyme test for glucose (2, 6), a practical distinction between glycosuria and other positive reducing reactions can be quickly made in most instances.

GLYCOSURIA

Although glycosuria is generally associated with the diabetic state, numerous other physiologic and pathologic conditions can produce detectable amounts of glucose in the urine (Table 1).

The physiologic glycosurias are uncommon and of slight degree. Some cases of glycosuria of pregnancy are of diagnostic importance, serving as an indicator of incipient diabetes mellitus. In other instances, this may be the first sign of serious obstetrical difficulty, while more frequently it may only be an inconsequential phenomenon in pregnancy (8).

The most frequent types of pathologic glycosurias exhibit concentrations of blood glucose above the level of renal tubular reabsorption. The common denominator in each of these conditions is disease affecting one or more organs involved in glucose metabolism. A group of conditions of related etiology and growing prevalence are the iatrogenic glycosurias owing to the administration of one of many hormonal and other agents which are active in glucose metabolism. These materials act by either inducing excess glycogenolysis, blocking glycogen formation, or interfering with glucose metabolism. Other iatrogenic glycosurias are the result of damage to organs involved in glucose metabolism (e.g., hepatotoxins).

The second group of glycosurias are the result of renal tubular abnormality or disease. The blood glucose level is normal but renal tubular reabsorption is impaired. The lesion may be found in an essentially benign familial form or may be associated with an aminoaciduria arising from defective tubular aminoacid transport. Rarely, nephritis or nephrosis exhibits a glycosuria resulting from a tubular defect (4). Recent studies indicate that hypoparathyroidism leads to decreased tubular reabsorption of glucose, and the occurrence of renal glycosuria in hypercalcemic sarcoidosis or vitamin D intoxication has been postulated to represent feedback parathyroid hypofunction (9). Exogenous agents, notably the heavy metals, can produce tubular lesions with associated glycosuria. This manifestation of tubular damage occurs more often in infancy or early childhood.

On rare occasions, glycosuria has been reported in disease states where the involved organs do not play a large role in glucose metabolism. The mechanism for these cases is not known, but it has been reported in diphtheria and other acute infectious diseases, myocardial infarction, and some gastrointestinal disorders.

TABLE 1—POSITIVE BENDICT REACTIONS (After D'Agostino (3))

I. Glycosuria
   A. Physiologic
   B. Pathologic
      1. Hyperglycemic
         a. diabetes mellitus
         b. endocrinopathic origin
            1. pituitary
            2. adrenal
            3. thyroid
            4. pancreas
         c. non-endocrine origin
            1. liver
            2. muscle
            3. nervous system
            4. neonatal dysmaturity
         d. iatrogenic
            1. metabolic
               a. glucagon
               b. alloxan
               c. adrenocorticotropin
               d. corticosteroids
               e. thyroid hormone
               f. somatotropin
               g. epinephrine
               h. morphine
               i. curare
               j. dehydroascorbic acid
               k. reserpine, chlorpromazine and others
               l. estrogen-progesterone ovulatory suppression
              m. anesthesia with ether, chloroform or cyclopropane
         2. toxic
            a. phlorizine
            b. ACTH
            c. corticosteroids
            d. adrenalin

TABLE 1 (CONT'D) POSITIVE BENDICT REACTIONS (After C' Agostion (3))

      e. pilocarpine, atropine, ergotamine
      f. succinic and maleic acid
      g. chlorothiazide and others
      h. lead, mercury, chromium, iodine, boric acid and carbon tetrachloride
  2. Renal tubular (low TmG)
    a. renal diabetes
    b. conditions associated with defective tubular amino acid transport
    c. nephrosis, interstitial nephritis or acute glomerulonephritis
    d. parathyroid hypofunction
    e. toxic tubular nephropathy
      1. lead, mercury, cadmium, uranium
      2. certain phenolic compounds
      3. potassium ferrocyanate
      4. degraded tetracycline
  3. Idiopathic

II.   Mellituria
  A. Hereditary
    1. Galactose
    2. Fructose
    3. Pentose
    4. Lactose
      a. essential
      b. lactase deficiency
  B. Neonatal
    1. Physiologic lactosuria
    2. Disease related mellituria
      a. acute gastroenteritis
      b. steatorrhea
      c. neonatal jaundice
      d. infectious (or toxic) hepatitis
      e. sepsis
      f. hiatus hernia
      g. pyloric stenosis
  C. Lactation lactosuria ("hyperfunctioning breast")
    1. Antepartum
    2. Postpartum

III.   Pseudomellituria
  A. Metabolite
    1. Ascorbic acid
    2. Glucuronic acid
    3. Homogentisic acid
    4. Uric acid
    5. Creatinine
  B. Medication
    1. Unmodified
      a. ascorbic acid
      b. isoniazide
      c. tetracycline
      d. penicillin
      e. cycloserine
      f. sulfame thoxypyridiazine and others
      g. strophanthin and other cardiac glycosides
      h. nitrofuran
      i. chlorothiazide group
    2. Modified

TABLE 1 (CONT'D) POSITIVE BENDICT REACTIONS (After C' Agostion (3))

3. Conjugate (glucuronic acid) reaction
   a. chloral hydrate
   b. phenacetin
   c. salicylates
   d. p-aminosalicylic acid
   e. chloramphenicol
   f. p-aminobenzoic acid
   g. probenecid

MELLITURIA

With the exception of sucrose which has no reducing activity, all of the natural sugars found in the human diet and metabolism can cause a positive Benedict's test if they are excreted in significant amounts in the urine. Hereditary defects involving galactose, fructose, pentose and lactose have been described. Lactosuria may be essential, or associated with reduced intestinal lactase and increased permeability of the gastro-intestinal mucose to lactose.

In the neonatal period, mellituria (lactosuria, fructosuria or galactosuria) may be isolated or mixed, and accompany a variety of disease conditions. Occasionally, a normal newborn infant may exhibit lactosuria.

Lactosuria may be encoutered in the late stages of pregnancy, or during the period of lactation, and is thought to result from hyperfunctioning breast tissue.

PSEUDOMELLITURIA

This term is reserved for those noncarbohydrate substances capable of giving a positive reducing test. These may be ingested materials, normal metabolites produced endogenously, or drugs and their excretory products.

Among the natural metabolites capable of producing a positive reducing test, uric acid and creatinine are usually listed. In our experience with Benedict's test, this phenomenon has not bee encountered, even with the hyperuricuria of chronic myelogenous leukemia in the early stages of treatment or the hyper-creatininuria of severe muscle disease.

Urinary ascorbic acid is a good reducing agent. If the tissues are saturated with ascorbic acid, significant amounts may be excreted. A continued heavy dietary intake will lead to positive reducing tests. With high tissue levels of ascorbic acid, ovulation, or infectious processes such as scarlatina, measles and tuberculosis may lead to urinary ascorbic acid excretion of similar magnitude.

Glucuronic acid gives a positive reducing test. Most natural urinary metabolites containing glucuronic acid are ethers and are not easily decomposed to yield their glucuronic acid. The few that exist in the hydrolyzable ester from do not contribute enough glucuronic acid to cause a positive reaction. Bilirubin diglucuronide is the only ester of glucuronic acid that might produce a positive test. This would require a massive bilirubinuria.

The only natural metabolite that consistently gives a positive reducing test is homogentisic acid, and this appears in the urine in significant amounts only in the hereditary condition alkaptonuria. The black color appearing in the test solution as the copper precipitate settles slightly, allows for the immediate identification of this substance.

Almost all pseudomellituria is the result of drug administration. Many compounds have been described as giving positive tests, most of which are listed in Table 1, and others will be added to such lists in the future. The theoretical possible ways in which this may occur are: 1) the drug may appear in the urine unaltered and it may have reducing activity; 2) a metabolite of the drug may have reducing activity while the administered drug does not; 3) a drug metabolite in the urine may decompose during Benedict's test to give off one or more simpler substances that have reducing power. In this last category, the single important example is glucuronic acid which is conjugated to many drugs as an ester. The linkage is hydrolyzed by the strong alkali during the Benedict's test, and the released glucuronic acid produces a positive reaction. Although glucuronate esters are formed with many common drugs, this mode of detoxication is never the principle one (10). Generally, less than 20% of any drug appears as the glucuronate ester. However, a large dose of a drug, or abnormalities in liver function, may increase the amount of glucuronide, and its appearance in the urine will be reflected in a positive Benedict's test.

MODIFIED BENEDICT'S TEST

Principle

Soluble cupric ions, in a strongly alkaline solution, react with various urinary compounds that take up oxygen when heated. The cupric ions are reduced to cuprous ions which form insoluble yellow (hydrated) and red precipitates of cuprous oxide. While the method is not specific for glucose, it is the substance most frequently encountered in reacting urines.

Reagents

1. *Benedict's Reagent* (1). One hundred gm of sodium carbonate (anhydrous), ACS, and 173.0 gm of sodium citrate · $2H_2O$ reagent grade, are dissolved in 700 ml of heated distilled water in large beaker. In a separate beaker, 17.3 gm of cupric sulfate · $5H_2O$, ACS, are dissolved in 100 ml of distilled water. The latter solution is slowly added with continuous stirring to the still hot alkali solution. The mixture is cooled and diluted to 1 liter. The reagent keeps indefinitely in clear plastic bottles at room temperature. Prepared 5-ml volumes of reagent may be conveniently dispensed and stored in rubber stoppered test tubes.

Procedure

1. Four-tenths ml (8 drops) of urine are added to 5.0 ml of Benedict's reagent in a pyrex test tube and mixed.

2. The tube is placed uncapped in a suitable boiling water bath for *exactly* 5 minutes. (The prepared test may stand at room temperature before heating for a long period of time without affecting the result.)

3. The tube is removed from the water bath and examined for the presence of a diffuse precipitate.

4. No change in the reagent, the presence of color change without turbidity, or the appearance of a white precipitate are regarded as negative results. Mild reduction of the copper produces a yellow precipitate which appears green in the blue copper solution. Greater amounts of precipitate lead to less residual blue color and are perceived as yellow. Still greater reducing activity

produces some red precipitate, and mixtures of this and the yellow pigment leads to a brown or orange color. In cases where minimally significant reducing activity is present, the turbidity only appears after cooling.

5. The results are recorded semiquantitatively according to the color change (glucose standards in urine):

50 mg	Transparent blue-green	Negative
100 mg	Opaque blue-green	Trace
200 mg	Opaque green	1+
300 mg	Opaque green	1+
500 mg	Yellow green	2+
700 mg	Yellow green	2+
1.0 gm	Olive	2+
1.3 gm	Tannish green	3+
1.6 gm	Tan (no green tint)	3+
1.9 gm	Yellow brown	4+
3.0 gm	Orange brown or red	4+

6. Higher concentrations of glucose can be measured by reducing the amount of urine added to the reagent. Smaller concentrations of glucose and other sugars can be measured by increasing the amount of urine. This latter step is only recommended as a screening test in the newborn period where urines are dilute and other potential reducing substances are not likely to be present.

Discussion

The original test has been modified over the years in order to give greater uniformity to the results in the hands of a large number of different individuals and to allow for the performance of a great number of tests in a short period of time. Reaction in a boiling water bath for 5 minutes has been substituted for direct boiling over a flame. The test is slightly more sensitive than the commercially available tablet variant (Clinitest ®, Ames Company, Elkhart, Indiana), but with modern reagent dispensing system, it is no less convenient to perform in a fixed laboratory area.

Sources of Error

Chloroform and formaldehyde, sometimes used as preservatives, are reducing substances.

Range of Values

It is generally assumed that normal persons excrete less than 100 mg of reducing substance (glucose equivalents) in each 100 ml of urine. These levels should give a negative Benedict's test (no precipitate). The exact range of reducing activity in normal urine is not known but is probably one-tenth of this level.

Resume of Clinical Interpretations

The single most important compound to identify among the many reducing substances is glucose. For practical purposes, there should be a semiquantitative correspondence between Benedict's test and the more sensitive glucose oxidase test papers (Clinistix®, Ames Company, Elkhart, Indiana, or Tes-Tape®, Eli Lilly Company, Indianapolis, Indiana). If some other carbohydrate is the source of reaction, thin layer chromatography can precisely identify the type of mellituria (7).

Many of the conditions associated with mellituria and the compounds that react in Benedict's test are listed in Table 1.

REFERENCES

1. Benedict, J. R.: The detection and estimation of glucose in urine. J.A.M.A., *57*:1193-1195, 1911.
2. Comer, J. P.: Semiquantitative specific test paper for glucose in urine. Analyt. Chem., *28*:1748-1750, 1956.
3. D'Agostino, S.: Mellituria e pseudomellituria provocate da medicamenti. Rass. Clin. Ter. Sci. Affini (Roma), *63*:149-157, 1964.
4. Doolan, P. D., Morris, M. D., and Harper, H. A.:

Aminoaciduria in an elderly man with the nephrotic syndrome and in a young man with a variant of the Fanconi syndrome. Ann. Int. Med., *56*:448-456, 1962.

5. Flint, Austin: Manual of Chemical Examination of the Urine in Disease, New York, D. Appleton, 1870, pp. 14, 36-39.

6. Leonard, J. R.: Evaluation of enzyme tests for urinary glucose. J.A.M.A., *163*:260, 1957.

7. Morris, M. D., and Quittner, H.: In, Sunderman, F. W., and Sunderman, F. W., Jr. (eds.): Clinical Pathology of Infancy. Springfield, Thomas, 1967, pp. 185-189.

8. Piver, M. S.: Fetal outcome in nondiabetic glucosuria of pregnancy. Obstet. Gynec., *30*:576-579, 1967.

9. Transbøl, I., and Halver, B.: Relation of renal glycosuria and parathyroid function in hypercalcemic sarcoidosis. J. Clin. Endocrin., *27*:1193-1196, 1967.

10. Williams, R. T.: Detoxication Mechanisms: The metabolism and Detoxication of Drugs, Toxic Substances and Other Organic Compounds, 2 Ed. New York, J. Wiley & Sons, 1959.

The Clinical Interpretation of Measurements of Urine and Serum Proteins in Kidney Diseases

F. WILLIAM SUNDERMAN, JR., M.D., and JOHN SAVORY, PH.D.

INTRODUCTION

The traditional concept that glomerular capsular fluid is a protein-free ultrafiltrate of plasma has been refuted by recent investigations, and it is now clearly established that plasma proteins with molecular weights less than 200,000 are normally subject, to a limited extent, to glomerular filtration and tubular reabsorption (3, 58, 62, 66). Relatively minor increases above the renal clearances for plasma proteins can result in massive proteinuria. Hence, increased excretion to protein in urine usually occurs early in the course of renal diseases, and ultimately results in alterations in the concentrations of the serum proteins (24, 62).

QUANTITATIVE MEASUREMENTS OF NORMAL URINE PROTEINS

Current interest in quantitative methods for determination of proteins in urine from healthy subjects has been stimulated by the revised regulations of the Food and Drug Administration regarding clinical trials of new drugs (84). The protocols for many clinical trials currently specify analyses of urine protein, inasmuch as increased excretion of protein in urine is one of the most dependable indications of nephrotoxicity. Unfortunately, the methods which are employed for measurements of urine protein are often imprecise (63), and may be subject to interference from drugs and drug metabolites. As examples of drug interference, colorimetric determinations of protein by the Folin-Lowry phenol reaction may be affected by streptomycin, sulfonamides, salicylates, p-aminosalicylic acid, phenacetin and chlorpromazine (29). Similarly, turbidimetric estimations of protein by the sulfosalicylic acid procedures are subject to interference from organic iodine compounds, and from 1-butyl-3-carboxyphenylsulfonylurea, an excretory product of tolbutamide (29).

The most sensitive methods for determination of urine protein involve drying specimens of urine upon strips of filter paper, and staining the dried proteins with amido black (36, 60) bromphenol blue (81) or light green (82) dyes. The dye which becomes bound to the proteins is either estimated directly by densitometry, or is eluted and measured by colorimetry. Although interference from drugs is apparently not a serious problem with the dye-binding methods, such methods are prone to marked day-to-day variability, and are inconvenient for routine use in clinical laboratories. Moreover, the dye-binding methods are subject to systematic errors owing to differences in the relative affinities of the protein fractions for amido black or bromphenol blue (76).

Several investigators have employed the biuret reaction for quantitative measurements of proteins in pathological urine (17, 24, 31, 32, 37, 38, 80), since the biuret reaction is relatively specific for proteins and yields equivalent chromogenicity with albumin and globulin fractions (33). The biuret reaction has been reported by Piscator (54) to be applicable to measurements of protein in normal urine, and has been used by him for the detection of renal toxicity in industrial workers who are exposed to cadmium (55, 56). The Piscator procedure (54) has been modified in our laboratory in order to improve its sensitivity and precision, and to minimize interference from drugs and pigments (68). Our modified biuret procedure (68) is described in Section B-I of this Chapter.

The normal values for urine protein which were obtained in our laboratory are contrasted in Table 1 with the values reported by previous investigators. The range of protein concentrations which was observed (3 to 12 mg per 100 ml) agrees with the findings of most previous authors. It may be noted that the ranges of protein excretions which have been obtained by the Folin-Lowry phenol reaction have, in general, been higher than the ranges obtained by the other methods of analysis. The finding that

TABLE 1—NORMAL VALUES FOR EXCRETION OF PROTEIN IN URINE

Authors	Year	Method of Quantitation	No. of Subjects	Urine Protein mg/100 ml	(Mean and Range) mg/day
Morner (49)	1895	Gravimetry		(2- 8)	
Gunton + Burton (25)	1947	Surface activity	100 ♂	3.7(0-12)	
Tarnoky (79)	1951	Surface activity	42	5.6(2-12)	
Rigas + Heller (64)	1951	Refraction gradient scanning	15		39(30- 50)
Boyce *et al.* (8)	1954	Biuret reaction	13		45(42- 53)
Melo *et al.* (47)	1959	Folin-Lowry reaction	15 ♂		126(90-168)
Coye + Rosandich (16)	1960	Folin-Lowry reaction	10 ♂	3.4(1- 7)	55(22-130)
Piscator (54)	1962	Biuret reaction	22	5.5(3-12)	
Tidstrom (81)	1963	Bromphenol blue	29 ♂		36(9- 73)
			29 ♀		29(10- 80)
Saifer + Gerstenfeld (67)	1964	Folin-Lowry reaction	8		194(S.D.±53)
Jorgensen (35)	1967	Folin-Lowry reaction	17 ♂		122(91-158)
			18 ♀		115(85-145)
DeLuna + Hulet (41)	1967	Folin-Lowry reaction	46	11.4(4-25)	140(77-263)
Hemmingsen + Skov (28)	1968	Folin-Lowry reaction	49		216(38-394)
		Nitrogen analyses	49		96(2-190)
Savory *et al.* (68)	1968	Biruet reaction	14 ♂	6.4(3-12)	79(48-150)
			14 ♀	6.0(4-10)	76(40-131)

there was no significant difference between normal excretion of urine protein in male and female adults is consistent with the observations of Tidstrom (81) and Jorgensen (35).

Quantitative measurements of urine proteins by sensitive methods, such as the authors' biuret procedure (68), are primarily useful as a means of detecting nephrotoxicity (1, 54, 71, 83). The methods also have clinical applications as a quantitative means of assessing orthostatic (39, 40) and exercise-induced (9, 15, 16, 58) proteinuria. Moreover, the investigations of Harlan and co-workers (25) indicate that quantitative measurements of urine protein may be valuable as an index of immunologic rejection in patients who have received renal transplants.

Fractionations of Urine Proteins

Electrophoretic fractionations of urine proteins were first described in 1939 by Hesselvik, (30) and have been studied by numerous subsequent investigators (8, 10, 11, 12, 13, 20, 21, 46, 51, 64, 66, 70, 86, 88). In order to separate urine proteins electrophoretically, the proteins may first be concentrated by precipitation, dialysis and lyophilization, ultra-filtration, or gel-filtration (48, 52, 57). Electrophoretic patterns obtained with proteins from normal urine reveal traces of pre-albumin components and a well-defined albumin peak with mobility identical to that of serum albumin. The globulin fractions which are derived from serum are poorly separated in electrophoretograms of normal urine proteins, owing in part to the presence of mucoproteins which originate in the urinary tract, and which obscure the demarcation between alpha-1, alpha-2, and beta globulins (20, 21, 64, 66, 78, 86). In addition to the mucoproteins and the globulin fractions with mobilities similar to those of serum globulins, a "post-gamma" globulin fraction has been found in certain pathological urines by Butler and Flynn (12).

The method for electrophoretic fractionations of urine proteins which is employed in our laboratory is described in Section B-IV of this Chapter. Fractionations of protein in urine collections from 28 healthy adults yielded a mean percentage of albumin of 37.7 (standard deviation = ±5.8) with a range from 27 to 50%. Albumin excretions in urine were computed by multiplying the total protein values (determined by the biuret procedure) by the percentages of albumin (measured by electrophoresis). The mean excretion of albumin was 29.0 mg per day (standard deviation = ±12.0) with a range from 19 to 52 mg per day. These normal values for urine albumin are compared in Table 2 with the values reported by investigators who have employed a variety of electrophoretic techniques and various methods for quantitation of total protein. It may be noted that the mean percentage of urine albumin obtained in our laboratory agrees closely with the mean percentages of albumin previously reported by Rigas and Heller (64), Boyce and co-workers (8), McGarry and co-workers (46), and Poortmans and Jeanloz (58).

In most cases of pathological proteinuria, the percentage of albumin becomes increased (10, 70, 88), For example, the percentages of albumin which have been reported in 13 patients with nephrotic syndrome have ranged from 55 to 92% (10, 70, 88). Similar percentages of albumin have been observed in glomerulonephritis, hypertensive nephrosclerosis

TABLE 2—NORMAL VALUES FOR EXCRETION OF ALBUMIN
IN URINE BASED UPON ELECTROPHORETIC FRACTIONATIONS

Authors	*Year*	*Method of Electrophoresis*	*No. of Subjects*	*Urine Protein % of total*	*(Mean and Range) mg/day*
Rigas + Heller (64)	1951	Tiselius	15	36(S.D.$\pm$5)	15(S.D.$\pm$2)
Boyce *et al.* (8)	1954	Tiselius	13	38	17
McGarry *et al.* (46)	1955	Tiselius	7	39(32-54)	
Webb *et al.* (87)	1958	Tiselius	11	23(13-27)	31(15-45)
		Filter paper	11	27	36
Hemmingsen + Skov (28)	1968	Acrylamide gel	49	53(22-77)	
Poortmans + Jeanloz (58)	1968	Immunodiffusion	6	40	13(9-22)
Savory *et al.* (68)	1968	Cellulose acetate	28	38(27-50)	29(18-52)

and most other renal diseases (10, 70, 88). The studies Boyce and co-workers (8) and of Wolvius and Vershure (88) indicate that the mean percentages of albumin in obstructive pyelonephritis and calculous disease may be lower than in intrinsic diseases of the kidney. Butler and Flynn (11, 13) have reported that an increased proportion of urinary alpha-2 globulin usually occurs in renal tubular disorders. Despite these observations, our experience supports the conclusions of several investigators (10, 70, 88) that, excepting for mutiple myeloma and Franklin's disease, electrophoretic fractionations of urine proteins have limited value in differential diagnosis.

URINE PROTEINS IN
MULTIPLE MYELOMA
AND FRANKLIN'S DISEASE

Recent studies in our laboratory of a patient with multiple myeloma are illustrated in Figure 1, as an example of the clinical usefulness of urine electrophoresis in this disorder. Electrophoretic fractionation of the patient's serum proteins revealed hypoalbuminemia and borderline diminution in gamma globulin. No myeloma globulin was detected in the serum electrophoretogram. Measurements of the patient's serum immunoglobulins by immunodiffusion are indicated by the stippled columns in Figure 1, and are contrasted with our normal values (hatched columns). The patient's serum contained a diminished concentration of IgG and low normal concentrations of IgA and IgM. Electrophoresis of urine proteins revealed a spike-like protein peak with mobility similar to gamma globulin. The heat precipitation test of Putnam and co-workers (61) (described in Section B-II of this Chapter), demonstrated that the urine proteins consisted predominently of Bence-Jones protein. Thus, this patient is an example of multiple myeloma with Bence-Jones proteinuria, in the absence of detectable myeloma globulin in the sermu. Although this situation was formerly believed to be uncommon, Osserman and Takatsuki (50) and Paraskevas (53) have reported that Bence-Jones proteinuria without myelomaglobulinemia occurred in approximately 23% of patients with multiple myeloma.

Recent investigations have demonstrated that the Bence-Jones proteins in multiple myeloma consist of "light chain" polypeptides of the immunoglo-

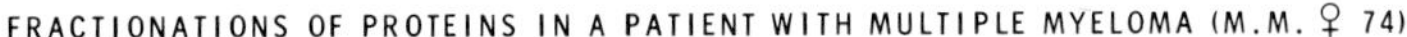

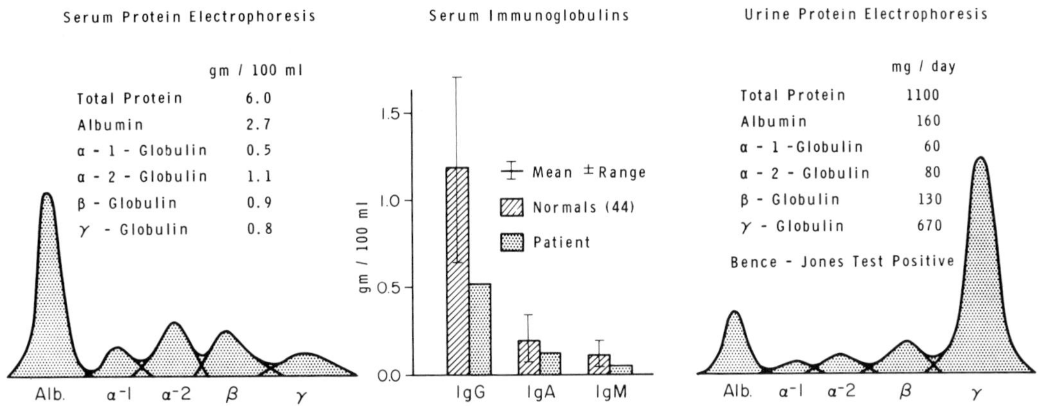

Fig. 1. Fractionations of serum and urine proteins in a patient with multiple myeloma (see text).

bulins (6, 50, 89). The light chains in multiple myeloma are present in urine either in the form of monomers with molecular weights of approximately 22,000 or as dimers with molecular weights of approximately 44,000 (6, 26). Whereas the light chains which are excreted in trace amounts in the urine of normal subjects are a mixture of "kappa" and "lambda" antigenic varieties (77, 85), the Bence-Jones proteins in multiple myeloma are almost always entirely kappa or entirely lambda in their antigenic constitution (26, 89). However, an unusual patient with multiple myeloma who excreted both kappa and lambda light chains has been reported by Rosen and co-workers (65).

Harrison and co-workers (26) have shown that the renal clearance of proteins in myeloma, as in other disorders, is inversely related to the molecular size of the proteins. Therefore, the high clearances of Bence-Jones proteins are consistent with their small molecular radii (27). Bence-Jones proteins in urine from 9 patients with multiple myeloma

who were studied by Harrison and associates (26) had electrophoretic mobilities varying from alpha-2 to gamma globulins. In 11 patients with Bence-Jones proteinuria studied in our laboratory, the Bence-Jones proteins have migrated as either beta or gamma globulins.

The electrophoretic pattern of urine proteins in patients with Franklin's disease ("heavy chain" disease) also reveals a homogeneous peak which resembles the peaks seen in multiple myeloma (18, 19, 50). The urine protein in Franklin's disease consists of "heavy chains" of the immunoglobulins, which give a negative Bence-Jones test and do not react antigenically with kappa or lambda antisera. The molecular weight of the urine protein is approximately 70,000, and the sedimentation constant is approximately 3.7 S. Serum protein electrophoresis in Franklin's disease usually reveals a paraglobulin peak with mobility identical to that of the abnormal urine protein (18, 19, 50).

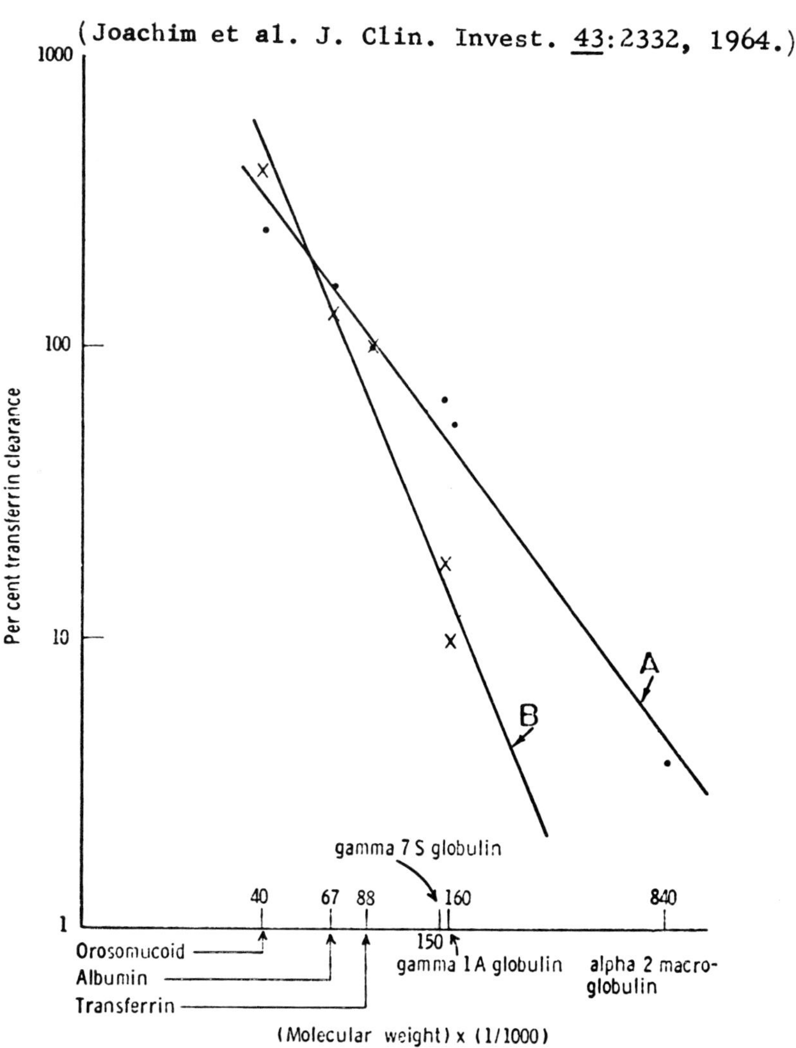

Fig. 2. Graphical method of expressing the "selectivity" of proteinuria (see text). (Reproduced with permission (34).)

IMMUNOLOGICAL STUDIES OF URINE PROTEINS

Immunological studies of urine proteins are becoming increasingly valuable as guides to prognosis in diseases affecting the renal glomerulus (7, 14, 34, 42, 43, 44, 45, 58, 72). Immunoelectrophoretic fractionations of urine proteins have demonstrated the presence in normal urine of at least 25 constituents of the serum proteins (3, 4, 5, 58, 59, 77). By means of immunodiffusion (14, 34, 42, 72) or gel filtration (23, 27, 42, 69), estimations can be made of the renal clearances of serum proteins of varying molecular weights. Such measurements provide an index of the relative "selectivity" of proteinuria. In this connotation, the term "selectivity" has been defined as the slope of the line relating the logarithims of the relative renal clearances of the

NEPHROTIC SYNDROME AND CHRONIC GLOMERULONEPHRITIS

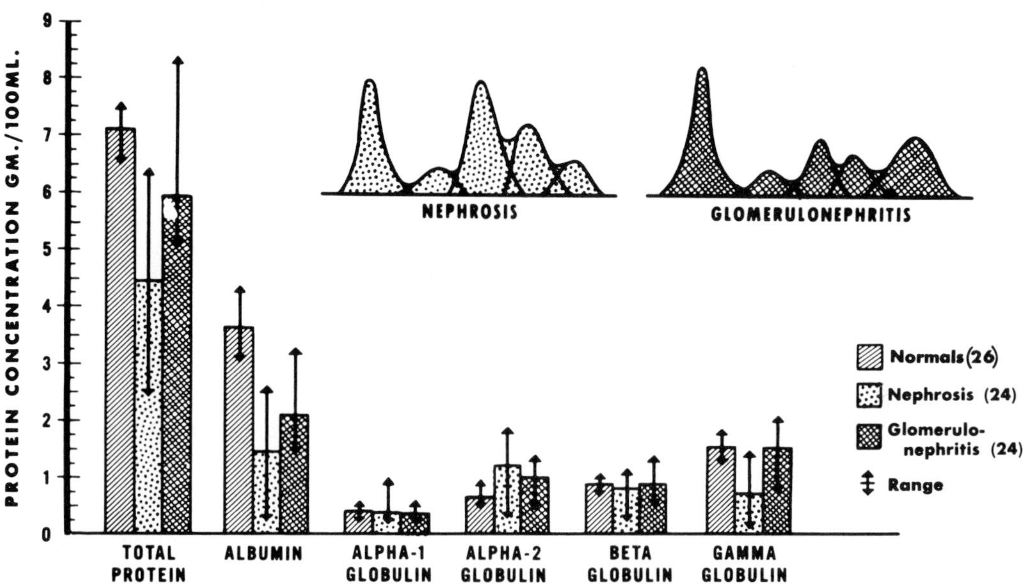

Fig. 3. Electrophoretic fractionations of serum proteins in 24 patients with nephrotic syndrome and 24 patients with chronic glomerulonephritis (see text).

serum proteins to the logarithims of their molecular weights (14, 34, 72). When very small amounts of high molecular weight proteins such as gamma globulins and alpha-2 macroglobulin are excreted in the urine, the slope is steep, as indicated by line B in Figure 2, and the proteinuria is termed "selective." When larger amounts of the macromolecular proteins are present in the urine, the slope is relatively more flat, as indicated by line A in Figure 2, and the proteinuria is termed "unselective." This technique provides a graphic means of expressing the permeability of the renal glomerulus to proteins ranging in size from orosomucoid (molecular weight = 40,000) to alpha-2 macroglobulin (molecular weight = 840,000). According to Joachim and associates (34), and Cameron and White (14), steroid sensi-

tive patients with nephrotic syndrome typically have "selective" proteinuria, and steroid-insensitive patients with nephrotic syndrome usually have "unselective"proteinuria.

ALTERATIONS OF SERUM PROTEINS IN KIDNEY DISEASES

As previously mentioned in the Introduction to this chapter, pathological proteinuria ultimately produces alterations in the concentrations of the serum proteins. Therefore, electrophoretic fractionations of serum proteins are frequently valuable in assessing the type and severity of renal diseases (24, 51, 73, 74, 75).

In Figure 3, the results of electrophoretic fractionations performed in our laboratory upon serums from 26 normal subjects (the hatched columns) are compared with data obtained with serums from 24 patients with the nephrotic syndrome (the stippled columns) and 24 patients with chronic glomerulonephritis (the cross-hatched columns). Typical electrophoretic patterns for the two groups of patients are illustrated at the top of Figure 3. In the patients with the nephrotic syndrome, there was a great increase in the mean concentration of serum alpha-2 globulin, associated with profound decreases in the mean concentrations of albumin and gamma globulin. In several instances, the concentrations of gamma globulin approached the values encountered in hypogammaglobulinemia. In our experience, these electrophoretic patterns of serum proteins in nephrotic syndrome are virtually characteristic, the only similar findings being observed in patients with exudative enteropathy (73, 74).

In contrast to the pattern observed in the nephrotic syndrome, electrophoretic frantionations of serum proteins in patients with chronic glomerulonephritis reveal diminished mean concentration of albumin and slightly increased mean concentration of alpha-2 globulin (Fig. 3). The concentrations of the other globulin fractions are usually normal in chronic glomerulonephritis. Although not shown in Figure 3, the electrophoretic patterns of proteins obtained in our laboratory in serums from patients with chronic pyelonephritis were essentially the same as in chronic glomerulonephritis.

CONCLUSION

In 1870, Basham (2) made the following statement in his textbook on renal diseases; "In a pathological sense the presence of albumen in the urine occupies the very highest place of importance. Its connection with . . . one of the most fatal classes of disorders entitles it to precedence before all other substances foreign to healthy urine." Although the techniques for the measurements of urine proteins have been improved from the primitive methods which were described in Basham's text, the clinical importance of proteinuria in relationship to the diagnosis and prognosis of renal diseases has remained undiminished.

BIBLIOGRAPHY

1. Axelsson, B., and Piscator, M.: Renal damage after prolonged exposure to cadmium. Arch. Environ. Health., *12:*360-373, 1966.
2. Basham, W. R.: Renal Diseases: A Clinical Guide to Their Diagnosis and Treatment. Philadelphia, H. C. Lea Co., 1870, 304 pp.
3. Berggard, I.: Studies on the plasma proteins in normal human urine. Clin. Chim. Acta, *6:*413-429, 1961.
4. Berggard, I.: On a γ-globulin of low molecular weight in normal human plasma and urine. Clin. Chim. Acta, *6:*545-549, 1961.
5. Berggard, I., Cleve, H., and Bearn, A. G.: The excretion of five plasma proteins previously unidentified in normal human urine. Clin. Chim. Acta, *10:*1-11, 1964.
6. Bernier, G. M., and Putnam, F. W.: Myeloma proteins and macroglobulins: Hallmarks of disease and models of antibodies. Progr. Hemat., *4:*160-186, 1964.
7. Blainey, J. D., Brewer, D. B., Hardwicke, J., and Soothill, J. F.: The nephrotic syndrome. Diagnosis by renal biopsy and biochemical and immunological analyses related to the response to steroid therapy. Quart. J. Med., *29:*235-256, 1960.
8. Boyce, W. H., Garvey, F. K., and Norfleet, C. M., Jr.: Proteins and other biocolloids of urine in health and in calculous disease. I. Electrophoretic studies at pH 4.5 and 8.6 of those components soluble in molar sodium chloride. J. Clin. Invest., *33:*1287-1297, 1954.
9. Bozovic, L., Castenfors, J., and Piscator, M.: Effect of prolonged heavy exercise on urinary protein excretion and plasma renin activity. Acta Physiol. Scand., *70:*143-146, 1967.
10. Broch, O. J., and Brodwall, E.: Urinary proteins in renal diseases. Acta Med. Scand., *160:*353-361, 1958.
11. Butler, E. A., and Flynn, F. V.: The proteinuria

of renal tubular disorders. Lancet, *2:*978-980, 1958.

12. Butler, E. A., and Flynn, F. V.: The occurence of post-gamma protein in urine: a new protein abnormality. J. Clin. Path., *19:*172-178, 1961.

13. Butler, E. A., Flynn, F. V., Harris, H., and Robson, E. R.: A study of urine proteins by two-dimensional electrophoresis with special reference to the proteinuria of renal tubular disorders. Clin. Chim. Acta, *7:*34-41, 1962.

14. Cameron, J. S., and White, R. H. R.: Selectivity of proteinuria in children with the nephrotic syndrome. Lancet, *1:*463-465, 1965.

15. Castenfors, J., Mossfeldt, F., and Piscator, M.: Effect of prolonged heavy exercise on renal function and urinary protein excretion. Acta Physiol. Scand., *70:*194-206, 1967.

16. Coye, R. D., and Rosandich, R. R.: Proteinuria during the 24-hour period following exercise. J. Appl. Physiol., *15:*592-594, 1960.

17. Foster, P. W., Rick, J. J., and Wolfson, W. Q.: Studies in serum proteins. VI. The extension of the standard biuret method to the estimation of protein in urine. J. Lab. Clin. Med., *39:*618-623, 1952

18. Franklin, E. C., Lowenstein, J., Bigelow, B., and Meltzer, M.: Heavy chain disease-a new disorder of serum γ-globulin. Amer. J. Med., *37:*332-350, 1964.

19. Franklin, E. C., Meltzer, M., Guggenheim, F., and Lowenstein, J.: An unusual micro-gamma-globulin in the serum and urine of a patient. Fed. Proc., *22:*264, 1963.

20. Grant, G. H.: The proteins of normal urine. J. Clin. Path., *10:*360-368, 1957.

21. Grant, G. H.: The proteins of normal urine. II. From the urinary tract. J. Clin. Path., *12:*510-517, 1959.

22. Gunton, R., and Burton, A. C.: On the concentration of protein in samples of normal urine measured by its surface activity. J. Clin. Invest., *36:*892-898, 1947.

23. Hardwicke, J.: Estimation of renal permeability to protein on Sephadex G-200. Clin. Chim. Acta, *12:*89-96, 1965.

24. Hardwicke, J., and Squire, J. R.: The relationship between plasma albumin concentration and protein excretion in patients with proteinuria. Clin. Sci., *14:*509-530, 1955.

25. Harlan, W. R., Jr., Holden, K. R., Williams, G. M., and Hume, D. M.: Proteinuria and nephrotic syndrome associated with chronic rejection of kidney transplants. New Eng. J. Med., *277:*769-776, 1967.

26. Harrison, J. F., Blainey, J. D., Hardwicke, J., Rowe, D. S., and Soothill, J. F.: Proteinuria in multiple myeloma. Clin. Sci., *31:*95-110, 1966.

27. Harrison, J. F., and Northam, B. E.: Low molecular weight urine protein investigated by gel filtration. Clin. Chim. Acta, *14:*679-688, 1966.

28. Hemmingsen, L., and Skov, F.: The protein and LDH isoenzyme pattern of normal human urine determined by polyacrylamide gel disc electrophoresis. Clin. Chim. Acta, *19:*81-87, 1968.

29. Henry, R. J.: Clinical Chemistry: Principles and Technics. New York, Harper and Row, 193-197, 1964.

30. Hesselvik, L.: An electrophoretic study of normal and pathological body fluids. Acta Med. Scand., *101:*461-464, 1939.

31. Hiller, A., Greif, R. L., and Beckman, W. W.: Determination of protein in urine by the biuret method. J. Biol. Chem., *176:*1421-1429, 1948.

32. Hiller, A., McIntosh, J. F., and Van Slyke, D. D.: The excretion of albumin and globulin in nephritis. J. Clin. Invest., *4:*235-251, 1927.

33. de la Huerga, J., Smetters, G. W., and Sherrick, J. C.: Gravimetric standardization of the biuret reaction. In, Sunderman, F. W., and Sunderman, F. W., Jr. (eds.): Serum Proteins and the Dysproteinemias. Philadelphia, J. B. Lippincott Co., p. 62, 1964.

34. Joachim, G. R., Cameron, J. S., Schwartz, M., and Becker, E. L.: Selectivity of protein excretion in patients with the nephrotic syndrome. J. Clin. Invest., *43:*2332-2346, 1964.

35. Jorgensen, M. B.: A gel filtration method for the determination of protein in normal urine. Acta Med. Scand., *181:*153-162, 1967.

36. Kaltwasser, F., Walters, P., and Pieper, J.: Kolorimetrische Mikromethode zur Bestimmung des Gesamteiweisses in eiweissarmen Flussigkeiten. Clin. Chim. Acta, *15:*347-351, 1967.

37. Kibrick, A. C.,: Extended use of the Kingsley biuret reagent. Clin. Chem., *4:*232-236, 1958.

38. Lauritsen, O. S.: Estimation of protein concentration in urine and solutions of albumin and globulin. Scand. J. Clin. Lab. Invest., *19:* (Suppl 100), 147-148, 1967.

39. Lecocq, F. R., McPhaul, J. J., and Robinson, R. R.: Fixed and reproductible orthostatic proteinuria. Ann. Int. Med., *64:*557-569, 1966.

40. Levitt, J. I.: The prognostic significance of proteinuria in young college students. Ann. Int. Med., *66:*685-696, 1967.

41. Luna, M. B. de, and Hulet, W. H.: Urinary protein excretion in healthy infants, children and adults. Abstracts of the American Society of Nephrology (Los Angeles Meeting), p. 16, October, 1967.

42. MacLean, P. R., and Petrie, J. J. B.: A comparison of gel filtration and immunodiffusion in the determination of selectivity of proteinuria. Clin. Chim. Acta, *14:*367-376, 1966.

43. MacLean, P. R., and Robson, J. S.: Unselective proteinuria in acute ischaemic renal failure. Clin. Sci., *30:*91-102, 1966.

44. MacLean, P. R., Robson, J. S.: A simple method for determining the selectivity of proteinuria. Lancet, *1:*539-542, 1967.

45. Maiorce, R., Scarpioi, L., Cambi, V., Carrara, G.

C., and Dall'Aglio, P.: Urinary protein clearances in chronic renal diseases with and without uremia. Clin. Chim. Acta, *16:*253-257, 1967.

46. McGarry, E., Sehon, A. H., and Rose, B.: The isolation and electrophoretic characterization of the proteins in the urine of normal subjects. J. Clin. Invest., *36:*832-844, 1955.

47. Melo, E. H. L., Mariani, I., Martirani, I., and Cintra, A.B.U.: Protein, hexose and hexosamine in the nondialyzable fraction of the filtered urine in normal young men. J. Lab. Clin. Med., *54:*739-745, 1959.

48. Miyasato, F., and Pollak, V. E.: Serum proteins in urine: an examination of the effects of some methods used to concentrate the urine. J. Lab. Clin. Med., *67:*1036-1043, 1966.

49. Morner, G. K. A. H.: Untersuchungen über die Proteinstoffe und die eiweissfällenden Substanzen des normalen Menschenharns. Skand. Arch. Physiol., *6:*332-437, 1895.

50. Osserman, E. F., and Takatsuki, K.: Plasma cell myeloma: gamma globulin synthesis and structure. Medicine, *42:*357-384, 1963.

51. Owen, J. A., and Rider, W. D.: Electrophoretic analysis of serum and urinary proteins in the diagnosis of myelomatosis. J. Clin. Path., *10:*373-378, 1957.

52. Palmer, D. A., and Peters, T., Jr.: Optimal conditions for dialysis of spinal fluid and urine in the routine laboratory. Amer. J. Clin. Path., *47:*824-826, 1967.

53. Paraskevas, F.: Gamma globulins, antibodies and myeloma patients. Clin. Biochem., *1:*135-153, 1967.

54. Piscator, M.: Proteinuria in chronic cadmium poisoning. II. The applicability of quantitative and qualitative methods of protein determination. Arch. Environ. Health, *5:*325-332, 1962.

55. Piscator, M.: Proteinuria in chronic cadmium poisoning. III. Electrophoretic and immunoelectrophoretic studies on urinary proteins from cadmium workers, with special reference to the excretion of low molecular weight proteins. Arch. Environ. Health, *12:*335-344, 1966.

56. Piscator, M.: Proteinuria in chronic cadmium poisoning. IV. Gel filtration and ion exchange chromatography of urinary proteins from cadmium workers. Arch. Environ. Health, *12:*345-359, 1966.

57. Pollak, V. E., Gaizutis, M., and Rezaian, J.: Serum proteins in urine: examination of new method for concentrating urine. J. Lab. Clin. Med., *71:*338-344, 1968.

58. Poortmans, J., and Jeanloz, R. W.: Quantitative immunological determination of 12 plasma proteins excreted in human urine collected before and after exercise. J. Clin. Invest, *47:*386-393, 1968.

59. Poortmans, J. R., Jeanloz, R. W., and Schmid, K.: α_2-HS-Glycoprotein levels of normal human plasma and urine. Clin. Chim. Acta, 17:305-306, 1967.

60. Poortmans, J. R., and van Kerchove, E.: Dosage de la proteinurie: comparaison de deux methodes. Clin. Chim. Acta, *8:*485-488, 1963.

61. Putnam, F. W., Easley, C. W., Lynn, L. T., Ritchie, A. E. and Phelps, R. A.: The heat precipitation of Bence-Jones proteins. I. Optimum conditions. Arch. Biochem. Biophys., *83:*115-130, 1959.

62. Rather, L. J.: Filtration, resorption and excretion of protein by the kidney. Medicine, *31:*357-380, 1952.

63. Rennie, I. D. B., and Keen, H.: Evaluation of clinical methods for detecting proteinuria. Lancet, *2:*489-492, 1967.

64. Rigas, D. A., and Heller, C. G.: The amount and nature of urinary proteins in normal human subjects. J. Clin. Invest., 30:853-861, 1951.

65. Rosen, B. J., Smith, T. W., and Bloch, K. J.: Multiple myeloma associated with two serum M components, *b*G-type K and γA-type L. New Eng. J. Med., *277:*902-907, 1967.

66. Rowe, D. S., and Soothill, J. F.: Serum proteins in normal urine. Clin. Sci., *21:*75-85, 1961.

67. Saifer, A., and Gerstenfeld, S.: Photometric determination of urinary proteins. Clin. Chem., *10:*321-334, 1964.

68. Savory, J., Pu, P. H., and Sunderman, F. W., Jr.: A biuret method for determination of protein in normal urine. Clin. Chem., *14:*1160-1171, 1968.

69. Schubert, G., Doleschel, W., and Auerswald, W.: The information value of Sephadex G-150 gel filtration concerning the molecular sizes of serum and urinary proteins. Wien. Klin. Wschr., *78:*629-633, 1966.

70. Sellers, A. L., and Marmorston, J.: Electrophoretic study of human urinary protein in disease. J. Lab. Clin. Med., *47:*248-254, 1956.

71. Smith, J. C., Wells, A. R., and Kench, J. E.: Observations on the urinary protein of men exposed to cadmium dust and fume. Brit. J. Indust. Med., *18:*70-78, 1961.

72. Soothill, J. F., and Hendrickse, R. G.: Some immunological studies of the nephrotic syndrome of Nigerian children. Lancet, *2:*629-632, 1967.

73. Sunderman, F. W., Jr.: Studies of the serum proteins. VI. Recent advances in clinical interpretation of electrophoretic fractionations. Amer. J. Clin. Path., *42:*1-21, 1964.

74. Sunderman, F. W., Jr., and Jonhson, M. W.: Studies of the serum proteins. VII. Sucrose gradient electrophoresis. Amer. J. Clin. Path., *45:*381-397, 1967.

75. Sunderman, F. W., Jr., and Sunderman, F. W.: Clinical applications of the fractionation of serum proteins by paper electrophoresis. Amer. J. Clin. Path., *27:*125-158, 1957.

76. Sunderman, F. W., Jr., and Sunderman, F. W.: Studies of the serum proteins. IV. The dye-binding of purified serum proteins separated by continuous-flow electrophoresis. Clin. Chem., 5:171-185, 1959.
77. Takatsuki, K., and Osserman, E. F.: Demonstration of two types of low molecular weight γ-globulins in normal human urine. J. Immunol., 92:100-107, 1964.
78. Tamm, I., and Horsfall, F. L., Jr.: A mucoprotein derived from human urine which reacts with influenza, mumps and Newcastle disease viruses. J. Exper. Med., 95:71-97, 1952.
79. Tarnoky, A.: "Apparent protein" in human urine; some surface film measurements. Biochem. J., 49:205-209, 1951.
80. Thieler, H., and Anger, G.: Vergleinchende quantitative Harnproteinbestimmung mit der Biuret-Methode und der Kupfer-Folin-Reaktion nach Lowry. Klin. Wschr., 44:464-467, 1966.
81. Tidstrom, B.: Quantitative determination of protein in normal urine. Scand. J. Clin. Lab. Invest., 15:167-172, 1963.
82. Trotter, M. D., and Fairburn, E. A.: Subclinical proteinuria in dermatological outpatients. Lancet, 2:231-233, 1967.
83. Tsuchiya, K.: Proteinuria of workers exposed to cadmium fume. Arch. Environ. Health, 14:875-880, 1967.
84. U.S. Department of Health, Education and Welfare (Food and Drug Administration): Clinical testing, Synopsis of the new drug regulations. Int. J. Clin. Pharm., 1:35-39, 1967.
85. Vaughan, J. M., Jacox, R. F., and Gay, B. A.: Light and heavy chain components of gamma globulins in urines of normal patients and patients with agammaglobulinemia. J. Clin. Invest., 46:266-279, 1967.
86. Walravens, P., Laterre, E. C., and Heremans, J. F.: Studies on tubular proteinuria. Clin. Chim. Acta, 19:107-120, 1960.
87. Webb, T., Rose, B., and Sehon, A. H.: Biocolloids of normal human urine. Canad. J. Biochem. Physiol., 36:1159-1166, 1958.
88. Wolvius, D., and Verschure, J. C. M.: The diagnostic value of the protein excretion pattern in various types of proteinuria. J. Clin. Path., 10:80-83, 1957.
89. Zawadzki, Z. A., Edwards, G. A.: M-components in immunoproliferative disorders. Amer. J. Clin. Path., 48:418-430, 1967.

Methods for Measurement and Fractionation of Proteins in Urine and Serum

JOHN SAVORY, Ph.D., F. WILLIAM SUNDERMAN, Jr., M.D., and PIN H. PU, M.D.

INTRODUCTION

This section describes the techniques which are currently employed in the authors' laboratory for: I) determination of total proteins in urine: II) detection of Bence-Jones protein in urine; III) ultrafiltration of urine proteins preparatory to electrophoretic fractionation; IV) fractionation of proteins in urine and serum by cellulose acetate electrophoresis; V) measurements of serum immunoglobulins by radial immunodiffusion, and VI) determination of total serum proteins.

I. DETERMINATION OF TOTAL PROTEINS IN URINE (10)

Principle

After centrifugation of urine to remove sediment, the protein is precipitated from duplicate 20 ml samples of urine by addition of an equal volume of cold ethanolic phosphotungstic acid. After 15 minutes in an ice bath to ensure complete precipitation, the protein precipitates are separated by centrifugation and washed with cold ethanol. Protein from one of the duplicate samples is dissolved in 4 ml of biuret reagent. Protein from the second sample is dissolved in 4 ml of an alkaline tartrate reagent which is identical to the biuret reagent, excepting that copper sulfate has been omitted. After 20 minutes at room temperature, the differential absorbance of the 2 samples is measured at 540 mμ.

Reagents

1. *Ethanolic Phosphotungstic Acid.* Into a 1 liter beaker are transferred 50 ml of concentrated hydrochloric acid (sp. gr = 1.19), 60 ml of distilled water, and 770 ml of 95% (v/v) ethanol. Fifteen gm of phosphotungstic acid are added and dissolved. The solution is filtered and stored in the refrigerator.

2. *Ethanol,* absolute, stored in the refrigerator

3. *Sodium chloride solution,* 0.85% (w/v).

4. *Biuret Reagent.* Nine and six-tenths gm of potassium sodium tartrate (KNaC$_4$H$_4$O$_6$ · 4H$_2$O) are dissolved in 400 ml of distilled water in a 2-liter

graduate cylinder with ground-glass stopper. Two and four-tenths gm of cupric sulfate pentahydrate ($CuSO_4 \cdot 5H_2O$) are added and dissolved. Three hundred and sixty ml of 2.5 N sodium hydroxide are added slowly, followed by one gm of potassium iodide. The solution is diluted to 1500 ml with distilled water. The reagent is stored in a plastic bottle, and is stable for several months at room temperature.

5. *Alkaline Tartrate Reagent.* This solution is prepared in exactly the same manner as the biuret reagent, excepting that the cupric sulfate is omitted.

6. *Protein Standards.* The concentration of protein nitrogen in a sample of pooled human serum is determined by the Kjeldahl procedure (12). The total protein concentration is calculated using the factor of 6.54 gm of protein per gm of nitrogen (13). The serum protein standard is stored in small ampoules at -15°C. An appropriate dilution of the protein standard is made with 0.85% (w/v) sodium chloride solution to achieve a final concentration of 10 to 15 mg of protein per 100 ml. The dilute protein standard is stored at 4°C, and is stable for 1 week.

Special Apparatus

Centrifuge tubes, 50 ml, with ground-glass stoppers (Cat. No. 45168, Kimble Glass Co., Toledo, Ohio). These tubes fit centrifuge cups No. 367, with rubber cushions No. 575, metal shields No. 572, and trunnion rings No. 366, International Equipment Co., Boston, Mass.

Procedure

1. The volume of the 24-hour collection of urine is measured. Fifty ml of urine are centrifuged at 2000 rpm for 15 minutes. The supernatant urine is de-

canted into a beaker and is used for the analysis.

2. The protein concentration in the centrifuged urine sample is estimated by means of "Albustix" test strips (Ames Co.). If the "Albustix" reaction is "negative" or "trace," 20 ml of urine are taken for analysis. If the "Albustix" test gives quanitative reactions of 1+, 2+, 3+, and 4+, the following volumes of urine should be taken: 10 ml, 5 ml, 2 ml and 0.5 ml, respectively. The requisite volumes of urine are transferred into duplicate 50 ml centrifuge tubes, and are diluted (if necessary) to 20 ml with 0.85% (w/v) sodium chloride solution.

3. Into 2 additional pairs of 50 ml centrifuge tubes are transferred (in duplicate) 20 ml of sodium chloride solution (blank samples), and 20 ml of dilute protein standard solution (standard samples). The centrifuge tubes are placed in an ice bath for 5 to 10 minutes.

4. Twenty ml of cold ethanolic phosphotungstic acid reagent are added to all of the tubes. The contents of the tubes are mixed and the tubes are allowed to stand in the ice bath for 15 minutes.

5. The tubes are centrifuged at 2000 rpm for 15 minutes. The supernatants are discarded by decantation, and the tubes are inverted to drain onto filter paper.

6. Ten ml of cold ethanol are added to the tubes, and the protein pellets are dispersed by means of a "Vortex" rotary mixer. The tubes are centrifuged at 2000 rpm for 10 minutes, and the ethanol is discarded by decantation. The tubes are again inverted to drain onto filter paper.

7. Four ml of biuret reagent are added to 1 of each pair of duplicate tubes. Four ml of alkaline tartrate reagent are added to the remaining tubes. The protein precipitates are dissolved by agitation with a "Vortex" rotary mixer.

8. The tubes are allowed to stand at room temperature for 20 minutes. The contents of each tube are transferred to a Coleman spectrophotometer cuvet (19 mm diameter). An adapter is placed at the bottom of a Coleman cuvet holder, in order that the optical density of a 4 ml volume can be measured.

9. A Coleman spectrophotometer is adjusted to zero optical density at 540 mμ, using the cuvet which contains the blank sample and alkaline tartrate reagent. The optical densities of the remaining samples are then measured and recorded.

Calculations

$$\text{Protein conc. (mg/100 ml)} = \frac{\text{O.D.}_U - (\text{O.D.}_{UB} + \text{O.D.}_{RB})}{\text{O.D.}_S - (\text{O.D.}_{SB} + \text{O.D.}_{RB})} \times \text{std. conc.}$$

O.D._U = absorbance of urine sample treated with biuret reagent.

O.D._{UB} = absorbance of urine sample treated with alkaline tartrate reagent.

O.D._S = absorbance of protein standard treated with biuret reagent.

O.D._{SB} = absorbance of protein standard treated with alkaline tartrate reagent.

O.D._{RB} = absorbance of blank sample treated with biuret reagent.

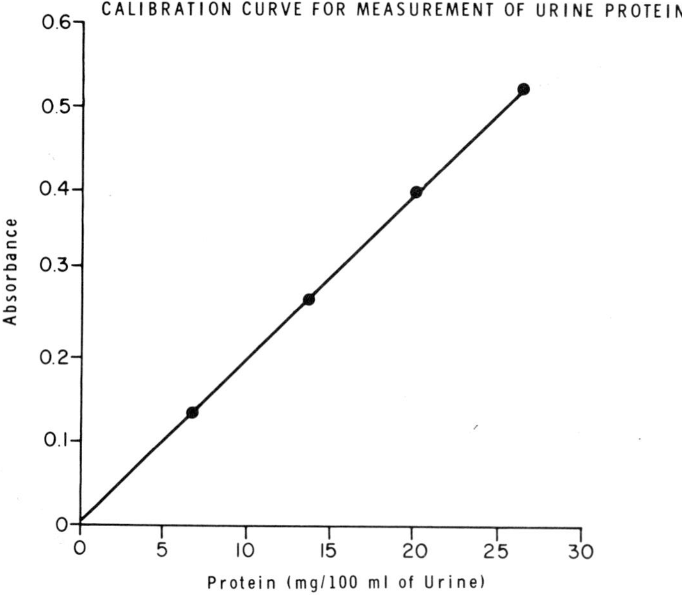

Fig. 1. Calibration chart for measurements of urine proteins by the biuret procedure. Protein concentration is expressed in mg per 100 ml of urine.

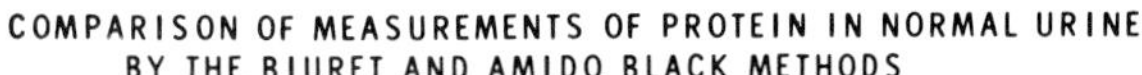

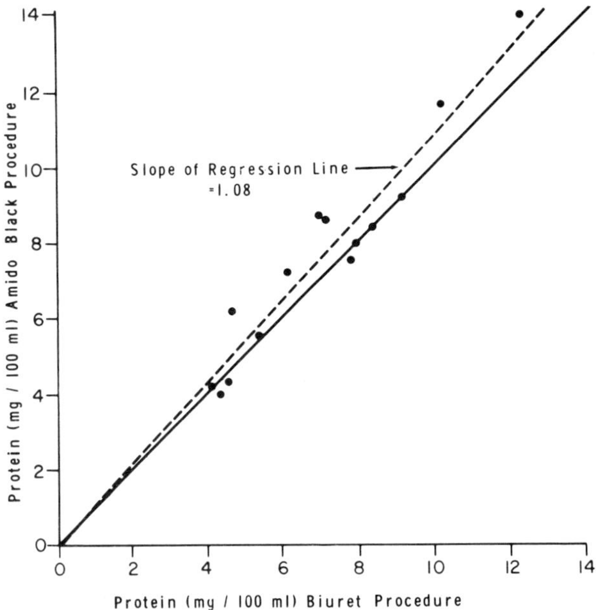

Fig. 2. Comparison of measurement of protein concentrations in 24-hour urine collections from 14 healthy adults by the biuret procedure and by the amido black procedure of Kaltwasser and associates (3). The interrupted line indicates the calculated regression line, and the solid line represents the theoretical relationship of x = y.

Discussion

The *limit of detection* for urine protein (i.e., the protein concentration which gives a corrected absorbance value of 0.01) is 0.5 mg per 100 ml. As illustrated in Figure 1, the calibration curve is linear with protein concentrations ranging up to at least 27 mg per 100 ml. The *coefficient of variation* of duplicate analyses of 24-hour urine collections from 28 healthy adults was 4.2%, (mean concentration = 6.2 mg per 100 ml; standard deviation of duplicates = ±0.26). *Measurements of recovery* of serum protein added to 7 normal urine samples in a concentration of 15 mg per 100 ml averaged 103% (standard deviation = ± 3) with a range from 98 to 109%.

Preservation of Urine Specimens

Urine specimens are stored in a refrigerator at 4 to 10°C during the 24-hour collection period, and until the time of analysis. No preservative is added. The stability of urine protein concentration was studied by repeated analyses of a specimen of urine which was kept for one month at 4 to 10°C. Protein determinations were performed 3 times each week for 4 weeks. The 12 measurements yielded a mean protein concentration of 39.3 mg per 100 ml (standard deviation = ± 0.5), with a range from 38.5 to 40.5. No consistent increase of decrease in protein concentration was observed during the period of observation.

The stability of protein concentration in urine which was kept frozen at -15°C

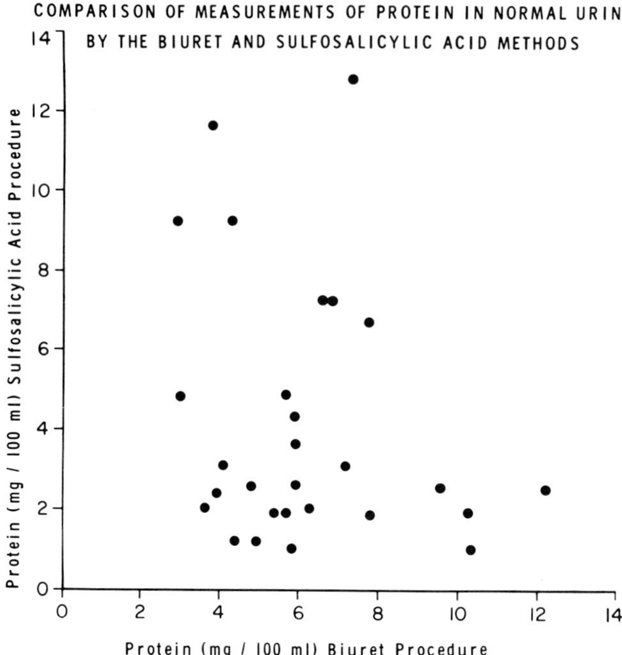

Fig. 3. Comparison of measurements of protein concentrations in 24-hour urine collections from 28 healthy adults by the biuret procedure and by the sulfosalicylic acid method of Poortmans and van Kerchove (8).

was investigated by performing 5 replicate analyses of a specimen of urine before and after freezing for one month. The mean protein concentration was 40.5 mg per 100 ml before freezing, and 40.7 mg per 100 ml after freezing.

Comparisons with other Methods

Concentrations of protein in 24-hour urine collections from 14 healthy adults were measured by the biuret procedure and by the amido black method of Kaltwasser and associates (3). As shown in Figure 2, urine protein measurements by the amido black method averaged 8% higher than by the biuret procedure. The correlation coefficient was 0.96, and the standard error of estimate was 0.77. Protein concentrations in 24-hour urine collections from 28 healthy adults were measured by the biuret procedure and

by the sulfosalicylic acid method of Poortmans and van Kerchove (8). As shown in Figure 3, there was apparently a random scattering of results of protein measurements by these 2 techniques. The absorbances which were obtained with normal urine by use of the sulfosalicylic acid method ranged from 0.005 to 0.045. Therefore, it is apparent that the sulfosalicylic acid method was not sufficiently sensitive to permit quantitative measurements of protein in normal urine.

Normal Values for Urine Protein

Twenty-four hour collections of urine were obtained from 14 male and 14 female adults who were judged to be healthy on the basis of medical history and physical examination. The mean concentration of urine protein in the males was 6.4 mg per 100 ml (range = 3 to 12), and the mean concentration in the females was 6.0 mg per 100 ml (range = 4 to 10). The mean excretion of urine protein in the males was 79 mg per day (range 48 to 150), and the mean excretion in the females was 76 mg per day (range 40 to 131). There was no significant difference between the urine protein concentrations and excretions in the 2 sexes, as determined by Student's "t" test. Frequency distribution graphs for urine protein in the combined group of 28 healthy adults are illustrated in Figure 4. The urine protein concentrations (mg per 100 ml) are plotted in the graphs on the left side on the figure, and the urine protein excretions (mg per day) are plotted on the right side of the figure. As shown in Figure 4, the logarithmic distribution graphs alhered more closely to the Gaussian conformation than did the arithmetic graphs. Therefore, the ±2 standard deviation limits computed after logarithmic transformations are recommended for use as the normal ranges of values.

Search for Interfering Drugs and Pigments

In an endeavor to detect sources of interference, the biuret procedure was employed for measurements of protein in 24-hour collections of urine from patients on the medical, surgical, pediatric and psychiatric services of the hospital. Systematic search failed to reveal any interference from pigments, including porphyrins and bilirubin, or from a wide variety of drugs, including antibiotics, sedatives, analgesics, vitamins tranquillizers and roentgenographic contrast media.

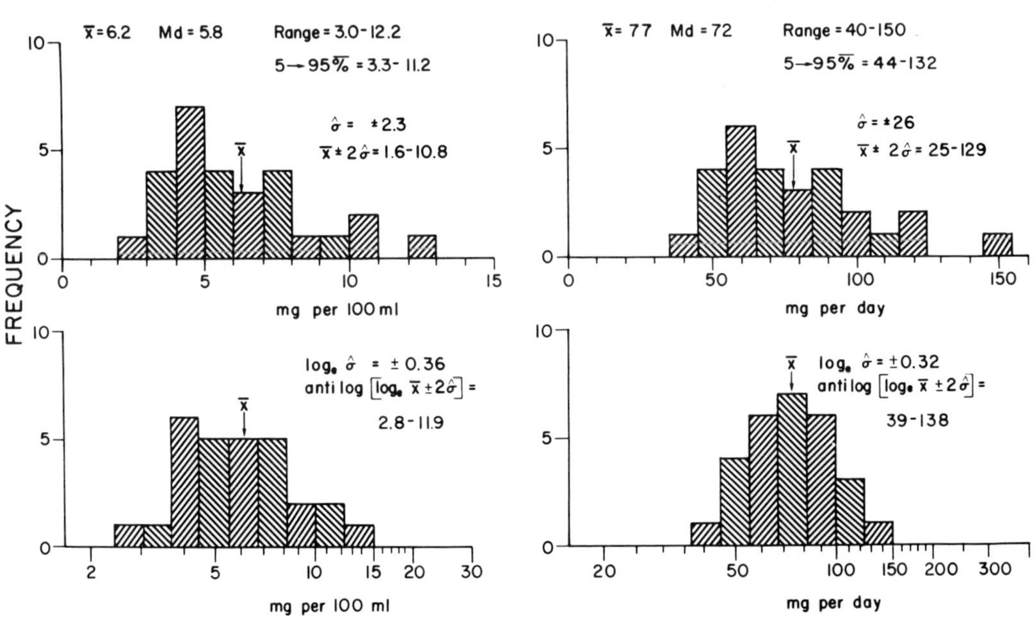

Fig. 4. Frequency distribution graphs for protein excretion in 24-hour urine collections from 28 healthy adults ($\overline{X}$ mean; Md. = median; and $\hat{\sigma}$ = standard deviation.) The abscissae in the upper graphs are arithmetic, and the abscissae in the lower graphs are logarithmic.

II. DETECTION OF BENCE-JONES PROTEIN IN URINE
(Method of Putnam *et al.* (9))

Principle

The most characteristic property of urine Bence-Jones protein is its precipitation on heating at temperatures as low as 46 to 52°C, with redispersion on boiling and reprecipitation on cooling. Putnam and co-workers (9) have systematically studied the optimum conditions for detection of Bence-Jones protein with respect to temperature, pH, protein concentration, and electrolyte composition and concentration. The heat test which was described by Putnam and co-workers involves experimental conditions which produce maximum precipitation of a wide variety of Bence-Jones proteins, without precipitation of normal serum proteins.

Procedure

1. To 4 ml of filtered urine is added 1 ml of acetate buffer (2 M, pH 4.9). This gives a final pH of 4.9 ± 0.1 with urine samples in the normal pH range. The pH of the buffered urine is tested with a pH meter.

2. The buffered urine is heated for 15 min at 56° in a water bath. Any precipitation is indicative of Bence-Jones protein.

3. The same tube is heated for 3 min in a beaker of boiling water, and the contents of the tube are observed while in the boiling bath. Any decrease in the amount of precipitate, or clearing of the opacity, is considered confirmatory of Bence-Jones protein.

Discussion

Verification of the excretion of Bence-Jones protein may be performed by electrophoresis, as described in Section IV. Demonstration of a sharply demarcated band of protein in the globulin region of the electrophoretic pattern constitutes positive identification. Ultracentrifugal demonstration of a urine protein with a sedimentation constant of 3.65 or lower, and immunological identification by gel diffusion are additional means of confirming the presence of Bence-Jones protein.

III. ULTRAFILTRATION OF URINE PROTEINS
(Method of Kaplan and Johnston (4)

Principle

Collodion bags are employed for the concentration and enrichment of urine proteins as a preliminary step to electrophoretic fractionation. Ultrafiltration is achieved by maintaining a constant reduced pressure (50 cm Hg) in the suction vessel. Ultrafiltration is continued until a protein concentration of 3 to 9 gm per 100 ml is achieved.

Reagents

1. *Sodium chloride solution,* 0.85%, (w/v).

Special Apparatus

1. *Ultrafiltration apparatus* (Carl Schleicher and Schuell Co., Keene, New Hampshire, Cat. "CBA").

2. *Collodion bags* 8 ml capacity (Carl Schleicher and Schuell Co., Cat # "CB").

3. *Manometer, manostat and filtration pump,* to maintain a constant suction of 50 cm Hg).

4. *Refrigerated bath,* 0 to 4°C.

Procedure

1. Urine is centrifuged and the protein concentration is measured as described in Section I.

2. The ultrafiltration apparatus is assembled as illustrated in Figure 5. The collodion bag is soaked for at least 1 hour in sodium chloride solution in order to elute traces of methanol in which the bag is stored. The collodion bag is pushed for about 1 cm of its length over the plastic sleeve of the inner glass tube, and is tightly fastened to the latter by aid of the outer tube. The parts thus assembled are then inserted vertically into the suction vessel which has been partially filled with sodium chloride solution. The level of sodium chloride solution inside the suction vessel should not exceed the lower edges of the inner and outer glass tubes (Figure 5). The ultrafiltration apparatus is attached to a ring stand and is immersed in a refrigerated bath at 0 to 4°C.

3. Eight ml of urine are pipetted through the inner glass tube into the collodion bag. The side-arm of the suction flask is attached to the vacuum system. The suction is adjusted to 50 cm Hg.

4. Ultrafiltration proceeds at a rate of 2 to 3 ml per hour, and is continued until the volume of sample has a protein concentration of 3 to 9 gm per 100 ml. The final volume is seldom critical, since a wide range of protein concentrations is satisfactory for electrophoretic fractionation. The final sample usually has a volume in the range of 20 to 50 μl, and can be removed from the bottom of the bag by means of a disposable 50μl

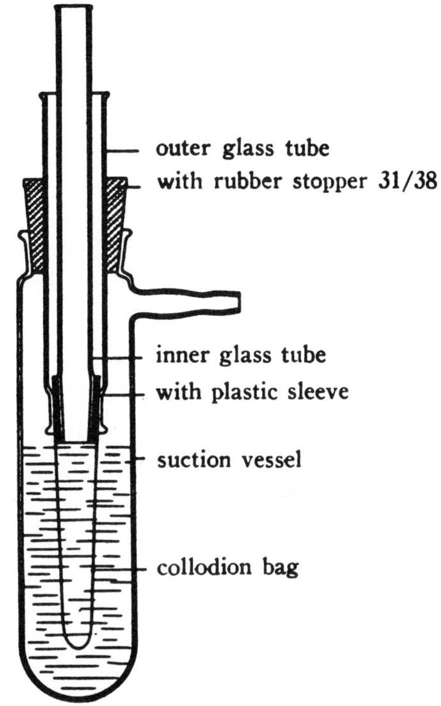

Fig. 5. Ultrafiltration apparatus for concentration of urine proteins preparatory to electrophoretic fractionation.

micropipet.

5. The sample in the micropipet may be sealed with plastic putty and kept frozen until electrophoresis is performed.

6. The collodion bag is removed from its holder and is soaked in a 6 molar solution of urea for 1 hour. The bag is placed in a large beaker of distilled water overnight, and thereafter is stored in 20 percent (v/v) methanol.

Discussion

Vacuum ultrafiltration has been found by Kaplan and Johnston (4) to produce minimal denaturation of proteins. The method is relatively rapid, and is more convenient than lyophilization or chromatography upon Sephadex. The progress of the ultrafiltration can readily be followed by inspection, and the conical tip of the collodion bag provides a simple means of collecting the small volume of protein concentrate. Urine samples are ultrafiltered at 0 to 4°C rather than at room temperature in order to prevent the rapid growth of bacteria.

IV. FRACTIONATION OF PROTEINS IN URINE AND SERUM
BY CELLULOSE ACETATE ELECTROPHORESIS
(Method of Williams (14))

Principle

Electrophoretic fractionations of serum and urine proteins are performed upon a cellulose acetate membrane. The separated protein fractions on the membrane are stained with Ponceau S dye. The stained membrane is evaluated with an automatic densitometer which plots a graph of optical densities along the band of separated proteins. The area under the optical density curve for each protein fraction is measured and is assumed to be proportional to the relative concentration of that fraction.

Reagents

1. *Barbital buffer,* pH 8.6 ionic strength 0.075.

2. *Ponceau S dye.* Three gm of trichloroacetic acid and 3 gm of sulfosalicylic acid are dissolved in distilled water in a 100 ml volumetric flask. Two tenths gm of Ponceau S dye is added, and the solution is diluted to 100 ml.

3. *Acetic acid,* 5% (v/v).

4. *Clearing solution.* Twenty ml of glacial acetic acid are added to 80 ml of methanol.

5. *Methanol,* anhydrous.

Special Apparatus (Beckman Instrument Co., Spinco Division, Palo Alto, Calif.)

1. *Microzone electrophoresis chamber and sample applicator.*

2. *Regulated D. C. power supply.*

3. *Cellulose acetate membranes,* 14.5 cm by 5.7 cm, prepared with 2 rows of holes to fit the bridge of the electrophoresis chamber.

4. *Flat-tipped acid-proof forceps* for handling the membranes.

5. *Five stainless-steel trays*

6. *Two glass plates,* 2½" X 6¼".

7. *Squeegee*

8. *Ventilated oven* at 75°C.

9. *Plastic envelopes,* to protect the completed membranes.

10. *Microzone densitometer.*

11. *Parafilm* (Marathon Division, American Can Co., Menasha, Wisconsin).

Procedure

1. Barbital buffer is poured into the electrophoresis chamber to the level indicated on the side of the buffer compartments.

2. One hundred ml of barbital buffer are placed in a stainless steel tray.

3. A cellulose acetate membrane is floated on the surface of the barbital buffer so that the liquid enters from the underside of the membrane and displaces air. Uniform wetting of the membrane is essential, and trapped air pockets should be avoided.

4. The membrane is submerged quickly in the buffer, blotted gently between a pair of blotters, and fitted onto the electrophoresis chamber so that the two ends of the membrane make contact with buffer in the chamber.

5. A drop of serum or urine concentrate is placed on a piece of Parafilm.

6. The drop is touched with the

platinum loop of the sample applicator (which picks up approximately 0.2μl of sample).

7. The sample is transferred to the membrane by placing the applicator in the central position of the electrophoresis chamber, and depressing the tip to make contact with the membrane. Eight positions are available for application. One application per position is usually adequate for serum but it may be necessary to make as many as three applications for a urine sample. The tip is rinsed carefully after application of each sample.

8. Electrophoresis is carried out with a constant potential of 250 v. for 20 minutes. The starting current is usually 3 to 5 ma. and increases to 5 or 6 ma. by the end of 20 minutes.

9. The wet membrane is stained for 10 minutes in a tray containing 100 ml of Ponceau S solution.

10. The membrane is washed with agitation in a series of three 4-minute rinses of 5% acetic acid in order to remove all excess dye.

11. The membrane is dehydrated by immersion in 200 ml of anhydrous methanol for exactly 1 minute. It is then placed in the methanol-acetic acid clearing solution; positioned upon a glass plate, and removed after exactly 45 seconds of immersion. Excess solution is removed by gently applying a squeegee to the surface of the membrane.

12. The glass plate with membrane attached is dried for 3 minutes at room temperature, and then is heated in a drying oven for 20 minutes at 70° to 80°.

13. The membrane is peeled away from the glass plate and is mounted in a plastic envelope. The membrane is scanned in a microzone densitometer fitted with 520 mμ interference filters.

14. Gaussian curves are construced for each protein fraction by extrapolating the descending slopes of each peak to the base line in such a way that the triangular areas above and below the points of intersection are approximately equal.

15. Perpendicular lines are dropped through the intersections of the Gaussian curves and extended to intercept the densitometer integration record. The areas subtended by the Gaussian curves are tabulated from the corresponding sections of the integration record.

16. The percentage distribution of the protein fractions is calculated by dividing the areas subtended by the individual Gaussian curves by the total area subtended by the electrophoretic pattern, and multiplying by 100. The concentrations of the protein fractions are computed by multiplying the concentration of total protein by the percentages corresponding to each fraction.

Computer Program

In the authors' laboratory, a computer program has been devised in order to expedite computation of electrophoretic fractionations. An IBM card is key-punched with the patient's name and hospital number, together with a tabulation of the raw data from the densitometer intergration record. By use of an IBM 1440 computer system, the results of the fractionation are calculated in the same manner as the customary manual computation. The following steps constitute the program:

1) Read the IBM "result" card.

2) Add the integration values of albumin, alpha-1, alpha-2, beta, and gamma globulins to obtain the "sum."

3) Divide the integration values of albumin, alpha-1, alpha-2, beta and gamma globulins by the "sum" to obtain

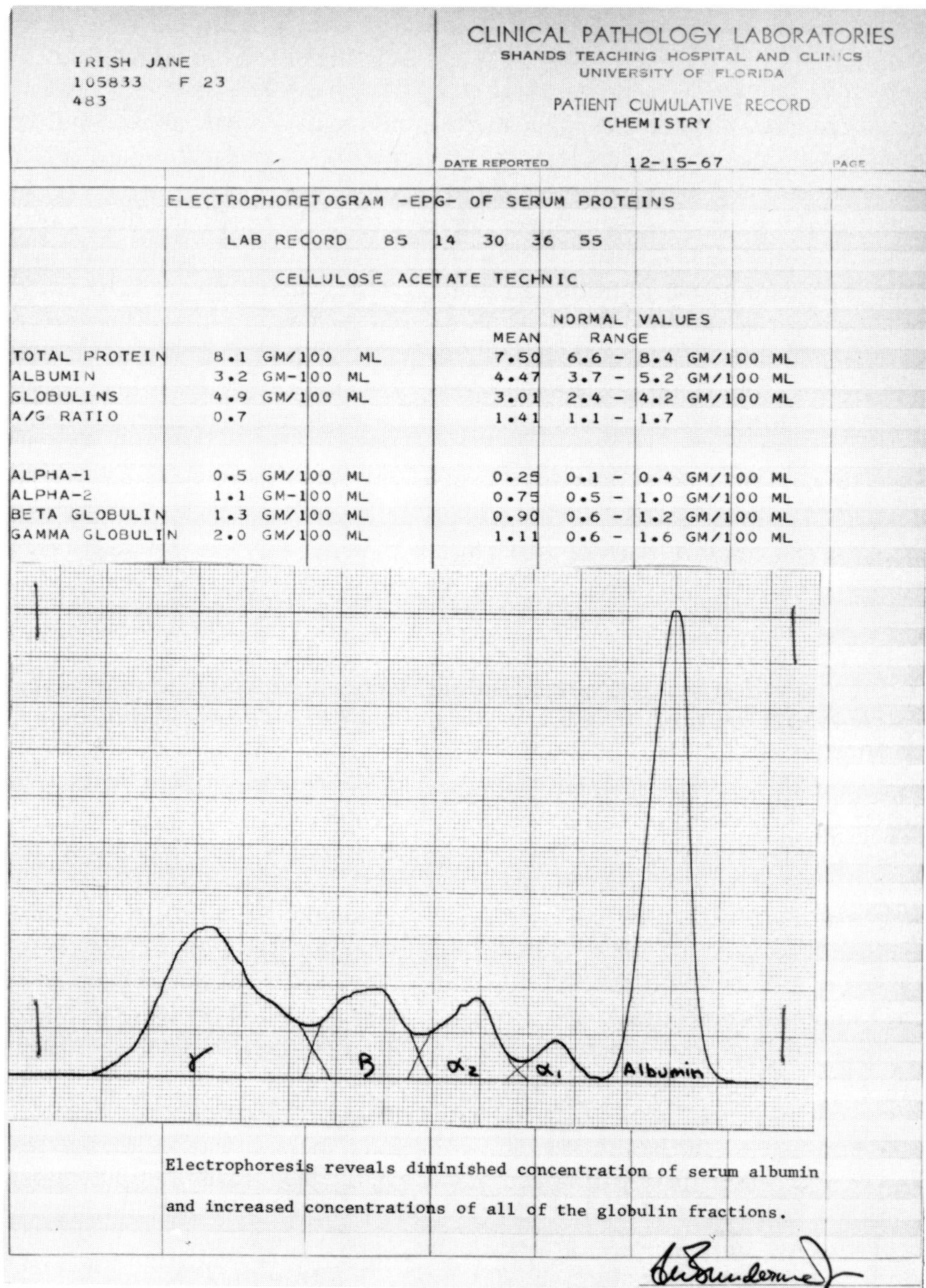

Fig. 6. An example of computer-assisted reporting of electrophoretic fractionations of serum proteins.

the ratio of each value of the "sum."

4) Multiply each ratio by the total protein concentration to obtain the concentrations of albumin, alpha-1, alpha-2, beta and gamma globulins.

5) Add the concentrations of the individual globulin fractions to obtain the concentration of total globulins.

6) Divide the concentration of albumin by the concentration of total globulins to obtain the "A/G ratio."

7) Print the results as illustrated in Figure 6, together with the normal values for electrophoretic fractionation which have been stored in the computer's memory.

8) As illustrated in Figure 6, a Xerox copy of the original electrophoretic tracing is stapled to the computer print-out, together with the clinical pathologist's interpretation. This record constitutes the report which is sent to the patient's hospital chart.

Discussion

The use of cellulose acetate membranes as the supporting medium for protein electrophoresis has several advantages over the use of filter paper. There is no albumin-trailing; the regularity of pore size results in sharp resolution of protein fractions in a short period of time; protein staining is more stoichiometric and more reproducible; the membrane is easily rendered transparent, thereby increasing the accuracy of densitometry; and wet cellulose acetate membrane has a greater tensile strength. In direct densitometry of transparent cellulose acetate membranes, there is little deviation from the Beer-Lambert Law with optical densities as great as 1.0.

TABLE I—NORMAL VALUES FOR ELECTROPHORETIC FRACTIONATIONS OF SERUM PROTEINS (9)

Protein	Protein Concentration (gm/100 ml)		
	Mean Std. Dev.		Range
Total protein	7.50 ± 0.37		6.6 – 8.4
Albumin	4.47 ± 0.36		3.7 – 5.2
α_1 -Globulin	0.25 ± 0.06		0.1 – 0.4
α_2 -Globulin	0.75 ± 0.13		0.5 – 1.0
β Globulin	0.90 ± 0.13		0.6 – 1.2
γ Globulin	1.11 ± 0.24		0.6 – 1.6

The values obtained in our laboratory for electrophoretic fractionations of proteins in serums of 20 healthy adults are listed in Table I. As discussed in Section A of this chapter, electrophoretic fractionations of proteins in urine from healthy adults reveal a distinct albumin fraction and poorly demarcated globulin and mucoprotein components. The mean percentage of albumin in urine from 28 healthy adults was 37.7 (standard deviation = ± 5.8) with a range from 27 to 50%. The mean excretion of albumin was 29.0 mg per day (standard deviation = ± 12.0) with a range from 18 to 52 mg per day.

V. DETERMINATION OF SERUM IMMUNOGLOBULINS BY RADIAL IMMUNODIFFUSION
(Lou and Shanbron's modification (5) of the methods
of Mancini and co-workers (6), and Fahey and McKelvey (1))

Principle

Immunodiffusion plates are prepared using agar gel which contains antibodies to one of the human immunoglobulins, IgA, IgG, or IgM. Six sample wells are punched in the agar. When a sample well is filled with serum (or standard), the antigens in the serum diffuse into the agar and form a precipitin ring. The diameter of the precipitin ring is related to the concentration of the protein being tested. Three standards are tested on each immunodiffusion plate in order that a standard curve can be plotted. The concentration of the specific protein in the unknown serum is estimated by reference to the standard curve.

Reagents and Special Apparatus

1. *Immunoglobulin Standard Solutions*

A) *IgA Standards:* Serum samples containing 90, 250 and 450 mg IgA per 100 ml.

B) *IgG Standards:* Serum samples containing 300, 780 and 1560 mg IgG per 100 ml.

C) *IgM Standards:* Serum samples containing 20, 50 and 116 mg IgM per 100 ml.

Reference samples of serum for immunoglobulin assays may be purchased from Hyland Laboratories, Los Angeles, California. These reference samples are standardized against immunochemically pure preparations of the specific proteins. However, the protein concentrations as assayed by Hyland Laboratories are based upon the factor of 6.25 gm of protein per gm of nitrogen, rather than the more accurate nitrogen factor of 6.54 (13). Therefore, the assayed values

for protein concentration should be multiplied by 6.54/6.25 (= 1.046) in order that analytical results may correlate with measurements of total proteins and electrophoretic fractions, as described in Sections I, IV, and VI.

2. *Agar immunodiffusion plates,* each containing a specific antibody against IgA, IgG, IgM may be purchased from Hyland Laboratories, or they may be prepared by the method of Fahey and McKelvey (1). Each agar diffusion plate should be fitted with a plastic cover. The agar diffusion plates are stored at 4° and are stable for several months.

3. *Viewbox with magnifier,* for measuring the diameter of precipitin rings to within = 0.1 mm.

Procedure

1. The agar diffusion plate is allowed to equilibrate at room temperature (for measurements of IgA or IgM) or at 37° (for measurement of IgG).

2. , Serums and 3 standards are transferred into the sample wells of the agar diffusion plate by use of capillary pipets. The pipet tip is touched to the bottom of the well and the sample is allowed to flow into the well by gravity. The sample wells should be filled exactly level with the surface of the agar.

3. The plastic cover is placed on the agar diffusion plate and the plate is placed in a covered Petri dish which contains moistened filter paper.

4. The agar diffusion plates for measurement of IgA or IgM are incubated at 25° for 16 hours. Plates for measurements of IgG are incubated at 37° for 4 hours.

5. After incubation, the diameter of each precipitin ring is measured by placing the diffusion plate (with cover removed) on the viewer. One side of the ring is aligned with the zero mark on the measuring grid. The diameter of the precipitin ring is estimated to the nearest 0.1 mm. Alternatively, a dissecting microscope with a stage micrometer or eye piece reticle may be used.

6. If the diameter of the precipitin ring of the serum exceeds that of the most concentrated standard, the sample is diluted with saline and the test is repeated.

Calculations

Using semi-logarithmetic graph paper, the diameters of the precipitin rings of the standard samples are plotted on the (arithmetic) abcissa against the concentrations of the standards on the (logarithmic) ordinate. The concentration of the immunoglobulin in the unknown sample is determined by reference to the standard curve.

Discussion

Normal values for serum immunoglobulins determined in our laboratory with serums from 40 healthy adults are listed in Table II.

TABLE II—NORMAL VALUES FOR
SERUM IMMUNOGLOBULINS

Protein	Protein Concentration (mg/100 ml)		
	Mean	*S.D.*	*Range*
IgA (γA)	184 $\pm$	80	60 – 345
IgG (γG)	1176 $\pm$	286	620 – 1700
IgM (γM)	101 $\pm$	47	30 – 190

VI. DETERMINATION OF TOTAL SERUM PROTEINS
(Method of de la Huerga, Sherrick and Smetters (2))

Principle

Serum proteins react with copper sulfate and sodium hydroxide to form a violet-colored "biuret" complex. The intensity of the violet color is proportional to the concentration of protein.

Reagents

1. *Biuret reagent* (see Section "I")

2. *Biuret "blank" reagent* (see Section "I")

3. *Protein standard.* Protein nitrogen in pooled serum is analyzed by the Kjeldahl procedure, (see Section "I"). Ampoules containing approximately 1 ml of pooled serum are frozen, and one ampoule is thawed on each day of analysis.

Procedure

1. Six ml of biuret reagent are added to three 19 mm Coleman cuvets.

2. One hundred μl of serum; 100 μl of protein standard, and 100 μl of water (reagent blank) are added to separate cuvets. The contents are mixed and are allowed to stand at room temperature for 20 minutes.

3. The spectrophotometer is adjusted to zero optical density at 540 mμ with a

cuvet filled with water. The optical densities of the unknown, standard and blank samples are measured.

4. A correction of lipemic or icteric serum is made by preparing a "serum blank" using 6 ml of the biuret "blank" reagent in lieu of the biuret reagent. The optical density of this "serum blank" is subtracted from that obtained with the biuret reagent.

Calculations

$$\text{Total protein (gm/100 ml)} = \frac{\text{O.D. serum} - \text{O.D. reagent blank}}{\text{O.D. std.} - \text{O.D. reagent blank}} \times \text{conc. of std.}$$

Discussion

Beer's law is obeyed with concentrations of total serum proteins from 2 to 16 gm per 100 ml. The mean concentration of total proteins (using the N factor of 6.54) in serums from 20 healthy adults has been found to be 7.50 ± 0.37 gm per 100 ml, with a range from 6.6 to 8.4 gm per 100 ml.

REFERENCES

1. Fahey, J. L., and McKelvey, E. M.: Quantitative determination of serum immunoglobulins in antibody-agar plates. J. Immunol., *94*:84-90, 1965.
2. de la Huerga, J., Smetters, G. W., and Sherrick, J. C.: Colorimetric determination of serum proteins: The biuret reaction. In, Sunderman, F. W., and Sunderman, F. W., Jr. (eds.): Serum Proteins and the Dysproteinemias. Philadelphia, J. B. Lippincott Co., pp. 52-62, 1964.
3. Kaltwasser, F., Walters, P., and Piper, J.: Kolorimetrische Mikromethode zur Bestimmung des Gesamteiweisses in eiwassarmen Flussigkeiten. Clin Chim. Acta, *15*:347-351, 1967.
4. Kaplan, A., and Johnstone, M.: Concentration of cerebrospinal fluid proteins and their fractionation by cellulose acetate electrophoresis. Clin. Chem., *12*:717-727, 1966.
5. Lou, K., and Shanbron, E.: Immuno-diffusion techniques in clinical medicine. II. Raidal Immuno-diffusion. J. Amer. Med. Assn., *200*:323, 1967.
6. Mancini, G., Carbonara, A. O., and Heremans, J. F.: Immunochemical quantitation of antigens by single radial immuno-diffusion. Immunochemistry, *2*:235-254, 1965.
7. Piscator, M.: Proteinuria in chronic cadmium poisoning. Arch. Environ. Health, *5*:325-332, 1962.
8. Poortmans, J., and van Kerchove, E.: Dosage de la proteinurie: comparison de deux methodes. Clin. Chim. Acta, *8*:485-488, 1963.
9. Putnam, F. W., Easley, C. W., Lynn, L. T., Ritchie, A. E., and Phelps, R. A.: The heat precipitation of Bence-Jones proteins. I. Optimum conditions. Arch. Biochem. Biophys, *83*:115-139, 1959.
10. Savory, J., Pu, P. H., and Sunderman, F. W., Jr.: A biuret method for determination of protein in normal urine. Clin. Chem. *14*:1160-1171, 1968.
11. Savory, J., and Sunderman, F. W., Jr.: Electrophoretic fractionations of the serum proteins. In, Faulkner, W. R. (ed.): Handbook of Clinical Laboratory Data, 2nd ed. Chemical Rubber Co., Cleveland, 1968, 14:1160-1171, 1968.
12. Sunderman, F. W.: Micro-Kjeldahl procedure for determination of serum protein nitrogen. In, Sunderman, F. W., and Sunderman, F. W., Jr. (eds.): Serum Proteins and the Dysproteinemias. Philadelphia, J. B. Lippincott Co., pp. 46-49, 1964.
13. Sunderman, F. W., Jr.: The nitrogen content of the serum proteins. In, Sunderman, F. W. and Sunderman, F. W., Jr. (eds.): Serum Proteins and the Dysproteinemias. Philadelphia, J. B. Lippincott Co., pp. 36-39, 1964.
14. Williams, F. G., Jr.: Microzone elctrophoresis of serum proteins. In, Sunderman, F. W. and Sunderman, F. W., Jr. (ed.): Serum Proteins and the Dysproteinemias. Philadelphia, J. B. Lippincott Co., pp. 125-130, 1964

Enzyme Tests in Renal Diseases

J. HENRY WILKINSON, D.Sc., Ph.D.

The kidney is a rich source of enzymes and in view of the spectacular progress which has been made in the past decade in diagnostic enzymology, it is not surprising that much attention has been paid to the behavior of serum and urinary enzymes in diseases of the urinary system. Some renal enzymes of diagnostic interest are listed in Table 1.

TABLE I—ENZYMES OF THE
RENAL PARENCHYMA

Aspartate transaminase	Asp T (GOT)
Alanine transaminase	Ala T (GPT)
Alkaline phosphatase	
Acid phosphatase	
Lactate dehydrogenase, principally anodic isoenzymes	
"2-Hydroxybutyrate dehydrogenase"	

SERUM ENZYMES IN RENAL DISEASE

Although there had been a number of earlier reports of raised serum enzyme levels in renal diseases (24, 43, 45, 49), the first extensive study was that of West and Zimmerman (44), who observed elevated serum lactate dehydrogenase activities in 43 of 71 patients with various kidney disorders. In confirmation of earlier reports (6, 26, 48), the serum aspartate transaminase (glutamate-oxaloacetate transaminase,

GOT) was found to be normal in all except 6 of 63 patients. In 5 of the patients with elevated values, there was extra-renal pathology which might have been responsible for the transaminase elevations.

The incidence of abnormal serum lactate dehydrogenase activities was found to be similar in the various groups of diseases studied. These included benign and malignant nephrosclerosis, acute and chronic glomerulonephritis, acute and chronic pyelonephritis, acute renal failure and systemic lupus erythematosus (44). Though there appeared to be no obvious relationship between the serum lactate dehydrogenase and the degrees of azotemia, proteinuria or hypercholesterolemia, West and Zimmerman (44) found a statistically significant inverse correlation between the serum enzyme level and the serum albumin content. This recalls the earlier observations of Vorhaus and Kark (39) who found elevated serum cholinesterase levels in patients with the nephrotic syndrome, though they are decreased in hypoalbuminemia due to other causes.

The occurrence of raised serum lactate dehydrogenase activities in renal disease has since been confirmed (36), but their incidence generally appears to be appreciably less than that found by West and Zimmerman (44). In a series of 19 patients with renal parenchymal diseases investigated in the writer's laboratory (35), only four exhibited raised serum lactate dehydrogenase levels, and of these two had only marginal elevations and one of the others had extra-renal disease which might have been contributory. The serum transaminase was normal in every case.

As shown in Table 1, the kidney is a rich source of alkaline phosphatase, but elevation of the serum level of this enzyme has only rarely been found in renal disease. Raised values, however, are encountered in most cases of renal infarction along with increased levels of lactate dehydrogenase and aspartate transaminase (16, 20, 21, 38). A rise in the serum lactate dehydrogenase has also been reported after experimental renal infarction and ischemia in dogs and rabbits (4, 25). An acute episode resulting in the destruction of an appreciable quantity of renal cells would be expected to lead to release of their enzymes into the circulation in much the same manner as the cardiac enzymes after an episode of myocardial infarction.

The serum levels of certain enzymes which do not occur in the kidney may be increased in renal disease if they are normally excreted in the urine. Amylase is such an enzyme and its serum level has been demonstrated to be increased in renal failure (22).

While the serum lactate dehydrogenase is increased in renal disease more frequently than any other serum enzyme, it is now well established that elevations occur only in a relatively small proportion of patients. Except in renal infarction, the serum levels of other enzymes are almost invariably normal, unless there is concurrent disease of another organ. The general conclusion

therefore is that serum enzyme tests are of little diagnostic value in renal disease.

URINARY ENZYMES IN RENAL DISEASE

Considerable attention has recently been paid to the determination of urinary enzymes in patients with diseases of the urinary tract. In 1959, Dr. Rosalki and I (36) reported increased lactate dehydrogenase and aspartate transaminase activities in the urines of patients with tubular necrosis, acute and subacute glomerulonephritis and the nephrotic syndrome. Our findings were soon confirmed by others (7, 8, 15, 32, 34, 40). A great deal of information has since been obtained concerning the practical aspects of urinary enzyme determination and this will be briefly considered before discussing the diagnostic applications.

DETERMINATION OF URINARY ENZYME ACTIVITY

In general, methods which have been successfully employed for the determination of enzymes in serum have also been applied to their assay in urine, but several additional factors must be borne in mind. Some of these are listed in Table 2. Since much of the work has been carried out on lactate dehydrogenase, this enzyme will be taken as an example, but my remarks apply equally to other enzymes.

The urine must be fresh as enzyme activity diminishes on storage. Dr. Rosalki and I (36), found that 24-hour specimens could be collected by storing the daytime samples in a refrigerator and adding them to the overnight specimen. Assay of individual samples gave values which on summation closely approxi-

<sub>TABLE II—PROBLEMS IN THE
DETERMINATION OF URINARY ENZYMES</sub>

1. Presence of erythrocytes, leukocytes, casts, etc.
2. Bacterial infection or contamination
3. Storage or specimens
4. Effect of dilution
5. Presence of inhibitors, e.g., urea, oxalate, phosphate, peptides

mated to that of the complete 24-hour specimen, but it is essential that the final assay be carried out within a few hours of completion of the collection. Urinary enzyme assay has since been greatly simplified by using the 8-hour overnight specimen (40), and this seems now to have become standard practice.

Red and white blood cells are rich sources of lactate dehydrogenase and other enzymes and it is therefore essential to centrifuge the urine prior to enzyme assay and to examine the deposit. The hemoglobin content of the supernatant should also be measured by one of the sensitive *o*-tolidine procedures, and if values greater than 5 mg/100 ml are obtained, the sample is unsuitable for diagnostic purposes.

Since urine contains substances which inhibit enzymes, it is desirable to dialyse it before carrying out the enzyme assay. This is especially important in the case of alkaline phosphatase for inorganic phosphate behaves as a competitive inhibitor (23), and for lactate dehydrogenase particularly when lactate is used as substrate (11). Among the diffusible substances which might interfere are urea (31, 33, 47), oxalate (19, 29, 30), and certain peptides (37, 42).

Determination of lactate dehydrogenase with pyruvate as substrate is less susceptible to urinary inhibitors than when lactate is used because the reaction rate is about three times as great with pyru-

vate, and urinary volumes of about 0.2 ml or 0.3 ml rather than 1 ml can be used in each 3 ml assay volume. Similar results have been obtained in comparative studies with undialyzed urine using pyruvate as substrate and dialyzed urine with lactate (17), but it is probably desirable to use dialyzed urine irrespective of the substrate chosen.

Unpublished work by Mr. Y. Fujimoto in the writer's laboratory has shown that dialysis of lactate dehydrogenase preparations treated with urea does not restore the enzyme activity to the control value, and furthermore that the inhibitory effect of urea is greater at $37°$ than at the usual temperature $(25°)$ used for enzyme assay. It is probable therefore that storage of urine in the bladder may lead to irreversible loss of enzyme activity, and dialysis may thus be only of theoretical rather than practical significance.

A further problem incidental to dialysis is the loss of activators. This is important in the case of alkaline phosphatase, and it is essential to add Mg^{2+} ions before performing the enzyme determination on the diffusate.

URINARY ENZYMES IN RENAL DISEASE

The upper limits of normal for some urinary enzymes are listed in Table 3.

Much interest was stimulated by the suggestion of Wacker and Dorfman (40) that the urinary lactate dehydrogenase might be used as a screening test for malignant diseases of the urinary tract, but these and other investigators have since confirmed that elevated levels occur in various non-malignant renal diseases (1, 7, 8, 15, 34, 36, 40, 41). The Boston group later reported that the urinary alkaline phosphatase was of

TABLE III
NORMAL LIMITS FOR URINARY ENZYMES

Enzyme	Substrate	Normal Limit
Lactate dehydrogenase	Pyruvate	13.4 micromolar units/24 hr.(36)
		11.1 micromolar units/24 hr.(34)
		3.6 micromolar units/8 hr.(18)
	Lactate	0.99 micromolar units/8 hr.(11)
		1.37 micromolar units/8 hr.(15)
Alkaline phosphatase	p-Nitrophenyl phosphate	7,650 spect. units/8 hr.(3)
		9,343 spect. units/8 hr.(14)
	Phenyl phosphate	11 King-Armstrong units/24 hr.(5)

value in differentiating malignant tumors of the urinary tract from benign space-occupying lesions (2). Several other investigators, however, have observed normal excretion of one or other or both of these enzymes in proven cases of malignant disease, and their reliability as a screening procedure is therefore by no means absolute (12, 18, 28).

Increased urinary lactate dehydrogenase is found in a substantial proportion of patients with non-neoplastic diseases of the urinary tract including acute and chronic glomerulonephritis, chronic pyelonephritis, the nephrotic syndrome, acute renal failure, diabetic glomerulosclerosis, malignant hypertension, renal tuberculosis, renal cysts, renal calculi, prostatic hypertrophy, cystitis and other conditions (see review (46)). High levels occur in carcinoma of the kidney, the bladder and the prostate (12, 15, 18, 27,

28, 40), but the urinary values frequently return to normal after successful treatment (18).

Dr. Pauline Emerson made serial studies of the serum and urinary lactate dehydrogenase in a patient with chronic renal failure who underwent renal transplantation. Though the presence of numerous blood cells precluded urinary enzyme determination during the first five weeks after the operation, impending rejection was prefaced by a rise in both serum and urinary enzymes. These fell after a further course of immunosuppressive therapy, but unfortunately complications developed and the patient died from a cerebral hemorrhage (17).

As mentioned above, experience with the urinary alkaline phosphatase has been somewhat mixed. While Amador, Zimmerman and Wacker (2) found this enzyme to be raised in a higher proportion of patients with carcinoma of the kidney as compared with other malignant diseases of the urinary tract, Dubach (38) concluded that the increased activity has no differential diagnostic significance at the present time, though the finding of normal values may indicate the absence of a carcinoma.

Butterworth, Moss and their colleagues (5) studied the serial alkaline phosphatase excretion in a number of patients with acute renal failure, and found that the onset of diuresis was characterized by sharply oscillating increases in the urinary output of the enzyme.

The urinary alkaline phosphatase and lactate dehydrogenase are also elevated after renal infarction (21), but as raised levels have been observed after myocardial infarction (10, 15) and cirrhosis (9), their role in the diagnosis of renal infarction is somewhat limited.

SOURCE OF URINARY ENZYMES

The value of urinary enzymes in diagnosis depends upon knowledge of their origin and much of the information available at present is rather conflicting. Dr. Rosalki and I suggested that in renal parenchymal diseases the urinary lactate dehydrogenase probably originates in the damaged kidney, and also that the low enzyme activity found in normal urine could possibly be accounted for by "wear and tear" breakdown of renal cells (36). The absence of a direct relationship between the urinary and serum enzyme levels is not consistent with the alternative suggestion that the urinary enzyme originates in the plasma (7, 8).

The isoenzyme patterns of urinary lactate dehydrogenase resemble those of the erythrocyte in exhibiting a predominance of the anodic components, but urines containing appreciable numbers of leukocytes may show increased quantities of the cathodic isoenzymes. This observation has been interpreted as indicating that the lactate dehydrogenase found in urine reflects the nature of the main cellular constituents of the urinary deposit (13). Such an explanation, however, cannot be regarded as conclusive owing to the similarities of the isoenzyme patterns of the renal cortex and medulla, erythrocytes and normal urine. Another difficulty is that urea differentially inhibits the cathodic isoenzymes (30, 31, 33, 47), and it is possible that in concentrated urines the isoenzyme patterns may be considerably distorted by the high urea concentrations.

SUMMARY AND CONCLUSIONS

Although raised serum lactate dehydrogenase levels have been detected in the sera of patients with renal disease, the elevations seem to be slight and somewhat erratic. A raised serum aspartate transaminase activity rarely occurs and can nearly always be attributed to disease of some organ other than the kidney.

The urinary lactate dehydrogenase, aspartate transaminase and alkaline phosphatase is increased in most acute and chronic renal parenchymal diseases as well as in other disorders of the urinary tract. Urinary enzyme determinations, however, appear to have little value at present in the differential diagnosis of diseases of the urinary system. It seems that any advance in this field must await the accumulation of more information concerning the effects of other urinary constituents on the enzyme activities.

REFERENCES

1. Amador, E., Dorfman, L. E., and Wacker, W. E. C.: Urinary alkaline phosphatase and LDH activities in the differential diagnosis of renal disease. Ann. Int. Med., *62*:30-40, 1965.
2. Amador, E., Zimmerman, T. S., and Wacker, W. E. C.: Urinary alkaline phosphatase activity. I. Elevated urinary LDH and alkaline phosphatase activities for the diagnosis of renal adenocarcinomas. J. A. M. A., *185*:769-775, 1963.
3. Amador, E., Zimmerman, T. S., and Wacker, W. E. C.: Urinary alkaline phosphatase activity. II. An analytical validation of the method. J. A. M. A. *185*:953-957, 1963.
4. Bett, M. M., Skaggs, J. D., Johnston, G., and Hershey, F. B.: Lactic dehydrogenase of dog plasma and urine following renal injury. Surg. Forum, *9*:65-67, 1959.
5. Butterworth, P. J., Moss, D. W., Pitkanen, E., and Pringle, A.: Patterns of urinary excretion of alkaline phosphatase in acute renal disease. Clin. Chim. Acta, *11*:212-219, 1965.
6. Chinsky, M., Shmagranoff, G. L., and Sherry, S.: Serum transaminase activity: Observations in a large group of patients. J. Lab. Clin. Med., *47*:108-118, 1956.
7. Coltorti, M., Ascione, A., Giusti, G., and Di Simone, A.: Eliminazione urinaria di alcuni in soggetti a reno integro ed in nefropatici: correlazione con l'entita della proteinuria. Rif. Med., *47*:1313-1318, 1962.
8. Crockson, R. A.: Lactic dehydrogenase in renal

disease. Urinary concentrations and relative clearances. Lancet, *1*:140-142, 1961.

9. Dietz, A. A., and Hodges, L. K.: Correlation of the activities of the phosphatase of the urine and serum of normal and cirrhotic persons. Clin. Chim. Acta, *15*:393-402, 1967.

10. Dietz, A. A., Hodges, L. K., and Foxworthy, D. T.: Correlation of serum and urinary enzyme activity in patients with acute myocardial infarction. Clin. Chem., *13*:359-370, 1967.

11. Dorfman, L. E., Amador, E., and Wacker, W. E. C.: Urinary lactic dehydrogenase activity. III. An analytical validation of the assay method. J. A. M. A., *184*:1-6, 1963.

12. Dubach, U. C.: Diagnostischer Wert von Enzymbestimmungen im Urin bei Tumoren des Urogenitalsystems. Oncologia, *19*:254-258, 1965.

13. Dubach, U. C.: On the origin on lactic dehydrogenase isoenzymes in urine. Helv. Med. Acta, *33*:139-150, 1966.

14. Dubach, U. C., and Padlina, G.: Aktivität der alkalischen Phosphatase im Urin. Klin. Wschr., *44*:180-186, 1966.

15. Dubach, U. C., and Rediger, R.: Die Lactatdehydrogenase-Aktivität im Urin bei urologischen und medizinischen Krankheiten. Urol. Int., *17*:65-83, 1964.

16. Duggan, M. L.: Acute renal infarction. J. Urol., *90*:669-676, 1963.

17. Emerson, P. M.: A study of lactate dehydrogenase isoenzymes in tissue extracts and body fluids and their diagnostic import. M. D. thesis, University of London, 1965.

18. Emerson, P. M., Morgan, M. N.: Lactate dehydrogenase in urinary tract disease. Brit. J. Urol., *38*:551-555, 1966.

19. Emerson, P. M., Wilkinson, J. H., and Withycombe, W. A.: Effect of oxalate on the activity of lactate dehydrogenase isoenzymes. Nature, *202*:1337-1338, 1964.

20. Frahm, C. J., and Folse, R.: Serum oxalacetic transaminase levels following renal infarction. Report of a case and experimental observations following ligation of the renal arteries. J. A. M. A., *180*:209-211. 1962.

21. Gault, M. H., and Steiner, G.: Serum and urinary enzyme activity after renal infarction. Canad. M. A. J., *93*:1101-1105, 1965.

22. Heifetz, C. J., Probstein, J. G., and Gray, S. H.: Clinical studies on blood diastase. II. Significance of increased blood diastase. Arch. Int. Med., *67*:819-827, 1941.

23. Hilliard, S., O'Donnell, J. F., and Schenker, S.: On the nature of the inhibitor of urinary alkaline phosphatases. Clin. Chem., *11*:570-574, 1965.

24. Hsieh, K. M., and Blumenthal, H. T.: Serum lactic dehydrogenase levels in various disease states. Proc. Soc. Exp. Biol. Med., *91*:626-630, 1956.

25. Kemp, E., and Laursen, T.: Investigation of the excretion of enzymes in urine. Scand. J. clin. Lab. Invest., *12*:463-471, 1960.

26. LaDue, J. A., and Wróblewski, F.: The significance of the serum glutamic oxalacetic activity following acute myocardial infarction. Circulation, *11*:871-877, 1955.

27. Macalalag, E. V., Jr., and Prout, G. R., Jr: Confirmation of the source of elevated urinary lactic dehydrogenase in patients with renal tumor. J. Urol., *92*:416-423, 1964.

28. Mirabile, C. S., Bowers, G. N., Jr. and Berlin, B. B.: Urinary lactic dehydrogenase: a report based on 250 hospitalized patients. J. Urol., *95*:79-82, 1966.

29. Novoa, W. B., Winer, A. D., Glaid, A. J., and Schwert, G. W.: Lactic dehydrogenase V. Inhibition by oxamate and by oxalate. J. Biol. Chem ., *234*:1143-1148, 1959.

30. Plummer, D. T., and Wilkinson, J. H.: Organ specificity and lactate dehydrogenase activity. 2. Some properties of human-heart and liver preparations. Biochem. J., *87*:423-429, 1963.

31. Plummer, D. T., Wilkinson, J. H., and Withycombe, W. A.: The effect of urea on the activities of lactate dehydrogenase preparations. Biochem. J., *89*:48P. 1963.

32. Pojer, J. Mojzis, A., and Tovarek, J.: Activité enzymatique de l'urine au cours des néphropathies. Rev. franç. Études Clin. Biol., *5*:919-921, 1960.

33. Richterich, R., Burger, A., and Weber, H.: Die Inaktivierung der Lactat-Dehydrogenase durch Harnstoff. I. Selectiv Hemmung her electrophoretisch langsam wandernden Isoenzyme. Helv. Physiol. Pharmacol. Acta., *20*:C78, 1962.

34. Riggins, R. S., and Kiser, W. S.: A study of lactic dehydrogenase in urine and serum of patients with urinary tract disease. J. Urol., *90*:594-601, 1963.

35. Rosalki, S. B.: Studies on serum and urinary enzymes with particular reference to serum transaminases in infectious mononucleosis and lactic dehydrogenase in renal disease. M. D. thesis, University of London, 1961.

36. Rosalki, S. B., and Wilkinson, J. H.: Urinary lactic dehydrogenase in renal disease. Lancet, *2*:327-328, 1959.

37. Schoenenberger, G. A., and Wacker, W. E. C.: Peptide inhibitors of lactic dehydrogenase (LDH). II. Isolation and characterization of peptides I and II. Biochemistry, *5*:1375-1379, 1966.

38. Sheinin, J., and Cohen, L.: Serum enzymes and diagnosis of acute myocardial infarction. Postgrad. Med., *36*:594-601, 1964.

39. Vorhaus, L. J., and Kark, R. M.: Serum cholinesterase levels in health and disease. Amer. J. Med., *14*:707-719, 1953.

40. Wacker, W. E. C., and Dorfman, L. E.: Urinary lactate dehydrogenase activity. I. Screening

method for detection of cancer of kidneys and bladder. J.A.M.A., *181*:972-978, 1962.

41. Wacker, W. E. C., Dorfman, L. E., and Amador, E.: Urinary lactic dehydrogenase activity. IV. Screening test for detection of renal disease dissociated and in association with arterial hypertension. J. A. M. A., *188*:671-676, 1964.

42. Wacker, W. E. C., and Schoenenberger, G. A.: Peptide inhibitors of lactic dehydrogenase (LDH). I. Specific inhibition of LDH-M-4 and LDH-H-4 by inhibitor peptides I and II. Biochem. Biophys. Res. Comm., *22*:291-296, 1966.

43. Wacker, W. E. C., Ulmer, D. D., and Vallee, B. L.: Metalloenzymes and myocardial infarction: II. Malic and lactic dehydrogenase activities and zinc concentrations in serum. New Engl. J. Med., *255*:449-456, 1956.

44. West, M., and Zimmerman, H. J.: Serum enzymes in disease. IV. Lactic dehydrogenase and glutamic oxalacetic transaminase levels in renal disease. J. Lab. Clin. Med., *52*:185-192, 1958.

45. White, L. P.: Serum enzymes. I. Serum lactic dehydrogenase in myocardial infarction. New Eng. J. Med., *255*:984-988, 1956.

46. Wilkinson, J. H.: Diagnostic significance of enzyme determinations in urine. In, Aebi, H., Mattenheimer, H., and Schmidt, F. W., (ed): Enzymes in Urine and Kidney. Berne, Huber, pp 207-236, 1968.

47. Withycombe, W. A., Plummer, D. T., and Wilkinson, J. H. Organ specificity and lactate dehydrogenase activity. Differential inhibition by urea and related compounds. Biochem. J., *94*:384-389, 1965.

48. Wróblewski, F., and LaDue, J. S.: Serum glutamic oxalacetic transaminase as an index of liver-cell injury from cancer. Cancer, *8*:1155-1163, 1955.

49. Zimmerman, H. J., and Weinstein, H. G.: Lactic dehydrogenase activity in human serum. J. Lab. Clin. Med., *48*:607-616, 1956.

Measurement of Urinary Lactate Dehydrogenase

J. HENRY WILKINSON, D.Sc., Ph.D.

INTRODUCTION

Serum enzyme tests have not proved of such wide applicability in renal diseases as in disorders of the liver and other organs, but attention has recently been directed towards the excretion of enzymes, particularly lactate dehydrogenase, in the urine. Significant amounts of this enzyme have been shown to be excreted in a number of diseases of the urinary tract, and some of the problems involved in its determination are discussed in this section.

Principle

Lactate dehydrogenase (LDH) activity may be determined spectrophotometrically in either of two ways, according to the direction of the reaction:

$$CH_3CHOHCOO^- + NAD \rightleftarrows CH_3COCOO^- + NADH_2$$

$$\text{Lactate} \qquad\qquad \text{Pyruvate}$$

Lactate (1-3) or pyruvate (4,5) may be used as substrate with nicotinamide adenine dinucleotide, NAD, or its reduced form $NADH_2$, respectively. Optimal conditions (pH, substrate and conezyme concentrations), however, are quite different for the two reactions. When the reaction is carried out from left to right, there is a gradual increase in the extinction (absorbance) at $340m\mu$; a fall in extinction occurs when the reaction is performed in the opposite direction.

In applying these methods to the determination of LDH activity in urine, it has to be borne in mind that urine normally contains substances (6), such as urea (7) and certain polypeptides (8), which might inhibit the enzyme. It is therefore desirable to dialyze the urine to remove such substances before determining enzyme activity. When lactate is used as substrate, there is evidence of non-specific reduction of NAD, but the interfering substance is also removed by dialysis (6).

The method described below is based upon that of Kubowitz and Ott (4) and depends upon the reduction of pyruvate with $NADH_2$ as coenzyme.

Reagents

1. *Phosphate Buffer, 0.067M.* Sφrensen phosphate buffer, pH 7.4, is prepared by dissolving 2.560 gm of reagent grade potassium dihydrogen phosphate (KH_2PO_4) and 19.230 gm of reagent grade disodium hydrogen phosphate dihydrate ($Na_2HPO_4 \cdot 2H_2O$) or 17.060 gm of anhydrous Na_2HPO_4 in deionized or distilled water and making up the volume to two liters. The pH is checked at 25°C. The solution is prepared freshly each month and stored at 4°C. in a refrigerator. It should be discarded if any turbidity develops.

2. *$NADH_2$ Solution.* Five mg (conveniently from a pre-weighed vial) are dissolved in 5 ml of phosphate buffer. This solution should be prepared freshly each day; any surplus should be discarded.

3. *Sodium pyruvate, 0.022M* Fifty mg of sodium pyruvate are dissolved in 20 ml phosphate buffer. The solution is divided into 2 ml aliquots and stored frozen. Under these conditions, it is stable for one week. Surplus solution should be discarded and should never be refrozen.

4. *Dichromate Reference Blank.* A 0.001 M stock solution (29 mg potassium dichromate in 100 ml water containing two drops concentrated sulfuric acid) is diluted to 0.0001 M with water.

Special Apparatus

The procedure can be carried out in almost any spectrophotometer equipped with adequate temperature control in the cuvette housing and capable of operating at 340 mμ, but it is recommended that an instrument capable of recording extinction changes with time be used. Among those found satisfactory are several also fitted with an automatic cell changer, e.g., the Gilford cell positioner and absorbance indicator attached to a Beckman DU spectrophotometer equipped with thermospacers, or preferably a double beam instrument such as the Unicam SP 800 recording spectrophotometer, etc.

Procedure

1. *Preliminary Treatment of Urine.* An eight-hour overnight specimen can be collected without preservative. Alternatively, a 24-hour specimen may be preserved with thymol or toluene, but the daytime samples must be refrigerated and added to the overnight sample. In either case, the urine must be kept in the refrigerator until analysis is begun within six hours of the completion of collection. After measuring the total volume, a portion of the urine is centrifuged and the sediment examined for cells, casts, etc. A 25-ml sample of the supernatant is then dialyzed for two hours against 3 liters of distilled water, after which the water is changed and dialysis continued for a further two hours. The total volume (v) of the dialyzed urine, together with 2-5 ml water washings, is then measured.

2. *LDH Determination.* Into an 85 x 15 mm disposable glass test tube is pipetted:

Phosphate buffer 2.4 ml
$NADH_2$ solution 0.3 ml
Dialyzed urine   0.2 ml

The solution is mixed by "flipping" the tube with the fingers — a Vortex mixer should not be used as the possible introduction of small air bubbles might cause difficulty during the spectrophotometry. The tubes are placed in a 30°C water bath for 15 minutes to enable non-specific oxidation of $NADH_2$ to be completed.

The lamp of the spectrophotometer is

switched on and the instrument prepared for use. The monochromator is adjusted to 340 mμ and water at 30° is circulated through the thermospacers. If a recording instrument is used, the calibration should be checked at this stage. The reference cuvette with a 1 cm light path is filled with 0.0001 M dichromate reference blank and after about ten minutes, the galvanometer or recorder is adjusted to zero. When read against this reference blank, reaction mixtures containing urine should give initial readings of about 0.6.

One-tenth ml of sodium pyruvate is then pipetted into each of four 1 cm cuvettes (three in the case of a non-recording spectrophotometer) and the contents of each tube are added to one of the cuvettes. Mixing is effected by covering the cuvettes with Parafilm and gently inverting. The cuvettes are then placed in the carrier and readings are commenced within one minute of adding substrate to the first cuvette. A stop-watch should be used for timing the readings if a recording instrument is not available. Readings are taken at accurately timed intervals (15 sec., 20 sec., or 30 sec., according to the instrument) over a total period of about five minutes. In the manual instrument with three simultaneous determinations, specimen 1 is read at 0, 1, 2, 3, and 4 minutes, specimen 2 at 20, 80, 140, 200, and 260 seconds, and specimen 3 at 40, 100, 160, 220, and 280 seconds. At least three readings should be obtained during the linear (zero order) phase of the reaction. Such timing is obtained automatically when a recording spectrophotometer is used.

Calculation of LDH Activity

The fall in optical density per minute is calculated or read from the recording. One spectrophotometric unit of LDH activity produces a fall in the optical density of 0.001 per minute per ml urine in a reaction volume of 3 ml Thus:

$$\text{LDH Activity} = \frac{\text{Fall in O.D. per minute}}{0.001} \times \frac{1}{0.2} \times \frac{v}{25} \text{ spec. units per ml}$$

$$\text{or } \frac{\Delta\text{O.D.}}{0.001} \times \frac{v}{5} \times V \text{ spect. units per specimen}$$

where V ml is the volume of the 8-hour or 24-hour specimen.

Spectrophotometric units per ml can readily be converted into micromolar (International) units per liter simply by multiplying by a factor of 0.48, i.e., one spect. unit per ml = 0.48 micromolar unit per liter.

This factor is derived as follows:
With a 1 cm light path, the molecular extinction of $NADH_2$ at 340 mμ is 6.22 X 10^6, hence the consumption of 1 micromole in a volume of 1 ml would produce a change of 6.22 in the O.D. In the method described, a volume of 3 ml is used, so under these conditions utilization of 1 micromole would lead to a fall of 2.07 in the O.D. One liter of solution (serum, urine, etc.) containing 1 micromolar unit of LDH activity would thus produce a change of 2.07 O.D. per minute or 2070 spectrophotometric units, i.e.,

$$1 \text{ spectrophotometric unit per ml} = \frac{1}{2.07} = 0.48 \text{ micromolar units per liter}$$

$$\text{Thus, LDH activity} = \Delta\text{O.D.} \times \frac{v}{5} \times V \times 0.48 \text{ micromolar units per specimen.}$$

If measurement of the urinary activity is inconveniently slow, the determination can be repeated using 0.5 ml urine and 2.1 ml phosphate buffer, and the calculation adjusted accordingly.

Discussion

The method described is a modification of that used clinically by the writer and his colleague in 1959 (9). This method is less sensitive to the presence of inhibitors than the alternative procedure which uses lactate as substrate. The reaction rate is about three times as fast with pyruvate as substrate as with lactate, (10), a circumstance which enables smaller volumes of urine to be employed, and hence smaller amounts of inhibitors are introduced into the reaction mixture. Some investigators have shown that the pyruvate reaction gives the same results with undialyzed urine as with dialyzed specimens, (11) but others find slightly higher values after dialysis (12). Dialysis, however, is essential when lactate is used as substrate (6, 13).

The International Union of Biochemistry (14) recommends that all enzyme activities be determined at 30° whenever possible, but the method gives valid results at other temperatures. Each laboratory should standardize its reaction temperature and avoid the use of corrections. The is particularly important for LDH which consists of five isoenzymes with different temperature coefficients.

The effects of changes in the concentrations of buffer, coenzymes, and substrate have been investigated by Henry and his co-workers (15), and their suggestions have been incorporated in the method described.

The presence of large numbers of red and white cells in the sediment may lead to high urinary LDH levels which are difficult to control. If the supernatant contains significant mounts of hemoglobin, a correction can be applied by measuring the LDH activity of an aqueous hemolysate of the patient's erythrocytes containing the same concentration of hemoglobin as the urine.

Jösch and Dubach (16) have recently shown both clinically and experimentally that the urinary excretion of LDH and other enzymes depends upon the state of diuresis. While the enzyme *concentration* is greater in antidiuresis, the total activity excreted per unit time is greater in diuresis. The state of diuresis must therefore be taken into account when using urinary enzyme determinations for clinical or diagnostic purposes.

Human lactate dehydrogenase occurs in five distinct isoenzymes, the proportions of which vary according to their tissue or origin (17). A close correlation has been observed between the isoenzyme patterns of the urinary enzyme and the presence of red or white blood cells in the sediment. (18)

Sources of Error

The principal sources of error in the determination of urinary enzymes fall into two categories: (a) those inherent in enzyme determination, and (b) those due to other urinary components:

1. *Improperly Cleaned Glassware.*

Traces of heavy metals, especially mercury, act as enzyme "poisons."

2. *Variation of Temperature, pH and Timing.* Since enzyme determination involves measurement of reaction rates, errors in timing must be avoided, and during manual operation timing errors due to technician fatigue are liable to occur. The effect of temperature changes is large and variable and the use of temperature controlled cuvette housings is strongly recommended.

3. *Instability of NADH$_2$* (19, 20). During storage, inhibitors of alcohol dehydrogenase and LDH develop in samples of NADH$_2$. This is especially the case when solutions of the coenzyme are stored; such solutions should be used only on the day of preparation.

4. *Vigorous Shaking of Reaction Mixtures.* Trouble may be experienced as the result of fine air bubbles being trapped as the result of over-vigorous mixing.

5. *Storage of Specimens of Urine.* Prolonged storage even at 4° leads to loss of activity, (21) and enzyme determination should therefore be performed within a few hours of completion of urine collection. Bacterial contamination may lead to spuriously raised levels, and the use of strong acids as preservatives causes denaturation of the enzyme protein.

6. *Enzyme Inhibitors.* Urine normally contains inhibitors of LDH activity, some of which can be removed by dialysis (see above), but highly concentrated urines may contain sufficient urea (>0.8M) to react irreversibly with the enzyme. In such cases, activity cannot be restored by dialysis.

Range of Values

Owing to the different methods which have been employed, there is considerable discrepancy between the various normal ranges reported in the literature. A selection is listed in Table 1. It is therefore essential for any laboratory contemplating the introduction of this procedure to establish its own normal range.

RÉSUMÉ OF CLINICAL INTERPRETATIONS

Although one of the first evaluations of urinary LDH in diseases of the urinary tract established that elevated levels occur in glomerulonephritis, the neph-

TABLE 1
NORMAL UPPER LIMITS FOR URINARY LACTATE DEHYDROGENASE
(Determined at 25°C. unless otherwise stated.)

Substrate	Spectrophotometric	Micromolar Units	Reference
Pyruvate	30,000/24 hrs.	14.4 /24 hr.	9
	23,000/24 hrs.	11.0 /24 hr.	22
	–	3.6 / 8 hr.	11
	–	0.017/Kg body wt./hr.	12
Lactate	2,050/ 8 hr.	1.0 / 8 hr.	6
	2,923/ 8 hr.	1.4 / 8 hr.	13
	16,000/ 8 hr. (37°C.)	7.7 / 8 hr. (37°C.)	23

rotic syndrome and other non-malignant conditions (9), the test has been recommended as a screening procedure for neoplastic diseases of the kidney and bladder (3). While it has been confirmed that a high proportion of patients with malignant diseases of the kidney, bladder, and prostate do indeed excrete increased amounts of the enzyme in the urine, several investigators found normal levels in a number of patients known to have such neoplasms (11, 22-24).

High levels have been reported in papilloma of the renal pelvis, carcinoma of the bladder and prostate, and in hypernephroma, but increased output was also found in pyelonephritis, acute glomerulonephritis, renal stone, cystitis and many other inflammatory states (11, 22-24).

It must be borne in mind that increases in the urinary LDH may also occur in non-renal diseases, for example, transient high values have been reported after episodes of myocardial infarction (12, 13).

Urinary enzyme determination seems to have little value for the differential diagnosis of benign and malignant conditions of the urinary tract. While high values usually suggest the presence of urinary tract disease, they do not give much indication of its nature. Further investigation from both the enzymatic and clinical points of view is needed before the full significance of urinary enzyme test can be established.

REFERENCES

1. Von Euler, H., Adler, E., and Hellstrom, H.: Uber die Komponenten der Dehydrasesysteme. XII. Mechanismus der Dehydrierung von Alkohol und Triosephosphaten und der Oxydoreduktion. Z. Physiol. Chem., *241*:239-272, 1936.
2. Wacker, W. E. C., Ullmer, D. D., and Vallee, B. L.: Metalloenzymes and myocardial infarction II. Malic and lactic dehydrogenase activities and zinc concentrations in serum. New Eng. J. Med., *255*:449-456, 1956.
3. Wacker, W. E. C., and Dorfman, L. E.: Urinary lactic dehydrogenase activity. I. Screening method for detection of Cancer of kidneys and bladder. J. A. M. A., *181:*972-978, 1962.
4. Kubowitz, F., and Ott, P.: Isolierung und Kristallization eines Garungsfermente aus Tumoren. Biochem. Z., *314*:94-117, 1943.
5. Wroblewski, F., and LaDue, J.S.: Lactic dehydrogenase activity in blood. Proc. Soc. Exp. Biol. Med., *90*:210-213, 1955.
6. Dorfman, L. E., Amador, E., and Wacker, W. E. C.: Urinary lactic dehydrogenase activity III. An analytical validation of the assay method. J.A. M.A., *184*:1-6, 1963.
7. Withycombe, W. A., Plummer, D. T., and Wilkinson, J. H.: Organ specificity and lactate-dehydrogenase activity. Differential inhibition by urea and related compounds. Biochem. J., *94*:384-389, 1965.
8. Schoenenberger, G. A., and Wacker, W. E. C.: Peptide inhibitors of lactic dehydrogenase (LDH) II. Isolation characterization of peptides I and II. Biochemistry, 1375-1379, 1966.
9. Rosalki, S. B., and Wilkinson, J. H.: Urinary lactic dehydrogenase in renal disease. Lancet, 2:327-328, 1959.
10. Wilkinson, J. H.: An Introduction to Diagnostic Enzymology. Baltimore, Williams, and Wilkins, 1962, pp. 144-146.
11. Emerson, P. M.: Personal communication.
12. Dietz, A. A., Hodges, L. K., and Foxworthy, D. T.: Correlation of serum and urine enzyme activity in patients with acute myocardial infarction. Clin. Chem., *13*:359-370, 1967.
13. Dubach, U. C., and Rediger, R.: Die Lactatdehydrogenase — Aktivitat im Urin bei urologischen und medizinischen Krankheiten. Urol. Int., *17*:65-83, 1964.
14. Enzyme Nomenclature. Recommendations, 1964, of the International Union of Biochemistry. New York, Elsevier, 1965.
15. Henry, R. J., Chiamori, N., Golub, O. J., and Berkman, S.: Revised spectrophotometric methods for the determination of glutamic-oxaloacetic transaminase, glutamic-pyruvic transaminase, and lactic acid dehydrogenase. Amer. J. Clin. Path., *34*:381-398, 1960.
16. Jösch, W., and Dubach, V. C.: Einfluss der Diurese auf die Enzymurie. Clin. Chim. Acta, *15*:325-330, 1967.
17. Wilkinson, J. H.: Isoenzymes, Philadelphia, Lippincott, 1966.
18. Dubach, U. C.: On the origin of lactic dehydrogenase isoenzymes in urine. Helv. Med. Acta, *33*:139-150, 1966.
19. Fawcett, C. P., Ciotti, M. M., and Kaplan, N. O.:

Inhibition of dehydrogenase reactions by a substance formed from reduced diphosphopyridine nucleotide. Biochim. Biophys. Acta, *54*:210-212, 1961.

20. Dalziel, K.: An inhibitor of liver alcohol dehydrogenase in preparations of reduced diphosphopyrideine nucleotide. Nature (London), *191*:1098, 1099, 1961.

21. Plummer, D. T., and Leathwood, P. D.: Some properties of lactate dehydrogenase found in human urine. Biochem. J., *103*:172-176, 1967.

22. Riggins, R. S., and Kiser, W. S.: A study of lactic dehydrogenase in urine and serum of patients with urinary tract disease. J. Urol., *90*:594-601, 1963.

23. Mirabile, C. S., Bowers, G. N., Jr., and Berlin, B. B.: Urinary lactic dehydrogenase: A report based on 250 hospitalized patients. J. Urol., *95*:79-82, 1966.

24. Dubach, U. C.: Diagnostischer Wert von Enzymbestimmungen im Urin bei Tumoren des Urogenitalsystems. Oncologia, *19*:254-258

Alterations of Uric Acid in Serum and Urine in Kidney Diseases

ROBERT E. ZIPF, M.D., and BERNARD J. KATCHMAN, Ph.D.

At some point in time, in the early development of the anthropoids, there occurred one of many mutations in purine catabolism. This change led to the disappearance of uricase in the tissues; as a consequence, all mankind is victim to a species-wide inborn error of metabolism that has abolished the main pathway for degradation of uric acid. The renal mechanisms for the regulation of uric acid excretion were not affected. Therefore, the efficient tubular reabsorption of the filtered urate continued, even though uricase was no longer available in the liver to effect the conversion to allantoin. The absence of uricase in the tissues permits an accumulation of uric acid which inevitably results in a large body pool or body burden of uric acid (1).

A steady state of this body pool of uric acid is established under these circumstances by the brisk rate of uric acid clearance. Uric acid is filtered through the glomeruli very rapidly. It is likely that most of the urate is reabsorbed in the proximal convoluted tubules and recycled since the rate of reabsorption exceeds 15 mg per minute per 1.73 M^2 (2, 3). The quantity of uric acid appearing in the urine thus depends very largely, under ordinary circumstances, upon the rate of tubular excretion of uric acid by the organic acid system. Uric acid secretion proceeds at a less active rate of about 0.5 mg per minute.

The reabsorbed urate is recycled and recirculated through the kidneys for further renal elimination. When the diet is low in proteins and purines, the mean rate of elimination in the urine is approximately 500 mg per 24 hours. The remainder of the urate formed daily is excreted by the gut. Crone and Lassen (4), using the enzymatic method, found that the urinary endogenous uric acid excretion in normal subjects on a purine-free diet was 401 ± 42 mg in 53 males and 321 ± 34 mg in 18 females.

When on a regular diet, adults excrete from 500 to 1000 mg of uric acid per 24 hours. Ingested purines contribute from 200 to 500 mg of this total amount. In the newborn, there is high elimination of uric acid.

Sunderman and Boerner (5) have noted the daily excretion of uric acid to be from 500 to 1000 mg; this rate of excretion is confirmed by Hawk *et al.* (6). Davidsohn and Wells (7) reported a value of from 400 to 1000 mg per 24 hours. Colton and Ward (8) reported the normal adult ordinarily makes about 600 to 1200 mg of uric acid per day while excreting the same amount via the kidneys and gastrointestinal tract.

The renal regulator of uric acid excretion appears to be a complete filtration of plasma urates through the glomerular membrane (9). There follows a 90 to 95% reabsorption of the urate load submitted to the proximal convoluted tubules (9). There are data that, in addition to the two processes, there is also tubular excretion of urate in the distal convolutions (10). The glomerular filtration for urates is from 5 to 6 mg per minute (2, 11). Berliner concluded that the reabsorption capacity of the tubules is so extensive that under physiological conditions it is never excreted. Therefore, T_{max} per se has no regulating influence on the concentration of plasma urate or the excretion of uric acid (2, 11). The daily extrarenal excretions of uric acid are estimated to be: gastric juice, 40 to 70 mg; feces, 30 mg; and sweat, 6.0 mg.

Allantoin is the chief end product of purine metabolism in most mammals. It was isolated from human urine for the first time in 1909 by Wiechowski (12) who extracted 10 mg from a 24-hour urine specimen. This led to an early conclusion that man, like other mammals, can oxidize uric acid to allantoin. Now, however, it is assumed that the urinary allantoin is derived from preformed allantoin in the diet (13). However, work done by Sorensen in 1960, using ^{14}C tagged uric acid demonstrated that there is a significate conversion of uric acid to allantoin in man (9).

SERUM URIC ACID

The formation of uric acid results from:

1. The breakdown of ingested preformed nucleic acid and nucleotides: the exogenous uric acid.
2. The breakdown of tissue nucleoproteins and nucleotides: the endogenous uric acid.
3. The synthesis of purines from glycine and other nitrogen and carbon-containing compounds.

Preformed purines are ingested primarily as nucleoproteins, which are combinations of proteins, predominantly of basic character, with nucleic acids. It is the purines guanine and adenine that are the uric acid precursors (14).

The degradation of ingested nucleoproteins involves several steps, each requiring a separate enzyme system. Whether the nucleic acids originate from food or from tissue nucleoprotein, the pattern of their breakdown is similar.

The use of isotopic uric acid has made it possible to determine the total body content of uric acid. Wyngarden (15) found the average uric acid pool in

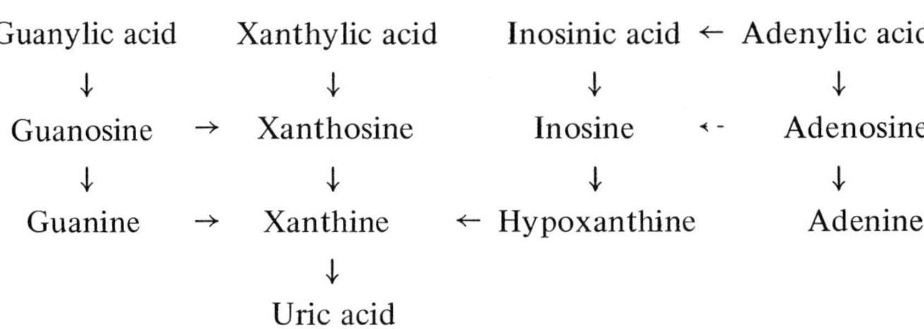

Fig. 1. The catabolic pathways of adenylic and guanylic acids in man.

normal males was 1125 mg of which 45 to 83% was replaced daily by newly formed non-labeled uric acid. He found the average uric acid production was 750 mg per day. In the normal female, the average uric acid pool was 651 mg, with a daily uric acid turnover of 501 mg. An elevated uric acid pool can be regarded as a new biochemical criterion for the diagnosis of certain diseases. This evaluation appears to be far more accurate than the concentration of uric acid in plasma.

Increase in Serum Uric Acid
1. Gout
2. Impaired kidney function (uremia)
3. Increased destruction of nucleo-proteins
   a. leukemia
   b. polycythemia
   c. infectious disease
   d. hypoparathyroidism
   e. psoriasis

Decrease in Serum Uric Acid
1. Severe liver disease, acute yellow atrophy
2. Renal tubular dysfunction
3. Hepatolenticular degeneration (Wilson's disease)
4. Fanconi's syndrome
5. Acromegaly
6. Insulin reduction (temporary reduction only)
7. Drugs
   a. atophan
   b. cinchophen
   c. dicumarol
   d. cortisone
   e. probenecid
   f. phenylbutazone
   g. salicylates
   h. sulphoxyphenylpyrazolidine
   i. thiophenylpyrazolidine

SUMMARY

Uric acid is formed in the body by the breakdown of nucleoproteins and nu-

TABLE I—THE CONCENTRATION OF URIC ACID IN PLASMA
AS DETERMINED BY DIFFERENT METHODS (9)

| Method | Males | | Females | | Reference |
	Number of observations	Uric Acid mg per 100 ml	Number of observations	Uric Acid mg per 100 ml	
Colorimetric	63	4.4 ± 0.09	37	4.0 ± 0.11	Jacobson (16) 1938
Titrimetric	33	7.4 (5.4−8.8)	37	6.3 (4.4−8.1)	Brøchner-Mortensen (17) 1940
Enzymatic-colorimetric	56	5.4 ± 1.4	51	4.1 ± 0.9	Yü and Gutman (18) 1952
Enzymatic-spectrophotometric	143	(5.04 (2.6−7.5))	157	3.84 (2.0−5.7)	Gjørup, Poulsen and Prætorius (19) 1955
Enzymatic-spectrophotometric	53	4.4 ± 0.4	18	4.1 ± 0.5	Crone and Lassen (4) 1956

cleotides which are derived from tissues or ingested food. Purine nucleotides are synthesized from glycine and a series of carbon and nitrogen-containing substances. It appears likely that formed purine nucleotides may escape obligatory incorporation into nucleic acids, and by shunting mechanisms become uric acid. There is little evidence to indicate the occurrence of allantoin production in man. It is believed allantoin results from preformed ingestion, and an increase has never been found to be present in man.

Elimination of uric acid takes place primarily through the urine. Smaller amounts appear in feces, saliva, and sweat. The functioning glomerulus allows passage of 100% of the uric acid. The proximal tubule reabsorbs 90 to 95% of the filterable urates. The distal tubules secrete and contribute the remaining urinary uric acid.

Neither serum uric acid determination of total urinary uric acid excretion appears sensitive to kidney disease. Because of the extremely capable reserve of the kidney, increased serum uric acid and decreased urinary uric acid is seen late in kidney disease and is preempted by increase in the blood urea nitrogen and creatinine. The additional information provided by the total body pool of uric acid may be more meaningful in the future as simple methods of measurement become routine.

The biological significance of uric acid formation and excretion is meager. The abnormalities of uric acid metabolism, serum and urinary uric acid excretion should be studied in depth. The simple method of analysis should make this a more practical aid in the diagnosis of disease.

REFERENCES

1. Gutman A. B.: The biological significance of uric acid. Harvey Lectures Ser., *60:*35-55, 1966.
2. Berliner, R. W., Hilton, J. G., Yu, T. F., and Kennedy, T. J.: The renal mechanism for urate excretion in man. J. Clin. Invest., *29:*396-401, 1950.
3. Yü, T. F., Berger, L., and Gutman, A. B.: Renal function in gout. II. Effect of uric acid loading on renal excretion of uric acid. Am. J. Med., *33:*829-844, 1962.
4. Crone, C., and Lassen, U. V.: Some uric acid values in normal subjects. Scand. J. Clin. Lab. Invest., *8:*51-54, 1956.
5. Sunderman, F. W., and Boerner, F.: Normal Values in Clinical Medicine. Philadelphia, W. B. Saunders, 1949, p 369.
6. Hawk, P. B., Oser, B. L., and Summerson, W. H.: Practical Physiological Chemistry. New York, McGraw-Hill Book Company, 1954, p 788.
7. Davidsohn, I., and Wells, B. B. (eds): Todd-Sanford Clinical Diagnosis by Laboratory Methods, 13th edition. Philadelphia, W. B. Saunders, 1962, p 25.
8. Colton, R. S., and Ward, L. E.: Uric acid, gout, and the kidney. Med. Clin. North Am., *50:*1031, 1966.
9. Sorensen, L. B.: The elimination of uric acid in man. Scand. J. Clin. Lab. Invest., *12:* (Supplement 54), 1960.
10. Yü, T. F., and Gutman, A. B.: Renal regulation of uric acid excretion in normal and gouty man: modification by uricosuric agents. Bull. New York Acad. Med., *34:*287-296, 1958.
11. Berliner, R. W., Kennedy, T. J., and Hilton, J. G.: Renal mechanisms for excretion of potassium. Am. J. Physiol., *162:*348-367, 1950.
12. Wiechowski, W.: Biochem. Ztschr., *19:*368, 1909.
13. Ackroyd, H.: Biochem. J., *5:*400, 1911.
14. Brown, G. B.: Cold Spring Harbor Symp. Quant. Biol., *13:*43, 1948.
15. Wyngaarden, J. B.: The effect of phenylbutazone on uric acid metabolism in two normal subjects. J. Clin. Invest., *34:*256-262, 1955.
16. Jacobson, B. M.: Uric acid in serum of gouty and non-gouty individuals: its determination by Folin's recent method and its significance in diagnosis of gout. Ann. Int. Med., *11:*1277-1295, 1938.
17. Brøchner-Mortensen, K.: Uric acid content in blood and urine in health and disease. Medicine, *19:*161-229, 1940.
18. Yü, T. F., and Gutman, A. B.: Gout, a derangement of purine metabolism. Advances in Internal Medicine, *5:*227, 1952.
19. Gjørup, S. H., Poulsen, H., and Praetorius, E.: The uric acid concentration in serum determined by enzymatic spectrophotometry. Scand. J. Clin. Lab. Invest., *7:*201-203, 1955.

The Measurement of Uric Acid in Serum and Urine

F. WILLIAM SUNDERMAN, M.D.

The early methods for estimating uric acid in biological fluids were gravimetric in which uric acid was precipitated either by ammoniacal silver nitrate and magnesium chloride (1) or by a saturated solution of ammonium chloride (2). Since the introduction of the micro-colorimetric method for uric acid by Folin in 1912 (3), most methods used routinely in clinical laboratories have been based upon the formation of a blue color when uric acid reacts with phosphotungstic acid. Uric acid reduces phosphotungst*ate* complexes to intensely colored phosphotungst*ite* complexes. Such reactions are not specific when applied directly to filtrates of blood or serum. Commonly used methods employing the phosphotungstic acid reaction include those of Folin (4, 5), Benedict (6), Newton (7), Brown (8), Kern and Stransky (9), Archibald (10), Henry (11), and Hausman *et al.* (12). The phosphotungstic acid methods differ primarily in the adjuvants which are added to intensify the color. Cyanide reagents are frequently employed to intensify the color of the phosphotungstite complex, but these have the disadvantage of high toxicity. Other reagents used to intensify the color include hydrazine sulfate (13) and hydroxylamine (14). Automated adaptations of the phosphotungstic acid methods have been evaluated by O'Sullivan, Francis, and Kantor (15), by Crowley (16), by Allan (17, 18), by Nishi (19), and by Rosenmund and Knob (20).

The estimation of uric acid in serum has certain deficiencies because of the presence of non-uric acid components in serum which react with uric acid reagents to produce spurious elevations. To achieve greater specificity and accuracy, a number of workers (21-24) have used methods employing uricase, a specific enzyme prepared from beef kidney that oxidizes uric acid to allantoin. The uricase method of Praetorius and Poulsen (15, 26), is based upon the observation that uric acid produces maximum absorption in the ultraviolet range between 290 mμ and 296 mμ at pH 9.4. This absorption band disappears after incubation with uricase, since allantoin does not absorb light at 292 mμ (27). The concentration of uric acid may be calculated from the difference in optical density before and after the action of uricase. Modifications of the uricase method have been described by

Feichtmeir and Wrenn (28); Dubbs, Davis, and Adams (29); and Liddle, Seegmiller, and Laster (27). Caraway and Marable (30) have recently described a colorimetric phosphotungstic acid reduction procedure for uric acid in which serum is incubated with uricase to destroy uric acid. Residual nonurate chromogens are subtracted from total chromogens to obtain the concentration of "true" uric acid. The authors state that this method is applicable to serums from patients with uremia or those receiving salicylates in which high concentrations of non-urate chromogens may be encountered. Caraway and Marable (30) report that traces of formaldehyde markedly inhibit uricase activity. An enzymatic method has been described by Lorentz and Berndt (31) based upon the liberation of peroxide by uricase, coupled with oxidation of a chromogenic O_2 acceptor by peroxidase. This method has the advantage of permitting measurements in the visible range of the spectrum. Morgenstern *et al.* (32) also devised a colorimetric enzymatic method based upon the formation of a neocuproine complex before and after uricase treatment of serum.

Reducing substances, such as glutathione, ergothioneine, thionine, tyrosine, ascorbic acid, salicylates, and glucose, are known to affect color development in the uric acid-phosphotungstate reaction. Some of these interfering substances, such as thionine, are contained in greatest concentrations in erythrocytes. Interference from these is obviously partially avoided when serum is used. Alvsaker (33) has reported that xanthine and hypoxanthine are present in normal serum in a total concentration ranging from 0.05 to 0.3 mg per 100 ml (expressed as uric acid equivalents) and that elevated concentrations of xanthine and hypoxanthine are found in acute gouty arthritis and leukemia. Xanthine and hypoxanthine react with colorimetric uric acid reagents but are not measured by uricase procedures.

Comparisons of values obtained by phosphotungstate procedures and by uricase procedures for the determination of "true" uric acid have been published by Johnstone (34), O'Sullivan *et al.* (15), and Paologgi and co-workers (35). In normal serums, the two methods agree closely, — the phosphotungstic acid procedures yielding values from 0.1 to 0.4 mg per 100 ml greater than the values obtained with the uricase method. In cases of gout, the serum values were elevated, but the non-uric acid reacting substances were normal. By way of contrast, both uric acid and non-uric acid reacting components were increased in uremic serums. Paologgi *et al.* (35) indicate that the Folin method gives higher values in hyper-uricacidemia and lower values in hypo-uricacidemia as compared to the Praetorius method.

In 1965, Buchanan, Isdale, and Rose (36) showed that non-urate chromogens which interfere with colorimetric methods for uric acid disappear from serums which have been stored frozen for three weeks. This observation has been confirmed by Boyle *et al.* (37) While storage of serum for three weeks may be practical for epidemiological studies, it is not feasible for routine analysis in clinical laboratories. Recently, Isdale, Buchanan and Rose (38) have found that heating of serum at 60°C for one hour in a rubber-stoppered test tube produces a decrease of non-urate chromogens to a level comparable to that following three week's storage. Control of temperature apparently is crucial, for heating serum to more than 62°C caused loss of uric acid through protein coagulation, while heating to 58°C or less required much longer than one hour. At 60°C, there was little difference in non-urate chromogen destruction between 50 and 70 minutes.

Three additional approaches in the methodology of uric acid have been described: (A) Bergmann and Dikstein (39, 40), isolate uric acid by selective precipitation as the mercuric salt and measure the absorbance of the redissolved uric acid at 290 mμ. This method lends itself to the application of chromatographic procedures. (B) Shapiro and co-workers (41) separate uric acid with an appropriate ion-exchange resin and determine the uric acid in the eluate by direct measurement of ultraviolet absorbance at 286 mμ. Sambhi and Grollman (42) modified the ion-exchange method of Shapiro *et al.* by the addition of N-ethylmaleimide to remove interfering chromogens. (C) Marymont and London (43) have described a direct ultraviolet absorption method not requiring uricase in which the serum proteins are coagulated by heat and the uric acid is extracted into water. The absorbance of the extract is measured at 295 mμ. The authors report excellent agreement with measurements made by phosphotungstic acid reduction; however, salicylates may be a source of interference.

TABLE I

COMPARISON OF URIC ACID MEASUREMENTS
IN 14 HUMAN SERUMS
BY DIFFERENT METHODS (28)
(mg per 100 ml)

Method	Mean Value	Standard Deviation
Brown (8)	5.88	2.00
Newton (7)	4.34	1.16
Kern and Stransky (9)	3.80	0.67
Folin (3)	4.71	1.35
Blauch and Koch (21)	3.75	1.17

Normal Values

In Table I are given values for the concentration of uric acid in human serum by five methods that are used in clinical laboratories. It is apparent that various methods yield different values. This fact should be taken into account in comparing results from different laboratories.

The concentration of uric acid in serum is approximately twice the concentration in the red cells. Thus, the concentration of uric acid in whole blood is considerably lower than the concentration in serum. Owing to the variability in the percentage of cells contained in whole blood, measurements of uric acid should always be made on serum. It is noteworthy that uric acid in the serum of males is slightly higher than in females (44) and also that the concentration may be increased in older age groups (45). The ranges of normal values for males and females are given in Table II. A brief summarization of normal values for uric acid in serum has been given by Caraway and Marable (30).

Precautions with Reference to Colorimetric Methods for Uric Acid

1. Local excesses of sulfuric acid may cause a diminution in the concentration of uric acid. Therefore, if Folin-Wu filtrates are used in making the analyses, it is important to shake the reaction mixture continuously during the slow addition of the sulfuric acid reagent. In addition, it is important that "half-strength" tungstic acid reagent be used in the preparation of the protein filtrates of serum.

2. Cyanide solutions should never be pipetted with the usual transfer pipet; either automatic pipets or burets should be used for measuring these solutions. If kept in the cold, cyanide solutions are

TABLE II

CONCENTRATION OF URIC ACID IN THE SERUM OF NORMAL PERSONS

(mg per 100 ml)

			Males			Females	
Author	*Method*	*No.*	*Mean*	*Range*	*No.*	*Mean*	*Range*
Gjørup, et al. (26)	Prætorius (18)	157	5.0	2.6–7.5	143	3.8	2.0–5.7
Alper and Seitchik (46)	Archibald (10)	95	5.4	3.8–7.1	48	4.0	2.6–5.4

usable for about two months (27). Before use, cold cyanide solutions should be brought to room temperature by immersion in a water bath at 25°C.

3. Blank values should be obtained with each set of analyses since these appear to vary with the age of the cyanide solution. Freshly prepared cyanide solutions are prone to give high blanks. Cyanide solutions that have stood for about two days give blanks of more constancy. The readings obtained with such aged cyanide solutions are about one-half of those obtained with freshly prepared solutions.

4. With most colorimetric methods, the proportionality between the concentration of uric acid in serum and the color intensity is linear up to 8 mg per 100 ml. If the value in serum exceeds 8 mg per 100 ml, it is suggested that calibration curves be used to compensate for deviations from Beer's law (14).

Choice of Method

For routine clinical purposes, the Brown (8) method remains our method of choice. The Archibald method (10) is also described since it does *not* employ cyanide solutions. The uricase procedure may be valuable for checking purposes.* The uricase method of Liddle, Seegmiller, and Laster (27) is also included in this chapter. The importance of using

------

*Satisfactory enzyme preparations may be obtained from the Worthington Biochemical Corporation, Freehold, New Jersey 07728.

serum blanks in the method of Liddle *et al.* has been emphasized by Klein and Lafebar (47). The suggestions of Klein and Lafebar are incorporated in the uricase method given in this chapter.

THE METHOD OF BROWN (8)

Principle

The color produced by the reduction of phosphotungstic acid by uric acid in a protein-free filtrate of serum is compared with that produced by standard solutions of uric acid.

Reagents

1. *Uric Acid Stock Standard (10 mg per 100 ml).* One-hundred mg of recrystallized uric acid are weighed and transferred to a one-liter volumetric flask. Three-tenths gm of lithium carbonate is dissolved in 100 ml of water and filtered. The lithium carbonate solution is heated to 60°C and poured on the uric acid. The mixture is shaken until all of the uric acid is dissolved (the solution may be slightly turbid). The flask is cooled under running water, and 20 ml of 40% formaldehyde (formalin) are added. The solution is diluted to about 500 ml, and 15 ml of normal sulfuric acid are added. The solution is mixed, diluted to the mark, and transferred to a dark-brown bottle. This solution should now be clear. It should be kept in a cool, dark place (refrigerator). (Approximately normal H_2SO_4 is obtained by

adding 30 ml of concentrated sulfuric acid to water and diluting to one liter.)

2. *Dilute Uric Acid Standard #1.* One ml of uric acid stock standard solution is transferred into a 50-ml volumetric flask and diluted to the mark with distilled water. This solution contains 0.002 mg per ml and is equivalent to 2.0 mg uric acid per 100 ml serum. 3.

3. *Dilute Uric Acid Standard #2.* Two ml of uric acid stock standard solution are transferred into a 25-ml volumetric flask and diluted to the mark with distilled water. This solution contains 0.008 mg per ml and is equivalent to 8 mg uric acid per 100 ml serum.

4. *Urea Solution, 50%, w/v.* Fifty gm of urea are dissolved in distilled water and diluted to the 100-ml mark. This reagent is stable at room temperature. Urea will cystallize out if placed in the refrigerator.

5. *Sodium Cyanide, 12%, w/v (Poison).* Twelve gm of sodium cyanide are dissolved in distilled water and diluted to 100 ml. This solution is placed in a dark bottle and kept in a refrigerator.

6. *Uric Acid Reagent (Phosphotungstic Acid).* Into a 500-ml round-bottom flask with a ground-glass neck (previously cleaned with dichromate-sulfuric acid cleaning solution) are placed 50 mg of sodium tungstate ($Na_2WO_4 \cdot 2H_2O$) and 10 gm of anhydrous disodium phosphate (or 18.9 gm of $Na_2HPO_4 \cdot 7H_2O$). One-hundred and fifty ml of water are added to the flask and the mixture is warmed until complete solution has taken place. Then 12.5 ml of concentrated sulfuric acid are added to the tungstate solution. The flask is fitted to a condenser (cleaned with dichromate-sulfuric aicd), and the mixture is refluxed for one hour. The mixture is cooled, transferred with rinsing to a 500-ml volumetric flask, and diluted to the mark. The reagent is stable indefinitely and should be practically colorless. If it becomes blue, or if the blank determination develops a color, a drop of bromine is added, and the solution is boiled to remove excess bromine.

Procedure

A protein-free filtrate of serum is prepared by adding 1 ml of serum to 4.5 ml of mixed tungstic acid reagent (8 ml of $N/12\ H_2SO_4$ and 1 ml of 10% sodium tungstate) and 4.5 ml of water. The resultant solution and precipitate are filtered or centrifuged. One ml of the filtrate is introduced into a cuvet graduated at 10 ml. Two ml of the cyanide solution are added to the tube by means of an automatic pipet. This is followed by the addition of 2.0 ml of urea solution and 1.0 ml of phosphotungtic acid reagent. The contents are mixed and the tubes are stoppered and kept at room temperature for 50 minutes. The contents are diluted to the 10-ml mark and readings are made with a photometer. A blank and 1.0 ml of standards #1 and #2 are treated in the same manner as the protein-free filtrate. The maxmum absorption is at approximately 690 mμ. Readings for the standards are plotted on graph paper, and the concentrations of uric acid in the samples may be read from this graph or calculated from the following equation:

$$\frac{\text{mg Standard per 100 ml}}{\text{O.D. Standard}} \times \text{O.D. Unknown} = \text{mg Uric Acid per 100 ml Serum}$$

THE METHOD OF ARCHIBALD (10)

Principle

The ability of uric acid to reduce the hexavalent tungsten of phosphotungstic acid to a lower valence with the formation of a blue color is employed in this method. Clouding, which has been a threat in phosphotungstic acid reduction methods for uric acid, is prevented by a mixture of glycerol, sodium silicate, and polyanethol sodium sulfonate. The reduction belongs to the class of incompletely defined oxidation-reduction reactions, and accuracy depends on precise observance of empirically fixed conditions.

Reagents

1. *Standard Solution of Uric Acid.* Approximately 0.5 gm of lithium carbonate, dissolved in 150 ml of hot water, is added with stirring to exactly 1 gm of uric acid. The solution is transferred with 300 ml of rinsings to a liter volumetric flask; 25 ml of 40% formaldehyde, then 3 ml of glacial acetic acid are added with mixing. After the liberated CO_2 has been removed from solution by shaking, water sufficient to bring the volume to one liter is added and the solution is mixed. This stock standard, if protected from light, is stable for at least one year.

2. *Dilute Working Standard of Uric Acid, 0.005 mg per ml.* One ml of stock standard solution is placed into a 200-ml volumetric flask and diluted to the mark with distilled water. This solution is prepared fresh on the day it is to be used.

3. *Polyanethol Sodium Sulfonate.* One gm of "Liquoid La Rochee" is dissolved in 50 ml of water. The solution is stored in a refrigerator. (This reagent is obtained from Hoffman-LaRoche, Inc.,

Nutley, New Jersey 07110.)

4. *Glycerine-silicate Reagent.* Ten gm of Merck's cystalline sodium silicate "soluble" are dissolved in 100 ml of hot water, then mixed with 20 ml of glycerine. Alternately, 130 ml of Merck's water-glass dissolved in 250 ml of water, and 85 ml of reagent-grade glycerine are mixed at room temperature and made up to 500 ml with water. If the solution prepared by either procedure is cloudy, it should be filtered through hardened paper and stored in a Pyrex container.

5. *Phosphotungstic Acid Solution.* Fifty gm of reagent-grade sodium tungstate, $(Na_2WO_4 \cdot 2H_2O)$; 400 ml of water; and 40 ml of 85% orthophosphoric acid are boiled under a reflux condenser for four hours, then made up to a volume of 500 ml with water and stored, protected from light.

6. *Sodium Hydroxide Solution, 0.5 N.*

Procedure

The protein-free serum filtrate is prepared by pipetting 1 ml of serum into a 25-ml Erlenmeyer flask and then adding 8 ml of distilled water and 0.4 ml of 0.5 N NaOH. The solution is mixed by swirling the flask for one minute. After mixing, 0.6 ml of the phosphotungstic acid solution is added. The first 0.3 may be added rapidly, but the last 0.3 ml must be added dropwise with constant mixing to insure complete precipitation of protein. (It is suggested that a buret be used for the addition of phosphotungstic acid.) After five minutes, the mixture is filtered through a Whatman #42 filter paper or centrifuged. To 5 ml of the filtrate are added 2.5 ml of glycerine-silicate reagent and 0.5 ml of polyanethol sodium sulfonate solution with constant mixing. Then, 0.5 ml of the phosphotungstic acid solution is added with instantaneous mixing. The tubes are allowed to stand for 15 minutes at room temperature and absorbance measurements are read at 700 mμ in a spectrophotometer. The color is stable for about 30 minutes. Five ml of the diluted standard and 5 ml of water are each treated in the same manner as the serum filtrate to provide a standard and a photometric blank, respectively.

Calculation

$$\text{Uric Acid in plasma or serum} = 5 \times \frac{\text{absorbance of unknown}}{\text{absorbance of standard}}$$
$$\text{(mg per 100 ml)}$$

URICASE METHOD FOR URIC ACID (30, 47)

Principle

The concentration of uric acid in serum is determined by measuring the optical density of buffered serum at 292 mμ before and after the action of uricase enzyme.

Reagents

1. *Glycine Stock Buffer (0.67 M, pH 9.4).* Twenty-five gm of glycine and 4.4 gm of NaOH pellets are dissolved in distilled water and diluted to 500 ml. Three ml of chloroform are added as a preservative. The solution is stored in a refrigerator.

2. *Glycine Working Buffer (0.067 M, pH 9.4).* Ten ml of stock buffer are diluted to 100 ml with distilled water. This solution is stable for one week at room temperature.

3. *Uricase Solution, Purified* (Worthington Biochemical Corporation, Freehold, New Jersey 07728). This preparation is purchased in 1-ml ampules, and is stored frozen. The ampule in daily use is kept at 6°C.

4. *Uric Acid Stock Standard (30 mg per 100 ml).* Thirty mg of Pfanstiehl uric acid are dissolved in ten ml of hot distilled water by the addition of 1 ml of a hot saturated solution of lithium carbonate. The solution is diluted to 100 ml with distilled water. The solution is stored in the refrigerator.

5. *Uric Acid Working Standard (1.2 mg per 100 ml).* One ml of stock standard is diluted to 25 ml with distilled water. This standard is used to check the calibration of the spectrophotometer and to assay the activity of the uricase solution.

Procedure

A. *Serum*

The analysis is made by measuring the change in O.D. at 292 mμ which results from uricase action in the assay cuvet. Additional control cuvets are needed to correct for changes in O.D. resulting from factors other than the enzyme reaction.

1. *Assay Cuvet.* To a 10 mm Beckman silica cuvet are added 3 ml of glycine buffer, 0.1 ml of serum, and 0.01 ml of uricase. The contents are mixed by covering the cuvet with Parafilm and inverting several times. The cuvet is immediately placed in the ultraviolet spectrophotometer. The O.D. is determined at 292 mμ initially and at 3, 25 and 30 minutes, respectively, after the addition of uricase. The 3-minute

reading is obtained to check the activity of the uricase. At 3 minutes, the change in O.D. should be more than 30% of the total change if the reaction is to be complete by 25 minutes. The 30-minute reading is obtained to ascertain that the reaction is complete. The O.D. at 30 minutes is the "Final O.D."

2. *Serum Blank Cuvet.* To a 10 mm cuvet are added 3 ml of glycine buffer and 0.1 ml of serum. Spectrophotometer readings are made in the same manner as for the "Assay Cuvet."

3. *Enzyme Blank Cuvet.* To a 10 mm cuvet are added 3 ml of glycine buffer and 0.010 ml of uricase. Spectrophotometer readings are made in the same manner as for the "Assay Cuvet." (The change in O.D. for the enzyme blank is usually negligible.)

4. *Reference Cuvet.* This cuvet serves only as a reference and is used to adjust the spectrophotometer to zero. The large amounts of nonurate material which are present in serum and which absorb at 292 mμ must be cancelled by substituting a reference cell of a corresponding optical density in place of the usual water-containing silica cuvet. Use of the reference cuvet should bring the initial O.D. in the assay cuvet to the range of 0.2 to 0.4. In practice, a pyrex with an O.D. approximately 0.85 greater than a silica cuvet may be used for this purpose. Alternately, reference cells may be improvised by using the frosted surface of a silica cuvet or by using a monel metal mesh placed in a silica cuvet.

Calculations

A solution of uric acid at pH 9.4 containing 1 mcgm per ml has an O.D. of 0.0745 in a silica cuvet wtih a 1.00 cm light path. Oxidation of uric acid by uricase abolishes this absorption completely. Therefore, the quantitiy of uric acid in the cuvet in mcgm equals

$$\frac{\Delta \text{O.D. uric acid}}{0.0745}$$

times the total volume of solution in the assay cuvet.

$$
\begin{aligned}
(1)\quad &\Delta\text{O.D. assay cuvet} &&= \text{Initial O.D.} - \text{Final} &&\text{O.D.}\\
(2)\quad &\Delta\text{O.D. enzyme blank} &&= \text{Final O.D.} - \text{Initial} &&\text{O.D.}\\
(3)\quad &\Delta\text{O.D. serum blank} &&= \text{Final O.D.} - \text{Initial} &&\text{O.D.}\\
&\Delta\text{O.D. uric acid} &&= (1) + (2) + (3)
\end{aligned}
$$

$$
\text{Uric acid in Serum (mg per 100 ml)} = \frac{\Delta\text{O.D. uric acid}}{0.0745} \times \frac{3.11}{0.1} \times \frac{1}{1000} \times 100
$$

$$
= \text{O.D. uric acid} \times 41.7
$$

B. *Urine*

1. The spectrophotometer is set at 292 mμ and is balanced with a reference cuvet filled with water.

2. Urine is diluted between 1:100 to 3:100 with distilled water to provide a satisfactory quantity of uric acid for assay.

3. To the assay cuvet are added 2 ml of glycine buffer (0.1M, pH 9.4) and 1.0 ml of diluted urine.

4. The optical density is read; if it is much lower than 0.100, then dilution is necessary so that the optical density is at least 0.100.

5. Precisely 0.01 ml of uricase enzyme is added. The procedure is continued in the same matter as for serum.

Calculation

$$\text{Uric acid in Urine} \atop \text{(mg per ml)} = \frac{\Delta \text{O.D.} \times 3.01}{0.0745 \times 1000} \times \text{dilution}$$

$$= \Delta \text{O.D.} \times 0.04 \times \text{dilution}$$

Precision and Accuracy

According to Liddle *et al.* (27), the standard deviation of 28 paired observations (range 138 to 1109 mg per 24 hours) for urine was ± 3.8 mg per 24 hours, and of 50 paired observations (range 4.7 to 12.24 mg per 100 ml) for serum was ± 0.043. The average recovery of added uric acid was 100.1 percent (range 99.3 to 101.1) in urine and 99.4% (range 98.3 to 100.8) in serum.

REFERENCES

1. Salkowski, E., and Ludwig, E.: Tierfelder's Handbuch der Physiologisch und Pathologisch Chemischen Analyze. Berlin, 1924, p. 709.
2. Hopkins, F. G.: On the estimation of uric acid in urine. A new process by means of saturation with ammonium chloride. Proc. Royal Soc. London, 52:93-99, 1893.
3. Folin, O., and Denis, W.: A new (colorimetric) method for the determination of uric acid in blood. J. Biol. Chem., 13:469-475, 1912-13.
4. Folin, O.: Standardized methods for the determination of uric acid in unlaked blood and in urine. J. Biol. Chem., 101:111-125, 1933.
5. Folin, O.: The preparation of sodium tungstate free from molybdate, together with a simplified process for the preparation of a correct uric acid reagent (and some comments). J. Biol. Chem., 106:311-314, 1934.
6. Benedict, S. R.: The determination of uric acid in blood. J. Biol. Chem., 51:187-207, 1922.
7. Newton, E. B.: A chromogenic tungstate and it's use in the determination of the uric acid in blood. J. Biol. Chem., 120:315-329, 1937.
8. Brown, H.: The determination of uric acid in human blood. J. Biol. Chem, 158:601-608, 1945.
9. Kern, A., and Stransky, E.: Study on the colorimetric determination of uric acid. Biochem. Z., 290:419-427, 1937.
10. Archibald, R. M.: Colorimetric measurement of uric acid. Clin. Chem., 3:102-105, 1957.
11. Henry, R. J., Sobel, C., and Kim, J.: A modified carbonatephosphotungstate method for the determination of uric acid and comparison with the spectrophotometric uricase method. Amer. J. Clin. Path., 28:152-160, 1957.
12. Hausman, E. R., Lewis, G. T., and MeAnally, J. S.: Determination of uric acid. A note, Clin. Chem., 3:657-658, 1957.
13. Patel, C. P.: A semi-micro method for determination of uric acid using EDTA-hydrazine. Clin. Chem., 13:700, 1967.
14. Sobrinho-Simoes, M.: A sensitive method for the measurement of serum uric acid using hydroxylamine. J. Lab. Clin. Med., 65:665-668, 1965.
15. O'Sullivan, J. B., Francis, J. O.'S., and Kantor, N.: Comparison of a colorimetric (automated) with an enzymatic (manual) uric acid procedure. Clin. Chem., 11:427-435, 1965.
16. Crowley, L. V.: Determination of uric acid. An automated analysis based on a carbonate method. Clin. Chem., 10:838-844, 1964.
17. Allan, R. D.: An automated modification of Eichhorn's uric acid method. J. Med., Lab. Technol. (London), 21:240-241, 1964.
18. Allan, R. D.: The simultaneous estimation of uric acid and urea with the autoanalyzer. J. Med. Lab. Technol. (London), 23:151-160, 1966.
19. Nishi, H. H.: Determination of uric acid. An adaptation of the Archibald method on the autoanalyzer. Clin. Chem., 13:12-18, 1967.
20. Rosenmund, H., and Knob, M.: Enzymatic and automatic colorimetrically determined values of uric acid in blood serum, Z. Rheumaforsch, 24:184-190, 1965.
21. Blauch, M. B., and Koch, F. C.: A new method for the determination of uric acid in blood with uricase. J. Biol. Chem., 130:443-454, 1939.
22. Mull, J. W.: Determination of uric acid in whole blood and serum. J. Lab. & Clin. Med., 28:1038-1042, 1942, 43.
23. Block, W. D., and Geib, N. C.: An enzymatic method for the determination of uric acid in whole blood. J. Biol. Chem., 168:747-756, 1947.
24. Leon, E.: Determination of uric acid in blood. Quaderni notriz. 10:63-75, 1947. (CA 43:7074a).
25. Praetorius, E.: Enzymatic determination of uric acid. Scand. J. Clin. Lab. Invest., 5:273-280, 1953.
26. Gjorup, S., Poulsen, H., and Praetorius, E.: The uric acid concentration in serum determined by enzymatic spectrophotometry. Scand. J. Clin. Lab. Invest., 7:201-203, 1955.
27. Liddle, L., Seegmiller, J. E., and Laster, L.: The enzymatic spectrophotometric method for deter-

mination of uric acid. J. Lab. and Clin. Med., *54*:903-913, 1959.

28. Feichtmier, T. V., and Wrenn, H. T.: Direct determination of uric acid uring uricase. Amer. J. Clin. Path., *25*:833-839, 1955.

29. Dubbs, C. A., Davis, F. W., and Adams, W. S.: Simple microdetermination of uric acid. J. Biol. Chem., *218*:497-504, 1956.

30. Caraway, W. T., and Marable, H.: Comparison of carbonate and uricase-carbonate methods for the determination of uric acid in serum. Clin. Chem., *12*:18-24, 1966.

31. Lorentz, K., and Berndt, W.: Enzymic determination of uric acid by a colorimetric method. Analyt. Biochem., *18*:58-63, 1967.

32. Morgenstern, S., Flor, R. V., Kaufman, J. H., and Klein, B.: The automated determination of serum uric acid. Clin. Chem., *12*:748-766, 1966.

33. Alvsaker, J. O.: Uric acid in human plasma. I. Investigations on the presence of purines in human blood. Scand. J. Clin. Lab. Invest., *17*:1-8, 1965.

34. Johnstone, J. M.: True uric acid values. J. Clin. Path., *5*:317-318, 1952.

35. Paolaggi, F. *et al.*: Comparative value of Folin's colorimetric method and Praetorius' enzyme method for the determination of uricemia and uraturia. Path. Biol. Semaine Hop., *12*:589-593, 1964.

36. Buchanan, M. J., Isdale, I. C., and Rose, B. S.: Serum uric acid estimation chemical and enzymatic methods compared. Ann. Rheum. Dis., *24*:285-288, 1965.

37. Boyle, J. A. *et al.*: Serum uric acid levels in normal pregnancy with observations on the renal excretion of urate in pregnancy. J. Clin. Path., *19*:501-503, 1966.

38. Isdale, I. C., Buchanan, M. J., and Rose, B. S.: Serum uric acid estimation. A modified chemical method. Ann. Rheum. Dis., *25*:184-185, 1966.

39. Bergmann, F., and Dikstein, S.: Quantitative determination of uric acid in biological fluids. J. Biol. Chem., *211*:149-153, 1954.

40. Bergmann, F., Dikstein, S., and Chaimouitz, M.: Notes on the quantitative determination of xanthines and uric acids in plasma. J. Biol. Chem., *230*:193-201, 1958.

41. Shapiro, B., Seligson, D., and Jessar, R.: Measurement of uric acid in biologic fluids using an ion-exchange separation. Clin. Chem., *3*:169-177, 1957.

42. Sambhi, M. P., and Grollman, A.: A simplified procedure for the routine determination of uric acid. Clin. Chem., *5*:623-633, 1959.

43. Marymont, J. H., Jr., and London, M.: Analysis on heat coagulated blood and serum. IV. Direct determination of uric acid by ultraviolet absorption. Clin. Chem., *10*:937-941, 1964.

44. Brochner-Mortensen, K.: The uric acid content in blood and urine in health and disease. Medicine, *19*:161-229, 1940.

45. Gephardt, M. C., Hanlon, T. J., and Matson, C. F.: Blood uric acid values as related to sex and age. JAMA, *189*:1028-1029, 1964.

46. Alper, C., and Seitchik, J.: Comparison of the Archibald-Kern and Stransky colorimetric procedure and the Praetorius enzymatic procedure for the determination of uric acid. Clin. Chem., *3*:95-101, 1957.

47. Klein, F., and Lafeber, G.J.M.: Improvements of the uricase-u.v. method for the determination of uric acid in serum and urine. Clin. Chim. Acta, *14*:708-710, 1966.

Chapter 21

Specific Ion Activity Determination for Measurement of Serum and Urine Electrolytes in Renal Disease

KURT M. DUBOWSKI, Ph.D.

INTRODUCTION

The kidneys play a primary role in the homeostasis of body water and electrolytes, as for example in the maintenance of body fluid isotonicity by the retention or elimination of water, controlled largely through the regulation of sodium excretion by the kidney. Because of this central role of the kidneys in water and electrolyte regulation, renal disease produces a large variety of electrolyte disturbances, the character and extent of which is further affected by such extrarenal factors as edema or dehydration.

Serum and urine electrolyte measurements are therefore of fundamental and critical importance for the prompt and correct diagnosis and treatment of renal disease, particularly the various types of renal insufficiency. They are of equal importance in the assessment and treatment of disturbances of renal function of extrarenal origin, e.g., in adrenal insufficiency, pituitary diabetes insipidus, hyperparathroidism, etc.

At the present state of knowledge, measurement of the following cations in serum and urine is of greatest significance in relation to renal disease: ammonium, calcium, hydrogen, magnesium, potassium, and sodium. The correspondingly most pertinent anion measurements are those of bicarbonate, chloride, phosphate, and sulfate. The present-day routine measurement of most of these substances in clinical laboratory practice is carried out almost exclusively by a relatively few instrumental methods of analysis representing acceptable compromises among economic and technological factors and the clinical requirements and limitations (time, sample size, etc.) Most of the major techniques involved, such as flame photometric determination of sodium and potassium in body liquids, atomic absorption spectrometry and titrimetric determination of calcium and magnesium, gasometric measurement of bicarbonate, and titrimetric and electrometric determination of chloride have been recently reviewed in detail (1) and hence will not be considered here.

However, many of the chemical and instrumental methods in common use for measurement of the electrolytes in biological liquids have such severe limitations for clinical applications as lack of specificity, sensitivity and freedom from interference by normal biological fluid constituents such as proteins, complexity and high acquisition and maintenance cost of the required instrumentation, narrow limits of acceptable concentration in the analyzed sample aliquot, instability of required reagents, overly great dependence on analyst judgment (e.g., of end-point color), and excessively great time requirements for completion of analysis as well as in technician working time. In contrast, potentiometric measurement of clinically significant anions and cations in biological liquids by means of ion-specific or ion-selective electrodes has none of these limitations and embodies a substantial number of additional theoretical and practical advantages. Perhaps the most notable and unique characteristic of ion-specific electrode potentiometry, compared with flame photometry, titrimetry, gasometry, and coulometry, is that *activity* is measured in contradistinction to the concentration values given by the other methods. However, concentration values can be obtained from electrode measurements directly by maintenance of constant ionic strengths, or indirectly by computations employing empirical activity coefficients. Activity values are considerably more basic than concentrations because thermodynamic events such as transport phenomena, complex formation, etc. are direct functions of activity, and their use in clinical and experimental medicine will undoubtedly assume increasing significance as our understanding of the biochemical mechanisms of electrolyte homeostasis and metabolism and their alteration expands.

Commercial ion-specific electrodes* are presently available for the measurement of every anion and cation mentioned above. Potentiometry is a most attractive technique for automated chemical analysis — possessing the inherent advantages of speed, simplicity of procedures and instrumentation, high precision and selectivity, small sample requirements, non-destruction of sample,

____

*This term will be employed throughout this chapter for simplicity, although it is recognized that in some instances, the electrodes are highly ion-selective rather than completely ion-specific.

ION-SELECTIVE ELECTRODES FOR CHEMICAL POTENTIOMETRY

Electrode Class	*Selectivity Determinants*	*Use*	*Manufacturer*
Glass Membrane • pH Type • Cation-Sensitive Type • Sodium-Sensitive Type	Composition of glass membrane	Univalent cations: H^+, Na^+, K^+, Ag^+, NH_4^+, Li^+	Beckman Corning Thomas
Liquid-Liquid Membrane	Liquid ion-exchanger; glass or plastic porous membrane	Divalent cations, some anions: Ca^{++}, Mg^{++}, Cu^{++}, Cl^-, ClO_4^-, NO_3^-	Corning Orion
Solid State • Synthetic Crystal Type • Precipitate-impregnated Membrane Type	Synthetic crystal type; type of precipitate imbedded in silicone rubber matrix	Chiefly anions: Cl^-, Br^-, F^-, I^-, $S^=$, $PO_4^=$, $SO_4^=$	Orion Pungor

etc. The ion-specific electrodes, therefore, lend themselves well to incorporation into automated analysis systems (2, 7).

Because of space and time limitations. this discussion is limited to measurement of sodium in biological liquids with sodium ion electrode. Analogous considerations and procedural details apply to the measurement of other cations and anions by potentiometry with ion-specific electrodes.

Principles

When a thin membrane of glass or certain other materials is interposed between two solutions, an electric potential difference is observed across the membrane, which depends upon the ions present in the solutions in a simple and reproducible manner (3). The potentiometric response, in glass electrodes, may be to H^+ ion or to other cations, such as Na^+, K^+, Li^+, NH_4^+, Ag^+, Ca^{++}, Mg^{++}, etc., depending upon the composition of the glass, which is the critical variable. The glass electrodes constitute one class of ion-specific electrode in common use, the others being liquid-liquid membrane electrodes, precipitate-impregnated membrane electrodes, and solid-state membrane electrodes.

The selectivity of various glasses for one cation relative to another apparently depends on the negative electrostatic field strength of the glass lattice, which in turn is a function of the unscreened charge on oxygen atoms. One member of the group of aluminosilicate glasses, NAS_{11-18} (Na_2O, 11 mole per cent; AL_2O_3, 18 mole % SiO_2, 71 mole %) has marked preference for Na^+ over K^+ and for practical purposes does not respond to changes in $[H^+]$ above pH5.

Potentiometric measurability of ion activity depends upon the proportionality of the system's free energy to the logarithm of the specific ion activity. The electrode is filled with a solution which has a fixed sodium ion activity, and an internal silver-silver chloride junction provides a stable potential between all internal surfaces. Thus, any changes in the electrode potential are due only to changes in sodium ion activity in the *sample* solution.

At appropriate pH, the developed electrode potential follows very closely the theoretical response described by the Nernst equation:

$$E_{obs} = E_o + \frac{2.303\ RT}{n\ F} \log (a_{Na^+}) \tag{I}$$

where E_{obs} = potential observed for any given Na^+ activity

E_o = potential of the standard state

R = universal gas constant in Joules per degree per mole

T = absolute temperature in degrees Kelvin

n = valence

F = Faraday constant in coulombs per equivalent

$\log (a_{Na^+})$ = logarithm of sodium ion activity

NOTE: $2.303 \dfrac{R}{F} = 0.1984$

Since activity (a_{Na^+}) is equal to concentration (C_{Na^+}) multiplied by the activity coefficient (γ_{Na^+}), the Nernst equation can be rewritten as follows to permit either activity or concentration measurements to be made when the mean ionic activity coefficient for sodium is known:

$$E_{obs} = E_o + \frac{2.303\ RT}{F}\ \log (\gamma_{Na^+}) + \frac{2.303\ RT}{F}\ \log (C_{Na^+}) \qquad (II)$$

More generally, the electrode response is given by:

$$E_{obs} = E_o + \frac{2.303\ RT}{F}\ \log (a_{Na^+} + Ka_{M^+}) \qquad (III)$$

where M = any univalent ion (e.g., K^+, NH_4^+. . .)

K = apparent selectivity for Na^+ over M^+, reciprocally expressed

NOTE: For NAS_{11-18} glass, at pH 7,

K = 0.001 when M^+ is potassium,

and the K^+ effect can therefore be neglected for sodium measurement.

Since standard solutions can be used to calibrate the system, E_o can be disregarded in practical calculations. Thus, at 25°C.,

$$0.1984 \times T = 59.15\ \text{millivolts} \qquad (IV)$$

which is the theoretical slope of E_{obs} versus $\log (a_{Na^+})$. Therefore, the potential changes approximately 59 mv for each decade change in Na^+ activity at 25°C., over the concentration range from 10^{-6} moles per liter to saturated solutions, at pH 5 to 13, in pure solutions of sodium salts.

At concentrations below 15 to 20 mEq sodium per liter, the potential response of the sodium ion electrode is virtually identical to concentration or activity. In suitably diluted and buffered unknown specimens, therefore, the sodium *concentration* can be determined from the observed millivolt reading by means of a semilogarithmic plot of concentration versus millivolts. With some expanded scale pH meters incorporating logarithmic millivolt scales, the sodium concentration can also be read directly from such scales after direct calibration of the meter with one or more standard solutions.

Reagents and Standard Solutions

1. *Sodium Chloride*, 0.1 M. Dissolve 5.845 gm of dry, desiccated reagent grade crystalline sodium chloride in distilled-demineralized water and dilute to 1 liter. Store in a polyethylene bottle.

2. *Sodium Stock Standard*, 1000 mEq per liter. Dissolve 58.454 gm of dry, desiccated reagent grade crystalline sodium chloride in distilled-demineralized water and dilute to 1 liter. Store in a polyethylene bottle.

3. *Sodium Working Standards*, 1.5, 10, 50, 100, 150, 200 mEq per liter. Dilute appropriate volumes of the sodium stock standard to 1 liter with distilled-demineralized water. Store in polyethylene bottles.

4. *"Tris" Buffer-diluent, pH 8.0.* Dissolve 12.12 gm of trishydroxymethyl-aminomethane in 1 liter of distilled-demineralized water. Add 4.3 ml conc. hydrochloric acid. Check the pH and, if necessary, adjust to pH 8.0 ± 0.1 with 1 N hydrochloric acid or with additional "Tris." Store in a polyethylene or a borosilicate glass bottle.

Special Apparatus

1. *Electrometer.* The resistance of the cation-specific glasses ranges from 10^5 to 10^{11} ohms. The electrometer used must therefore have an input impedance of at least 10^{12} and preferably 10^{14} ohms. With ideal electrode response to Na^+ only, the potential difference between a solution containing 140 mEq Na^+ per liter and one containing 141 mEq per liter is of the order of 0.18 mv, and this delineates the instrumental requirements for sensitivity, precision, drift-stability, and resolution. While vibrating reed electrometers meet all requisite characteristics, it is satisfactory and more practical to use high-precision pH meters with millivolt calibrations of the "expanded scale" type, readable to $\pm$ 0.2 mv, such as the Corning Model 12 Research pH Meter, the Orion Model 801 Digital Display pH Meter, the Radiometer pH Meter 22 with pHA 630 scale expander, etc.

2. *Reference Electrode.* A standard calomel reference electrode, such as Corning Catalog Number 476002, Arthur H. Thomas Co. Catalog Number 4857-F15, etc.

3. *Sodium Ion Electrode.* A sealed glass-membrane sodium ion electrode, such as Corning Catalog Number 476210 or Arthur H. Thomas Co. Catalog Number 4923-L10.

4. *Diluter.* A motor-driven automatic diluter-dispenser, such as York Instrument Corp. Model LD-1.

Procedure

The procedure described for sodium measurements in serum or urine with the sodium ion electrode is essentially that of Annino (5).

A. *Electrode Preparation and Care*

1. Before use, a new sodium ion electrode is dipped into 2% hydrofluoric acid for a few seconds, followed immediately with copious water rinsing, dipping into 0.1 N hydrochloric acid, and again copious rinsing with distilled-demineralized water.

2. If the electrode response time becomes excessive after prolonged service, reactivation is carried out by first removing any film of protein or dirt with a mild nonionic detergent, and then soaking the electrode in 0.1 N hydrochloric acid for at least 1 hour, followed by rinsing with distilled-demineralized water. If the electrode does not respond adequately to this treatment, it is reconditioned with hydrofluoric acid, as outlined under 1 above.

3. The new electrode, after conditioning, is soaked in 0.1 M aqueous sodium chloride for at least 24 hours prior to use. The electrode is also stored in this solution when not in use.

4. The calomel electrode is handled and used according to normal procedure and with the usual precautions against drying and contamination.

B. *Measurement of Urine Sodium Concentration*

1. The well-mixed urine specimen is diluted 1:10 with "Tris" buffer-diluent, e.g., 2.00 ml urine are mixed with 18.0 ml of buffer-diluent using the automatic diluter. Similar dilutions of 2 or more sodium standards in the expected sample

range are prepared. (Typically, nominal 100 and 200 mEq per liter standards are used.)

2. The sodium-ion and calomel reference electrode pair is immersed successively into at least 10 ml of 2 or more diluted standards and the resultant millivolt readings recorded. The electrodes are carefully dried (but not rinsed) between successive standard or sample measurements.

3. The electrode pair is then immersed into at least 10 ml of the diluted sample and the resultant millivolt measurement recorded.

4. Alternatively, with such instruments as the Corning Model 12 pH meter, the reading of the logarithmic cation activity-concentration scale is adjusted to correspond directly to the nominal concentration of a suitable diluted standard, after which diluted samples are measured and their sodium concentrations obtained directly from the instrument reading.

5. To avoid undesirable temperature effects, the diluted sample and standards are allowed to come to room temperature, and all samples are measured at approximately the same temperature at which the calibration was performed.

Discussion

The present state of theoretical and practical aspects of ion-selective electrodes has recently been reviewed in detail by Rechnitz (6). As noted by Rechnitz, a functioning glass electrode has a membrane structure which can be schematically represented as follows:

Internal Solution	Hydrated gel layer	Dry glass layer	Hydrated gel layer	External Solution

The hydrated glass surface undergoes cation exchange according to

$$Na^+_{Soln} + H^+_{glass} \overset{K_{ex}}{\rightleftharpoons} Na^+_{glass} + H^+_{Soln}$$

when the membranes are in contact with a solution containing sodium ions; anions are not exchanged. Greater quantities of metal ion are taken up than are required for simple monolayer coverage of the glass, indicating that metal ions diffuse into the hydrated layer. It is now recognized that hydrogen ions do not selectively *penetrate* the glass membrane of the pH electrode to yield the electrode potential. Similarly, in other ion-specific glass electrodes, while there is current flow during the potentiometric measurement and consequently a transport of charges across the glass membrane system, this takes the form of an ion-exchange process. No single sodium ion (for sodium silicate glass) moves through the entire thickness of the dry glass membrane, but rather the charge is transported by an interstitial mechanism where each charge carrier needs to move only a few atomic diameters before passing on its energy to another carrier (6). Typically, for the Na_{11-18} glass the selectivity for sodium over potassium ranges from $K_{Na^+/K^+} = 300$ at pH 7 to $K_{Na^+/K^+} = 14,000$ at pH 10 for a well-conditioned electrode. The general selectivity order for such glasses is $H^+>Na^+>Li^+> K^+$. There is no interference from proteins or uric acid. The response characteristics of the electrode improve with proper preconditioning; most commercial glass electrodes have very rapid reponse times following sufficient soaking.

Adequate buffering and reasonable dilution of samples was found necessary to obtain reproducible quantitative data (5, 7), and anionic buffers such as the "Tris" or triethanolamine systems are preferred for this purpose. With the the electrodes and buffering-diluting system described, the potentiometric response does not coincide quantitatively with that predicted from the Nernst equation for pure salt systems; but this deviation does not affect the accuracy of the results. Sodium ion electrode analysis typically yields an average difference between duplicate activity measurements of $\pm$ 0.3 mEq per liter and a standard deviation of $\pm$ 0.44 mEq per liter for electrometric sodium measurements in urine (4). There is no systematic difference in urine sodium concentrations determined by ion-specific electrode measurements and by internal-standard flame photometry on the same specimens (5, 7). Recoveries of added sodium from urine typically average 95 to 98% by electrometric measurement (5).

The method is equally adaptable to measurement of single specimens or large series of samples; a single measurement requires perhaps one-half minute. Automated systems incorporating the sodium ion electrode have been described (2, 7). Dilutions of urine from 1:10 to 1:100 have been successfully analyzed for sodium, as have undiluted specimens.

With the ready availability of digital-reading millivoltmeters, direct read-out of linearized sodium values in milliequivalents per liter is also practical at reasonable equipment cost.

Sources of Error

In addition to the several potential sources of difficulty noted above, which are obviated by appropriate dilution and buffering of unknown samples and reference standards, it should be noted that most types of sodium ion electrodes are extremely sensitive to silver and somewhat sensitive to lithium. Both of these ions should be absent from the samples, or diluted out. Influence of anions and of cations other than Na^+, Ag^+, Li^+, K^+, and H^+ is generally negligible. Dilution with water instead of buffer solutions leads to significant errors and measuring difficulties such as noise and instability.

Interference from potassium in urine is for practical purposes eliminated by buffering the sample to pH 8 (where the Na^+/K^+ selectivity is of the order of 1,000 to 5,000), which also eliminates the influence of H^+ activity since unknowns and standards are routinely measured at the same pH.

The electrode response time may become undesirably long if the electrode is not properly conditioned between measurements, e.g., allowed to dry; in which event continued drift during measurements may lead to appreciable errors. These are readily avoided by keeping the electrode immersed in 0.1 M sodium chloride solution when not in actual use.

REFERENCES

1. Sunderman, F. W., and Sunderman, F. W., Jr. (eds.): Clinical Pathology of the Serum Electrolytes, Springfield, Thomas, 1966.
2. Dahms, H.: Automated potentiometric determination of inorganic blood constituents (Na^+, K^+, H^+, Cl^-). Clin. Chem., *13*:437-450, 1967.
3. Eisenman, G., Bates, R., Mattock, G., and Friedman, S. M.: The Glass Electrode. New York, Interscience Publishers, 1966.
4. Moore, E. W., and Wilson, D. W.: The determination of sodium in body fluids by the glass electrode. J. Clin. Invest., *42:*293-304, 1963.
5. Annino, J. S.: Determination of sodium in urine by specific ion electrode. Clin. Chem., *13:*227-232, 1967.
6. Rechnitz, G. A.: Ion-selective electrodes. Chem. and Engr. News, *45:*146-158, 1967.
7. Jacobson, H.: Direct determination of sodium and potassium in the presence of ammonium with glass electrodes. Anal. Chem., *38:*1951-1954, 1966.

Chapter 22

Measurement of Aldosterone in Urine

BENJAMIN N. HORWITT, Ph.D.

INTRODUCTION

Many methods have been described for the quantitation of aldosterone. Even before the isolation of aldosterone by Simpson *et al.* (1, 2), bioassays had been described for mineral corticosteroid activity in blood and urine extracts. These were usually based on the estimation of excretion or retention of potassium or sodium. These were estimated either as inert (3, 4) or radioactive substances (5, 6). Simpson and Tait (7) developed a reasonably specific bioassay which was based on the degree of suppression of the urinary N^{24}/K^{42} ratio in adrenalectomized rats following injection of the radioactive isotopes. This assay proved very helpful in experiments which led to isolation of aldosterone (1, 2).

With the isolation and establishment of the aldosterone structure (8), information concerning physical and chemical properties of the free compound and its derivatives became available. This led to the development of chemical methods for the quantitative analysis of aldosterone. Since the amounts found in normal urines are in the order of micrograms per 24 hours, it is necessary that the chemical methods be sensitive and micro techniques be applied.

Various procedures have been described for the chemical assay of aldosterone in urine (9). In many of these methods, the end point depended on the reduction of tetrazolium salts and soda fluorescence.

Chemical methods require extensive purification and result in losses and variable recoveries. A partial correction for loss may be incorporated by using a single radioactive tracer. In such cases, the final chemical reaction may be relatively insensitive. In 1960, Kliman and Peterson (10) applied the principle of double isotope derivative technique of analysis to the measurement of aldosterone.

Principle

Extracts of urine are reacted with tritium labeled acetic anhydride to convert aldosterone to the tritium labeled diacetate. A measured amount of authentic aldosterone diacetate-^{14}C is added. The double labeled aldosterone is separated from contaminants by paper chromatography and chromic acid oxidation. The tritium and ^{14}C content of the purified steroid is counted in a liquid scintillation spectrometer. The amount of aldosterone present in the original extract is calculated from the determination of the amount of ^{14}C lost during purification, the yield of tritium radioactivity, and the specific acitivity of the tritium labeled acetic anhydride.

Reagents

1. *Hydrochloric Acid, 4N.*
2. *Sodium Hydroxide, 0.1N.*
3. *Acetic Acid, 0.1N.*
4. *Dichloromethane,* Spectro Grade.
5. *Benzene,* reagent grade.
6. *Cyclohexane,* reagent grade.
7. *Carbon tetrachloride,* reagent grade.
8. *Dioxane,* reagent grade, peroxide free.
9. *Pyridine, Anhydrous.* Is refluxed over barium oxide for 4 to 6 hours and is distilled in a "closed" system through a fractionating column. The middle fraction that boils at 115°C. is then collected.
10. *Acetic Acid, Purified.* Ten gm CrO_3 are added to a liter of reagent grade glacial acetic acid and refluxed for one hour. The contents are distilled twice, discarding first and last 100 ml each time.
11. *Ethanol, Purified.* To a liter of ethanol are added 0.5 gm 2,4 dinitrophenylhydrazine hydrochloride and 0.5 ml conc. HCl. The solution is permitted to stand in the dark at room temperature overnight and then distilled through a Vigreaux column, discarding the first 100 ml. The distillation is discontinued when a yellowish condensate is observed on the thermometer bulb. The distillation is repeated.
12. *Methanol, Purified.* The same procedure is used as for ethanol, Item 11.
13. *Chromic Oxide, 0.5%* in purified acetic acid. The solution is discarded when appreciable darkening occurs.
14. *Acetic Anhydride.* This is refluxed over calcium carbide for 4 to 6 hours and distilled through a fractionating column. The middle fraction boiling at 139°C. is collected.

15. *Aldosterone Diacetate for Reference Spots.* Thirty mg of aldosterone monacetate are transferred to a 50 ml g.s. tube and allowed to stand unstoppered in a vacuum desiccator over anhydrone for at least 2 hours. Seven ml anhydrous pyridine and 3.5 ml purified acetic anhydride are then added. The contents are mixed, tightly stoppered, and allowed to stand in a dark cupboard for 24 hours. The solution is evaporated under nitrogen in a 50°C water bath to a volume of 1 to 2 ml. Six ml purified methanol are added and the solution is evaporated to dryness. The evaporation is repeated with 6 ml of methanol until the pyridine odor disappears. The residue is dissolved in 10 ml purified ethanol and stored in a refrigerator. (10 μl = about 30 μg).

16. *Solvents for Chromatographic Systems.*

Solvents	Paper I	Paper II	Paper III
Cyclohexane	4 parts	4 parts	4 parts
Benzene	2 parts	- - -	3 parts
Methanol	4 parts	2 parts	4 parts
Water	1 part	1 part	1 part
Dioxane	- - -	4 parts	- - -

17. *Acetic Anhydride—^3H, 108 mC/mM in Benzene.* (Concentration, approximately 18%.)

18. *Scintillating Fluid, Stock Reagent.* One hundred gm 2,5-diphenyl-oxazole (PPO) and 1.25 gm 1,4-bis-2-(5 phenyloxazolyl) benzene are dissolved in 1 liter reagent grade toluene.

19. *Scintillating Fluid, Working Reagent.* Two hundred ml of reagent grade toluene are mixed with 155 ml stock reagent #18. Ten ml of the solution are transferred to a scintillation vial. Radio-

active counts should be same as the Packard Instrument Co. blank.

20. *Acetic anhydride—*[14]*C, 10 mC/ mM in Benzene.*

21. *Aldosterone Alcohol.*

22. *Aldosterone 21-acetate.*

23. *Toluene,* Reagent Grade.

24. *Benzene,* anhydrous purified as follows: Five gm barium oxide are added to 300 ml reagent grade benzene in a flask and refluxed for one hour. The benzene is distilled in a closed system fitted with an anhydrone trap. The first and last 50 ml of solvent are discarded. The purified benzene is stored in a desiccator.

25. *Ethanol, 20%.* Prepare 20% ethanol in distilled water made from purified ethanol (reagent #11).

26. *Carbon Tetrachloride,* reagent grade, redistilled.

27. *Methanol-dichloromethane Mixture.* One-hundred-and-sixty (160) ml of purified methanol (reagent #12) are mixed with 40 ml dichloromethane.

28. *Ethanol, 25%.* Prepare 25% ethanol in distilled water made from purified ethanol (reagent #11).

Special Apparatus

1. Liquid Scintillation spectrometer.
2. Paper chromatography equipment.
3. U-V lamp, short wave length.
4. Photography equipment for developing contact prints.
5. Dry box.

Procedure

Determination of Acetic Anhydride [3]*H Specific Activity.* To 0.5 mg cortisol in a glass-stoppered tube are added 0.030 ml of tritium labeled acetic anhydride and 0.025 ml anhydrous pyridine; the cortisol is dissolved. Mix by rotating tube carefully between palms. Stopper tightly and place in 37°C incubator. After 24 hours, 0.5 ml of 25% ethanol in water is added. Three ml of dichloromethane are added and tube shaken vigorously for 30 seconds. The upper ethanol-aqueous phase is removed by aspiration. Five-tenths ml water is added to wash the dichloromethane. The dichloromethane is dried in a nitrogen stream at 50°C. The cortisol acetate is chromatographed on Whatman No. 1 paper after application as a narrow stripe (15 cm long). Descending chromatography for 16 hours in the solvent system: Cyclohexane, benzene, methanol, and water (4:3:4:1) are used. The cortisol acetate area is located by photographing the paper using an ultra-violet lamp as a light source. The area is cut out, and the cortisol acetate is eluted from the paper with ethanol. The cortisol acetate is rechromatographed for 12 hours in the solvent system: Cyclohexane, methanol, water, and dioxane (4:2:1:4). The cortisol acetate is located and eluted as above. The eluate is transferred to a 50-ml volumetric flask and diluted to mark with ethanol. The cortisol content is determined by the means of absorbance at 242 mμ. The molar absorbance index for cortisol is 16,200. An aliquot is counted for tritium (high voltage), and the specific activity is expressed as c.p.m. per mμmole. For aldosterone diacetate, the value is multiplied by 2.

Preparation of Aldosterone Diacetate [14]C. One mC acetic anhydride ^{14}C in 4 μl benzene is transferred to a glass-stoppered tube containing 3.5 mg aldosterone with 110 μl dry benzene. Add 20 μl "cold" acetic anhydride and 75 μl purified pyridine. The tube is stoppered tightly and incubated at 37°C for 24 hours. After 24 hours, 0.5 ml 25% ethanol in water and 3 ml dichloromethane are added. The mixture is processed as described above, and the residue is chromatographed on Whatman No. 1 paper using solvent system I and 5 hours running time, and solvent system II and 8 hours running time. The steroid is eluted from the second paper and brought to a volume of 50 ml with purified ethanol. Ten μl are counted in the liquid scintillation spectrometer for ^{14}C (low voltage). On the basis of the counts, the solution is diluted with purified ethanol and "cold" aldosterone diacetate so that the final solution has 28,000 to 32,000 cpm per ml and approximately 30 μg aldosterone diacetate in 100 μl. This usually will require 4 ml of the aldosterone diacetate ^{14}C solution and 6 ml of the "cold" aldosterone diacetate (reagent #15) to be diluted to 50 ml with purified ethanol.

Processing of Urine

The urine should be collected so that the pH of the final 24-hour collection is between 4 and 6. If it cannot be analyzed immediately, the pH should be adjusted to 3-4 and stored in a refrigerator. Four-tenths percent of the 24-hour volume is adjusted to pH 1 with a pH meter by adding 4N HCl. The aliquot is kept between 4 and 15 ml. The acidified urine is transferred to an 8 oz. glass-stoppered bottle, graduated at 60 and 90 ml. If the aliquot was 10 ml or less, dichlormethane is added to the 60 ml mark; if it was over 11 ml, dichlormethane is added to the 90 ml mark. The bottle is shaken vigorously for about 30 seconds and then set aside in the dark for 24 hours. After 24 hours, the mixture is shaken vigorously for about 5 minutes. The upper aqueous phase is aspirated and discarded. The dichloromethane is washed with 1/10 volume 0.1N NaOH, the aqueous layer discarded, and the solvent washed with 1/10 volume 0.1N acetic acid. After removing the acetic acid, the dichloromethane is washed with 10 ml water, and the aqueous layer discarded. Measure and record the volume of dichloromethane remaining. The dichloromethane is evaporated to dryness.

By means of small amounts of purified methanol (total 4ml), the residue is transferred quantitatively to a 125-ml separatory funnel. Thirteen ml of water are added, and the aqueous alcohol is extracted with 40 ml cyclohexane. The upper cyclohexane phase is aspirated off and discarded. Be careful not to remove any of lower phase. Ninety ml dichloromethane are added to the funnel, the mixture shaken vigorously, and the dichloromethane phase drawn off into a flask and dried. The residue is transferred quantitatively with small volumes of methanol to an "acetylation" tube (6.5 ml conical ground glass stoppered tube 13 mm diameter x 90 mm long) and dried with the aid of nitrogen at 40°C. The walls of tube are rinsed with methanol to concentrate the extract in the tip. The tubes are stored in a vacuum desiccator overnight.

Acetylation

Acetylations are carried out in a "dry box." All micro pipettes used in this procedure are stored in a vacuum desiccator over anhydrone until ready for use. The pyridine is kept in a desiccator until ready for use.

The residue is dissolved in 30 μl of tritium labeled acetic anhydride. Twenty-five μl pyridine are added and the tube is stoppered tightly and rotated between palms to mix contents. The acetylation mixture is placed in an incubator at 37°C for 24 hours. After incubation, 0.1 ml of aldosterone diacetate-^{14}C is added. At same time, an equal amount of aldosterone diacetate-^{14}C is measured into a scintillation vial and counted to determine the number of counts added (see calculation). One-half ml of water and 5 ml carbon tetrachloride are added to acetylation mixture. The mixture is shaken, and the upper phase is removed by aspiration and discarded. Additional 0.5 ml water is added, and the washing repeated. The material is dried under nitrogen at 40°C. The walls are rinsed down with 0.5 ml methanol-dichloromethane reagent, dried, and process repeated using 2 ml of methanol-dichloromethane reagent.

Chromatography

1st Paper. The acetylated residue is dissolved in 100 μl methanol-dichloromethane reagent. The sample is applied as a stripe 1.5 cm long on Whatman No. 1 paper. The tube is rinsed 2 times with 100 μl portions of the solvent and the extract applied to the paper. Ten μl (30 μg) aldosterone diacetate (reagent #15) are applied to the paper as a reference. Solvent system for paper I is used. The paper is equilibrated for one hour at 25°C and then developed for 5½ hours. After the paper is dried, it is photographed using the U-V lamp as the light source. The paper and the photograph are placed in precise alignment, and an imprint of the steroid area is made by tracing the spot on the photograph and bearing down on the pencil. The spot is cut out and eluted with methanol. The eluates are dried under nitrogen at 50°C. The material is concentrated at bottom of tube by means of successive rinsings and dryings.

2nd Paper. The residue from the 1st paper is transferred to a second paper and developed with the solvent system cyclohexane-methanol, water, dioxane (4:2:1:4) for 8 hours. The steroid area is located, eluted, and dried in small glass-stoppered tubes as described for 1st paper.

Oxidation

To the dried eluate from the 2nd paper chromatography, 10 μl aldosterone diacetate reference solution (reagent #15) are added and dried. One-tenth ml chromium trioxide reagent is added. The tube is rotated to completely wet the residues and allowed to stand exactly 6 minutes from the time of addition of reagent. One ml of 20% ethanol in water and 10 ml dichloromethane are added, and the tube is shaken vigorously for 20 seconds. The aqueous layer is aspirated and discarded. The solvent is washed once more with 1 ml distilled water and dried in a stream of nitrogen at 50°C.

3rd Paper. The residue is applied to Whatman No. 1 paper as described above as a stripe of 1 cm and chromatographed for 8½ hours in the solvent system cyclohexane-benzene-methanol-water (4:3:4:1). As described above, the steroid area is located, cut out, and eluted directly into a scintillation counting vial. The eluate is dried at 50°C in a stream of nitrogen.

Counting and Calculation

Ten ml of scintillating fluid are added to the dried residue in the scintillation vials. The samples are assayed in a liquid scintillating Spectrometer for tritium and ^{14}C (Packard TriCarb 314A). All counts are corrected for background.

$$C_{hv} = \text{c.p.m. at high voltage (Tritium} + {}^{14}\text{C)}$$

$$C_{lv} = \text{c.p.m. at low voltage } ({}^{14}\text{C})$$

$$C_1 = \text{c.p.m. } {}^{14}\text{C added (high voltage)}$$

$$C_2 = \text{c.p.m. } {}^{14}\text{C added (low voltage)}$$

$$R = \frac{C_1}{C_2}$$

$$S = \text{Specific activity aldosterone diacetate,}$$
$$\text{c.p.m. } {}^{3}\text{H per m}\mu\text{mole, high voltage}$$

$$\text{Mol Weight} = \text{Molecular weight free steroid}$$

$$V_1 = \text{Volume extraction solvent}$$

$$V_2 = \text{Volume solvent recovered}$$

$$\mu\text{g Aldosterone per 24 hours} = \frac{(C_{hv} - C_{lv}R)}{S} \times \frac{\text{mol weight}}{1000} \times \frac{C_2}{C_{lv}} \times$$

$$\frac{V_1}{V_2} \times \frac{\text{24 hour vol.}}{\text{vol. urine extracted}}$$

Discussion

In common with radioactivity procedures in general, this method for the assay of aldosterone is extremely sensitive. This permits the use of less than one-tenth the volume of urine required for most previously published methods. Theoretically, the sensitivity of the method is limited only by the specific acitivity of the acetic anhydride. This may not be practical due to the presence of tritium labeled contaminants which may persist through the third paper chromatography. The small amount of urine permits almost quantitative extraction and recovery of the aldosterone up to the acetylation phase. The addition of labeled aldosterone diacetate ^{14}C acts as an indicator to locate chromatogram spots and corrects for losses for all steps beyond the acetylation step. Therefore, because of this built-in correction, one need not exercise any undue precautions in the technical procedures. Because of the correction for losses, the values obtained by the double isotope derivative procedure tend to give higher ranges than previously reported procedures. The use of the labeled tracer allows for elution of smaller areas of the chromatogram spots with resultant better specificity. The addition of radioactive aldosterone to the urine aliquot would permit correction for losses through the entire procedure. If ^{3}H-aldosterone were to be added to the urine to obtain a full recovery correction, the use of ^{14}C-acetic anhydride would be necessary and commercial supplies of this reagent are much more costly. It appears that it would be advantageous for a supply of high specific activity ^{14}C-aldosterone to be made readily available for use as an indicator so that the economical tritiated acetic anhydride may be used.

Sources of Error

The procedure, because of the recovery factor, is essentially error-free from the point beyond the acetylation step. The adjustment to pH 1 should be made with care. Hydrolysis at pH 0.5 or pH 1.5 results in lower recovery. Any loss of aldosterone during extraction from sample or on evaporation and transfer to acetylation tube could represent a source of error.

Acetylation with the tritiated acetic anhydride is subject to error if not carried out under strictly anhydrous conditions with anhydrous reagents. Any failure to completely acetylate the aldosterone in the residue is a source of error.

Exposure to the ultraviolet light to locate the aldosterone area on the papers after chromatography should be kept to a minimum. It is known that exposure to excessive ultraviolet light will lead to destruction of aldosterone. Should this destruction occur, it will lead to loss of radioactivity and inaccuracies in counting.

In common with other quantitations based on radioactivity, care should be exercised to prevent radio cross-contamination.

Range of Values

The normal range for urinary aldosterone by this procedure is 5 to 26 μg per 24 hours if the individual is on an adequate salt intake. It is generally agreed that the aldosterone excretion increases some five or sixfold in normal pregnancy. Since sodium restriction in normal individuals increases the urinary aldosterone, it is important that the intake of sodium be adequate if one intends to obtain a base line urinary aldosterone determination.

Clinical Correlation

While secretion of adrenocorticotropin (ACTH) by the pituitary is wholly responsible for the regulation of cortisol secretion, it affects the production of aldosterone to only a comparatively minor degree. As a result, frequently states of hyperadrenocortical function are not accompanied by excessive urinary aldosterone.

In Conn's syndrome, also known as "primary aldosteronism," an adenoma of the adrenal cortex is usually present. In general, these produce excessive amounts of aldosterone resulting in abnormally high values of urinary aldosterone.

Aldosterone excretion is increased secondarily in a number of conditions, in none of which is the adrenal cortex primarily at fault. Included in the category of secondary hyperaldosteronism are edematous states such as nephrosis, hepatic cirrhosis, and congestive heart failure. Malignant hypertension and renovascular hypertension also result in secondary aldosteronism.

REFERENCES

1. Simpson, S. A., Tait, J. F., Wettstein, A., Neher, R., and Reichstein, T.: Isolation of new crystalline compound from beef adrenal extracts with especially high activity on mineral metabolism. Experientia, *9*:333-335, 1953.
2. Simpson, S. A., Tait, J. F., Wettstein, A., Neher, R., Schindler, O., and Reichstein, T.: The constitution of aldosterone, a new mineral corticoid. Experientia, *10*:132-133, 1954.
3. Deming, W. B., and Luetscher, J. A., Jr.: Bioassay of desoxycorticosterone-like material in urine. Proc. Soc. Exp. Biol., *73*:171-175, 1950.
4. Spencer, A. G.: Biological assay of small quantities of desoxycorticosterone acetate. Nature, *166*:32-33, 1950.
5. Dorfman, R. I., Potts, A. M., and Feil, M.: The use of radio sodium for the detection of small quantities of desoxycorticosterone. Endocrinol., *41*:464-469, 1947.
6. Dorfman, R. I.: Adrenal cortical hormones. In, Emmens, C. W. (ed.): Hormone Assay. New York, Academic Press, 1950, pp. 325-362.
7. Simpson, S. A., and Tait, J. F.: A quantitative method for the bioassay of the effect of adrenal cortical steroids on mineral metabolism. Endocrinol, *50*:150-161, 1952.
8. Simpson, S. A., Tait, J. F., Wettstein, A., Neher, R., Schindler, O., and Reichstein, T.: The constitution of aldosterone. Helv. Chim. Acta, *37*:1200-1223, 1954.
9. Tait, S. A. S., and Tait, J. F.: Assay of aldosterone and metabolites. In, Dorfman, R. I. (ed): Methods in Hormone Reasearch, Vol. I. New York, Academic Press, 1962, pp. 265-336.
10. Kliman, B., and Peterson, R. E.: Double isotope derivative assay of aldosterone in biological extracts. J. Biol. Chem., *235*:1639-1648, 1960.

Comments on Methods for Measurement of Renin Activity in Plasma

PHILIP A. KHAIRALLAH, M.D., F. MERLIN BUMPUS, PH.D. and ROBERT R. SMEBY, PH.D.

If one assumes that the physiological action of renin is entirely through its product, angiotensin II, then it is more desirable to measure the peptide rather than the enzyme that produces it. Several procedures have been described for measurement of plasma angiotensin but all have proven to have very limited use largely because of their lack of sensitivity.

In general, incubation of plasma produces a mixture of angiotensin I and angiotensin II. The decapeptide is further converted to the biologically active octapeptide using the assay animal's own converting enzyme. Since angiotensin may be further degraded into inactive peptides and amino acids on incubation, the angiotensinases have to be removed, inhibited, or prevented from acting by protecting the angiotensin formed.

A technical limitation to the measurement of renin is the biological assay of angiotensin, thus the application of immunoassay or isotope dilution techniques to this problem may overcome this limitation.

Knowledge of absolute values of renin levels in peripheral or renal venous blood, while very necessary for an understanding of renal action, may prove misleading when applied to comparative studies of various diseased states. This results from the fact that angiotensin

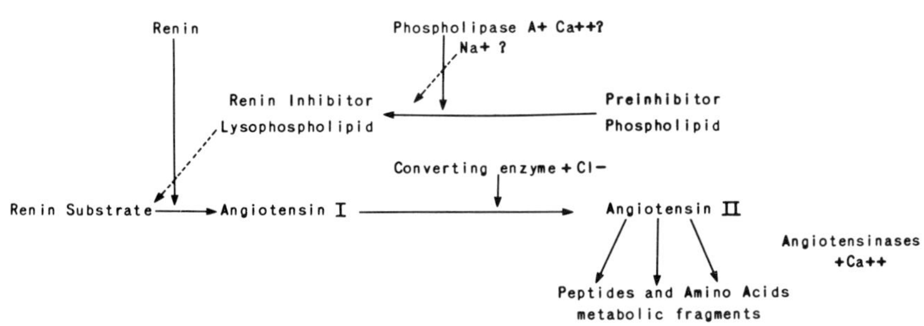

levels are not necessarily proportional to renin levels, being dependent upon variations in renin substrate, renin inhibitors, plasma angiotensinases and possibly the ability of various organs to destroy or rapidly remove the active hormone. It is possible that organ angiotensinases may play an important role in determining the level of plasma angiotensin. Many of the methods now being applied measure a composite of some of these variables and are described as measuring "renin activity" rather than "renin." All these procedures, while not ideal, have yielded useful information. One of the great limitations is that the results from various methods have been reported in units of activity which are difficult to interconvert. Examples of expressions of renin activity are listed in Table I.

TABLE I—EXPRESSIONS OF
PLASMA RENIN ACTIVITY

Helmer	Goldblatt units per L per hr.
Fitz	ng angiotensin per ml per hr.
Boucher	ng angiotensin per 100 ml per 3 hr.
Warzynski	ug angiotensin per L per 30 min.
Yoshinaga	ug angiotensin per L per 2 hr.

Although not all variations are shown here, these are representative of wide variance of terms used and clearly shows the difficulty in comparing results obtained in different laboratories. This variance of terms is decreasing and possibly will disappear in the future.

It has been impossible to evaluate objectively the methods which have been reported, especially since no one has had experience applying each method. For this discussion, each of the more recent assay techniques which have been reported since 1957 will be outlined.

The first of these came from the laboratory of Helmer and is outlined in Table II.

TABLE II—METHOD OF
HELMER AND JUDSON (9)

(1) Plasma from cooled, heparinized blood
(2) Dialyzed, pH 5.5, against cold running tap water, 18 to 20 hr.
(3) Made isotonic with NaCl, incubated 1 hr at 37°
(4) Liberated angiotensin assayed on:
    (a) Spirally cut strip of rabbit aorta or
    (b) Pithed, nephrectomized cat.

The renin reaction as carried out at renin and substrate concentrations occurring in plasma is probably not always a zero order reaction and in some instances is substrate limiting due to presence of NaCl during incubation. This has been substantiated by increase in "renin reactivity" in plasma obtained following nephrectomy (1, 3, 15). Helmer has used the first order rate constant to correct for limiting substrate. This criticism applies to most of the methods now being used. In the earlier method described by these authors, there was no means of inhibiting angiotensinase. In later modifications ethylenediamine tetraacetic acid (EDTA) or its sodium salt was used to eliminate this possible artefact.

Fasciolo and co-workers have applied the method outlined in Table III to numerous plasma samples.

TABLE III—METHOD OF FASCIOLO *ET AL.* (9)

(1) Plasma from heparinized blood
(2) Angiotensinase removed (pH 3.8, 25° for 30 min.)
(3) One-half deproteinized immediately (control)
(4) One-half incubated pH 5.1 (2 hr.), deproteinized with 4 volumes ethanol
(5) Supernate dried in rotary evaporator, extracted with ether
(6) Dissolved in water, saturated with NaCl, extracted 2 times with butanol
(7) Butanol phase extracted 3 times with 0.01 N HCl, then neutralized with NaOH
(8) Adsorbed on Aminex 50 W X2 resin, angiotensin eluted with 0.8 ml 1 M NaOH followed by 1.5 ml water
(9) Assayed in anesthetized rat

This is rather long, tedious method, and no figures are given for renin recovery. This method was modified (De Vito and Fasciolo (4)), incorporating the use of EDTA to inhibit angiotensinase. Here, the authors mentioned a recovery of about 60% of added angiotensin but do not state the amount of peptide used for recovery experiments.

Boucher *et al.* (2) incorporated the use of adsorption of angiotensin on Dowex 50 having shown that angiotensin adsorbed on the resin is not metabolized by angiotensinases.

TABLE IV—METHOD OF BOUCHER ET AL. (2)

(1) Plasma from blood collected 0 to 5° (EDTA)
(2) Incubated, pH 5.5 in presence of Dowex 50 W–X2 (NH$_4$+)
(3) Time of incubation 1, 2 and 3 hours
(4) Angiotensin eluted from resin with 0.1 N diethylamine followed by 0.2 N NH$_4$OH
(5) Dried, dissolved in 20% ethanol
(6) Assayed in nephrectomized rats

The authors claim excellent recovery with this procedure. They have also reported the possibility that renin inhibitors do exist in plasma. Additional substrate is not added to the plasma incubation mixture and in some cases substrate may bc a limiting factor. This is probably the most widely used method at the present time.

Yoshinaga *et al.* used a procedure very similar to that of Fasciolo *et al.*

TABLE V—METHOD OF YOSHINAGA ET AL.(17)

(1) Plasma separated from heparinized blood at room temperature
(2) Incubated 2 hrs. (pH 5.5)
(3) Extracted with butanol at pH 1.5, saturated with NaCl, 3 times
(4) 2 vol. petroleum ether added then extracted back with 1.7 volumes water
(5) Adsorbed on Dowex 50, eluted with 0.1 N NaOH
(6) Assayed in anesthetized rat

They report a recovery of added angiotensin of about 30 to 35%.

The method of Warzynski, Demerjian and Hoobler is probably less effective in removal of pre-existing pressor substances. They report variable recovery, but do not state the range of variation.

TABLE VI—METHOD OF WARZYNSKI, DEMERJIAN AND HOOBLER (16)

(1) Plasma from heparinized blood, plus equal volume of isotonic saline
(2) Incubated 30 min (pH 5.1)
(3) Precipitate formed on incubation removed by centrifugation
(4) Supernate saturated with NaCl (pH 2.0), extracted into butanol
(5) Evaporate solvent, redissolve in water
(6) Assay in rat

In an attempt to overcome the possibility of limited substrate in this incubation procedure, we have modified the renin assay of Helmer and Judson. It was found that in an environment of decreased ionic strength, the velocity of renin reaction was decreased. Under these conditions the concentrations of substrate found in human plasma were not limiting.

TABLE VII—METHOD OF PICKENS ET AL. (13) SEE ALSO METHODS MANUAL

(1) Plasma separated from heparinized blood (1 to 5°)
(2) Dialyzed against EDTA, then H$_2$O
(3) Incubated (pH 5.5) for 4 hrs., DFP added
(4) Deproteinized by heat
(5) Assayed in pentolinium treated rats

It has been found later that if heparin is used in high concentration, it acts as a competitive inhibitor to renin. However, when this anticoagulant is used at a concentration of 1-5 units per ml plasma, no renin inhibition was observed.

TABLE VIII—METHOD OF
GUNNELL'S ET AL. (8)

(1) Heparinized plasma dialyzed against running tap water overnight at room temperature, remove precipitate
(2) pH adjusted to 5.5
(3) Saturated NaCl added to make sample isotonic
(4) Incubated 37° C for 1 hr.
(5) Reaction stopped by cooling in ice bath
(6) Assayed in nephrectomized, ganglion blocked rat

This method is similar to the method of Helmer (9), except that no correction is used for limiting substrate. Also angiotensinases are not inactivated. This method is now commercially available through New England Nuclear Biomedical Assay Laboratories, Boston, Massachusetts.

All methods outlined above are described as measuring renin activity. Lever, Robertson and Tree have reported a procedure which more nearly measures "renin" concentration rather than "renin activity."

TABLE IX—METHOD OF LEVER,
ROBERTSON AND TREE (12)

(1) Renin adsorbed and eluted from DEAE cellulose with phosphate saline buffer pH 6
(2) Dialyzed at pH 3 (glycine–HCl saline buffer) to destroy substrate and angiotensinase
(3) Additional purification:
    (a) dialysis at pH 5.7, 0.15 M phosphate-saline
    (b) dialysis against distilled water 96 hr
    (c) remove precipitate
(4) Lyophylized, incubated with added substrate from 30 min to 96 hr
(5) Assayed in rat

The recovery of added renin is reported to be less than 40%, and probably would be even lower if this enzyme occurs in more than one active form in plasma. When the original results of these authors are presented as Lineweaver-Burk plots, the curves are non-linear; later results show linear curves. This abnormal curve might possibly be explained by substrate inhibition or by the presence of an inhibitor which combines with renin substrate.

They have defined a renin unit as "the quantity of renin which, when incubated with prepared ox substrate at pH 5.7 at 37° in a substrate concentration of 30 u/ml and a total volume of 5 ml, formed 0.1 ug angiotensin/ml of incubation mixture per hour." Thus, their results cannot be compared to any of the others.

The recently reported method of Lee, Cook and McKenzie (11) is a modification of this latter method.

For an ideal renin assay, it is desirable to have a system free of interferring substances and one measurable in terms of action upon a renin substrate. None of the above fulfill these criteria. Knowledge of the existance and amounts of these interferring substances is also necessary in studies on disease states.

At the present juncture, one cannot recommend any of these as being greatly superior. On the other hand, it would be most unwise if we were not to continue measuring renin and renin activity even though the methods are still very crude.

TABLE X

Author	Normal	Essential Hypertension
Helmer (10)	130–500	0–130
Fitz (6), using Helmer's method	300	0–3200
Genes (7), using Boucher's method	50	0–150
Warzynski (16)	340	0–3200
Yoshinaga (17)	50	0–270
Pickens (14)	70	0–60
Gunnell's (8)	75–275	0–400

Standardization on one method now may likely prove injurious to research in this field. Efforts must continue toward a better understanding of this system and the application of this knowledge to assay techniques.

The wide spread of values from the different methods utilized can be obtained by a review of the literature. To compare results the published data have been converted to ng angiotensin formed during 1 hr. incubation, in 100 ml plasma (Table X).

The results using the Lever method cannot be compared to any of the others, since purified renin and substrate are used instead of plasma.

The value obtained from use of any method is determined from its application. Despite the many deficiencies of the various methods, many useful results are being obtained from their application. Our final recommendations are

1) to continue to determine plasma renin levels,

2) to continue to search for improved methods, and

3) to use caution in the interpretation of results.

REFERENCES

1. Blaquier, P., Basso, N., and de la Riva, I.: Kinetics of renin — Renin substrate. Hypertension, *15*:109-113, 1967.
2. Boucher, R., Veyrat, R., deChamplain, J., Genest, J.: New procedures for measurement of human plasma angiotensin and renin activity levels. Canad. M. A. J., *90*:194-201, 1964.
3. Carretero, O., and Gross, F.: Evidence for humoral factors participating in the renin substrate reaction. Hypertension, *15*:115-126, 1967.
4. DeVito, E., and Fasciolo, J. C.: A method for the estimation of renin activity in plasma. Acta Physiol. Lat. Americana, *15*:129-137, 1965.
5. Fasciolo, J. C., DeVito, E., Romero, J. C., and Cucchi, J. N.: The renin content of the blood of humans and dogs under several conditions. Canad. M. A. J., *90*:206-209, 1964.
6. Fitz, A. E., and Armstrong, M. L.: Plasma vasoconstrictor activity in patients with renal, malignant and primary hypertension. Circulation, *29*:409-414, 1964.
7. Genest, J., deChamplain, J., Veyrat, R., Boucher, R., Tremblay, G. Y., Strong, C. G., Koiw, E., and Marc-Aurele, J.: Role of renin-angiotensin system in various physiological and pathological states. Hypertension, *13*:79-89, 1965.
8. Gunnells, J. C., Grim, C. E., Robinson, R. R., and Wildermann, N. N.: Plasma renin activity in healthy subjects and patients with hypertension. Arch. Int. Med., *119*:232-240, 1967.
9. Helmer, O. M., and Judson, W. E.: The quantitative determination of renin in the plasma of patients with arterial hypertension. Circulation, *27*:1050-1060, 1963.
10. Helmer, O. M.: Renin activity in blood from patients with hypertension. Canad. M. A. J., *90*:221-225, 1964.
11. Lee, M. R., Cook, W. F., McKenzie, J. K.: A sensitive method for assay of plasma renin activity. Circulation Res., *19*:260-268, 1966.
12. Lever, A. F., Robertson, J. I. S., and Tree, M.: The estimation of renin in plasma by an enzyme kinetic technique. Biochem. J., *91*:346-352, 1964.
13. Pickens, P. T., Bumpus, F. M., Lloyd, A. M., Smeby, R. R., and Page, I. H.: Measurement of renin activity in human plasma. Circ. Res., *17*:438-448, 1965.
14. Pickens, P. T., Dustan, H. P., Bumpus, F. M., and Page, I. H.: Measurement of plasma renin activity in hypertension. Hypertension, *13*:90-95, 1965.
15. Smeby, R. R., Sen, S., and Bumpus, F. M.: A naturally occuring renin inhibitor. Hypertension, *15*:129-133, 1967.
16. Warzynski, R., Demerjian, Y. and Hoobler, S.: A method for the determination of 'renin' in blood and some preliminary findings. Canad. M. A. J., *90*:225-226, 1964.
17. Yoshinaga, K., Aida, M., Maebashi, M., Sato, T. Abe, K., and Miwa, I.: Assay of renin in peripheral blood. A modification of Helmer's method for the estimation of circulating renin. Tohoku J. Exp. Med., *80*:32-41, 1963.

A Method for the Measurement of Renin Activity in Human Plasma

PHILIP A. KHAIRALLAH, M.D., F. MERLIN BUMPUS, PH.D. and ROBERT R. SMEBY, PH.D.

INTRODUCTION

Plasma renin blood levels theoretically increase in classical renal hypertension of the Goldblatt type and should be normal in essential hypertension. The recommended methods do not measure quantitative renin blood levels, but renin activity which is proportional to absolute renin blood levels as modified by inhibitors, accelerators, and conditions of incubation.

Principle

Plasma is dialyzed to remove all small molecules that may have pressor or depressor activity. This is necessary since the blood pressure response of the assay rat is non-specific and detects all pressor substances. Upon incubation of plasma, endogenous renin acts on endogenous substrate to yield angiotensin and in the absence of salt, endogenous substrate in plasma is in excess. The amount of angiotensin formed is proportional to the amount of endogenous renin activity when enzymes destroying angiotensin are inhibited.

The angiotensin formed is assayed by its pressor effect in a rat given a ganglioplegic agent to increase its sensitivity, and is compared to the pressor effect of known amounts of a standard angiotensin injected into the same rat.

Reagents

1. *Disodium EDTA* 2.2 gm per liter.
2. *Hydrochloric Acid* 1 N.
3. *Saline,* 9.0 gm NaCl per liter distilled H_2O.
4. *Sodium Hydroxide,* 1 N.
5. *Acetic acid,* 0.1%
6. *Diethyl ether.*
7. *Heparin,* 1000 u per ml.
8. *Isoamylethyl barbituric acid.* Na salt (Amytal), 20 mg per ml of saline.
9. *Atropine,* 0.65 mg tablet dissolved in 0.3 to 0.5 ml of saline.
10. *Pentolinium,* in 20% P.V.P. Dissolve 20 mg polyvinyl pyrrolidone (Type NP-K30 for General Aniline and Film Corporation, Dyestuff and Chemical Division, 140 West 51st Street, New York, New York 10020) in 100 ml distilled H_2O. Pentolinium tartrate tablets are mashed and dissolved in the 20% P.V.P. to a final concentration of 5 mg per ml.

Standard Solutions

Angiotensin Stock Solution. One vial (2.5 mg) angiotensin (Hypertensin, Ciba) is dissolved in one liter of 0.1% bacitracin solution in saline. Ten-ml batches are placed in vials and frozen as primary stock solution. One 10-ml vial is diluted to 75.8 ml with 0.1% bacitracin to give a stock solution containing approximately 330 ng per ml. This is standardized against a preparation of known activity obtained from Doctor D. R. Bangham, Director, Department of Biological Standards, National Institute for Medical Research, Mill Hill, London NW, England, to determine concentration of biologically active peptide.

Special Apparatus

1. Oxford Multiple Dialyzer, Model B, 16 sample size, Oxford Laboratories, San Mateo, California 94401.

2. Refrigerated centrifuge.

3. Condon's Rat blood pressure measuring manometer from

    C. F. Palmer (London), Inc.

    Myographic Works

    Effra Road

    Brixton, London, SW 2, England

4. Water bath

5. Kymograph

Procedure

One-tenth ml of heparin (1000 u per ml) is placed in a 30-ml syringe to just wet the sides. Approximately 20 ml of heparinized peripheral venous blood are drawn and cooled rapidly in a 50-ml polyethylene tube in ice. All steps of the procedure prior to incubation are done at 0 to 4°. Following centrifugation, the plasma is removed and its volume recorded. The pH is adjusted to 6.5 with 1 N HCl, plasma is dialyzed with stirring, against 5 liters of a solution of di-sodium ethylenediamine tetraacetic acid (EDTA, 2.2 gm per liter) for 24 hours and then against 5 liters of distilled water for a further 24 hours using Visking 20/100

dialysis tubing. Up to 16 samples can be dialyzed together. The volumes of the dialyzed plasma samples are measured and the heavy precipitate formed during dialysis removed by centrifugation. To the supernatant is added one drop of 1:20 solution of diisopropylfluorophosphate (DFP) in isopropyl alcohol, and the solution adjusted to pH 5.5 with HCl or NaOH. The volume (usually about 10 ml) is measured, transferred to a polyethylene tube, and incubated for 4 hours at 37°C. One ml of saline is added, the volume adjusted to 20 ml with distilled water, the pH brought to 5.0 with HCl, and the tube placed in boiling water for 10 minutes. The tube is capped by a glass sphere to prevent volume loss by evaporation and possible contamination. Immediately afterward, the sample is cooled in ice for 10 minutes and centrifuged in the cold. The supernate is adjusted to pH 7.2 with NaOH, and then to pH 6.8 by addition of 0.1% acetic acid. If the solution is cloudy it is recentrifuged. An aliquot, usually about 15 ml, is evaporated to dryness in open tubes under a stream of nitrogen at 80°. The residue is prepared for assay by redissolving in distilled water to 1/20 the volume before evaporation.

Animals weighing between 150 mg and 200 mg are anesthetized by intraperitoneal injection of 100 mg per kg sodium Amytal (isoamylethylbarbituric acid). Atropine (0.65 mg in 0.3 to 0.5 ml saline) a pentolinium (5 mg in 1 ml 20% polyvinyl-pyrrolidone) are given by subcutaneous injection. The trachea is intubated and both vagi are cut. The carotid artery is cannulated and connected to a mercury manometer. A fine cannula is placed in one femoral vein for injections. Blood pressure can also be measured by a pressure transducer and electrical recording.

Standard solutions of angiotensin are made by dilution with saline at the time of assay, of the stock solution to the following concentrations: 33.3 ng per ml, 16.7 ng per ml, and 8.3 ng per ml. Injections of 0.1 or 0.2 ml are given and washed through with saline so that the total volume injected is 0.25 ml. A three-point assay system is used. One-tenth ml of each of the standards is injected first, then an unknown and standard are alternated. One injection can be given every 5 minutes, since blood pressure responses usually return to base line in that time interval. Every hour, another three-point assay with standards is run. There usually is a slight increase in sensitivity of the rat after one hour, but this does not invalidate the assay. A straight line is obtained when dose of angiotensin is plotted on the logarithmic scale on semilog paper against response on the linear scale. Renin values expressed as nanograms angiotensin formed can then be determined.

Calculations

$$\text{Assay result (ng per ml)} \times \frac{20}{A} \times \frac{B}{C} \times \frac{D}{E} \times \frac{F}{G} \times \frac{100}{F}$$

A = Volume of concentrated sample
B = Total volume after protein precipitation
C = Aliquot taken for evaporation
D = Volume of plasma after dialysis
E = Volume incubated
F = Volume of total plasma sample
G = Volume placed in dialysis bag

Results are expressed in nanograms angiotensin formed in 100 ml plasma after 4 hours incubation.

Discussion

Evaluation of renin assay results must take into account plasma volume of the patient when the blood sample was drawn. Reduction of plasma volume by low sodium diet, diuretic drugs, hemorrhagic, etc. can elevate the renin activity level. Conversly, elevation of plasma volume by high sodium diet can depress the renin activity level (12). Physical activity prior to blood sampling will also effect the renin activity level (8). In general, ambulatory patients tend to have higher levels than patients confined to bed. Inability to control all of these factors has probably caused widening of the range of normal values in normal human subjects (30-400 ng per 100 ml per 4 hours). When these factors are rigidly controlled in dogs the range of normal values can be considerably narrowed (50-100 ng per 100 ml per 4 hours).

The renin assay may be of value in the diagnosis of primary and secondary aldosteronism. In primary aldosteronism, the renin level is usually in the low normal range, but on occasion it can be in the upper normal range (3). However, the renin level cannot be increased by sodium depletion and ambulation in the presence of an aldosterone producing tumor. In secondary aldosteronism, the renin levels are usually very high (4, 12).

Patients with hypertension due to renal artery stenosis sometimes have normal or elevated renin activity levels (1, 2, 6, 8, 9, 14). Thus, this condition cannot be diagnosed on the basis of renin assay alone. Both substrate and renin are elevated during normal pregnancy. The effect of contraceptive medication on renin activity levels has not been well studied but should not be ignored.

During incubation in a salt-free medium, the substrate concentration in human plasma is high enough to insure zero order kinetics of the renin reaction (13). However, this reaction is significantly accelerated in the presence of salt and substrate concentration in plasma will often be low enough to be rate limiting. Under these conditions, the reaction will follow first-order kinetics. Assays by others have been conducted under these conditions, and the results calculated using the first order rate constant.

During the course of an assay, the sensitivity of the assay rat can change. If standard samples are alternated with unknown samples, any change in sensitivity can be easily detected. If a new standard curve is determined after the sensitivity has changed, the assay can continue with the same animal.

Since hog renin reacts with human renin substrate at a very slow rate, commercial hog renin cannot be used as an assay standard for human renin. Further, it is not good practice to use hog renin as a quality control standard. Only renin prepared from human kidneys can be considered satisfactory for such purposes.

Sources of Error

1. It has been reported by some that high concentrations of heparin inhibit renin activity; thus a final concentration of 5 u per ml blood should be adhered to since no inhibition at this level has been reported (10, 13, 15).

2. Some of the enzymes metabolizing angiotensin require calcium ions. (11) Since the amount of angiotensin formed is used as a means of renin activity, the angiotensinases must be totally inhibited. Thus, dialysis against 2.2 gm per liter disodium EDTA is necessary. The other angiotensinases are inhibited by diisopropyl fluorophosphate (DEP).

3. Rats anesthetized with sodium amytal can be used up to 3 hours. With atropine and pentolinium, the basal mean blood pressure is very steady at about 50 to 70 mm Hg. As the rat begins to recover from anesthesia, the base line becomes unsteady and uneven. It is recommended that at this stage another rat be set up. If absolutely necessary to continue, one can slowly inject up to 4 mg Na amytal intravenously. After this, the rat has to be restandardized with angiotensin controls.

All rats used must be healthy. Occasionally, in late winter and early spring, rats develop bronchopenumonia diagnosed by wet rales that can easily be heard. These rats should not be used for assay.

4. Very rarely, about 1%, the sample injected into the rat gives a sharp depressor response followed by a pressor response. The cause of this is not known at present, and assays that show this are not valid. When this occurs, the sample is evaporated to dryness again under nitrogen at 80°, and the dry residue washed with ether. The ether is carefully removed by decantation, and the sample placed in a water bath at 37° for 10 minutes to remove the last traces of ether. The sample is then redissolved with distilled water to 1/20th of the

volume before evaporation and assayed again. With this procedure, the depressor material can be decreased or removed in about half of the cases.

5. Blood samples for renin assay should be taken from patients who are not receiving medication. The effect drugs have on renin activity levels is still not yet fully known. Patients of low sodium diets, or receiving diuretics have high levels of renin. High salt diets depress renin levels. Bedrest also lowers renin levels, while exercise increases it. Other changes have not yet been studied, but there is an indication that adrenalectomy can decrease substrate levels, thus giving apparent lower renin levels. Deoxcorticosterone reverses this.

Range of Values

(Diet not controlled, upright posture, average exercise.)

25	subjects, 35 determinations,	159 ± 68	ng per 100 ml plasma[5]
32,		60–500	ng per 100 ml plasma[14]
17	subjects, 27 determinations, (Smeby, not published).	30–380	ng per 100 ml plasma

REFERENCES

1. Brown, J. J., Davies, D. L., Lever, A. F., and Robertson, J. I. S.: Plasma renin concentration in human hypertension. I. Relationship between renin sodium and potassium. Brit. Med. J., *2*:144-148, 1965.
2. Brown, J. J., Davies, D. L., Lever, A. F., and Robertson, J. I. S.: Plasma renin concentration in human hypertension. II. Renin in relation to etiology. Brit. Med. J., *2*:1215-1219, 1965.
3. Conn, J. W.: Plasma renin activity in primary aldosteronism. Importance in differential diagnosis and research of essential hypertension. J. A. M.A., *190*:222-225, 1964.
4. Davis, J. O., Urquhart, J., and Higgins, J. T.: Renin angiotensin and aldosterone in experimental secondary hyperaldosteronism. Canad. M. A. J., *90*:245-248, 1964.
5. Del Greco, F., Simon, N. M., Goodman, S., and Roguska, J.: Plasma renin activity in primary and secondary hypertension. Medicine, in press, Nov. 1967.
6. Fitz, A. E.: Renal venous Renin (RVR) in Evaluation of renovascular hypertension. Clin. Res., *14*:376, 1966.
7. Genest, J., deChamplain, J., Veyrat, R., Boucher, R., Tremblay, G. Y., Strong, C. G., Koiw, E., and Marc-Aurele, J.: Role of the renin-angiotensin system in various physiological and pathological states. Hypertension, *13*:97-116, 1965.
8. Helmer, O. M.: Renin Activity in Blood from patients with hypertension. Canad. M. A. J., *90*:221-225, 1964.
9. Judson, W. E. and Helmer, O. D.: Diagnostic and prognostic values of renin activity in renal venous plasma in renovascular hypertension. Hypertension, *13*:79-89, 1965.
10. Kaneko, Y., Ikeda, T., Takeda, T., and Ueda, H.: Renin release during acute reduction of arterial pressure in normotensive subjects and patients with renovascular hypertension. J. Clin. Invest., *46*:705-716, 1967.
11. Khairallah, P. A., Bumpus, F. M., Page, I. H., and Smeby, R. R.: Angiotensinase with a high degree of specificity in plasma and red cells. Science, *140*:672-674, 1963.
12. Laragh, J. M., Cannon, P. J., and Ames, R. P.: Interaction between aldosterone secretion, sodium and potassium balance and angiotensin activity in man: Studies in hypertension and cirrhosis. Canad. M. A. J., *90*:248-256, 1964.
13. Pickens, P. T., Bumpus, F. M., Lloyd, A. M., Smeby, R. R., and Page, I. H.: Measurement of renin activity in human plasma. Circulation Research, *17*:438-448, 1965.
14. Pickens, P. T., Dustan, H. P., Bumpus, F. M., and Page, I. H.: Measurement of plasma renin activity in hypertension. Hypertension, *13*:90-96, 1965.
15. Sealey, J. E., Gerten, J. N., Ledingham, J. G. G., and Laragh, J. H.: Inhibition of renin by heparin. J. Clin. Endocr. and Metab., *27*:699-705, 1967.

Chapter 24

Identification and Quantitation of Formed Elements in the Urine

HERBERT DERMAN, M.D.

INTRODUCTION

"...from studying the composition of water as it flows downward toward the sea, many inferences may be made concerning the mountains in which the stream originated" (3).

A. IDENTIFICATION OF FORMED ELEMENTS
EXAMINATION OF URINARY SEDIMENT

Principles

Study of the urinary sediment still provides the simplest means of recognizing and following renal disease. Light microscopy and centrifugation effectively expose the formed elements which in turn mirror their origin in the genito-urinary tract.

Reagents

1. Sternheimer-Malbin stain (9)
   A. Solution I

Crystal violet	3.0	gm
Ethanol, 95%	20.0	ml
Ammonium oxalate	0.8	gm
Water, distilled q.s.	80.0	ml

   B. Solution II

Safranin O	0.25	gm
Ethanol, 95%	10.0	ml
Water, distilled q.s.	100.0	ml

   C. Three parts of Solution I are mixed with 97 parts of Solution II. The mixed solution is filtered and stored in a dropper bottle. The working stain is stable for 3 months. Solutions I and II are stable indefinitely in separate containers.

2. Sedi-Stain™ (Clay-Adams J-760 and J-762)

3. Krystranin™ (Scientific Products U2750)

4. Stain for lipoid bodies
   Sudan III saturated solution (1%)
   Ethanol 70%

5. Urofix Urine Preservative Tablets (A.S. Wolf, 1581 Third Ave., New York City, New York, 10028)

6. Formalin 10%

7. Cargille Urinary Preservative Tablets

Procedure: Collection of Specimen

The first morning specimen should be voided into a clean container and delivered promptly to the laboratory for examination. For routine admission urinalysis cleansing of the urethral meatus

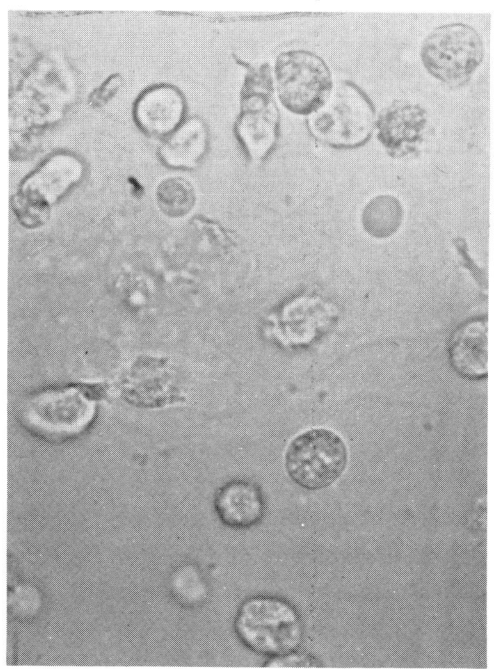

Fig. 1.   Red cells and many white cells. X500.

may not be critical. It is an important consideration in evaluating cases with abnormal findings. Refrigeration is recommended for any urine specimens which cannot be examined within 4 hours (11). Alternatively, a preservative in the form of 8 drops of 10% formalin per 30 ml of urine (12), Urofix or Cargille tablets, or a dash of sodium chloride crystals (8) may be used in the container.

Preparation of Sediment

1. The urine specimen is thoroughly mixed before a 12 to 15 ml aliquot is placed in a conical test tube.

2. The specimen is centrifuged for 3 minutes at moderate speed (2000 rpm) in an ordinary clinical centrifuge. Standardization of speed and duration of centrifugation permits rough comparisons to be made from specimen to specimen.

3. The supernatant urine is dis-

carded by complete inversion of the tube.

4. By vigorous "finger-flicking," the button of sediment is resuspended in the few drops of urine which drain back down the sides of the test tube.

5. A drop of sediment is aspirated with a rubber bulb dropping pipette. The drop is transferred to a clean 3 x1 glass slide and covered with a coverslip.

6. Sternheimer-Malbin stain is added to the reconstituted button of sediment in the proportion of one drop of stain to one drop of sediment. Sedi–Stain™ or Krystranin,™ may be substituted for Steinheimer-Malbin stain.

7. After the sediment is again sharply agitated by "finger-flicking," one drop of the stained material is placed under a coverslip alongside the previously mounted unstained sediment.

8. An entire coverslip is scanned using low power magnification and subdued light. Casts tend to congregate at

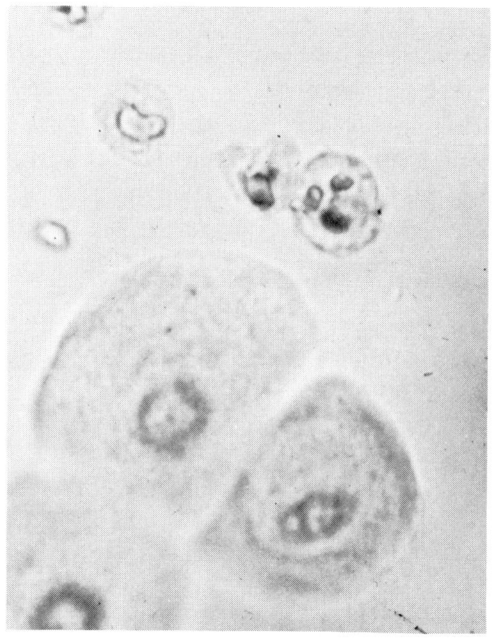

Fig. 2.   White cells and bladder epithelial cells. X500.

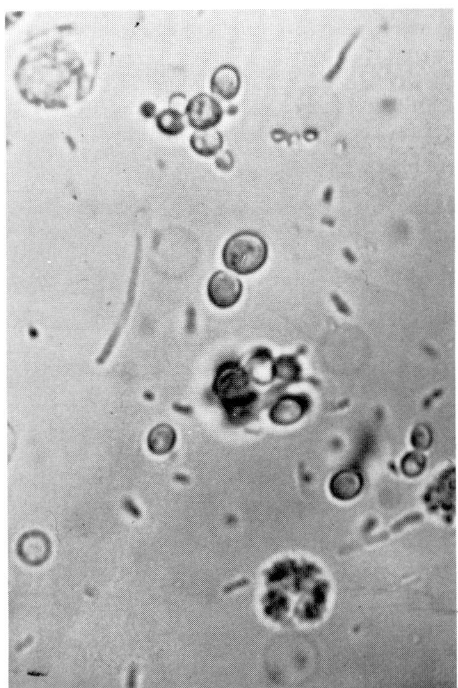

Fig. 3. Budding yeast cells, red cells, white cells, and bacteria. X500.

the edges of the coverslip. They are reported in terms of the average number in at least 10 low power fields of centrifuged sediment. Casts and their inclusions may be identified with high power and the assistance of the sediment stain.

9. Red cells, white cells, and epithelial cells are identified with high power magnification and reported as the average number in at least 10 high power fields of centrifuged sediment.

10. Miscellaneous objects in the sediment, such as mucus threads, bacteria, spermatozoa, and parasites, are reported as occasional, frequent or many, in centrifuged sediment.

11. Highly refractile droplets may occur free in the urine, as "oval fat bodies" or fatty casts. They are readily identified in subdued light and may be further examined by staining with Sudan III or by use of polarized light.

Classification of Casts (after Schreiner (8) and Moser (6,7)

1. Hyaline (transudation) casts
    a. Simple
    b. With inclusions
        1) red blood cells
        2) blood cast
        3) white blood cells
            a) purple or "dark-staining" WBC
            b) pale blue or "pale-staining" WBC (glitter cell)

        4) tubular epithelial cells
        5) bacterial
        6) crystals
        7) granular
        8) fatty inclusions or doubly refractile fat bodies
        9) bile-stained inclusions
        10) other

2. Epithelial (desquamation) casts
    a. Fresh cell cast
    b. Granular cast
        1) coarsely granular
        2) finely granular
    c. Waxy cast
    d. Fatty cast
    e. Tumor cell cast
    f. Broad or renal failure cast

3. Mucus casts

4. Casts of unusual composition
    a. Bence-Jones protein
    b. Amyloid
    c. Myoglobin
    d. Hemoglobin
    e. Dextran
    f. Globin
    g. Other

5. Pseudo casts
    a. Agglutinated red blood cells
    b. Agglutinated white blood cells
    c. Packed urates or other crystals
    d. Cells clinging to mucus thread

e. Bateria clinging to mucus
thread
f. Degenerated spermatozoa
g. "Fibrin" or mucus threads
6. Artefacts
a. Hair
b. Clothing fibers
c. Lubricating jelly or oil
d. Spores, hyphae and yeast
e. Vegetable fibers

Sources of Error

1. Random urine specimens passed during the day are subject to more variation than the "first morning specimen." The former are subject to dilution and the possibility of overlooking structures of low concentration. The latter comprise the equivalent of a standard specimen comparable from day to day, examination to examination, and, to a lesser degree, from patient to patient.

2. Unclean containers enhance the possibility of bacterial growth and the confusing presence of artefacts.

3. Delay in examination of the specimen permits lysis of formed elements in dilute urine or in alkaline urine.

4. Failure adequately to mix a urine specimen before removing an aliquot for examination may result in loss of the formed elements which settle to the bottom of the container.

5. Technical errors (1)
a. Drying of sediment.
b. Too much light in microscopic examination.
c. Use of high power only
d. Careless transfer of sediment.
e. Dirty equipment.
f. Scratches on slide or coverslip.
6. Failure to add preservative will result in lysis of formed elements by bacterial growth after 4 hours at room temperature.

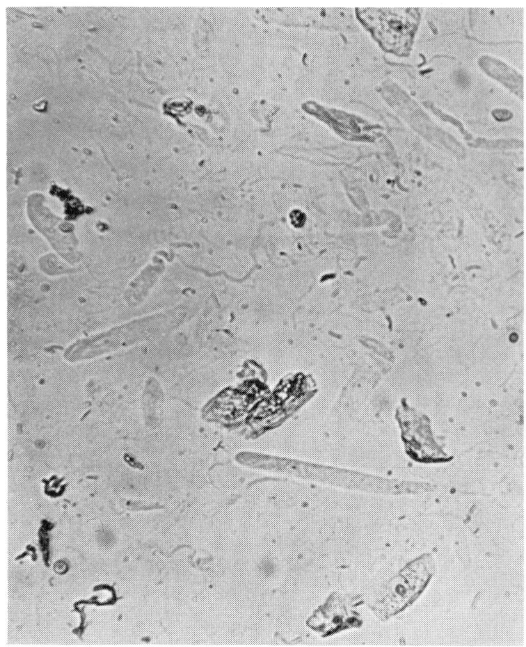

Fig. 4. Hyaline casts, cylindroids, mucus threads, and squamous cells. Unstained.. X125.

7. The sediment may be obscured by abundant amorphous precipitate. If the urine is alkaline, the amorphous phosphates can be removed by cautiously acidifying with 10% acetic acid before centrifugation. If the urine is acid, the amorphous urates can be dissolved by gently heating the specimen before centrifugation.

8. In the presence of gross blood or pus, the undiluted specimen should be examined microscopically because of the difficulty in finding casts in such specimens (2).

B. QUANTITATION OF FORMED ELEMENTS THE ADDIS COUNT (4, 6)

Principle

The rate of excretion of formed urinary elements is informative diagnostically and prognostically in renal disease. A timed urine specimen is col-

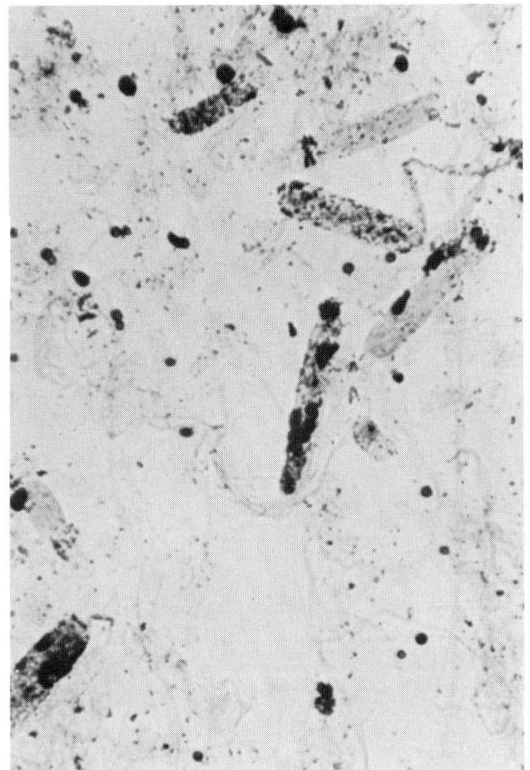

Fig. 5. Hyaline casts, cellular and granular casts, and mucus threads. S-M stain. X125.

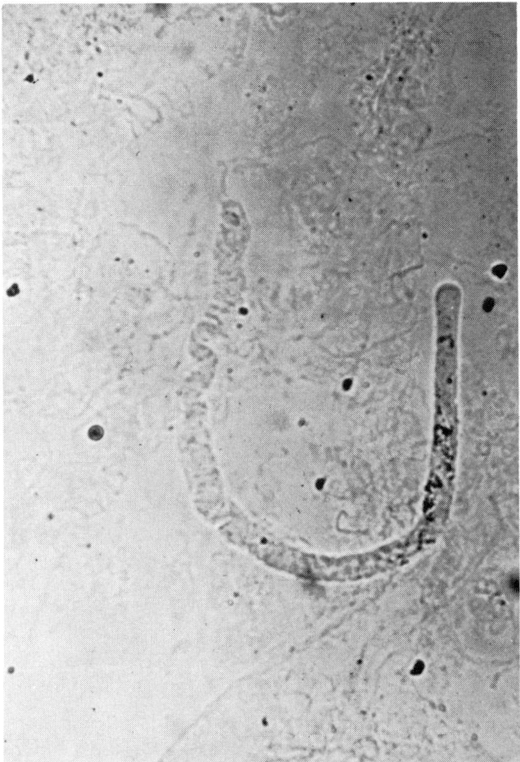

Fig. 6. Hyaline cast with convolutions. X125.

lected and the numbers of red cells, white cells, epithelial cells, and casts are expressed as 24-hour excretion rates.

Reagents

Formalin 10%

Special Apparatus

1. Hemocytometer, standard, colorless
2. Wide-mouth container, approximately 1000 ml.
   a. Cleaned, dried, and issued by Laboratory.
   b. Contains 1 ml of 10% formalin.
3. Centrifuge tube, 15 ml, graduated

Procedure: Specimen Collection

1. The patient is instructed to take no fluids of any kind after lunch on the day before the test. No restriction is placed on solid food.

2. At exactly 10 P.M., the bladder is completely emptied and the urine discarded.

3. All subsequent urine is voided directly into the laboratory-supplied, wide-mouth container.

4. The collection is ended at exactly 7 A.M. by voiding into the container.

5. The entire specimen is brought to the laboratory.

Laboratory Methodology

1. The urine pH and specific gravity are recorded.

2. If urates are present, they may be dissolved by immersing the container in warm water.

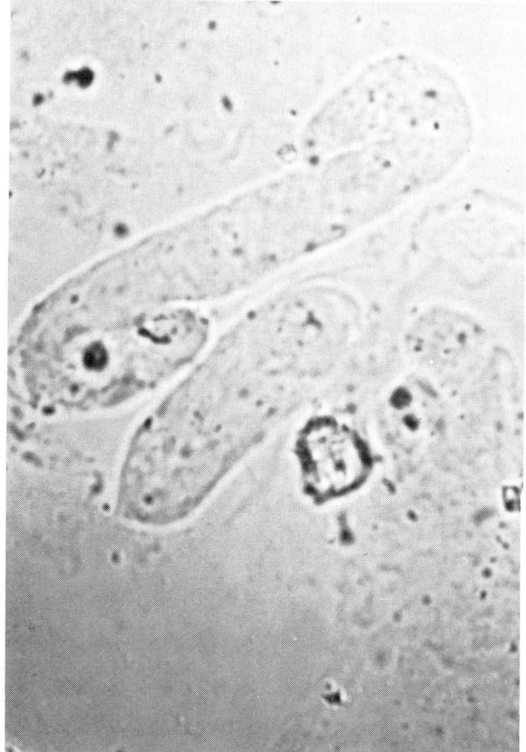

Fig. 7.   Hyaline casts. X250.

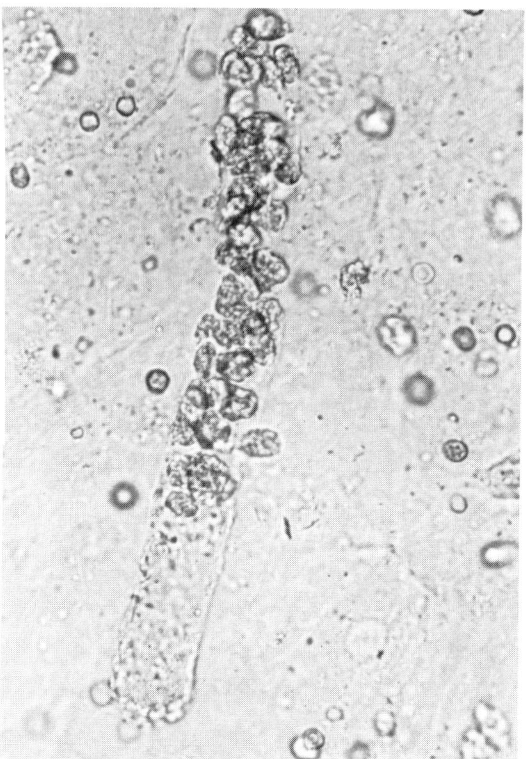

Fig. 8.   Mixed hyaline and epithelial cell inclusion cast. X500.

3. The urine is thoroughly mixed, and the total volume is carefully measured in a graduated cylinder. A drop of caprylic alcohol will prevent foaming.

4. The volume of urine produced per 1/5 hour during the nine hour collection period is obtained by dividing the total volume by 45. Lippman's nomogram (4) may be used in lieu of the calculation.

5. An aliquot equal to the 1/5 hour volume is transferred from the well-mixed specimen in the graduated cylinder to a 15 ml graduated centrifuge tube.

6. The aliquot is centrifuged for 5 minutes in an ordinary clinical centrifuge at 1700 to 2000 rpm.

7. The supernatant is withdrawn until only a volume of 0.5 ml remains. The sediment is *completely* resuspended by alternate aspiration and emptying with a rubber-bulb dropping pipette.

8. Drops of resuspended sediment are immediately placed in both counting chambers of a hemocytometer.

9. The number of casts is counted under low power in 6 large (1 x 1 mm) squares in each counting chamber.

10. The number of red blood cells is counted under high dry power in 1/5 of the vertically, finely-lined central section (0.2 x 3.0 mm) in each counting chamber.

11. The number of white blood cells and epithelial cells (but not squamous cells!) is counted under high dry power in the same area as for red cells in each of the counting chambers.

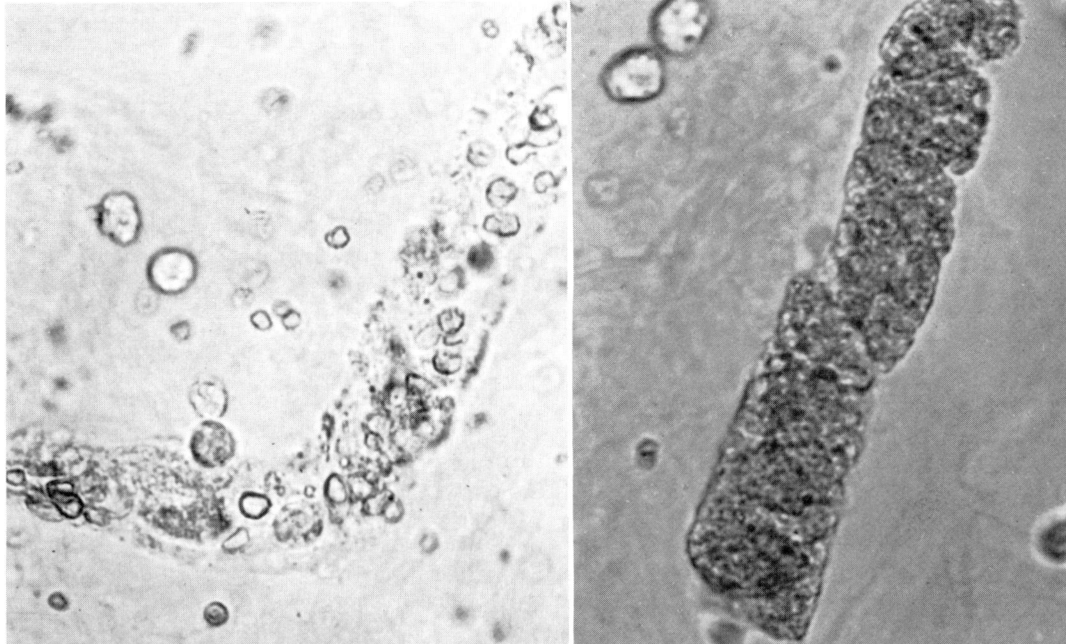

Fig. 9.   Mixed cellular cast. X500.   Fig. 10.   Coarsely granular cast. X500.

12. The hemocytometer chambers should be cleaned and re-charged 4 times to permit 10 counts to be averaged for casts, red blood cells, and white blood cells together with epithelial cells.

13. Calculations

   1) *Casts*

   Average of ten counts x 100,000 =
   24 hours excretion

   2) *Red blood cells*

   Average of ten counts x 1,000,000 =
   24 hour excretion

   3) *White blood cells and epithelial cells*

   Average of ten counts x 1,000,000 =
   24 hour excretion

Discussion

The uremic patient is unable to produce a concentrated urine. Fluid restriction in the face of renal insufficiency is therefore hazardous and should not be ordered. In children, a modified form of fluid restriction is advisable (10), e.g., no liquids after 5 p.m.

The quantitative Addis Count should be accompanied by a qualitative examination of the centrifuged urinary sediment to reveal elements too sparse to be found in the specific areas of the counting chamber.

The length of the collection time for an Addis count is not critical provided it is sufficiently long to enable reasonable accuracy. The necessary information is the rate of excretion. It is only necessary therefore to select a time interval longer than 4 hours (4) when the convenience and comfort of the patient and laboratory are best served. The recommended 9 hour period meets these criteria.

Sources of Error

1. Dilute urine causes lysis of red cells.

2. Alkaline urine causes dissolution of casts.

3. Thorough mixing of the total

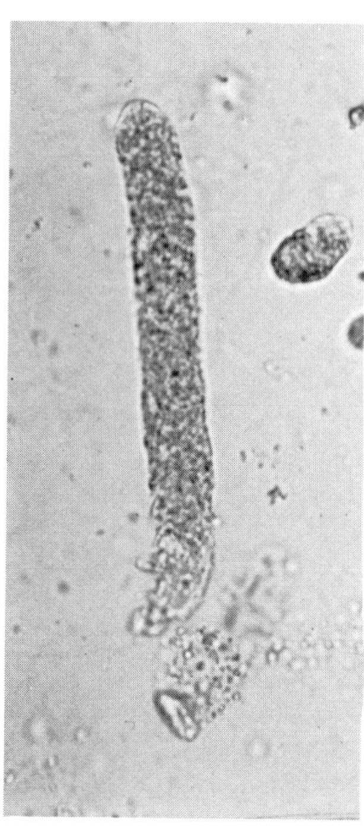

Fig. 11.   Finely granular cast. S-M stain. X250.

urine specimen before sampling is essential to prevent erroneous counts.

4. Exact measurement of the urine aliquot of the residual specimen after centrifugation is essential to avoid magnification of the least error.

5. Careful and consistent hemocytometer technique is needed for valid data.

6. A falsely low red cell and cast count may occur in patients on a salt-free diet (10).

Range of Values

The observation of more than one hyaline cast or red blood cell should be viewed with suspicion (4, 13).

Grateful acknowledgment for the photomicrographs is due Edward T. Doran.

REFERENCES

1. Hepler, O. E.: Manual of Clinical Laboratory Methods, 4th ed., revised. Springfield, Thomas, 1957, p. 19.
2. Kark, R. M., Lawrence, J. R., Pollak, V. E., Pirani, C. L., Muehrcke, R. C., and Silva, H.: A Primer of Urinalysis, 2d ed., corrected. New York, Hoeber, March, 1964, p. 62.
3. Lippman, R. W.: Urine and the Urinary Sediment, 2d ed. Springfield, Thomas, 1964, p. 4.
4. *Ibid.*, pp. 96-98, 103-106.
5. *Ibid.*, p. 54.
6. Moser, R. H.: Use of Sternheimer-Malbin staining technique in examination of urinary sediments. Part I. What's New (Abbott Laboratories), No. 218, Summer 1960.
7. *Ibid.*, Part II. No. 226, Oct.-Nov. 1961.
8. Schreiner, G. E.: The identification and clinical significance of casts. Arch. Int. Med., *99*:356-369, 1957.
9. Sternheimer, R., and Malbin, B.: Clinical recognition of pyelonephritis, with a new stain for urinary sediments. Amer. J. Med., *11*:312-323, 1951.
10. TM 8-227-6: Laboratory Procedures in Clinical Chemistry and Urinalysis. Department of the Army Technical Manual. January, 1964, p. 1–17.
11. Weller, J. M. and Greene, J. A., Jr.: Examination of the Urine. *A Programmed Text,* Part I. New York, Appleton-Century-Crofts, 1966, pp. 15 and 23.
12. *Ibid.*, Part III. P. 3.
13. *Ibid.*, p. 6.
14. *Ibid.*, p. 7.

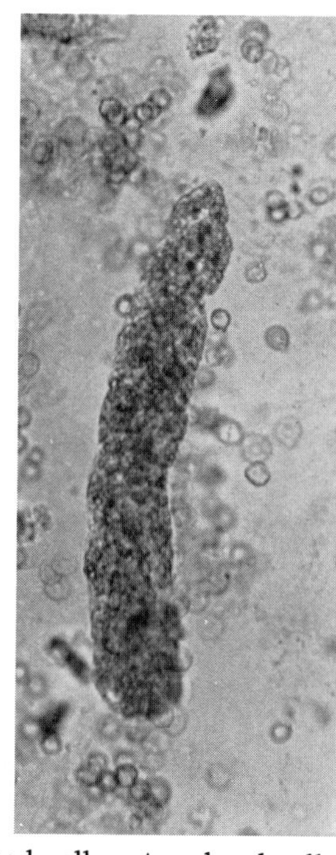

Fig. 12.   Red cell cast and red cells. S-M stain. X250.

Chapter 25

Cytologic Examination of Urine for the Diagnosis and Detection of Cancer

LEOPOLD G. KOSS, M.D.

INTRODUCTION

Cytologic examination of the urinary sediment is an excellent means of detection and diagnosis of cancer of the lower urinary tract (2,4,15,17). While a few authors have claimed considerable successes with the diagnosis of renal parenchymal cancer (9) this claim cannot be substantiated in our laboratories.

Principle

Proper collection and processing of the urinary sediment are essential elements of success. To this effect, urine must be fixed without delay. Knowledge of histology and cytology of the urinary tract in the absence of cancer is prerequisite for the identification of cancer cells.

Fixatives

The optimal fixative in the experience of this laboratory is a solution of 50% ethyl alcohol. Other fixatives such as propyl alcohol and acetone have been tried but they do not appear to offer any substantial advantages. Ether should not be used for the fixation of urine under any circumstances.

Special Appartus

Glass bottles with a capacity between 200 and 300 ml should be used. Gallon jugs and similar ungainly glassware are not recommended. Collection of large amounts of urine for cytologic evaluation is of no advantage.

Procedure

Bladder Urine. The bottles should be filled to about one-third capacity with the fixative and the *male patient* should void directly into the bottle. If a large quantity of urine is expected, the second portion of the first morning specimen is best suited for cytologic evaluation. In *female patients,* a catheterized specimen is preferable to a voided one in order to prevent contamination with vaginal contents.

If a separate evaluation of each kidney or ureter is required, the specimen may be obtained by ureteral catheterization. Each urinary specimen should be collected directly into the fixative.

Processing of Urinary Sediment in the Laboratory. The entire specimen is centrifuged for approximately 30 minutes at 1500 rpm using 50 ml tubes. The supernatant is discarded, leaving approximately 0.5 ml of liquid above the sediment. Two to three drops of Mayer's albumin solution is added to the sediment, and the suspension is mixed thoroughly. Four to six clean slides are covered with a thin layer of Mayer's albumin solution to facilitate adhesion of cells. The sediment is removed from the bottom of the centrifuged tube by means of a small spoon with a long handle, or a similar instrument (see Fig. 25$\frac{}{M}$2 in reference 5). The sediment is spread thinly and uniformly on the albuminized slides. Upon termination of this step, the edges of the slides are allowed to become dry. The slides are placed into Coplin jars containing 50% alcohol for an additional 30 minutes.

The slides are stained according to Papanicolaou. The following staining procedure has proved satisfactory in our experience (5).

1. The slide carrier is first placed in a staining dish containing 80% ethyl alcohol. Then the slides are removed from the alcohol fixative, appropriately identified with a diamond marking pencil and placed immediately in the carriers. Slides may remain in the 80% alcohol for as long a time as is required for filling the carrier.

2. Ethyl alcohol, 70%—5 dips (8 to 10 secs.)

3. Ethyl alcohol, 50%—5 dips (8 to 10 secs.)

4. Distilled water—5 dips (8 to 10 secs.)

5. Harris hematoxylin (without acetic acid)—6 mins.

6. Distilled water—5 dips (8 to 10 secs.)

7. Aqueous solution of hydrochloric acid (0.5%—3 to 5 dips (dip slowly—the number of dips depends on the strength of the hematoxylin).

8. Running tap water—5 dips

9. Ethyl alcohol, 50%—5 dips (8 to 10 secs.)

10. Ammonium hydroxide, 1.5%, in 70% alcohol—1 min.

11. Ethyl alcohol, 70%—5 dips (8 to 10 secs.)

12. Ethyl alcohol, 80%—5 dips (8 to 10 secs.)

13. Ethly alcohol, 95%—5 dips (8 to 10 secs.)

14. Orange G (1½ mins.)

15. Ethyl alcohol, 95%—5 dips (8 to 10 secs.)

16. Ethyl alcohol, 95%—5 dips

17. EA 65—1½ mins.

18. Ethyl alcohol, 95%—5 dips (8 to 10 secs)

19. Ethyl alcohol, 95%—5 dips (dip slowly) (8 to 10 secs.)

20. Ethyl alcohol, 95%—5 dips (dip slowly) (8 to 10 secs.)

21. Absolute ethyl alcohol—5 dips (8 to 10 secs.)

22. Absolute ethyl alcohol—5 dips (dip slowly) (8 to 10 secs.)

23. Equal parts of absolute ethyl alcohol and xylol—5 dips (8 to 10 secs.)

24. Xylol—5 dips (8 to 10 secs.)

25. Xylol—5 dips (8 to 10 secs.)

26. Xylol—5 dips (8 to 10 secs.)

27. Xylol—5 dips (8 to 10 secs.)

28. Xylol—5 dips (8 to 10 secs.)

29. Xylol—5 dips (8 to 10 secs.)

30. Xylol—5 dips (8 to 10 secs.)

A filtering device, such as the Millipore filter or Nuclepore filter, may be used for processing of urine sediment. The advantages of these devices lie in a greater concentration of the cells on the surface of the filter. The disadvantages are high cost and poor preservation of cell detail; the latter may prove critical in the evaluation of a difficult specimen. The writer does not recommend the use of any filtering devices.

Results

In the experience of the writer, virtually every primary cancer of the renal pelves, ureters, and the bladder yields diagnostic cells in the urinary sediment. Considerable experience is required in order to interpret the specimens adequately and in order to identify cancer cells. Particularly gratifying is the cytologic diagnosis of carcinoma of the urinary tract while still *in situ* (3,11-14,18). An important application of cytology is in the evaluation of industrial workers exposed to various bladder carcinogens (6).

The results are much less gratifying in primary cancers of the renal parenchyma. In fact, in the experience of this laboratory, only a few such tumors have shed identifiable cancer cells. An occasional Wilm's tumor may be identified in the urinary sediment (5). Metastatic cancers to the urinary tract may shed identifiable cancer cells (16).

Benign pathology of the urinary tract may at times reflect itself in the cell population. This is the case with malakoplakia (10) and herpes simplex. Inclusion bodies may also be observed in the urinary sediment in cases of lead poisoning (7) (the inclusion bodies are acid-fast) and in cytomegalic inclusion disease. The examination of the urinary sediment is a procedure of choice in the diagnosis of cytomegalic inclusion disease in adults and children (1).

Sources of Error

Inflammatory processes within the urinary tract, particularly with lithiasis, may result in significant cell abnormalities (5,8) that may be mistaken for cancer by inexperienced observers. It is critical to emphasize the fact that cellular make-up of catheterized specimens is quite different from that of voided specimens. Most diagnostic errors seen by this writer pertain to the misinterpretation of benign epithelial cells dislodged by the tip of a catheter in retrograde catheterization. A further source of error is inadequately fixed or processed material. Meticulous laboratory technique is required in order to achieve satisfactory diagnostic results.

REFERENCES

1. Bancroft, J., Seybolt, J. F., and Windhager, H. A.: Cytologic diagnosis of cytomegalic inclusion disease. Acta Cytol., *5*:182-186, 1961.
2. Deden, C.: Cancer cells in urinary sediment. Acta Radiol. Suppl., *115*:1-75, Figures 1-36, 1954.
3. Foot, N. C., and Papanicolaou, G. N.: Early renal carcinoma *in situ* detected by means of smears of fixed urinary sediment. J.A.M.A., *139*:356-358, 1949.
4. Foot, N. C., Papanicolaou, G. N., Holmquist, N. D., and Seybolt, J. F.: Exfoliative cytology of urinary sediments; review of 2829 cases. Cancer, *11*:127-137, 1958.
5. Koss L. G.: Diagnostic Cytology and Its Histopathologic Bases, 2nd. Ed. Philadelphia, J. B. Lippincott, 1968.
6. Koss, L. G., Melamed, M. R., Ricci, A., Melick, W. F., and Kelly, R. E.: Carcinogenesis in the human urinary bladder. Observations after exposure to para-aminodiphenyl. New Eng. J. Med., *272*:767-770, 1965.
7. Landing, B. H., and Nakai, H.: Histochemical properties of renal lead-inclusions and demonstration in urinary sediment. Amer. J. Clin. Path., *31*:499-503, 1959.
8. MacFarlane, E. W. E.: Some pathologic conditions affecting urine cytology. Acta Cytol., *7*:196-198, 1963.
9. Meisels, A.: Cytology of carcinoma of kidney. Acta Cytol., *7*:239-244, 1963.
10. Melamed, M. R.: The urinary sediment cytology in a case of malakoplakia. Acta Cytol., *6*:471-474, 1962.
11. Melamed, M. R., Grabstald, H., and Whitmore, Jr., W. F.: Carcinoma *in situ* of bladder: clinico-pathologic study of case with a suggested approach to detection. J. Urol., *96*:466-471, 1966.
12. Melamed, M. R., and Koss, L. G.: Developments in cytological diagnosis of cancer. Med. Clin. N. Amer., *50*:651-666, 1966.
13. Melamed, M. R., Voutsa, N. G., and Grabstald, H.: Natural history and clinical behavior of *in situ*

carcinoma of the human urinary bladder. Cancer, *17*:1533-1545, 1964.

14. Naib, Z. M.: Exfoliative cytology of renal pelvic lesions. Cancer, *14*:1085-1087, 1961.

15. Papanicolaou, G. N., and Marshall, V. F.: Urine sediment smears as diagnostic procedure in cancers of urinary tract. Science, *100*:519-520, 1945.

16. Piva, A., and Koss, L. G.: Cytologic diagnosis of metastatic malignant melanoma in urinary sediment. Acta Cytol., *8*:398-402, 1964.

17. Umiker, W.: Accuracy of cytologic diagnosis of cancer of the urinary tract. Acta Cytol., *8*:186-193, 1964.

18. Voutsa, N. G., and Melamed, M. R.: Cytology of *in situ* carcinoma of the human urinary bladder. Cancer, *16*: 1307-1316, 1963.

Chemical Analysis of Calculi from the Urinary Tract

JOHN T. McCALL, Ph.D., and LYNWOOD H. SMITH, M.D.

The composition of calculi from the urinary tract is useful information for the physician. Through accurate chemical analysis, with careful attention to the gross and microscopic appearances of the interior and exterior of the stone, the cause of the stone formation can usually be determined.

To provide adequate analysis of urinary calculi, a systematic approach is necessary. The use of chemical procedures which provide quantitative rather than qualitative analysis of the stone allows one to determine the major cystalloid content. When layers of different crystal structures are present, they can be analyzed separately to provide further information concerning the growth of the stone.

The techniques currently used at the Mayo Clinic for routine stone analysis are described. The Figure provides a flow diagram for the entire analysis.

Analytical Procedures

1. The gross appearance of the stone is observed, with special note being made of the color, consistency, and character of the surface. The stone is then cut in half with a scalpel or jewelers' saw if the size will allow, and the internal structure is observed. When the small size of a stone precludes this, careful crushing will allow inspection of the internal structure. The character and homogeneity of the crystalline structure is observed under a dissecting microscope, at a magnification of 20 to 30 times.

From these observations, one can usually recognize stones with mixed crystalline structure. It is important that adequate samples are taken from representative areas within the stone. When the stone appears to contain more than one type of crystal, samples are taken from each layer for analysis.

2. Representative parts of the stone are dried to constant weight at 105 C and weighed on an analytical balance.

3. *Qualitative Analysis for Carbonate.* After step 2, 2 ml of 6N HCl is added to the stone sample with stirring and gentle heating if necessary to allow dissolution of the stone. This is observed under the dissecting microscope. Effervescence indicates the presence of carbonate. No quantitative analysis of carbonate is made. The presence of material insoluble in acid may indicate an alkali-soluble crystalloid or the presence of large amounts of matrix.

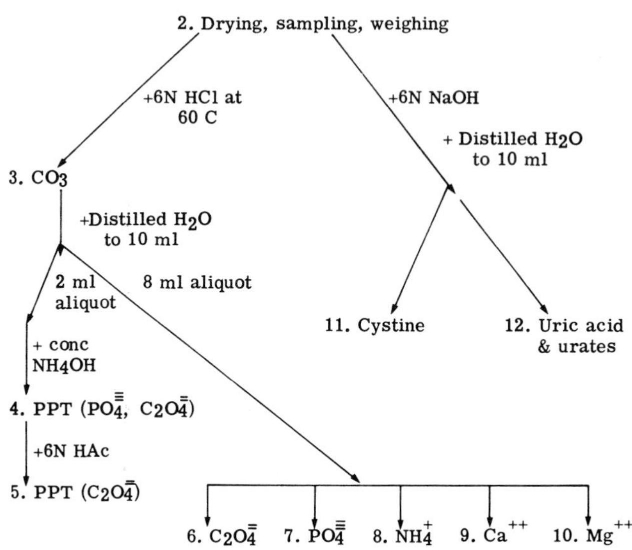

Fig. 1.   Flow sheet for analysis of calculi from urinary tract.

The solution is then brought to a volume of 10 ml by addition of distilled H_2O and is divided into aliquots of 2 and 8 ml.

4 & 5. Qualitative Analysis for Phosphate and Oxalate. To the 2-ml aliquot is added concentrated NH_4OH. A white precipitate indicates the presence of phosphate or oxalate or both. Then, 6N acetic acid (HAc) is added, which returns the phosphate into solution. The presence of a precipitate after acidification indicates oxalate. By observing the quantity of these precipitates, the dilutions necessary in the subsequent quantitative analyses for phosphate and oxalate can be estimated.

6. Quantitative Analysis for Oxalate. Depending on the quantity of the oxalate precipitate in step 5 (the smallest aliquot is taken for the heaviest precipitate), 0.5 ml to 2 ml of the 8-ml aliquot of the acid solution (step 3) is trans-

ferred to a 15-ml conical-tip centrifuge tube; excess Ca^{++} is added and the pH is adjusted to 4.5 (methyl orange) with NH_4OH. The tube is centrifuged for 5 minutes and the solution is decanted. The precipitate is resuspended in 2 ml of NH_4Ac-NH_4OH solution and centrifuged again. The supernatant solution is decanted, the tube is allowed to drain, the precipitate is dissolved in 6N HCl, and the volume is adjusted to 50 ml with distilled H_2O. The Ca^{++} content is determined by atomic absorption spectroscopy as described in step 9. The concentration of Ca^{++} is then divided by the gravimetric factor for calcium in calcium oxalate and the percentage content of oxalate is calculated.

7. Quantitative Analysis for Phosphate. If phosphate was detected in step 4, a 0.1-ml aliquot is used for this analysis; if no phosphate was detected, a 1.0-ml aliquot is used. The aliquot is added to a 25-ml volumetric flask containing 15 ml of distilled H_2O, 2 ml of ammonium molybdate reagent is added, the flask is swirled to mix the solutions, 2 ml of aminonaphtholsulfonic acid reagent is added, and the flask is swirled again. The flask then is filled to the mark with distilled H_2O and allowed to stand at room temperature for 20 minutes. The transmittance of the solution at 630 $m\mu$ is read on the Spectronic "20." A standard curve should be run with solutions containing 10 and 50 μg of phosphorus per 25 ml run through the procedure as outlined. Preparation of the necessary solutions is described in reference (1).

8. *Quantitative Analysis for Ammonia.* An aliquot (0.01 to 1.0 ml) of the acid solution (step 3) is put into a 50-ml volumetric flask and enough 6N NaOH is added to make the final solution 0.3N in NaOH (about 1 ml). Then, 1 ml of Nessler's solution (2) is added and the mixture is diluted to the mark. The absorbancy at 400 to 425 $m\mu$ is measured, and the ammonia concentration is calculated from a standard curve obtained by measuring the absorbancy of standard solutions prepared in the same manner. The final solution will be turbid if NH_4^+ or OH^- concentration is too high.

9. *Quantitative Analysis for Calcium.* The Perkin-Elmer Model 303 atomic absorption spectrophotometer is used for the calcium analysis (3). The analysis is performed using the 4227 angstrom resonance line. A 1-ml aliquot of the acid solution (step 3) is put into a 100-ml volumetric flask with 2 ml 6 N HCl. The flask is filled to the mark with distilled H_2O. This provides a 1:1,000 dilution which usually is within the range of the apparatus. Standards are used to plot a standard curve from which concentration in the solution can be determined.

10. *Quantitative Analysis for Magnesium.* The same atomic absorption spectrophotometer is used for the magnesium analysis, but the analysis is performed using the 2852-angstrom resonance line. A 1-ml aliquot of the acid solution (step 3) is placed in a 10-ml volumetric flask and diluted to the mark with distilled H_2O, giving a dilution of 1:100. Standards are used to plot the graph from which the concentration in the solution can be determined.

11. *Qualitative Analysis for Cystine.* A weighed portion of the stone is dissolved in 6N NaOH and diluted to 10 ml with distilled H_2O in preparation for steps 11 and 12.

To a 3-ml aliquot is added 0.5 ml of concentrated NH_4OH and then 2 ml of 5% sodium cyanide solution. These are mixed and allowed to stand for 10 minutes. Then 8 drops of freshly prepared 5% sodium nitroprusside solution is added. A permanent purplish red color indicates the presence of cystine (4), a yellow to tan color indicates a negative test.

12. *Qualitative Analysis for Urates and Uric Acid.* To another aliquot of the solution from step 11 (or to a small portion of pulverized stone) is added 1 ml of 2090 Na_2CO_3 and 2 ml of uric acid reagent (4). The presence of urate is indicated by the immediate formation of a deep blue color.

REFERENCES

1. Fiske, C. H., and Subbarow, I.: The colorimetric determination of phosphorus. J. Biol. Chem., *66*:375-400 (Dec.) 1925.
2. Koch, F. C., and McMeekin, T. L.: A new direct nesslerization micro-Kjeldahl method and a modification of the Nessler-Folin reagent for ammonia. J. Amer. Chem. Soc., *46*:2066-2069 (Sept.) 1924.
3. Willis, J. B.: Determination of calcium and magnesium in urine by atomic absorption spectroscropy. Anal. Chem., *33*:556-559 (Apr.) 1961.
4. Winer, J. H., and Mattice, Marjorie R.: Routine analysis of urinary calculi: A rapid, simple method using spot test. J. Lab. Clin. Med. *28*:898-904 (Apr.) 1943.

Identification of Crystals in the Kidney and Urine

FRANK B. JOHNSON, M.D.

It is difficult to recognize crystals in sections of kidney tissue, and at times in the urinary sediment, on the basis of morphology alone. The presence of protein or of mucus tends to modify normal crystalline configurations. Precise identification can be made by means of x-ray diffraction or infrared absorption. These techniques, however, require expensive equipment and considerable experience for interpretation. In addition, it is necessary to have several milligrams of the crystalline material in an isolated form for study.

A set of simple reactions that may be performed in any clinical laboratory is being developed. The present techniques are described in the section on Procedures but are subject to future modification. The most dependable technique is the one for the identification of calcium oxalate. This is based on the conversion of calcium oxalate to calcium carbonate by means of microincineration. The reliability of this procedure is fortunate, since the most commonly encountered crystals in sections of kidney tissue are calcium oxalate. These are seen in renal failure from various causes, ethylene glycol poisoning, diabetes mellitus, severe burns, primary oxalosis, and frequently in kidneys from patients on hemodialysis. Other conditions with characteristic crystals are hepatorenal syndrome, with amino acid crystals plus calcium oxalate; cystinosis, with cystine crystals; hyperparathyroidism, hypervitaminosis D, and heavy metal poisoning, with apatite crystals.

INTRODUCTION

Microscopic examination of sections of kidney tissue or of urinary sediment frequently reveals the presence of various crystals. In pathologic kidneys and urine, the crystals formed are often influenced by the presence of protein, so that the configuration of the crystals may be atypical for the pure substance. Spheroidal clusters of crystals are particularly difficult to identify by inspection. For these reasons, a set of simple tests for significant crystalloids is being developed.

Principle

Calcium oxalate, the most frequently encountered crystalline substance, is recognized by incineration and conversion to calcium carbonate, which yields bubbles on addition of acid. Apatite, unlike calcium oxalate, is only slightly birefringent and is positive for calcium with alizarin red S. It gives an insoluble, light-sensitive product on exposure to silver nitrate. Magnesium ammonium phosphate is alizarin negative but gives a similar product with silver nitrate. Uric acid and the urates give a blue precipitate with the ferric-ferricyanide reaction for strong reducing substances. Cystine causes the catalytic release of nitrogen in the iodine-azide reaction. Cystine, leucine, and tyrosine all give bubbles of nitrogen on exposure to nitrous acid.

Reagents

Acetic Acid, 2M

Acetic acid, glacial	12ml
Distilled water to	100 ml

Alizarin Red S Solution

Alizarin red S	2 gm
Distilled water	100 ml

Adjust solution to pH 4.1 to 4.3 by adding ammonium hydroxide drop by drop.

Ferric-Ferricyanide Reagent

Iron (ic) chloride	0.375 gm
Potassium ferricyanide K_3 Fe $(CN)_6$	0.050 gm
Distilled water	50 ml

Prepare this reagent just before use so that it is fresh.

Iodine-Azide Reagent

Sodium iodide	2 gm
Iodine	1.3 gm
Sodium azide	3 gm
Distilled water	100 ml

Silver Nitrate Solution

Silver nitrate	10 gm
Distilled water	100 ml

Nitrous Acid Reagent

Sodium nitrite	0.7 gm
Acetic acid, 2M	1.0 ml

Mix just before use.

Sulfuric Acid, Concentrated

Procedure

Urinary sediment or a paraffin section of kidney tissue is examined under the microscope, with both ordinary and polarized light. All commonly occurring urinary crystals except apatite are quite birefringent.

A portion of the sediment or one unstained hydrated section containing crystals is treated with 2 molar acetic acid. Evolution of bubbles indicates the presence of *carbonate apatite*. If the crystals remain undissolved and do not give bubbles, the test for calcium oxalate may be done as follows: An undeparaffinized slide bearing crystals or urinary sediment is placed on a piece of asbestos board measuring roughly 6 x 6 inches. The slide is heated directly with a high temperature burner of the Meeker type for five minutes. The slide is allowed to cool under the protection of a metal pie pan. The incinerated preparation is next covered with a cover slip, and the four corners are anchored with melted paraffin. Concentrated sulfuric acid is allowed to run between the slide and the cover while individual crystals are observed. The evolution of bubbles of gas from the crystals is indicative of the presence of *calcium oxalate* originally. Instead of sulfuric acid, alizarin red S solution can be run under the cover slip. Crystals that were *calcium oxalate* before incineration and were unstainable will not take a red coloration.

A fresh hydrated section or sample of sediment is layered with silver nitrate solution and covered with a cover slip and allowed to stand in bright sunlight or under a sun lamp for 30 minutes. A black reaction product is observed from crystals of *apatite, magnesium ammonium phosphate*, or mixtures containing either.

An additional specimen is examined for *urates* or *uric acid* after it has been covered with ferric-ferricyanide reagent. An immediate blue color is a positive reaction.

A sample is examined for *amino acid* crystals by allowing nitrous acid solution to run under its cover slip. Evolution of bubbles from the crystals is the positive reaction.

The amino acid cystine is detected on another specimen by allowing iodine-azide reagent to run under its cover. Evolution of bubbles from the crystals is the positive reaction. Cystine will also react with ferric-ferricyanide reagent.

REFERENCES

1. Councilman, W. T.: Description of the pathological histology of yellow fever. In, Sternberg, G.: Report on the Etiology and Prevention of Yellow Fever. Public Health Bull., *2*:151-153, 1890.
2. Daniels, R. A., Michels, R., Aisen, P., and Goldstein, G.: Familial hyperoxaluria: Report of a family, review of the literature. Amer. J. Med., *29*:820-831, 1960.
3. Dunn, H. G.: Oxalosis, report of a case with review of the literature. Amer. J. Dis. Child., *90*:58-80, 1955.
4. Johnson, F. B., and Pani, K.: Histochemical identification of calcium oxalate. Arch. Path. (Chicago), *74*: 347-350, 1962.
5. Lehr, D., and Antopol, W.: Specific morphology of crystals appearing in the urine during administration of sulfanilamide derivatives. Amer. J. Clin. Path., *12*:200-209, 1942.
6. Macaluso, M. P., and Berg, N. O.: Calcium oxalate crystals in kidneys in acute tubular nephrosis and other renal diseases with functional failure. Acta Path. Microbiol. Scand., *46*:197-205, 1959.
7. Morrin, P. F., Gedney, W. B., Barth, W., and Heptinstall, R. H.: Acute tubular necrosis - report of a case with failure to recover after 67 days of oliguria. Ann. Int. Med., *56*:925-930, 1962.
8. Papper, S., Belsky, J. L., and Bleifer, K. H.: Renal failure in Laennec's cirrhosis of the liver. I. Description of clinical and laboratory features. Ann. Int. Med., *51*:759-773, 1959.
9. Prien, E. L., Crabtree, E. G., and Frondel, C.: The mechanism of urinary tract obstruction in sulfathiazole therapy. Identification of crystals in tissue by polarized light. J. Urol., *46*:1020-1032, 1941.
10. Prien, E. L., and Frondel, C.: Crystallography of the urinary sediments with clinical and pathological observations in sulfonamide drug therapy. J. Urol., *46*:748-758, 1941.
11. Prien, E. L., and Frondel, C.: Studies in urolithiasis: I. The composition of urinary calculi. J. Urol., *57*: 949-994, 1947.
12. Smetana, H. F.: Nephrosis due to carbon tetrachloride, Arch. Intern. Med. (Chicago), *63*:760-777, 1939.
13. Weissman, M., Klein, B., and Berkowitz, J.: Clinical applications of infrared spectroscopy. Analysis of renal tract calculi. Anal. Chem., *31*:1334-1338, 1959.
14. Woods, W. W.: The changes in the kidneys in carbon tetrachloride poisoning and their resemblance to those in the "crush syndrome." J. Path. Bact., *58*:767-773, 1946.

Comments on the Quantitation of Bacilluria

CHARLES O. SENNETT, Jr., M.D.

In general, the presence of 100,000 or more bacteria per milliliter in properly collected urinc is considered to represent infection of the urinary tract (8,9). Less well known than the figure of 100,000 bacteria per ml is the fact that consistent finding of 10,000 to 100,000 bacteria per ml probably represents more than colonization of the distal urethra (4).

There is no biochemical procedure yet available that a clinical laboratory could use exclusively as a screening test without jeopardizing accuracy for speed or economy. In less than optimum conditions or massive screening, one or more of the indirect procedures may be indicated.

The Griess nitrite or modified rapid nitrite test (20,22,23,24) is based on the normal absence of nitrite in urine, unless infected with Gram-negative nitrate-reducing bacilli. This procedure yields a high percentage of false negative results, when compared with colony counts on specimens containing 100,000 or more bacilli per ml. Reports on the TTC (triphenyl tetrazolium chloride) test (5,18,20,23,25) are more favorable. Triphenyl tetrazolium chloride is reduced by actively respiring bacteria to insoluble triphenyl formazan. The cata-

lase (1) test ranges from the subjective recording of bubbles to timing flotation of urine-soaked discs in a tube of peroxide. Not all bacteria elaborate sufficient quantities of peroxidase, and false positive results can be expected from leucocytes and other cells. As with the other indirect methods, this approach should be limited to massive screening. Less useful are the more complicated enzyme studies, such as beta-glucaronidase (17), serum glutamic oxalacetic transaminase, and lactic dehydrogenase and lysozyme measurements.

The direct methods for the detection of bacilluria include the study of both wet and unstained dried films of uncentrifuged urine (20,21,27). While avoiding centrifugation and staining, this method is the least sensitive of the direct methods. Gram staining of centrifuged urine is advantageous, but at ordinary centrifuge speeds it is less sensitive than colony counting.

The reference procedure for the quantitation of bacilluria is colony counting of pour plates which have been inoculated with known dilutions of urine. This method has the principal advantage of beginning with a larger sample from which ten-fold dilutions using saline or liquid culture broth are made (6,26). Even this comparatively laborious approach is, at best, an approximation when taking into consideration the various factors which have a secondary influence on the numbers of organisms present (10). Briefly, these factors include increase or decrease of bacteria owing to one or more of the following circumstances (16):

a. Length of time urine remains in the bladder, or in a specimen bottle awaiting testing

b. Methods of collection:

(1) Where failure to cleanse periurethral surface leads to gross contamination; or, conversely,

(2) Over-zealous use of antiseptics which may inhibit colony development.

c. The inhibitory effects of urea and the presence of other bacteriostatic or bacteriocidal agents, such as antibotics.

The chore of making dilutions may be fairly well circumvented by various sampling devices, such as absorbent strips (12,19), small pipets, and calibrated loops (6,13,14). If these modifications are done carefully, good correlation with tube dilutions may be expected.

The calibrated loop inoculation of nutrient agar plates is one of the most practical compromises for hospital clinical laboratories. In special cases where immediate reports and staining reaction are required, microscopic examination is made of the Gram-stained urine sediment.

REFERENCES

1. Braude, A. I., and Berkowitz, H.: Detection of urinary catalase by disk flotation. J. Lab. Clin. Med., *57*(3):490-494, March 1961.
2. Brenner, B. M., and Gilbert, V. E.: Elevated levels of lactic dehydrogenase, glutamic-oxalacetic transaminase and catalase in infected urine. Am. J. Med. Sci., *245:*31-42, 1963.
3. Cohen, Stephen N., and Kass, E. H.: A simple method for quantitative urine culture. New Engl. J. Med., *277*(4):176-180, 27 July 1967.
4. Effersoe, P., and Jensen, E.: Urinary tract infection versus bacterial contamination. Lancet, *1:*1342, 1963.
5. Hnatko, S. I.: Uroscreen as a diagnostic aid in urinary tract infection. Lancet, *2:*964, 31 October 1964.
6. Hoeprich, P. D.: Culture of the urine. J. Lab. Clin. Med., *56*(6):899-907, December 1960.
7. Honeywell, K., *et al.:* A comparison of four tests for bacteriuria. Am. J. Med. Technology, *32:*207-209, May-June, 1965.
8. Kass, E. H.: Bacteriuria and the diagnosis of infections of the urinary tract. A.M.A. Arch. Intern. Med., *100*(5):709-714, November 1957.
9. Kass, E. H.: Pyelonephritis and bacteriuria, a major problem in Preventive Medicine. Ann. Int. Med., *56*(1):46-53, January 1962.
10. Kaye, D.: Antibacterial activity of human urine. J. Clin. Invest., *46*(6):1078, June 1967.
11. Kincaid-Smith, P., and Bullen, M.: Bacteriuria in pregnancy. Lancet, *1*(7382):395-399, 20 February 1965.
12. Mackey, J. P., and Sandys, G. H.: Laboratory diagnosis of infections of the urinary tract in general practice by means of dip-inoculum transport medium. Brit. Med. J., *2*(5473):1286-1288, 27 November 1965.
13. Mella, G. W., and Margileth, A. M.: Clinical experience with streak-plate urine cultures. Med. Ann. of the Dist. of Col., *35*(5):250-254, May 1966.
14. McGeachie, J., and Kennedy, A. C.: Simplified quantitative methods for bacteriuria. J. Clin. Path., *16*(1):32-38, January 1963.
15. Mou, T. W., and Feldman, H. A.: The enumeration and preservation of bacteria in urine. Am. J. Clin. Path., *35*(6):572-575, 1961.
16. Roberts, A. P., Robinson, R. E., and Beard, R. W.: Some factors affecting bacterial colony counts in urinary infection. Brit. Med. J., *1:*400-403, February 18, 1967.
17. Roberts, A. P., Frampton, J., Karim, S., Beard, R. W.: Estimation of beta-glucaronidase activity in urinary tract infection. New Engl. J. Med., *276*(26):1468-1470, 29 June 1967.
18. Ryan, W. L.: The use of triphenyltetrazolium in clinical microbiology. Am. J. Med. Technology, *31* (6):447-449, November-December 1965.
19. Ryan, W. L., Hoody, S., and Luby, R.: A simple quantitative test for bacteriuria. J. Urol., *88*(6):838-840, December 1962.
20. Sacks, T. G., and Abramson, J. H.: Screening tests for bacteriuria. J.A.M.A., *201*(1):79-82, 3 July 1967.

21. Schamadan, W. E.: Bacteriuria during pregnancy. Am. J. Obst. & Gyn., *89*(1):10-15, 1 May 1964.
22. Schaus, R.: Griess' Nitrite Test in diagnosis of urinary infection. J.A.M.A., *161*(6):528-529, 9 June 1956.
23. Simmons, N. A., and Williams, J. D.: A simple test for significant bacteriuria. Lancet, *1*:1377, 30 June 1962.
24. Sleigh, J. D.: Detection of bacteriuria by a modification of the nitrite test. Brit. Med. J., *1*:765-767, 20 March 1965.
25. Smith, L. G., and Schmidt, J.: Evaluation of three screening test for patients with significant bacteriuria. J.A.M.A., *181*(5):431-433, 4 August 1962.
26. Truant, J. P.: Evaluation of various methods used for the detection of significant bacteriuria in humans. Henry Ford Hospital Med. Bull., *12*(2):237-250, June 1964.
27. Turner, G. C.: Bacilluria in pregnancy. Lancet, *2*:1062-1064, 11 November 1961.
28. Urquhart, G., and Gould, J. C.: Simplified technique for counting the number of bacteria in urine and other fluids. J. Clin. Path., *18*(4):480-482, July 1965.
29. Weiser, O. L., and Emerson, J. S.: Selective screening for quantiative urine cultures. Am. J. Clin. Path., *45* (5):649-650, May 1966.

Quantitative Measurements of Bacilluria

CHARLES O. SENNETT, Jr., M.D., and PHYLLIS WARREN, B.S.

INTRODUCTION

The necessity for quantitating bacteriuria results from the variable amount of contamination from the urethra and perineum, particularly in the female. Other variables such as urine concentration, bacteriostatic or bactericidal substances, and methods of urine collection, have prompted numerous studies (1,5,6,9,11,19,20,23,35,36,42) to ascertain the best method to detect significant infection of the urinary tract. From the many procedures devised, a modified loop inoculation of blood agar plates has been selected as the most practicable compromise for hospital clinical laboratories.

Principle

Quantitative bacterial counts on urines (clean-catch voided or catheterized specimens) are helpful in the diagnosis and treatment of urinary tract infections. The calibrated loop methods have been shown (2,17,48) to be both accurate and practical, and are often used in clinical laboratories which offer a 24-hour service. Comparisons have been made by a number of workers (17,26,27,44,46) between the calibrated loop method and various other methods of quantitating viable organisms per ml of urine. From these studies results obtained using calibrated bacteriological loops, are comparable to both the pour plate method and the tube dilution method. The latter methods are somewhat more accurate than the calibrated loop method; however, this method best suits the purposes of a busy clinical laboratory. A calibrated bacteriological loop is employed to inoculate and streak plates containing standard and/or differential culture media. The plates are incubated, the number of colonies present estimated, and the number of bacteria per ml of urine reported. This method is considered to be an excellent screening procedure and most accurate when counts of 10^5 or greater bacteria per ml are observed.

Special Apparatus

1. Calibrated bacteriological loop

    a. 0.01 ml capacity (4 mm inside diameter) (Arthur H. Thomas Co., Phila.)

2. Sheep blood agar plate
3. Incubator, 37° C

Procedure

1. Using a flame-sterilized and cooled

4 mm platinum loop, which delivers 0.01 ml, one loopful of a well-mixed uncentrifuged urine specimen is inoculated on a blood agar plate.

2. The plate is streaked over its entire surface, using either the calibrated loop (after reflaming), a sterilized bent wire, or similar instrument.

3. The plate is incubated overnight at 37°C and read.

4. The colonies are counted and this colony count multiplied by 100 (0.01 ml used) to give the number of bacteria per ml of urine. As an example, 500 colonies would represent 50,000 bacterial cells actually present per ml of urine.

5. If no growth has occurred in 24 hours, the plates are reincubated for an additional 24 hours, and if still negative, it is reported as "no growth after 48 hours."

Discussion

Beginning with early Public Health studies of water and milk supplies, a variety of direct and indirect methods (22,26,45) of quantitating bacteria present in urine and other fluids have been described. It is widely accepted that the true count of 100,000 or more bacteria per ml even on a single sample, is significant. Repeated finding of more than 10,000 bacteria per ml of urine may represent something more than normal colonization of the distal urethra. These figures must be interpreted by the clinician treating the patient. It is the responsibility of the laboratory to see that reasonably accurate values are reported. Of the direct methods available for indicating the number of organisms in urine, the basic or reference procedure is colony counts of pour plates inoculated with known dilutions of specimen (1,2,14,15,21,28,33).

Microscopic examination of sediment

(13,31) for bacteria offers the advantage of speed and knowledge of the Gram stain reaction. Study of both wet and unstained dried smears of uncentrifuged urine has been reported (24, 29, 30, 37, 47). While avoiding centrifugation and staining, this method becomes the least sensitive of the direct methods of quantitating bacteriuria. Other indirect methods, such as the Griess nitrite test (8,18,38,39,41,43), the TTC test (7,10,14-16,34) or triphenyltetrazolium chloride, and enzyme tests, such as peroxidase (4,25) and beta-glucuronidase (3,32), all show a corresponding wide range of reliability, are quite laborious, and vary in difficulty of performance.

Source of Error

1. Failure to mix the urine specimen properly.

2. Failure to protect the calibrated loop, resulting in changes in diameter, and therefore inaccurate sampling of the urine specimen.

3. Failure to cool inoculating loop adequately after flaming.

4. Inadequate streaking of inoculate onto the media surface.

REFERENCES

1. Annon.: Detection of asymptomatic bacteriuria. Canad. M. A. J., *93*: 666-667, 1965.
2. Bailey, W. R., and Scott, E. G.: Diagnostic Bacteriology, 2nd ed. Chapter X. St. Louis, C. V. Mosby Co., 1966.
3. Bank, N., and Bailine, S. H.: Urinary beta-glucuronidase activity in patients with urinary tract infection. New Eng. J. Med., *272*: 70-75, 1965.
4. Braude, A. I., and Berkowitz, H.: Detection of urinary catalase by disk flotation. J. Lab. Clin. Med., *57*: 490-494, 1961.
5. Bulger, R. J., and Kirby, W.: Simple tests for significant bacteriuria. Arch. Int. Med., *112*:742-746, 1963.

6. Cohen, S., and Kass, E. H.: A simple method for quantitative urine culture. New Eng. J. Med., *277*:176-180, 1967.

7. Constable, P. J.: The Triphenyltetrazolium Chloride Test in general practitioner antenatal care. Lancet, *2*:195-196, 1966.

8. DeShan, P. W., *et al.*: The Griess Test as a screening procedure for bacteriuria during pregnancy. Obstet. & Gyn., *27*:202-205, 1966.

9. Deutch, M., and Jesperson, H. G.: The detection of significant bacteriuria. Acta Med. Scand., *175*:191-196, 1964.

10. Eliot, C. R., and Pryles, C. V.: Observations on the use of triphenyltetrazolium for the detection of bacteriuria. Pediatrics, *34*:421-422, 1964.

11. Fairley, K. F., and Barraclough, M.: The value of a chemical screening test for urinary infection. Med. J. Australia, *1*:93-94, 1966.

12. Fairley, K. F., and Barraclough, M.: Leukocyte excretion rate as a screening test for bacteriuria. Lancet, *1*:420-421, 1967.

13. Goss, L. B., *et al.*: Asymptomatic bacteriuria of pregnancy and detection by a simple stain. Amer. J. Obst. & Gyn., *87*:493-498, 1963.

14. Guze, L. B., and Kalmanson, G. M.: Observations on the use of the Triphenyl Tetrazolium Test to determine significant bacteriuria. Amer. J. Med. Sci., *246*:691-694, 1963.

15. Hinton, N. A., and van der Hoeven, E.: The detection of significant bacteriuria: An assessment of the Tripenyltetrazolium Chloride Reduction Test. Canad. M. A. J., *93*:639-642, 1965.

16. Hnatko, S. I.: Uroscreen as a diagnostic aid in urinary tract infection. Lancet, *2*:964, 1964.

17. Hoeprich, P. D.: Culture of the urine. J. Lab. Clin. Med., *56*:899-907, 1960.

18. Kahler, R. L., and Guze, L. B.: Evaluation of the Griess Nitrite Test as a method for the recognition of the urinary tract infection. J. Lab. Clin. Med., *49*:934-937, 1957.

19. Kass, E. H.: Bacteriuria and the diagnosis of infections of the urinary tract. A. M. A. Arch. Int. Med., *100*:709-714, 1957.

20. Kass, E. H.: Pyelonephritis and Bacteriuria, a major problem in Preventive Medicine. Ann. Int. Med., *56*:46-53, 1962.

21. Kaye, D.: Antibacterial activity of human urine. J. Clin. Invest., *46*:1078, 1967.

22. Kincaid-Smith, P., Bullen, M., Mills, J., Fussell, U., Huston, N., and Goon, F.: The reliability of screening tests for bacteriuria in pregnancy. Lancet, *2*:61-62, 1964.

23. Kincaid-Smith, P., and Bullen, M.: Bacteriuria in pregnancy. Lancet, *1*:395-399, 1965.

24. Kunin, C. M.: The quantitative significance of bacteria visualized in the unstained urinary sediment. New Eng. J. Med., *265*:589-590, 1961.

25. Montgomerie, J. Z., Kalmanson, G., and Guze, L. B.: The use of the Catalase Test to detect significant bacteriuria. Amer. J. Med. Sci., *251*:184-187, 1966.

26. Mou, T. W., and Feldman, H. A.: The enumeration and preservation of bacteria in urine. Am. J. Clin. Path., *35*:572-575, 1961.

27. Parker, R. H., Nord, N. M., Croft, G. F., and Hoeprich, P. D.: Reliability of a commercial triphenyltetrazolium chloride reduction test for detecting significant bacteriuria. Amer. J. Med. Sci., *251*:260-265, 1966.

28. Pinkerton, J., Roberts, A. P., and Hurley, R.: The relation between bacteriuria and urinary tract infection in pregnant women. Lancet, *2*:59-61, 1964.

29. Pryles, C. V., and Steg, N.: Specimens of urine obtained from young girls by catheter versus voiding. A comparative study of bacterial cultures, Gram stains, and bacterial counts in paired specimens. Pediatrics, *23*:441-452, 1959.

30. Rehm, R. A.: The stained urine smear. A comparison of centrifuged with uncentrifuged specimens. Ohio State Med. J., *60*:139-140, 1964.

31. Rehm, R. A., and Fishman, A.: The value of the urine smear in detecting bacteriuria. J. Urol., *89*:930-932, 1963.

32. Roberts, A. P., Frampton, J., Karim, S., and Beard, R. W.: Estimation of beta-glucuronidase activity in urinary tract infection. New Eng. J. Med., *276*:1468-1470, 1967.

33. Roberts, A. P., Robinson, R. E., and Beard, R. W.: Some factors affecting bacterial colony counts in urinary infection. Brit. Med. J., *1*:400-403, 1967.

34. Ryan, W. L.: The use of triphenyltetrazolium in clinical microbiology. Amer. J. Med. Tech., *31*:447-449, 1965.

35. Ryan, W. L., Hoody, S., and Luby, R.: A simple quantitative test for bacteriuria. J. Urol., *88*:838-840, 1962.

36. Sacks, T. G., and Abramson, J. H.: Screening tests for bacteriuria. J. Amer. Med. Assoc., *201*:79-82, 1967.

37. Schamadan, W. E.: Bacteriuria during pregnancy. Am. J. Obst. & Gyn., *89*:10-15, 1964.

38. Schaus, R.: Griess' Nitrite Test in diagnosis of urinary infection. J. Amer. Med. Assoc., *161*:528-529, 1956.

39. Simmons, N. A., and Williams, J. D.: A simple test for significant bacteriuria. Lancet, *1*:1377, 1962.

40. Simon, H. B., Dickstein, H., and Dunbar, K.: Laboratory aids in diagnosis of significant urinary tract infection. N. Y. State J. Med., *64*:255-258, 1964.

41. Sleigh, J. D.: Detection of bacteriuria by a modification of the Nitrite Test. Brit. Med. J., *1*:765-767, 1965.

42. Slowinski, E. J., and Smith, L. G.: A ten-second colorimetric test for asymptomatic bacteriuria in

pregnancy — The office use of the Griess Test. Amer. J. Obst. & Gyn., *94*:906-909, 1966.

43. Smith, L. G., Thayer, W. R., Malta, E. M., and Utz, J. P.: Relationship of the Griess Nitrite Test to bacterial culture in the diagnosis of urinary tract infection. Ann. Int. Med., *54*:66-72, 1961.

44. Sonnenwirth, A. C.: Chapter 31, Gradwohl's Clinical Laboratory Methods and Diagnosis, 6th ed. St. Louis, C. V. Mosby Co., 1963.

45. Standard Methods for examination of water and wastewater. Ed. XII. Part VII: Routine bacteriologic examination of water to determine its sanitary quality. Amer. Public Health Assoc., Inc., N. Y., 1965.

46. Truant, J. P.: Evaluation of various methods used for the detection of significant bacteriuria in humans. Henery Ford Hosp. Bull., *12*: 237-250, 1964.

47. Turner, G. C.: Bacilluria in pregnancy. Lancet, *2*:1062-1064, 1961.

48. Urquhart, G., and Gould, J. C.: Simplified technique for counting the number of bacteria in urine and other fluids. J. Clin. Path., *18*:480-482, 1965.

49. Williams, J. D., Leigh, D. A., and Rosser, E. I.: The organization and results of a screening program for the detection of bacteriuria of pregnancy. J. Obstet. Gynaec. Brit. Comm., *72*:327-335, 1965.

Chapter 28

Fluorescent Dye Staining of Mycobacterium Tuberculosis

GEORGE P. BLUNDELL, Ph.D., M.D.

INTRODUCTION

Tuberculosis of the urinary system is accepted as a secondary process, with the primary lesion being in the respiratory system, cervical lymph nodes or gastro-intestinal system. Thus, while it is possible for tuberculosis to be most extensive in the kidney and bladder, it is frequently part of a generalized diseminated form of the disease. Grossly, the kidney can appear swollen early in the disease process or eventually present as a fibrous sac containing caseous material. The degree of tissue destruction and the range of histopathological reaction may be as varied as in the lungs and other organs of the body. Lesions, therefore, can occur as minute, discrete tubercles or as large confluent tubercles, or, since the disease in the kidney is usually due to hematogenous spread, there may develop massive, infarct-like lesions secondary to obliterative tuberculous arteritis and the resulting obstruction of the blood supply.

Within this spectrum of renal tuberculosis, the etiologic agent, *Mycobacterium tuberculosis* may be as elusive as it is in other tissues. If the tubercle bacilli are present in urine, the problem of collecting them in sufficient number to identify them is as difficult as their visualization within tissues.

The initial means of staining and viewing the bacilli under the microscope was through the use of the Ziehl stain reported 85 years ago (39) or one of its modifications. Aniline dyes other than fuchsin have also been used to successfully stain tubercle bacilli. Thirty years ago (14), there was devised a new technic which offers numerous advantages over the Ziehl-Neelsen method and which can be used in conjunction with it. This technic is known as fluorochroming.

THE PRINCIPLE OF FLUORESCENT STAINING

Initially, bacteriologists encountered difficulty in recognizing the tubercle bacillus because of its apparent lack of affinity for aqueous solutions of stains. Even with the Ziehl-Neelsen technic, the intensity of the staining or the amount of dye retained in the bacillus may not be sufficient for visualization of the microorganism. Everyone who uses the technic, however, is accustomed to searching for red bacilli, seen in contrast against a blue or green background depending on the counter-stain employed.

Those who gained experience over the years with the Ziehl-Neelsen stain feel insecure with other staining methods.

The most valuable of the "new" staining technics is that of fluorescent staining or fluorochroming. The fluorochromes of choice are Auramine and Rhodamine. As with any fluorescent dye, they can be activated by a high intensity light source so that a minute amount of the dye can be detected as a brilliant active color. While a bright-field condenser may be used, it is customary to employ a dark-field condenser in the staining technic so that the brilliantly stained object appears even brighter against the dark background. A counterstain is not necessary unless the specimen tends to autofluoresce excessively.

The value of Auramine-Rhodamine is that as fluorescent compounds they absorb energy from a high intensity light source, and in a fraction of a second reemit it as a color with a slightly shorter wave length. The light from the lamp activates with the wave length of that portion of the spectrum which comprises the color of the fluorescent dyes or fluorochromes in use. In order to select the proper wave length for the yellowish-red of Auramine-Rhodamine, and to eliminate unwanted light, appropriate filters must be placed between the ultraviolet light source and the stained bacillus.

This activation of fluorochromes is in sharp contrast to the light transmission of the aniline dye fuchsin. The bacillus stained with fuchsin is viewed with a bright-field condenser. The intensity of redness depends in a large measure on the quantity of fuchsin which has penetrated and been retained by the bacillus. The tubercle bacillus stained with Auramine-Rhodamine, in contrast, is almost like a light bulb which becomes a luminous object when electricity enters it. The fluorochromes absorb energy and reemit it so it may be visualized. As with the filaments of the light bulb, the fluorochromes become energized, and within a relatively short time will have adsorbed and reemitted so much energy it is consumed, and its light or fire is "quenched" or used up. Before this "quenched" stage is reached, a trained observer has seen the Auramine-Rhodamine stained tubercle bacillus.

The advantage of the fluorescent method is that the tubercle bacillus is seen as a bright yellowish-red object against a dark background. It is visualized so readily it tends to "jump out at you."

THE DEVELOPMENT OF THE FLUORESCENT METHOD

The application of any use of fluorescence in microscopy requires that the microscopist be experienced in recognizing autofluorescence of artefacts or of the object under study. It is always important, therefore, to determine if an object can be recognized in its unstained state, when examined by a fluorescent miscroscope. The tubercle bacillus does autofluoresce. This observation was first recorded by Kaiserling in 1917 (19). The danger is not in this property, but rather that small bacillus-like artefacts may also autofluoresce.

In fluorescent microscopy, it must always be kept in mind that the microscopist is seeking a particular discrete object. A trained observer knows and recognizes a tubercle bacillus by its shape and size and markings. This capability is essential whether tubercle bacilli are being sought with the auramine-rhodamine stain or the Ziehl-Neelsen stain. Artefacts are a potential pitfall with either technique.

Many objects in a smear of sputum or a section of tissue may autofluoresce or stain with fluorochromes in addition to the tubercle bacillus. It is interesting that the same year Hagemann (14) first reported the use of auramine as a fluorochrome selective for tubercle bacilli, Herrmann (16) reported the use of potassium permanganate to reduce unwanted background fluorescence. This compound acts primarily to quench the auramine in objects other than the tubercle bacillus. The length of time the permanganate is applied is critical. It may even be used instead of an acid solution to "decolorize" the tubercle bacilli. Keller (20) was also an early participant in the application of fluorescence to the study of the tubercle bacillus.

Richards and Miller (29) were active in introducing the method to the United States. They assembled a useful and relatively inexpensive fluorescent microscope by using filters marketed by the Reichert Company in Europe, a low voltage high amperage filament lamp, and the instruments and lamp housing available through the Spencer Lens Company in the United States.

It can be safely stated that many bacteriology laboratories in this country purchased this equipment and arranged to keep it in a small, dark, windowless room. The principal advantage readily apparent at that time was that the staining procedure with fluorochromes was not as messy as was the case with the Ziehl-Neelsen stain. The major disadvantage was that the microscopist, with years of experience in searching for "red" bacilli, felt insecure with the method.

The use of double fluorochromes followed Hagemann's report, with Schallok (30) in 1940 recommending the use of thiazol yellow in addition to auramine. The German investigators had thus presented information that: 1) tubercle bacilli were autofluorescent; 2) and could be stained with the fluorescent dye, auramine. They further presented 3) potassium permanganate as a compound to lessen background staining, and 4) recommended the use of more than one fluorochrome for staining tubercle bacilli. At this time, their contributions were interrupted by World War II.

The use of double dyes was next modified by Graham (12) working at the New York State Hospital in Ithaca, a hospital which no longer has tuberculous patients to house. He added rhodamine to auramine and so introduced the dye combination recommended for use today. Two Australian workers further refined Graham's work, with Hughes (18) adopting it and adding acridine yellow, while Matthaei (25) found auramine and rhodamine satisfactory but in higher concentrations. Ten years later, Kuper and May (23) in England modified Matthaei's procedure into the one used today.

The major value of the addition of rhodamine to auramine is that rhodamine provides a longer examining time than auramine alone as it is not quenched as readily as auramine. The slight addition of red color has very likely subconsciously made the color more acceptable to those accustomed to the Ziehl-Neelsen stain.

Thirty years have passed since the first use of auramine for staining the tubercle bacilli. This dye alone was tried by many bacteriologists who concluded it was essentially on an equal with the Ziehl-Neelsen stain. At the end of the first half of this period, the combination of auramine-rhodamine began to be recognized as superior to auramine alone. The first fifteen years, therefore, were devoted to the development of a satisfactory dye combination and the adoption of the two dyes into general use.

The following fifteen years have seen a greater adoption of the fluorochroming method because of the improvement in instrumentation. The competitive improvement in the fluorescent microscope came about largely through the interest in and widespread adoption of the fluorescent antibody technique of Coons (5). As laboratories acquired the very superior fluorescent microscopes developed for fluorescent antibody procedures, these instruments were available for other uses and so the direct fluorochroming or staining of acid-fast bacilli in the bacteriology laboratory became a bonus of the activities in the serology laboratory.

The emphasis of these stages in the development and adoption of the fluorescent staining method does not mean that there was no significant activity in the intervening years. Lind, in 1949 (24), even surveyed the methods as other laboratories had applied it and found that most laboratories had discarded it. McClure (26) attributed this dissatisfaction to the use of auramine alone rather than auramine-rhodamine.

Another part of the transition in the application of fluorochroming has been the recognition of its value and emphasis on its use in examining histologic sections of tissue. Initially, the average bacteriology laboratory applied fluorochromes to cultures of tubercle bacilli and sputa from patients suspected of being tuberculous. Gradually, it has been given an accepted place in the routine examination of tissues suspected of being tuberculous. Finke (8) had reported from the start in 1939, the staining of tubercle bacilli in tissues.

Tanner reported a large series in 1941 (32) and later with McDonald (33) reported on the application of the stain to granulomatous prostatitis. Others reporting on their experiences with tissues were Gray (13) and the very comprehensive paper by McClure (26), both in 1953. The more recent papers include those of Kuper and May (23) who revised the stain concentrations and procedure, and Braunstein and Andriano (4) in the United States, and Wellman and Teng (37) in Canada. Subsequently, several groups in Michigan presented their support of the method. They are: Truant, Brett, and Thomas (34), de Groat and White (6), and Hertz, Pawlecki, and Green (17). Koch and Cole (21), Yamaguski and Braunstein (38) and Silver, Sonnenwirth and Alex (31) and Gillissen (11) further reinforce the advantages of auramine and rhodamine for both tissues and smears.

Reagents

The reagents required for fluorochroming are few, and are limited to those stains and chemicals incorporated in the staining solutions. These may be listed as follows for the fluorescent staining:

(1) Auramine O
(2) Rhodamine B
(3) Glycerol (used for stain solutions and with immersion objective)
(4) Phenol crystals
(5) Potassium permanganate
(6) Ethyl alcohol
(7) Hydrochloric acid
(8) Distilled water.

There will be needed in addition, for the Ziehl Neelsen control or confirmation stain the following:

(9) Basic fuchsin
(10) Tergitol-7

Additional substances are required for the concentration of urine specimens:

(11) Aluminum potassium sulfate
(12) Human serum

The reagents listed above are for phenolized solutions, which are considered critical compounds in the staining of acid-fast microorganisms. From the time of the introduction of fluorescent compounds it was recognized that aqueous solutions of fluorochromes alone could stain the tubercle bacillus. This has recently been confirmed by Mr. Marvin H. Palmer (28) who has found that an aqueous solution of uranin stains acid-fast mycobacteria.

Uranine is a commercial grade of sodium fluorescein, available from the Fischer Scientific Company. It is used by public health engineers as a coloring compound to trace ground water supplies.

Standard Solutions

A. *Fluorochroming Solutions* (after Kuper and May (23), 1960).

The *auramine-rhodamine stain* is prepared as follows:

    1. Auramine O . . . . . .1.5 gms
    2. Rhodamine B . . . 0.75 gm
    3. Glycerol . . . . .75.0 ml
    4. Phenol crystals liquified
       at 50°C . . . . .10.0 ml
    5. Distilled water: . . .50.0 ml

Though all of the dye may not appear to dissolve, mixing is done thoroughly and then the stain is filtered through glass wool and stored in a glass bottle.

The *decolorizing solution* of acid-alcohol is prepared as follows:

    1. Hydrochloric acid
       (concentrated) . . . . .0.5 ml
    2. Ethyl alcohol (70%)99.5 ml

The solution for *counterstaining* or reducing background staining is prepared as follows:

    1. Potassium
       permanganate: . . . .0.5 gms
    2. Distilled water: . .100.0 ml

B. *Fuchsin-Tergitol Acid-fast Stain:* (A modification of the Kinyoun-Ziehl-Neelsen stain after Muller and Chermock (27).

    1. Basic fuchsin: . . . . 4.0 gm
    2. Absolute alcohol: .75.0 ml
    3. Phenol: . . . . .25.0 ml
    4. Distilled water:. . .510.0 ml
    5. Tergitol No. 7: . 4.0 drops

The basic fuchsin is dissolved in the alcohol. The phenol is liquified at 56° and added to the alcoholic solution of fuchsin. This is placed in the 37° incubator overnight. The following day the water and Tergitol are added. The solution is more satisfactory if maintained at 37°C in the incubator. It should be filtered prior to use.

The *declorizing solution* may be the same as for the auramine-rhodamine stain.

Counterstains may be either of methylene blue or fast green. These solutions are prepared as follows:

(a)   1. Methylene blue: . . 0.5 gm
       2. Distilled water: . .100.0 ml
       3. Acetic acid: . . . . . . .0.5 ml
or (b) Loeffler's alkaline methylene
       blue stock solution:
       1. Methylene blue: . 1.48 gm
       2. 95% ethyl alcohol 100.0 ml

Final dye solution:
    1. Potassium hydroxide (10%
       aqueous solution) .0.07 ml
    2. Distilled water: . . .70.0 ml
    3. Stock solution of
       methylene blue: . .30.0 ml

C. *Fast Green:*
  (a) 1. Fast Green: . . . . . 3.24 gm
      2. Ethyl alcohol: . . .360.0 ml
      3. Sulfuric acid: . . . .180.0 ml
      4. Distilled water: 1,530.0 ml
or (b) 1. Fast Green (saturated
         alcoholic solution . .1.5 ml
      2. Distilled water: . . .98.5 ml

D. *Uranine* (sodium fluorescein) solution of Palmer:
      1. Uranine: . . . . 0.5 gm
      2. Hemagglutinin buffer,
         pH 7.3 . . . . 4.3 gm
      3. Distilled water: . .500.0 ml

E. *Precipitating Reagent for Urine Concentration:*
      1. Aluminum potassium
         sulfate, reagent grade 10 gm
      2. Sterile distilled
         water . . . . .100.0 ml
         Dissolve by heating.

F. *Film for Photography:*
      Agfa CT 18
      Orange and red colors are reproduced effectively with this film.

Special Apparatus

The special items of equipment for fluorescent staining are principally those related to the light source and the microscope.

It may be noted, however, that in order to fluorochrome specimens there is needed the usual equipment available in the microbiology and histology laboratories for the preparation of slides and stains. These include: glass microscopic slides, coverslips, Erlenmeyer flasks for preparing staining solutions, graduate cylinder, scales or balance, staining rack, and incubator.

The examination of the stained smears requires the availability of a high intensity light source, collecting lens, primary or exciter filter, dark-field condenser, various objectives, secondary or barrier filter, and eye pieces.

1. *Lamp*

The majority of microscopes in use at the present time are designed primarily for use with the fluorescent antibody (FA) technique. A high intensity lamp is required because the object to be examined is usually coated with a monomolecular layer of antiserum in which fluorescein is incorporated. This lamp is the Osram HBO-200, which costs about $56.00 and has a life of approximately 80 hours. If this lamp is available in the laboratory, it is certainly satisfactory and convenient to use.

A less powerful lamp is also satisfactory. An object subjected to fluorochroming or fluorescent staining, in contrast to fluorescent antibody (FA) staining, retains a greater quantity of the fluorescent dye than is the case with the thin coating of fluorescein-coupled antibody. In this country, the G. E. 397-AH 4 Mercury Arc Lamp, 100 watt, 103 volt, ultraviolet lamp is used extensively. It costs $16.00 and usually has a life of over 100 hours. It is available in a convenient lamp housing manufactured by the American Optical Company.*

Other lamps available include the Xenon high pressure burner XBO-162. It supplies light with a 6000° K color temperature and up to 1200 mu UV and IR rays. There is also available a GE 6v/18A ribbon-filament lamp which has a consumption of 108 W. Some laboratories have modified carbon arc lights for their use as well as other high intensity light sources. Sodium lamps and mercury

---

*AO Spencer 390B Mercury Arc Illuminator Reactance Transformer No. 397.

lamps for street lighting use have also been employed.

2. Filters

The wave length required to excite the fluorescence of auramine is approximately 4320 Å and of rhodamine 5560 Å. This was determined by Matthaei (25) and also reported by Kuper and May. For this fluorescence to occur, the critical filter becomes the exciter or primary filter. Initially, a solution of copper sulfate ammonia liquid served as an exciter filter.

At the present time, there are used a BG12, or Corning 5113, or 5850, or 5030 or Wratten blue-violet C-5. The secondary or barrier filter is a complementary filter which eliminates unwanted ultraviolet and serves to darken the background. Satisfactory filters may be a Kodak Wratten No. 8 or G (15G) or an OG 1. Filter combinations may be determined by referring to the transmission charts listed in the *Handbook for Chemistry and Physics* (15). The secondary or barrier filter may be eliminated with the use of a dark field condenser.

3. Condenser

The advantages of a dark-field condenser for use in fluorescent microscopy were first reported in 1936 by Barnard and Welch (2). Many investigators use bright field condensers and find them satisfactory with the proper combination of exciter or pass and barrier filters. The author prefers a dark-field condenser. One of the disadvantages is that the usual dark-field condenser requires the use of an immersion liquid. Glycerol is satisfactory for this purpose. This does slow the microscopist in the examination of specimens and does require additional effort in the cleaning of the condenser and microscopic slides. In other words, it

is messy. Leitz has available a dry dark-field condenser which avoids the use of an immersion liquid. Proper alignment or centering of the condenser is essential for good results.

4. Objectives

The objectives may be those ordinarily in use. These may include approximately 25x, 40x, and a 100x oil immersion. Screening is performed satisfactorily with the high dry objective. The oil immersion objective may be used to confirm the organism seen with the high dry objective by examining its morphology in greater detail.

5. Eyepieces

The eyepieces used in the fluorescent microscope are even more a matter of personal preference than the objectives. Most pathologists use 10x widefield objectives. 5x or 8x are equally satisfactory.

Procedure

The staining procedure for the auramine-rhodamine fluorescent stain is similar to that of the Ziehl-Neelsen technique. It may be applied to smears from any source whether it be cultures or sputum or urine or comparable material. Smears are made of a satisfactory thickness or thinness and are heat fixed. Coverslipping is not necessary following staining.

Sections of tissue must be deparaffinized and passed through decreasing concentrations of alcohol to water prior to staining, and following staining the water must be removed to permit coverslipping, with Fluormount by E. Gurr.

The steps in the staining procedure are as follows:

(1) Apply auramine-rhodamine fluorescent stain for 10 to 15 minutes.

(2) Heat is not essential. The author

prefers passing the Bunsen burner flame under the smears several times so that a minimal steaming is noted. The slides may be placed in a Coplin jar of stain at either 37°C or 56°C, or stained over a steaming water bath.

(3) The smears are washed in water for a minute or two. This also may be in a Coplin jar.

(4) Decolorization with acid alcohol requires 2 to 3 minutes. 0.52 HCl in ethyl alcohol is satisfactory for tissues. Some authors prefer to have sodium chloride in the solution and so use HCl 0.5 ml, 99.5 ml or 70% alcohol and 0.5 gm of NaCl.

(5) Smears are finally rinsed in running water for approximately 2 minutes.

(6) Smears showing a pronounced background fluorescence and tissues should have the non-acid fast bacillus fluorescence quenched by applying the potassium permanganate solution for 2 minutes, followed by 2 minutes of washing in water.

(7) Smears are allowed to dry at 37° C, while tissues must be dehydrated and coverslipped.

Known positive controls of smears and tissues must be prepared in parallel, with each staining of unknown specimens.

While experience is being gained with the method, or as a standard procedure, each specimen found to contain acid fast bacilli by the auramine-rhodamine stain, may be restained with the Ziehl-Neelsen method for confirmation.

It has been noted by numerous authors that acid fast bacilli in the same specimen may be stained by the fluorescent method and then restained by the Ziehl-Neelsen method. This sequence of fluorescent staining first and then Ziehl-Neelsen is the preferred way, but the reverse is also possible.

Fusillo (10) has proposed performing both staining procedures initially in sequence as follows:

1) The Smear is flooded with Auramine-O solution for 15 minutes; 2) washed with tapwater; 3) decolorized in acid-alcohol; 4) washed with tapwater; 5) stained with Kinyoun stain for 5 minutes; 6) flooded with acid-alcohol to remove the excess stain; 7) washed with tapwater; 8) stained with Methylene blue for 2 minutes; 9) washed with tapwater; 10) allowed to dry at 37°C and read.

This staining sequence is possible. The smear is examined with fluorescent microscopy. Once an auramine-rhodamine-stained bacillus is identified, the incandescent lamp is moved into position and the bacillus is observed for Ziehl-Neelsen staining. The modern fluorescent microscopes with both light sources attached make this change of lighting very simple.

The dual staining procedure of Fusillo is not 100% reproducible, but is certainly deserving of further evaluation.

If the fluorescent stained bacilli fade from being examined too long under the high intensity light source, or following prolonged storage, they may be restained successfully.

It was noted with the first trials of auramine and rhodamine that the dyes would stain tubercle bacilli without the inclusion of phenol or glycerol in the staining solution. This observation has never been fully exploited.

The recent observation of Mr. Marvin T. Palmer that water soluble sodium fluorescein selectively stains various Mycobacteria could lead to a revision of the concept of acid-fastness as it is now employed.

A final recommendation in regard to the use of the microscope is the advantage of not using it in a brightly lighted room. The microscope can be shielded by a light weight wooden frame covered with black cloth, or in a slightly darkened room, or in a completely blacked out or windowless room. By reducing the light in the room, eye strain is minimized.

The processing of urine for the isolation and identification of acid fast bacilli has always been troublesome because it has been customary to examine a large volume 24 hour specimen of urine. Ellner and Elbogen (7) have recently recommended the use of only the entire morning specimen. This is a sensible modification as most of the daytime specimen is greatly diluted. The urine is concentrated by adding 1.0 ml of human serum to each 100 ml of urine, mixing and then adding 1 ml of alum solution per 100 ml of urine. The specimen is mixed and stored at 5°C overnight. The following morning the supernatant is removed and the remainder of the specimen centrifuged. The sediment is examined by smear and culture.

Discussion

Almost thirty years after the initial report of the fluorochrome staining of the tubercle bacillus, the procedure has attained wide acceptance and use as a routine diagnostic procedure. This is attributed to: 1) the use of the two dyes auramine and rhodamine, and 2) the use of modern fluorescent microscopes.

The two dyes are satisfactory because auramine provides brightness and sharpness to the tubercle bacillus, and the rhodamine provides a redness with better contrast and does not quench as readily as auramine and so provides a longer time for examination. This is a distinct advantage over auramine alone.

The stain solutions are stable and have been found to retain their effectiveness for at least two months. Any stain retained for that period of time should be discarded and a new stain solution prepared.

In contrast to this stability of the stain solution, the stained bacterial smears are satisfactory for examination when kept at room temperature for four months. Tissue sections, however, should be examined within one to four days of the time they are stained. In any event, both types of specimens may be restained effectively.

Basically, two types of decolorizing procedures are a part of fluorescent acid-fast staining. The first procedure is that of using acid alcohol. In addition, it is possible to decolorize or quench background fluorescence with potassium permanganate. If no permanganate is used, background fluorescence remains. Hughes prefers to retain background fluorescence as negative specimens which are then less tedious to examine. If the permanganate follows acid alcohol and is applied for 1/2 minute the fluorescence is removed from tissue sections. Permanganate for 1 minute alone accomplishes essentially the same result. Permanganate applied for 4 minutes or longer causes the tubercle bacilli to lose some of their brilliance.

The early papers devoted much attention to the type of lamp which was satisfactory as well as to the filters and optics of the microscope. Today, excellent microscopes are readily available so that any detailed discussion of microscopes becomes superfluous. A stand may be taken, however, on recommending the use of a dark-field condenser. Those laboratories using Leitz equipment could gain by acquiring the dry condenser and so avoid using an immersion liquid. It should also be noted that where an immersion liquid is used, glycerol is satisfactory.

All microscope users must keep constantly in mind the criticalness of maintaining precise alignment of the optics for maximal sharpness of detail and brightness of the object to be viewed. Care must be given to the centering of the lamp, the mirror, the condenser as well as the objectives.

Those readers who are reassured by a statistical accounting of the effectiveness of the fluorescent stain are referred especially to several reports. Wellman and Teng concurred with the observations of von Haebler and Murray (35) that acid fast bacilli will be missed with the Ziehl-Neelsen stain 3 times compared with fluorescent stain. McClure, Wellman and Teng, and Koch and Cote recommended its use in examining suspected cases of sarcoidosis.

Sources of Error

There are always numerous sources of error in any procedure. These could be related to improperly prepared stain, use of stain older than two months, prolonged exposure to potassium permanganate, over-exposure to ultraviolet light, improper alignment of the microscope, and faulty selection of filter as well as other errors.

None of these are considered continuous, repetitious mistakes.

The one pitfall which must be guarded against is accepting artefacts as tubercle bacilli. This problem is just as critical with the Ziehl-Neelsen stain. In each procedure, a specific *object,* the tubercle bacillus, is being stained. As with any laboratory procedure, training and experience in the technique are necessary. The slender, discrete bacillus, which may show barring and beading must be carefully identified. Amorphous objects or crystals or granules are not to be accepted as bacilli.

RESUME

Numerous authors have listed the advantages of the auramine-rhodamine stain for the identification of tubercle bacilli. These include the facts that compared to the Ziehl-Neelsen stain auramine-rhodamine

(1) Offers better contrast.

(2) Requires less time for scanning.

(3) Scanning can be conducted with the high dry objective and so no immersion liquid is required.

(4) Has a staining time that is shorter.

(5) Is a cleaner or less messy stain.

(6) Provides for the identification of bacilli in a larger number of cases, especially in specimens containing very few bacilli.

(7) Is acceptable to those who are color blind for red.

(8) May be restained with satisfactory results.

(9) Eye strain is less.

REFERENCES

1. Alexander-Jackson, E.: A differential triple stain for demonstrating and studying non-acid fast forms of the tubercle bacillus in sputum, tissue and body fluids. Science, *99*: 307-308, 1944.
2. Barnard, J. E., and Welch, F. V., XIV: Fluorescence microscopy with high powers. J. Roy. Micr. Soc., *56*: 361-364, 1936.
3. Bogen, E.: Detection of tubercle bacilli by fluorescence microscopy. Am. Rev. Tuberc., *44*: 267-271, 1941.
4. Braunstein, H. and Adriano, S.M.: Fluorescent stain for tubercle bacilli in histologic sections. Am. J. Clin. Path., *36*: 37-40, 1961.
5. Coons, A. H., Creech, H. J., and Jones, R. N.: Immunological properties of an antibody-containing a fluorescent group. Proc. Exp. Biol. & Med., *47*: 200-202, 1941.

6. deGroat, A., and White, M.: Observations on fluorescent staining for the detection of acid-fast organisms in sputa and tissues. J. Mich. State Med., Soc., *63:* 34-36, 1964.

7. Ellner, P. D., and Elbogen, S.: Modern methods in tuberculosis bacteriology for the general hospital. Am. J. Clin. Path., Tech. Sec. *48:* 435-440, 1967.

8. Finke, L.: Ueber den Fluoreszenzmikroskopischen Nachweis von Tuberkelbazillen in Ausstrichen und Gewebeschnitten. Arch. fuer Hygiene und Bakteriologie, *123:* 381-392, 1939.

9. Freiman, D. G., and Mokotoff, G. F.: Demonstration of tubercle bacilli by fluorescent microscopy. Am. Rev. Tuberc. *48:* 435-442, 1943.

10. Fusillo, M. D., and Burns, H. D.: Simultaneous auramine and Kinyoun stain for screening smears for acid-fast bacilli. Am. J. Clin. Path., In Press.

11. Gillissen, G.: Die Fluorescenserologische Darstellung Von Mydobakterien. Zbl. Bakt. (orig)., *188:* 81, 1963.

12. Graham, C. F.: Fluorescence microscopy of Mycobacterium tuberculosis. Am. Rev. Tuberc., *48:* 421-434, 1943.

13. Gray, D. F.: Detection of small numbers of mycobacteria in sections by fluorescence microscopy. Am. Rev. Tuberc., *68:* 82-95, 1953.

14. Hagemann, P. K. H.: Fluoreszenzfaerbung von Tuberkelbakterien Mit Auramin. Muench. med. Wschr., *85:* 1066-1068, 1938.

15, *Handbook of Chemistry and Physics,* 42 Edition. Chemical Rubber Publishing Company, Cleveland, Ohio, 1960-1961, pp. 2967-2999.

16. Hermann, W.: Der Nachweis von Tuberkelbazillen Mit Dem Fluoreszenz Mikroskop. Dtsch. med. wschr., *64:* 1354-1356, 1938.

17. Hertz, C., Pawlecki, S. A., and Green, R. A.: Fluorescent staining and microscopy for detection of acid-fast bacilli. University of Michigan Med. Center J., *32:* 196-199, 1966.

18. Hughes, G. C.: An improved stain for fluorescence microscopy. Tubercle, *27:* 91 - 92, 1946.

19. Kaiserling, C.: Ueber die Unterscheidung der Tuberkelbazillen Mit Dem Fluoreszenzmikroskop. Z. Tuberk., *27:* 156, 1917. (Referred to by Ellinger, P.: Fluorescence microscopy in biology. Biol. Rev., *15:* 323-350, 1940 pp. 336).

20. Keller, C. J.: Vereinfachter Nachweis von Tuberkelbazillen im Fluoreszenzlicht. Muenchen, med. Wschr., *52:* 2024, 1938.

21. Koch, M. L., and Cote, R. A.: Comparison of fluorescence microscopy with Ziehl-Neelson stain for demonstration of acid-fast bacilli in smear preparations and tissue sections. Am. Rev. Resp. Dis., *91:* 283-284, 1965.

22. Korn, R. J., Kellow, N. F., Heller, P., Chomet, B., and Zimmerman, H. J.: Hepatic involvement in extrapulmonary tuberculosis. Am. J. Med., *27:* 60-72, 1959.

23. Kuper, S. W. A., and May, J. R.: Detection of acid-fast organisms in tissue sections by fluorescence microscopy. J. Path. & Bact., *79:* 59-68, 1960.

24. Lind, H. E.: Limitations of fluorescent microscopy for the detection of acid-fast bacilli. Am. J. Clin. Path., *19:* 72-75, 1949.

25. Matthaei, E.: Simplified fluorescence microscopy of tubercle bacilli. J. Gen. Microbiol., *4:* 393-398, 1950.

26. McClure, D. M.: The development of fluorescent microscopy for tubercle bacilli and its use as an adjunct to histological routine. J. Clin. Path., *6:* 273-281, 1953.

27. Muller, H. E. and Chermock, R. L.: A rapid staining technique for acid fast organisms. J. Lab. Clin. Med. *30:* 169-171, 1945.

28. Palmer, Marion H.: Personal Communication.

29. Richards, O. W., and Miller, D. K.: An efficient method for the identification of *M. tuberculosis* with a simple fluorescent microscope. Am. J. Clin. Path., Tech. Suppl. No. 5, 1-8, 1941.

30. Schallock, G.: Vereinfachter Nachweis von Tuberkelbazillen In Histologischen Schnitten Durch Die Fluoreszenz Methode Nach Hagemann., Muench. med Wschr., *87:* 102-103, 1940.

31. Silver H., Sonnenwirth, A. C., and Alex, N.: Modifications in the fluorescence microscopy technique as applied to identification of acid-fast bacilli in tissues and bacteriological material. J. Clin. Path., *19:* 583-588, 1966.

32. Tanner, F. H.: Fluorescence microscopy for demonstrating *M. tuberculosis* in tissues. Proc. Staff Meet. Mayo Clinic, *16:* 839-842, 1941.

33. Tanner, F. H., and McDonald, J. R.,: Granulomatous prostatitis. A histologic study of a group of granulomatous lesions collected from prostate glands. Arch. Path., *36:* 350-354, 1943.

34. Truant, J. P., Brett, W. A., and Thomas, W. Jr.: Fluorescence microscopy of tubercle bacilli stained with auramine and rhodamine. Henry Ford Med. Bull., *10:* 287-296, 1962.

35. von Haebler, T. Jr., and Murray, J. F.: Fluorescence microscopy as a routine method for detection of *M. tuberculosiss* and *M. leprae*. S. African Med. J., *28:* 45-48, 1954.

36. Wagoner, G. P., Anton, A. T., Gall, and Schiff: Needle biopsy of the liver. VIII Experiences with hepatic granulomas. Gastroenterol. *25:* 487-494, 1953.

37. Wellmann, K. F., and Kie Pin Teng: Demonstration of acid-fast bacilli in tissue sections by fluorescence microscopy. Canad. M.A.J., *87:* 837-841, 1962.

38. Yamaguski, B. T., and Braunstein, H.: Fluorescent stain for tubercle bacilli in histologic sections. II, Diagnostic efficiency in granulomatous lesions of the liver. Am. J. Clin. Path., *43:* 184-187, 1965.

39. Ziehl, F.: Zur Faerbung der Tuberkel Bazillen. Deutsche med. Wchnschr., *8:* 451, 1882.

Immunopathogenesis of Renal Disease

W. T. KNIKER, M.D.

During the past fifty years, immunologically induced renal disease in a variety of experimental situations has been studied extensively. Application of newer research techniques has brought us to a fairly clear understanding of the pathogenesis of glomerulonephritis (22). Accumulating clinical observations suggest that many types of human glomerular disorders are on an immunologic basis since they share so many features with experimental models (18,7). Some shared features include: 1) the development of hypersensitivity to specific antigens in association with nephritis; 2) lowering of serum complement; 3) circulating antibodies to renal antigens; 4) localization of antibody (host gamma globulin) and complement in affected glomeruli; and 5) a spectrum of morphologic alterations indicative of glomerulitis. Recent studies by many investigators, particularly those of Dr. Frank Dixon and his colleagues, have elevated to dogma the concept that many, if not most, cases of human glomerulonephritis are induced immunologically by the same mechanisms that are operative in experimental nephritis.

Two distinct mechanisms by which an antibody response causes glomerulonephritis now are well recognized (22,7). In either case, an antigen-antibody reaction is localized along glomerular basement membrane where it initiates an inflammatory response. The clinical form or severity of the subsequent glomerulitis is not characteristic for either pathogenic mechanism. Both may have a mild, indolent course or one that is severe and rapidly progressive. Although the two mechanisms of nephritis cannot be differentiated on clinical grounds, they are easily distinguished from each other by immunofluorescence and by electron microscopy (22,7,10).

THE FIRST PATHOGENIC MECHANISM:
GLOMERULAR DEPOSITION OF CIRCULATING
ANTIGEN-ANTIBODY COMPLEXES

One pathogenic mechanism of glomerulonephritis depends upon the formation of antibodies to soluble antigens not of glomerular origin. When such antigen and antibody combine in the blood stream, soluble immune complexes begin to circulate (8,26). Some of these complexes may become trapped passively along the filtering surface of the glomerular basement membrane. The complexes, containing antibody, antigen, and complement, aggregate within the basement membrane and along its outer aspects. By fluorescence, the deposits are particulate, irregular, granular or lumpy,

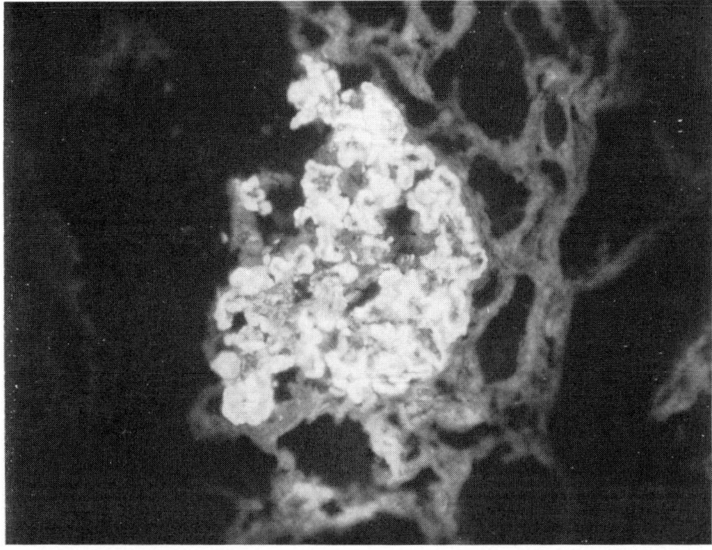

1a

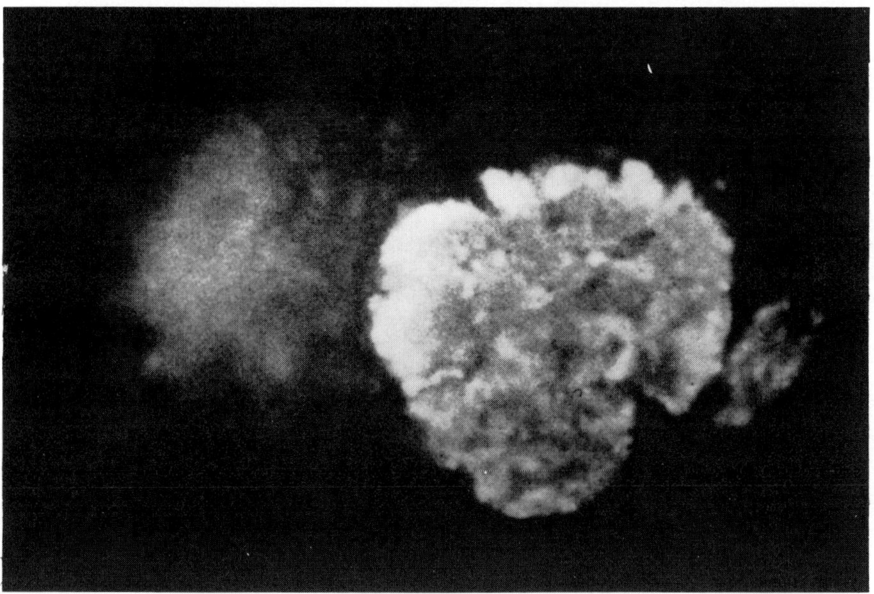

1b

Fig. 1. Immunofluorescent pattern of immune complex induced glomerulonephritis. Note the granular to lumpy fluorescent deposits irregularly spaced along the basement membrane of the representative glomerulus.

1a Chronic glomerulonephritis in rabbit following long-term circulation of bovine serum albumin (BSA)-antibody complexes. Stained with fluorescent antiserum to BSA.

1b Subacute glomerulonephritis in human. Stained with fluorescent antiserum to C'3 (third component of complement).

and may be distributed focally or diffusely (Fig. 1). By electron microscopy, such deposits can be seen to distort segments of the basement membrane and may protrude outward, pushing into the epithelial cells (Fig. 2).

When antibody meets antigen in the circulation, no glomerulitis will result unless resultant circulating complexes can penetrate the endothelial cell layer that lines the glomerular capillaries. Necessary for the deposition of complexes appear to be chemical mediators such as anaphylatoxin, histamine and serotonin that are released intravascularly by the interaction of immune complexes with complement, leucokytes and platelets (5,13,11). These released agents increase the permeability of the endothelial lining, permitting ingress of various macromolecules, including

TABLE 1—MEDIATION OF COMPLEX—INDUCED NEPHRITIS

1. Circulating antigen-antibody complexes
2. Passive deposition of complexes along glomerular basement membrane
   a. Vasoactive amines
   b. Hydrodynamic pressure
   c. Size of complexes
   d. Other factors?
3. Activation of complement (C′)
4. Release of chemotactic factors (C′5-6-7; C′3)
5. Accumulation of polymorphs with the release of lysosomal enzymes, peptides, etc.
6. Alterations in basement membrane and adjacent cells

antigen-antibody complexes (Table 1). Vascular localization of complexes is influenced also by their size. Only those complexes of intermediate size, formed in moderate antigen excess, are likely to be trapped in vessel walls (4). Other factors, such as hydrodynamic pressure

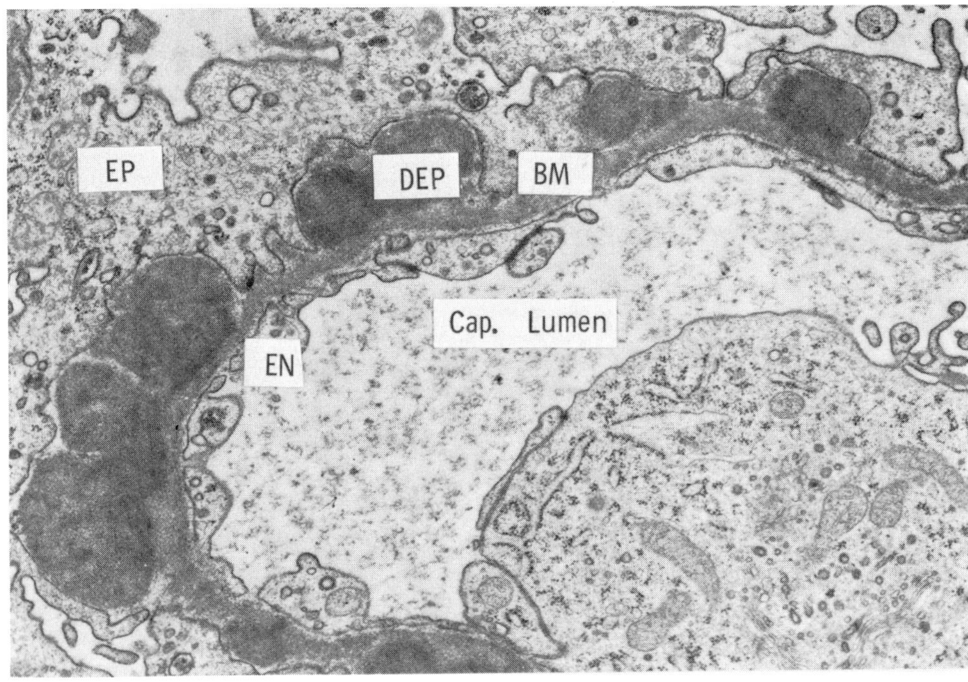

Fig. 2. Electron micrograph of rabbit glomerular capillary, demonstrating alterations in immune complex induced chronic glomerulonephritis. Cap. Lumen = capillary lumen. EN = Endothelial cell cytoplasm. BM = Basement membrane. DEP = Deposit. EP = Epithelial cell cytoplasm. (Courtesy of Dr. J. D. Feldman.)

TABLE 2—EXAMPLES OF COMPLEX-INDUCED NEPHRITIS

Experimental		*Human*
Animal Model	*Antigen*	
		A. *Acute*
Rabbit, serum sickness	Serum protein	Acute glomerulonephritis
Rabbit, chronic nephritis	Serum protein	Serum sickness
Rabbit, thyroiditis	Thyroglobulin	Anaphylactoid purpura
Rat, Heymann's nephritis	Prox. tub. cells	B. *Chronic*
NZB mice	Nucleoprotein	Subacute glomerulonephritis
Monkey	Strep. viridans	Chronic glomerulonephritis
Rabbit	E. coli	Membranous glomerulonephritis
Mouse	LCM virus	Lupus nephritis
		(Quartan) Malarial nephrosis

(13,9) and the character of antibody and antigen, undoubtedly play roles too (5,19).

As complexes accumulate along the basement membrane, complement is being activated continually (Table 1). The next important link in the chain of inflammation is the release of chemotactic factors; one is a trimolecular complex of C'5-6-7 (the fifth, sixth and seventh components of complement) and another appears to be a fragment of the C'3 (third component) molecule (25,24). These agents appear to be necessary for the attraction of polymorphonuclear neutrophiles (PMNs) into the area.

The function of the PMNs seems to be the removal and catabolism of the irritating immune complexes (3). Unfortunately, many PMNs are injured in the phagocytic process and there is a consequent discharge of lysosomal granules and their contents. It is this release of lysosomal cathepsins, other enzymes and cationic proteins that probably brings about the morphologic and pathphysiologic alterations typical of glomerulonephritis (3,21,12).

In Table 2 are listed examples of experimental glomerulonephritis known to be caused by deposited antigen-antibody complexes and examples of human glomerulonephritis believed to be caused by the same mechanism. For each animal model, the specified antigen can be found localized in the glomerular basement membrane along with host antibody and C'. Specific antigens have been demonstrated or strongly suspected in a few varieties of human nephritis: 1) streptococcal products in acute glomerulonephritis (2,1); 2) horse or bovine serum proteins in serum sickness (18); 3) nuclear antigens in lupus erythematosus (14); and 4) malarial protozoan antigen(s) in malarial nephrosis (Cited in 7). In the other examples of human nephritis with a deposited complex pattern of immunofluorescence, attempts to identify responsible exogenous or endogeneous antigens have proved unsuccessful so far.

THE SECOND PATHOGENIC MECHANISM ANTIBODY DIRECTED TO GLOMERULAR BASEMENT MEMBRANE ANTIGENS

In the second immunopathologic mechanism, antibodies that specifically react with antigenic components of the host's glomerular basement membrane

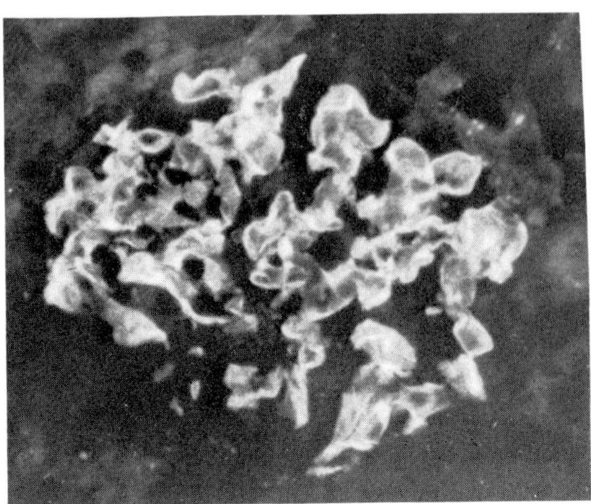

Fig. 3. Immunofluorescent pattern of nephrotoxic antibody induced glomerulonephritis. Rabbit had been injected intravenously with sheep antibody to rabbit glomerular basement membrane. Rabbit glomerulus stained with fluorescent antiserum to sheep gamma globulin. Note the linear, smooth, ribbon-like pattern of fluorescence along the glomerular basement membrane.

(gbm) are formed (22,15). As they circulate in the blood, such antibodies rapidly attach to the gbm. Because the antigenic sites are scattered uniformly along the basement membrane of all glomerular tufts, antibody and C′ are found in a smooth, continuous, ribbon-like linear pattern, as observed by fluorescence (Fig. 3). By electron microscopy, this immunologic reaction may not be detectable, although a thickening of the basement membrane along its inner aspect has been observed.

Once antibodies attach to gbm, C′ is activated and chemotactic factors are released, attracting PMNs to the site, just as was seen in complex induced nephritis (Table 3). Electron microscopic studies have shown that the PMN in the glomerular capillary lumen shoves aside the endothelial cell cytoplasm, to apply itself intimately against the naked basement membrane (6). In its attempt to

"get at" the antibody-gbm antigen reaction sites, the PMN apparently discharges lysosomal enzymes and proteins which bring about the inflammatory changes of glomerulitis (3,21,).

Experimentally, nephrotoxic serum nephritis can be induced two ways (Table 4). In one, antibody to gbm is produced in donor animals of species that are heterologous or homologous to that of the recipient. When the antibody is administered passively to the recipient animal, an immediate nephritis develops. Secondly, an animal can be actively immunized by gbm antigens from a variety of other animals. Produced antibodies, if they fix in his own glomeruli, may bring about autoimmune nephritis in the host (20,23). Of great fundamental importance is the recent observation by Lerner and Dixon that normal gbm products, excreted in the urine, can sensitize and cause autoimmune nephritis, following injection into the same animal that excreted the urine (16). Pathogenic nephrotoxic antibody can be eluted from nephritic kidneys at a pH of 3.2. This removed antibody later can be shown to fix specifically to gbm in vitro; it will induce nephritis when injected into new recipient animals *in vivo* (22,7,16).

TABLE 3—MEDIATION OF NEPHROTOXIC ANTIBODY —INDUCED NEPHRITIS

1. Antibody to glomerular basement membrane in circulation
2. Rapid fixation of antibody to antigenic sites along basement membrane
3. Activation of complement (C′)
4. Release of chemotactic factors (C′5-6-7; C′3)
5. Accumulation of polymorphs with the release of lysosomal enzymes, peptides, etc.
6. Alterations in basement membrane and adjacent cells

TABLE 4—EXAMPLES OF NEPHROTOXIC ANTIBODY-INDUCED NEPHRITIS

Experimental	Human

1. Passive administration of antibody to gbm
  a. Heterologous (Masugi)
  b. Homologous
	1. Goodpasture's syndrome

	2. Subacute glomerulonephritis

2. Immunization with gbm antigens
  a. Heterologous
  b. Homologous
  c. Autologous
	3. Chronic glomerulonephritis

	4. Immediate nephritis in renal allografts

In preliminary observations, Lerner *et al.* report that all cases of Goodpasture's syndrome, about half of the cases of subacute glomerulonephritis, and a smaller percentage of patients with chronic glomerulonephritis have a linear pattern of immunofluorescence in glomeruli (17). These findings strongly suggest that the patients' renal disease had been induced by auto-antibodies to their own gbm. In support of this notion was the finding that pathogenic antibody to gbm could be eluted from the kidneys in four of four cases of Goodpasture's syndrome, three of five cases of subacute nephritis, and two of twenty-nine cases of chronic glomerulonephritis. Some patients receiving renal allografts develop glomerulonephritis, showing the linear pattern of fluorescence, immediately after transplanting. This is not graft rejection. There is evidence to show that these individuals probably had auto-antibody (anti-gbm) induced nephritis originally, and that such antibodies rapidly fixed to and damaged the glomeruli of the donor kidney once it became exposed to the recipient's circulation (17). The mode of sensitization leading to auto-antibody induced glomerulonephritis in humans is obscure; one could speculate that either endogenous gbm antigens or exogeneous antigens cross-reacting with gbm might be responsible.

CONCLUSION

Many, if not most, cases of human glomerulonephritis appear to be caused by one of two possible immunologic mechanisms. In one case, circulating antigen-antibody complexes passively deposit and aggregate focally along the glomerular basement membranes. In the second case, autoimmune antibodies fix to antigenic sites uniformly spaced along glomerular basement membrane. In both cases, subsequent inflammation seems to be produced by common mediators, chiefly complement chemotactic factors and polymorphonuclear neutrophiles. Other mediators of inflammation, as yet not defined, probably are important.

The nature of offending antigens responsible for complex-induced nephritis remains unknown for most clinical examples of this mechanism. The mode of sensitization leading to antibodies directed against glomerular basement membrane and culminating in autoimmune glomerulonephritis in humans is obscure.

REFERENCES

1. Andres, G. A., Accinni, L., Hsu, K. C., Zabriskie, J. B., and Seegal, B. C.: Electron microscopic studies of human glomerulonephritis with ferritin-conjugated antibody. J. Exp. Med., *123*:399-412, 1966.
2. Andres, G. A., Seegal, B. C., Hsu, K. C., Rothenberg, M. S., and Chapeau, M. L.: Electron microscopic studies of experimental nephritis with ferritin-conjugated antibody. J. Exp. Med., *117*:691-704, 1963.
3. Cochrane, C. G.: Mediators of the Arthus and related reactions. Progress in Allergy., *11*:1-35, 1967.
4. Cochrane, C. G., and Hawkins, D.: Studies on cir-

culating immune complexes. III. Factors governing the ability of circulating complexes to localize in blood vessels. J. Exp. Med., *127*:137-154, 1968.

5. Cochrane, C. G., Hawkins, D., and Kniker, W. T.: Mechanisms involved in the localization of circulating immune complexes in blood vessels. Fifth Internat. Immunopathology Symposium, P. A. Miescher and P. Grabar (eds). New York. Grune and Stratton, Inc. pp. 32-48, 1967.

6. Cochrane, C. G., Unanue, E. R., and Dixon, F. J.: A role of polymorphonuclear leukocytes and complement in nephrotoxic nephritis. J. Exp. Med., *122*:99-116, 1965.

7. Dixon, F. J.: The pathogenesis of glomerulonephritis (editorial). Amer. J. Med. *44:*473, 1968.

8. Dixon, F. J.: The role of antigen-antibody complexes in disease. Harvey Lect., *58*:21-52, Academic Press, New York, 1962-1963.

9. Germuth, F. G., Jr., Kelemen, W. A., and Pollack, A. D.: Immune complex disease. II. The role of circulating dynamics and glomerular filtration in the development of experimental glomerulonephritis. Johns Hopkins Med. J., *120*:252-261, 1967.

10. Kniker, W. T.: Immunofluorescent methods in the diagnosis of renal disease. (Published elsewhere in this volume.)

11. Kniker, W. T.: The role of vasoactive amines in the pathogenesis of complex-induced chronic glomerulonephritis. Feder. Prac., 27:409, 1968.

12. Kniker, W. T., and Cochrane, C. G.: Pathogenic factors in vascular lesions of experimental serum sickness. J. Exp. Med., *122*:83-98, 1965.

13. Kniker, W. T., and Cochrane, C. G.: The localization of circulating immune complexes in experimental serum sickness. The role of vasoactive amines and hydrodynamic forces. J. Exp. Med., *127*:119-136, 1968.

14. Koffler, D., Schur, P. H., and Kunkel, H. G.: Immunological studies concerning the nephritis of systemic lupus erythematosus. J. Exp. Med., *126*:607-624, 1967.

15. Krakower, C. A., and Greenspon, S. A.: Localization of the nephrotoxic antigen within the isolated renal glomerulus. Arch. Path., *51*:629-639, 1951.

16. Lerner, R. A., and Dixon, F. J.: The induction of acute glomerulonephritis in rabbits with soluble antigens isolated from normal homologous and autologous urine. J. Immun., *100*:1277, 1968.

17. Lerner, R. A., Glassock, R. J., and Dixon, F. J.: The role of antiglomerular basement membrane antibody in the pathogenesis of human glomerulonephritis. J. Exp. Med., *126*:989-1004, 1967.

18. Michael, A. F., Drummond, K. N., Vernier, R. L., and Good, R. A.: Immunologic basis of renal disease. Pediat. Clin. of North Amer., *11*:685-721, 1964.

19. Pincus, T., Christian, C. L., and Haberkern, R. C.: Chronic glomerulonephritis induced by daily injection of bovine serum albumin (BSA)-character of antibodies (abs). Feder. Proc., *26*:702, 1967.

20. Steblay, R. W.: Glomerulonephritis induced in sheep by injection of heterologous glomerular basement membrane and Freund's complete adjuvant. J. Exp. Med., *116*:253-272, 1962.

21. Thomas, L.: The role of lysosomes in tissue injury. In: Zweifach, B. W., Grant, L. and McCluskey, R. T. (ed.): The Inflammatory Process, pp. 449-463, New York, Academic Press, 1965.

22. Unanue, E. R. and Dixon, F. J.: Experimental glomerulonephritis: Immunological events and pathogenetic mechanisms. Advances in Immunology (ed. Dixon, F. J., and Humphrey, J. H.), New York, Academic Press, *6*:1-90, 1967.

23. Unanue, E. R., Dixon, F. J., and Feldman, J. D.: Experimental allergic glomerulonephritis induced in the rabbit with homologous renal antigens. J. Exp. Med., *125*:163-176, 1967.

24. Ward, P. A.: A plasmin-split fragment of C'3 as a new chemotactic factor. J. Exp. Med., *126*:189-206, 1967.

25. Ward, P. A., Cochrane, C. G., and Muller-Eberhard, H. J.: Further studies on the chemotactic factor of complement and its formation in vivo. Immunology, *11*:141-153, 1966.

26. Weigle, W. O.: Fate and biological action of antigen-antibody complexes. Advances in Immunology (ed. W. H. Taliaferro, and J. H. Humphrey). New York, Academic Press, *1*:283-318, 1961.

Immunofluorescent Methods in the Diagnosis of Renal Diseases

WILLIAM T. KNIKER, M.D.

INTRODUCTION

For the understanding of pathogenic mechanisms in experimental renal diseases (1) and for the diagnosis of a variety of renal disorders (2, 3), the fluorescent antibody technique has proven to be of great value. The finding of localized antibody and complement (C') in human renal biopsies provides unique information as regards pathogenesis, management, and prognosis. Laboratories seeking to provide comprehensive diagnostic services should be able to apply immunofluorescent techniques to specimens of kidney obtained by percutaneous or open renal biopsy.

The fluorescent antibody method, first described in 1941 by Coons *et al*, depends upon the fact that antibody globulin can be linked chemically with a fluorochrome dye and still retain its immunological activity (4). The dye, when activated by ultraviolet light, acts as a marker to reveal sites of combination of labelled antibody with its corresponding antigen. Fluorescent antibody, therefore, can be used as a sensitive and specific histochemical reagent to detect antigens or antibodies on the tissue or cellular level. Modifications of the basic techniques and their application to a variety of problems have been discussed in thorough reviews (5–8).

Principle

The immunofluorescent (IF) technique rests entirely upon the principle that antigens react directly and specifically with antibodies having a complementary configuration. As this principle is applied in immunofluorescence, fluorochrome-labelled antibodies in solution deposit in those areas of tissue sections or cells where antigen is present. Subsequent washing removes labelled antibodies and inert proteins that did not fix. The specifically labelled antigen-antibody complexes can be visualized easily by microscopy employing ultraviolet excitation of the fluorochrome dye linked to fixed antibody.

Basic to all methods is the employment of an appropriate fluorochrome-labelled antibody. Certain criteria should be met: a) The fluorochrome ought to emit a high intensity of fluorescence distinct from the blue region of the spectrum, where tissue autofluorescence is common under ultraviolet light. Fluorescein derivatives that fluoresce green (9, 10) and lissamine rhodamine B200 that fluoresces orange (11) have been most popular. b) The immunologic activity and specificity of the antibody must be high, as determined by serologic and immunoelectrophoretic techniques. c) Non-specific fluorescence, removable by dialysis, chromatography, or tissue powder absorption, should be minimal.

Choice of IF methods depends upon the immunological reactants sought in the studied specimens. To detect antigens two approaches can be used. The direct method is the simplest: fluorochrome–labelled specific antibody reacts with antigen in the specimen. In the indirect method, non-labelled antibody is permitted to react with antigen in the material. After washing, the addition and fixation of labelled anti-globulin specific for that antibody identifies the tissue antigen-antibody complexes.

Antibodies in a specimen may be detected by the "sandwich" technique. A slide is flooded with a solution containing the appropriate antigen. After washing away unbound antigen, fluorescent antibody directed against the antigen combines with those antigen molecules complexed to antibody, thereby identifying foci of antibody in the specimen.

Only the direct method for detection of antigen will be outlined in this section, since this technique is adequate for diagnostic IF applications in clinical renal disorders. Methods of antibody production, characterization, purification, and conjugation with fluorochromes will not be discussed because commercially prepared fluorescent antibodies, satisfactory for clinical laboratory use, are available.

Reagents and Materials

1. *Staining dishes with covers* (minimum of 5).

2. *Ten-place slide racks* (minimum of 2).

3. *Physiologic phosphate* (0.01M) buffered saline (0.15M). Eighty gm of NaCl and 13.8 gm of NaH_2PO_4 are diluted to 10 L with distilled water, adjusting the pH to 7.0 with 7.0 ± ml of 40% NaOH.

4. *Anhydrous ethyl ether.*

5. *Absolute (dehydrated) ethyl alcohol.*

6. *Ethyl alcohol, 95%.*

7. *Gauze Sponges,* 4 x 4 inch.

8. *Fluorescein isothiocyanate conjugated antibodies to human serum proteins.* Labelled antibodies to gamma globulin (HGG) and to the third component of C′ (BIC/BIA globulin) are mandatory. Antibodies to fibrin-fibrinogen; albumin; or transferrin are useful as controls. These can be obtained for a number of suppliers, including:

Colorado Serum Company, Denver, Colorado

Fisher Scientific Company, Med. Lab. Division, Pittsburgh, Pennsylvania

Hoechst Pharmaceuticals, Cincinnati, Ohio

Hyland Laboratories, Los Angeles, California

Immunology, Inc., Glen Ellyn, Illinois

Microbiological Associates, Washington, D. C.

Pentex, Inc., Kankakee, Illinois

The Sylvana Company, Millburn, New Jersey

9. *Medicine dropper.*

10. *Mounting solution,* consisting of one part buffered saline solution and nine parts glycerol.

11. *Thin coverslips* (20 mm square or 20 x 30 mm).

12. *Twenty-place cardboard slide trays.*

Special Apparatus

1. Cryostat with microtome inside, preferably of stainless steel parts.

2. Serofuge (Adams) or centrifuge capable of 2500 rpm.

3. Staining chamber in which 20 to 40 3 inch slides can be placed horizontally. A tightly fitting cover is necessary to maintain humidity provided by wet gauze or sponge.

4. A standard research microscope with dark field condenser is basic. Objectives may be achromatic or apochromatic; high-power immersion objectives require an internal diaphragm. For fluorescence activation, a high power ultraviolet light source is essential. The HBO-200 (Osram), AH-6 (General Electric), and the ME/D (Mazda) 250 watt mercury vapor lamps are satisfactory.

Two types of filters must be used. The first (exciter) filter, which blocks all wavelengths except ultraviolet and dark blue, is placed between the light source and microscope slide. Between the light source and exciter filter a condensing lens and heat absorbant (distilled water; heat resistant filter; etc.) are necessary. The second (barrier) filter is placed between the microscope slide and eyepiece; it permits the passage of visible fluorescence but not ultraviolet light. Many paired combinations of filters may be used; the following are illustrative:

Exciter Filter	*Barrier Filter*
5-58, half-thickness (Corning)	OG − 4 (Zeiss)
OG − 2 (Zeiss)	Wratten 2B (Kodak)
5840, half-thickness (Corning)	Wratten 2B (Kodak)
Wratten 18A (Kodak)	Wratten 2B (Kodak)

5. Photomicrography of IF material with standard equipment is possible using high speed flims. Black and white (Polaroid, ASA 3000) and color (Anscochrome, ASA 200) exposure times vary between 10 and 90 seconds, depending upon field brilliance and the degree of magnification.

Procedure

The methods outlined were learned or developed in the laboratory of Dr. C. G. Cochrane, Division of Experimental Pathology, Scripps Clinic and Research Foundation, La Jolla, California. The fixing and staining method is a modification of the procedure described by Coons and Kaplan (9).

A. *Preparation of Specimen of Study.*

To preserve its morphology as well as its immunologic reactivity, the fresh renal specimen should be frozen rapidly. A needle biopsy specimen is laid lengthwise on the flat bottom of a molded "cup" of aluminum foil, containing 1.5 to 2.0 ml of lukewarm liquid 7% gelatin in water. The cup is floated on the surface of liquid nitrogen or a slush of butyl alcochol and solid CO_2 contained in a wide mouthed thermos. Once the specimen-in-gelatin is frozen, the cup is stored in a plastic air-tight container at -20°C. Kidney slices, 1 to 2 mm thick, that are obtained at open biopsy or autopsy, are placed against the inner wall of a test tube which is then immersed in the freezing solution. The tube should be sealed with a rubber stopper to avoid entry of freezing solution. The frozen tissue subsequently is stored in the closed tube at -20°C. Sections of kidney may be cut from the frozen "blocks" using a microtome in a cryostat cabinet at -15 to -20°C. A section, cut to 4 to 7 micra thickness, is flattened against a cold microscopic slide. It is further flattened and held in place by the warmth of a finger pressed against the underside of the slide. If the slides are not processed immediately they should be stored at 4°C in a moist environment for no longer than 36 to 48 hours.

B. *Fixation and Staining (Direct Technique)*

Slides bearing sections are convenitently processed in staining racks which can be transferred successively to appropriate staining dishes.

1. Mild fixation is necessary to prevent loss of water-soluble antigens. One can use an equal mixture of absolute ethyl alcohol and anhydrous ethyl ether at room temperature for 10 minutes. This is followed by 95% ethyl alcohol for 10 minutes.

2. To remove the alcohol, the slides are washed twice for 5 minutes (10 minutes, total) in cold buffered saline.

3. The top surface of each slide is dried with gauze leaving an island of wetness over the tissue. The slide is placed horizontally in the staining chamber and 1 to 2 drops of appropriate fluorescent antibody applied to the wet tissue. (Note: Sections should not be allowed to dry.) The fluorescent antiserum should have been just centrifuged at 2500 rpm for at least 5 minutes. Only the supernatant should be applied to the tissues, since sediment that accumulates with time greatly magnifies non-specific fluorescence. The staining time should be in the range of 15 to 30 minutes; a longer period increases background fluorescence. To avoid evaporation, high humidity is maintained inside the chamber during staining.

4. After staining, excess fluorescent antiserum is shaken off each slide before its replacement in a slide rack. The slides are washed for 10 minutes in cold buffered saline with two changes, one at 1 minute and the other at 5 minutes.

5. Each slide is dried as before and a drop of glycerol-saline mounting solution is put on the tissue. After mounting a coverslip, being careful to avoid air bubbles, the slide is stored in a slide holder at 4°C, for up to several months.

Note: Up to 20 slides (back-to-back) in a single rack can be processed in about 90 minutes. A maximum of 40 slides can be handled efficiently by beginning a second rack 10 minutes after the first. The fixatives should be replaced after each twenty slides.

C. *Microscopy*

A liberal amount of glycerol-saline or non-fluorescent immersion oil should be placed between the condenser and undersurface of the studied slide. The condenser and optical system are adjusted until a sharp circle of transmitted fluorescence shares the focal plane of the tissue being examined. If localized areas of brilliant fluorescence, typical of the fluorochrome employed, are observed, their location, pattern and intensity are noted.

Sources of Error

Analysis of renal specimens stained with fluorescent antisera requires great care as there are many possible sources of error. Difficulties in interpretation arise mainly from two factors. One is non-specific staining, caused by impurity or non-specificity of the labelled antibody; excessive amounts of labelled non-antibody proteins; or enhanced "stickiness' or adsorptive properties of studied tissues for labelled proteins. Adequate controls are required to permit proper interpretations. Useful controls include: 1) Partial inhibition (blocking) of fluorescence by prior application of unlabelled antibody; 2) The use of unrelated fluorescent antisera; 3) Absorption of fluorescent antibody by homologous antigen before staining; and 4) Comparison of positive slides with similarly stained sections known not to contain the antigen.

A second major source of difficulty is autofluorescence, induced in various extracellular components and intracellular structures by ultraviolet light. One may see a diffuse background glow that obscures specific fluorescence or may observe bright focal fluorescence. Autofluorescence can be recognized easily when it's color differs from that typical for the fluorochrome employed. In the kidney, autofluorescence is always present in the walls (elastin) of arteries and is occasionally seen in tubular epithelial cells.

Discussion and Clinical Interpretation

One of the hallmarks of immunologically induced experimental renal disease is the aggregation of antibody (gamma globulin) and C' (BIC globulin) along the glomerular basement membrane (gbm). Such deposition of immune reactants can be brought about two ways; each has a distinctive pattern of immunofluorescence (1, 12). In the first case, exemplified by serum sickness, circulating antigen-antibody complexes passively deposit along glomerular basement membranes. It is important to realize that the antigen and antibody need not be related immunologically to the kidney. Complexes localize by virtue of their size (13) and their ability to induce increased permeability in the endothelium of glomerular capillaries (14). Such complexes deposit in a random fashion throughout the glomeruli, the aggregates appearing to be focal and particulate, and granular to lumpy.

In the second case, antibody directed against gbm antigens is administered in-

travenously. Upon reaching the kidney, these "nephrotoxic" antibodies bind specifically to gbm of all glomerular tufts. In this Masugi model, the heterologous gamma globulin (nephrotoxic antibody) and host C' deposit diffusely in a smooth, linear, ribbon-like fashion. Recently, similar pathogenic mechanisms and IF patterns have been demonstrated in a variety of experimental situations, including examples of true autoimmunity to endogenous gbm antigens (12).

Extensive studies of renal tissues from patients with kidney disease have shown the both of the above described IF patterns are found. Each has been associated with certain disorders. The granular-lumpy pattern is typical for poststreptococcal acute glomerulonephritis, serum sickness, the nephritis associated with "collagen" diseases (i.e., lupus erythematosus), and malarial nephrosis (2, 3, 14, 15). The linear pattern is characteristic of Goodpasture's syndrome and rapidly rejecting renal allografts. (2, 12, 16).. Either IF pattern may be seen in subacute glomerulonephritis. In chronic glomerulonephritis, particularly with glomerulosclerosis, a distinctive IF pattern may be impossible to recognize. Absence of deposited HGG and C' in renal specimens is a strong argument against many diagnoses and against an immunologic basis of glomerular disease.

Fibrin (or fibrinogen) may be found localized in glomerular walls, Bowman's space, and along the basement membranes of Bowman's capsule and the tubules in some nephritides, toxemia of pregnancy and anaphlactoid purpura (2, 17). The significance of fibrin deposition is not yet clear. None of the other serum proteins are found along the gbm to any degree in experimental or clinical renal disorders. Any of the serum proteins may be found deposited irregularly in glomerular capillary lumens, beneath the endothelium, in the mesangium or in urinary casts.

In the evaluation of presumed immune complex induced renal disease, many attempts have been made to identify offending antigens at the sites of HGG and C' localization (12). Although nucleoprotein, malarial antigen, and streptococcal products have been implicated as antigenic components of deposited immune complexes in lupus erythematosis, malarial nephrosis, and acute glomerulonephritis respectively, the fact remains that the nature of offending antigens and mode of sensitization for most nephritides remain quite obscure.

REFERENCES

1. Unanue, E. R., and Dixon, F. J.: Experimental glomerulonephritis: Immunologic events and pathogenetic mechanisms. In, Advances in Immunology, *6*:1-90. New York, Academic Press, 1967.
2. Michael, A. F., Drummond, K. N., Vernier, R. L. and Good R. A.: Immunologic basis of renal disease. Ped. Clin. N. Amer., *11*:685-721, 1964.
3. Koffler, D., and Paronetto, F.: Immunofluorescent localization of immunoglobulins, complement, and fibrinogen in human diseases. II. Acute, subacute, and chronic glomerulonephritis. J. Clin. Invest., *44*:1665-1671, 1965.
4. Coons, A. H., Creech, H. J., and Jones, R. N.: Immunological properties of an antibody containing a fluorescent group. Proc. Soc. Exp. Biol., *47*:200-202, 1941.
5. Coons, A. H.: Fluorescent antibody methods. In, Danielli, J. F. (ed.): General Cytochemical Methods. New York, Academic Press, 1958, *1*:400-422.
6. Mellors, R. C.: Fluorescent-antibody method. In, Mellors, R. C. (ed.): Analytical Cytology (2nd ed.) New York, McGraw-Hill, 1959, pp. 1-67.
7. Beutner, E. H.: Immunofluorescent Staining: the fluorescent antibody method. Bacteriol. Reviews, *25*:49-76, 1961.
8. Holborow, E. J.: Fluorescent antibody techniques. In, AcKroyd, J. F. (ed.):Immunological Methods. Philadelphia, F. A. Davis, Co., 1964, pp. 155-174.
9. Coons, A. H., and Kaplan, M. H.: Localization of antigen in tissue cells. II. Improvements in a method for the detection of antigen by means of fluorescent antibody. J. Exp. Med., *91*:1-13, 1950.
10. Riggs, J. L., Seiwald, R. J., Burckhalter, J., Downs, C. M., and Metcalf, T. G.: Isothiocyanate compounds as fluorescent labelling agents for immune serum. Amer. J. Path., *34*:1081-1097, 1958.
11. Chadwick, C. S., McEntegart, M. G., and Nairn, R. C.: Fluorescent protein tracers; a trial of new fluorochromes and the development of an alternative to fluorescein. Immunology, *1*:315-327, 1958.
12. Dixon, F. J.: The Pathogenesis of glomerulonephritis (editorial). Amer. J. Med., *44*:473-498, 1968.
13. Cochrane, C. G., Hawkins, D., and Kniker, W. T.: Mechanisms involved in the localization of circulating immune complexes in blood vessels. In, Grabar, P., and Miescher, P. (eds.): Fifth International Immunopathology Symposium. New York, Grune and Stratton, Inc., 32-48, 1967.
14. Kniker, W. T., and Cochrane, C. G.: The localization of circulating immune complexes in experimental serum sickness. The role of vasoactive amines and hydrodynamic forces. J. Exp. Med., *127*:119-136, 1968.
15. Koffler, D., Schur, P., and Kunkel, H. G.: Immunological studies concerning the nephritis of systemic lupus erythematosis. J. Exp. Med., *126*:119-136, 1968.
16. Lerner, R. A., Glassock, R. J., and Dixon, F. J.: The role of antiglomerular basement membrane antibody in the pathogenesis of human glomerulonephritis. J. Exp. Med., *126*:989-1004, 1967.
17. McCluskey, R. T., Vassalli, P., Gallo, G., and Baldwin, D. S.: An immunofluorescent study of pathogenic mechanisms in glomerular diseases. New Eng. J. Med., *274*:695-701, 1966.

Chapter 30

Radioisotope Scanning Techniques in the Diagnosis of Renal Disease

AUGUST MIALE, Jr., M.D., and JOSEPH S. BURKLE, M.D.

INTRODUCTION

Renal photoscanning has become an accepted routine procedure in the diagnosis of renal disease. Tauxe has stated that "potentially the greatest customer of the diagnostic radioisotope laboratory is the nephrologist" (1). Techniques, instrumentation and diagnostic accuracy have evolved considerably since the early reports (2, 3, 4, 5, 6). Since two forms of the basic instrumentation are available in current practice, the methodology for uses of each will be presented. One is based on the original concept in scanning instruments utilizing the principle of point-by-point survey of an organ or area (7). This is done by moving a detector probe composed of a relatively small sodium iodide crystal and focusing collimator systematically over the body surface on a raster mechanism. The relative concentration of radioactivity is converted to light and recorded on x-ray film as an image of actual organ size or radioisotope distribution. This is known as rectilinear scanning. The other concept, scintillation camera scanning, was introduced by Anger (8, 9) and involves the use of a large-diameter stationary detector and multihole straight-bore collimator. Becuase of the inherent design of the scintillation camera, it is possible to study three separate aspects of renal function and anatomy sequentially during a single study using three different radiopharmaceuticals. These include: a) renal size, configuration and position: b) renal tubular function, and c) renal blood flow distribution. This device views the entire organ at once, in contrast to the point-by-point survey of rectilinear scanning. Imaging data are presented on an oscilloscope face and accumulated on high-speed Polaroid film. The scan image is reduced in size by a factor of 8. Many publications support the clinical applicability and diagnostic reliability of this instrument (10, 11, 12). Other designs of scintillation camera instruments have only recently been introduced commerically, so that little published data are available which describe their uses in comparable clinical settings.

Principle

Radiolabelled tracers concentrate in renal tissues so that they can be detected, and the distribution is visually portrayed by suitably designed instruments (5, 13). The nature of the carrier molecule will determine the characteristics of localization, e.g., radiomercury (^{203}Hg) labelled chlormerodrin (RMC) behaves like the parent non-radioactive chlormerodrin (Neohydrin). In pharmacological doses, this drug produces diuresis. In trace amounts, no diuresis is produced, but approximately 5-10% of the labelled material remains as a stable salt attached to sulfhydryl enzyme systems, primarily in cortical renal tubular cells. In the normal kidney, radioactivity is distributed evenly throughout the renal parenchyma, reflecting the structural integrity of the kidney.

Radioiodine labelled sodium ortho-iodohippurate (ROIH) behaves like para-aminohippurate (1). It is rapidly concentrated from blood into proximal tubular cells and rapidly secreted into urine. This produces a transient rapid rise in radioactivity with a peak at 4-5 minutes, normally followed by a precipitous loss of activity over the next 30 minutes. This pattern of uptake and excretion can be monitored with suitable detectors and presented in analog display on a strip chart. This tracing is called a renogram. A full discussion of the clinical applications of the renogram has been published recently by Taplin (14). Rapid sequential photoscans can also be made with the scintillation camera at short intervals to depict the regional intrarenal radioisotope distribution and total activity with respect to time. This spatial display of actual events in the kidney can then be interpreted in combination with the time-concentration curve tracing using either ROIH or RMC. The latter produces data which can be used as an independent comparison of renal blood flow (15).

An additional aspect of renal diagnosis includes the visualization of regional renal blood flow by sequential imaging of concentrated high-activity, short-lived, gamma-emitting externally detectable isotopes, such as ^{99m}Technetium (sodium pertechnetate, PTc) injected intravenously.

Details of scintillation camera and rectilinear scanner design, and physical principles are reviewed extensively by Anger (9) and by Beck (16).

Radiopharmaceuticals

1. Radiomercury (^{203}Hg) labelled chlormerodrin (Neohydrin) solution for I.V. use, 100 microcuries/ml (approx.).

2. Radioiodinated (^{131}I) sodium ortho-iodo-hippurate solution for I.V. use, 100 microcuries/ml (approx.).

3. Sodium pertechnetate (^{99m}Tc) solution for I.V. use, 2-4 millicuries/ml, obtained separately or prepared by eluting a radiomolybdenum (^{99}Mo) column.

These materials are available from several commercial radiopharmaceutical suppliers, but specific authorization is required in the form of a U. S. Atomic Energy Commission license or license from individual state licensing authorities where applicable.

Special Materials
A. Rectilinear Scanning

1. X-ray film (24 x 17-inch Kodak Blue Brand or DuPont Cronex I). Use the type specifically recommended by the manufacturer of the rectilinear scanner.

2. Teledeltos or other paper for dot positioning readout.

B. Scintillation Camera

1. Polaroid film pack, type 107 (ASA 3000).

2. Strip chart paper.

C. Both

1. Syringes (1.0, 10.0 and 20.0 ml, plastic or glass, disposable type).

2. Needles (19 or 20 gauge, disposable).

3. Plastic disposable gloves.

Special Apparatus

1. Rectilinear scanner (Picker, Nuclear-Chicago, Baird-Atomic Corp., etc.) equipped with either 3-inch or 5-inch sodium iodide crystal detector.

2. Anger-type scintillation camera with dual ratemeter and dual strip chart recorded modifications (Nuclear-Chicago, PhoGamma III).

Procedure

A. Rectilinear Scanning

1. No patient preparation is necessary.

2. 100-200 microcuries of RMC are injected I.V.

3. Scanning can begin in 30-60 minutes, depending on the rate of clearance of the labelled material from the blood. If necessary, the procedure can be delayed as long as twenty-four hours, since sufficient radioactivity is usually retained for this length of time.

4. The patient is comfortably settled in the prone position. A pillow under the abdomen will often increase comfort and avoid unnecessary motion by the patient. The patient is instructed to lie as still as possible and to breathe quietly. Appropriate sedation is justified in children or hyperkinetic adults when cooperation appears unpredictable. Optimal diagnostic information from the radioactivity administered is obtainable only when motion is minimal.

5. With the analyzer set for the ^{203}Hg photopeak (279 Kev, with an 80 Kev window setting), the moveable probe is positioned over the renal area and the highest count rate located. The photorecording circuitry, speed and field limits are adjusted appropriately, according to the specifications of the individual instrument (see respective instruction manuals). Suitable landmarks can be placed on the film or dot paper if desired. Scanning is started from below the kidney to minimize pickup from radioactivity collecting in the bladder urine during the course of the procedure.

6. After the area of interest has been scanned, the x-ray film is developed and inspected to confirm that a technically satisfactory image has been recorded. When evidence of motion, poor positioning or inappropriate settings is present, the scan is repeated.

B. Scintillation Camera Scanning

1. a. Adequate hydration of the patient is necessary for the renogram phase of the triple isotope study to insure urine flow, and may be obtained by giving water (10 to 20 ml per Kg of body weight) orally or I.V. as glucose or saline from 1 to 2 hours prior to the study. In certain patients this volume of fluid may be contraindicated, and the dose should be altered accordingly.

b. 150 microcuries of RMC is injected I.V. The analyzer photopeak is set for 279 Kev with a 25% window. If it is desired to obtain relative count data from both kidneys during this phase of the study, the crystal is electronically divided, the strip-chart recording begun 5 minutes after injection and continued for about 45-60 minutes.

c. 30-60 minutes after injection the patient is usually placed in the prone position as with the rectilinear study. However, because of the maneuverability of the camera detector head, the patient may be scanned while upright or supine. Under-table type rectilinear probes also allow scanning the patient in the supine position.

d. About 70,000 counts are recorded on the film (2-5 minutes) using the full crystal area with the 3-inch multihole (1000) collimator and appropriate dot intensity. Posterior and oblique projections are made routinely. The scan photos are labelled.

2. a. With the patient in the same position, the recording area of the 11-inch diameter crystal, which views both kidneys simultaneously, is divided by an electronic switch, so that right and left renal activity are recorded separately by the respective half of the crystal area.

b. The strip-chart recorder is started at 12 inches per hour and the analyzer photopeak reset to 364 Kev. Then 200 microcuries of ROIH are injected I.V.

c. Serial one-minute Polaroid exposures are made during the first 5 minutes, then one-minute exposures at 4-minute intervals for a total of thirty minutes, with the strip-chart running.

3. a. The collimator may be changed to a 1-3/4 inch multihole (4000) unit and the patient repositioned using the 279 Kev photopeak energy to reorient both kidneys within the field of the crystal, with one or two quick Polaroid prints as a final check. The original collimator can be left in place and used for this last phase; however, definition is slightly better with the 4000-hole unit.

b. After resetting the photopeak to 140 Kev, 10-15 millicuries of (PTc) are rapidly injected I.V. as a small bolus (1-5 ml) using a 20 ml syringe. A Polaroid photo is taken every three seconds for 8 exposures. Appropriate intensity settings are determined in advance by trial and error.

Discussion

A universal feature of these procedures is their high degree of safety and minimal discomfort to the patient. Allergy to iodide does not preclude use of (ROIH) since the quantity of iodide is small and allergic actions have not been reported. Radiation exposure is low and well below that received from other standard radiologic techniques. There are no specific contraindications to any of these studies provided the patient can tolerate transportation to the laboratory.

The bulk of experience in radioisotope renal scanning has been accumulated since 1960 using 3- or 5-inch diameter detector rectilinear scanners. These produce a single projection of the kidneys in about 15-30 minutes in most instances. The scintillation camera accumulates the data more rapidly and scans can be obtained in 2-5 minutes. This reduction in time and the maneuverability of the detector head make additional projections practical and enhance the diagnostic value of the procedure. The ability of the camera to record a readable image in a few seconds makes it feasible to visualize blood flow and tubular function as indicated by the respective tracers used.

The current applications of radioisotope techniques are listed in Table I. For additional details, see references 17-29.

TABLE I—USES OF RADIOISOTOPE SCANNING TECHNIQUES IN DIAGNOSIS OF RENAL DISEASE

1. Anatomical variations: size, configuration, position, congenital abnormalities.
2. Renovascular disease: infarcts, ischemia, renal artery occlusion.
3. Space-occupying lesions: cysts, tumors, abscesses.
4. Trauma.
5. Localization for renal biopsy.
6. Stasis of collecting system.
7. Homograft rejection.
8. Residual functional tissue in cystic disease.

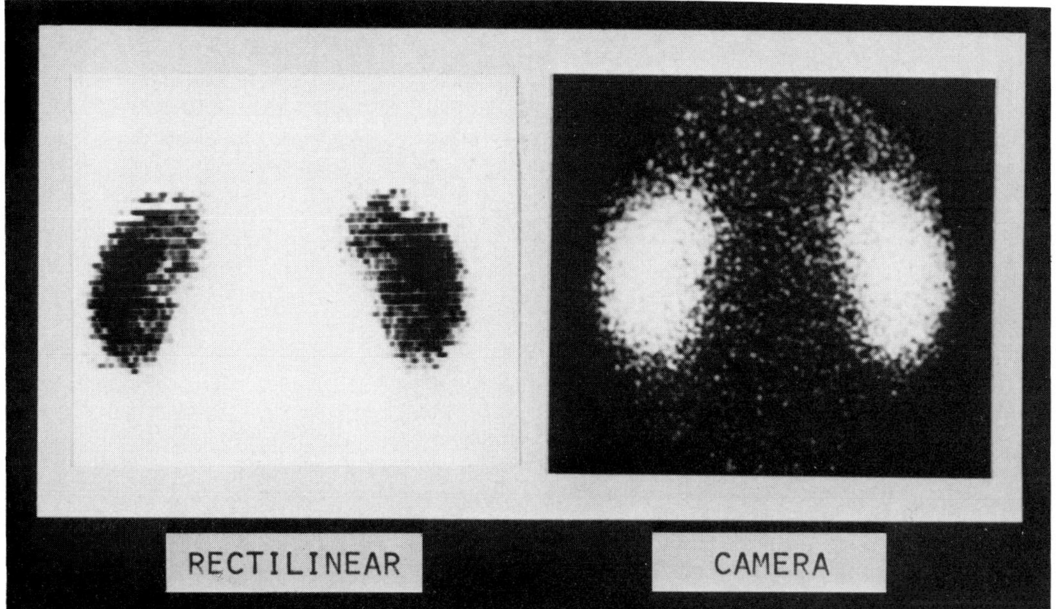

Fig. 1. Rectilinear scan (left) and scintillation camera study (right) of the same normal patient. The distribution of activity is homogeneous in all areas of both kidneys. There are some minor variations in the appearance of the activity seen in the right kidney on the rectilinear study, probably related to respiratory motion. With the patient in the prone position, the kidneys normally lie at approximately the same level.

Sources of error

Certain technical factors can be identified as causes of poor photoscans and thus lead to erroneous diagnosis. The more common errors include: use of outdated material or incorrectly calculated radioactive decay, extravasation of labelled material during injection, improper instrument set-up, improper positioning of the patient or of the detector probe, patient motion, high radioactivity room background (constant or intermittent), outdated x-ray film, poor developing technique, excessive main voltage variation, marginal "scalloping" in a rectilinear scan, and excessive background cut-off. This last factor tends to decrease the size of the kidney image. If the scintillation camera detector is not as close to the patient as possible, there is an unnecessary decrease in count rate. If too low over the back, bladder activity may be recorded later in the renogram phase (Part 2, pages 6 and 7)of the study and produce an appearance of prolonged urine retention. This artifact is easily detected, since it would be visible on the Polaroid prints as well.

Azotemia will impede the concentration of RMC and ROIH in the kidney, which generally results in a less well defined image. This can be overcome to some degree by larger doses of radioactivity, by waiting longer for blood background clearance or by increasing background suppression. One advantage of these techniques is that useful anatomical information can usually be obtained even in the presence of moderately severe azotemia and often in patients where the I.V.P. does not visualize. A useful change in the routine sequence of studies in severely azotemic patients is to perform the ROIH phase

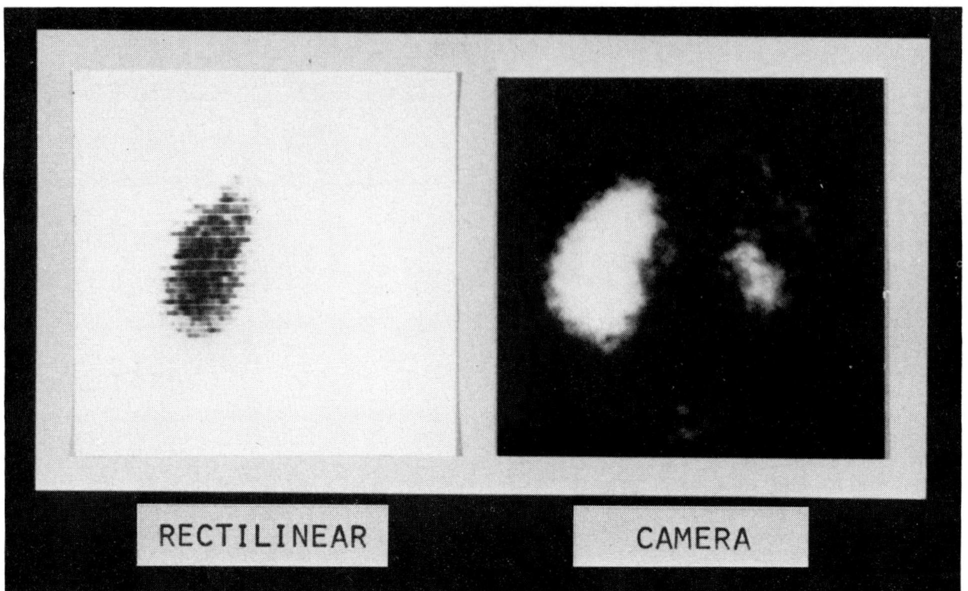

Fig. 2. Rectilinear scan (left) and scintillation camera study (right) of the same patient. The left kidney shows an essentially normal shape and size with a homogeneous distribution of activity. There is a small amount of activity seen in the area of the right kidney which represents a congenital hypoplastic kidney. The activity in this same area on the rectilinear scan is less well defined than on the camera study. This is due in part of the absence of background suppression in the camera study, which thereby increases the appearance of such areas of low concentration.

first, followed by PTc injection and lastly the RMC. If poor visualization is obtained with RMC, then additional views should be obtained the following day. Patients who have only recently undergone retrograde pyelography may have some residual ureteral spasm which causes an apparent pooling of ROIH in the renal pelvis or in the ureter itself. This is reflected by a prolongation of the renogram excretory phase and by collections of activity proximal to the site of obstruction.

PTc appearance in the kidney during the first or second circulations depends solely on blood flow, so that the presence of one or two kidneys, size, position and relative integrity can be judged remarkably accurately in the patient with acute renal shutdown. This rapid serial scanning with the scintill-ation camera for renal blood flow visualization requires injection of the material as a bolus. A smoothly executed injection with firm thrust of the syringe barrel with a free-flowing needle well placed in a suitable antecubital vein is very satisfactory. A Velcro cuff is sometimes helpful but not mandatory. Slowed circulation from heart failure or mechanical venous obstruction may prevent appearance of radiotracer in sufficient concentration for adequate diagnosis.

Clinical Interpretation

All the photoscan images produced in these studies are presented as positive activity on a negative background. The scanning image made with RMC provides direct information with regard to renal size, position and homogeneity of viable

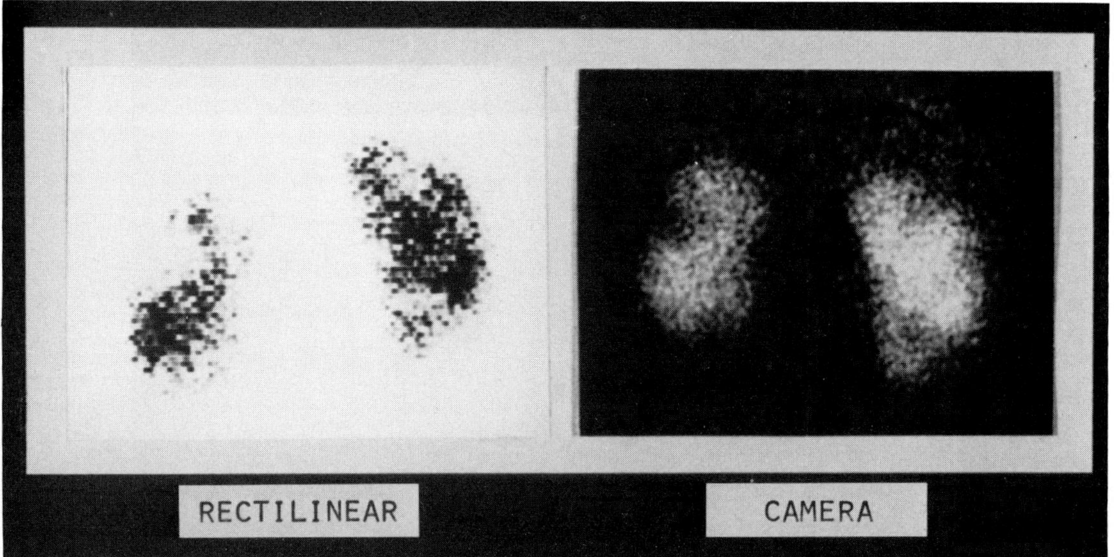

Fig. 3. Rectilinear scan (left) and scintillation camera study (right) of the same patient with polycystic renal disease, showing multiple areas of diminished uptake in both kidneys. The various defects seen in the camera study can also be defined in the rectilinear study indicating the close comparability of the diagnostic information available.

renal tissue (Fig. 1). In contrast, the intravenous pyelogram reflects the detailed anatomy of the calyces and collecting systems, but visualizes renal parenchyma poorly. Clinically significant obstruction of blood flow such as may be seen in congenital hypoplasia of a renal artery will result in a diffuse decrease in relative density of the affected side (Fig. 2). Space-occupying masses and areas of local ischemia due to chronic infection appear as marginal or intraparenchymal filling defects, local mottling or irregularity of distribution of activity (Fig. 3, 4, and 5).

The ROIH image can be evaluated in two ways. First, sufficient activity can be recorded soon after injection to provide an acutal scan of the kidneys based on the distruibution of the radioiodine label as is done with the RMC. Secondly, frequent short individual scan periods can reflect the dynamic changes in distribution within the kidney with respect to time. This is particularly valuable to visualize intracalyceal obstruction, hydronephrosis or cystic lesions (Fig. 6. 7 and 8).

The value of visualization of PTc flow through the kidney rests with the degree with which this represents renal blood flow. The resolution of photoscanning does not approach that available in standard angiography. However, the presence of clinically significant alterations in relative renal blood flow can be readily apparent in patients with hypertension (Fig. 9). This triple isotope approach should prove to be very valuable in screening hypertensive patients for correctable unilateral renal disease prior to aortography.

PTc will concentrate in renal carcinoma to a degree indistinguishable from normal renal tissue. By comparing the defect in a RMC scan caused by a tumor with the appearance of blood flow distribution, the distinction

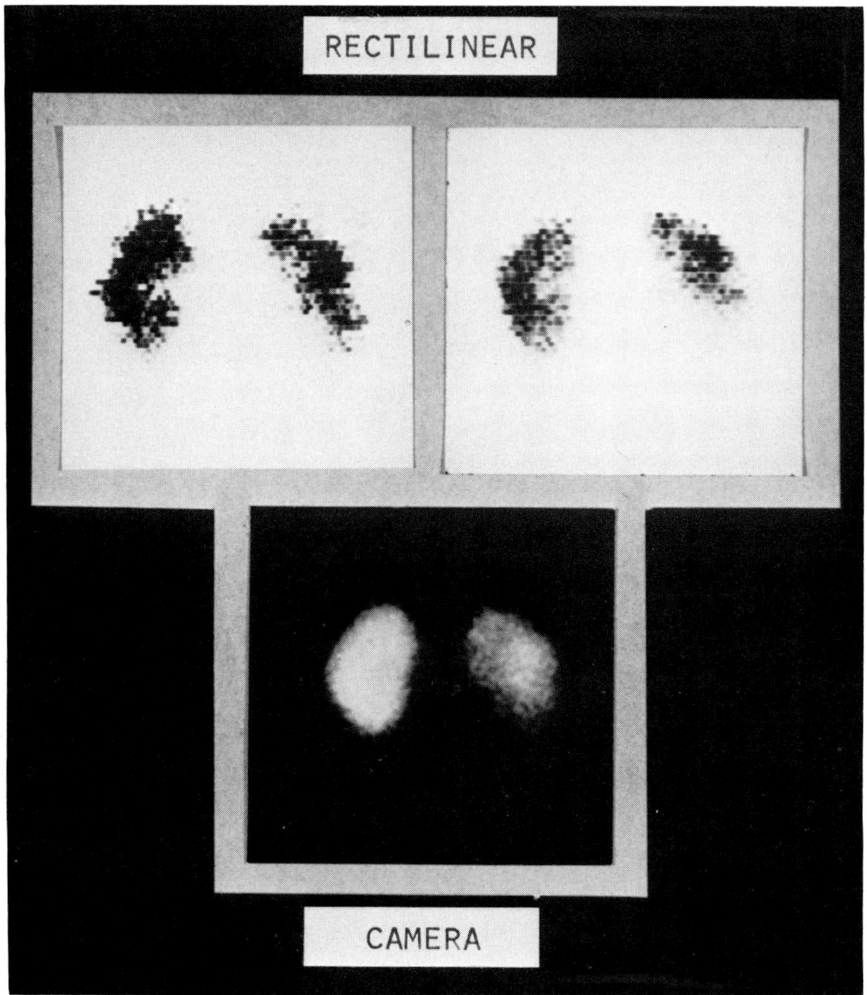

Fig. 4. Rectilinear scans (upper part) and scintillation camera study (lower) of the same patient. The two rectilinear studies shown were done sequentially under slightly different scanning conditions. The study on the left shows some motion artifact; the study on the right shows less motion artifact but reveals an area of diminished activity in the vicinity of the pelvis of the left kidney. This is not an uncommon finding in normal patients and represents a fortuitous passage of the focused scanning "plane" through the pelvic area of the kidney where there is less renal parenchyma to concentrate RMC. The right kidney, on the other hand, shows a definite patchy decrease in RMC uptake at the lower pole. A similar pattern is seen in the scintillation camera study. This patient had chronic pyelonephritis of the right kidney producing irregularities in the distribution of RMC activity. The left kidney appears normal.

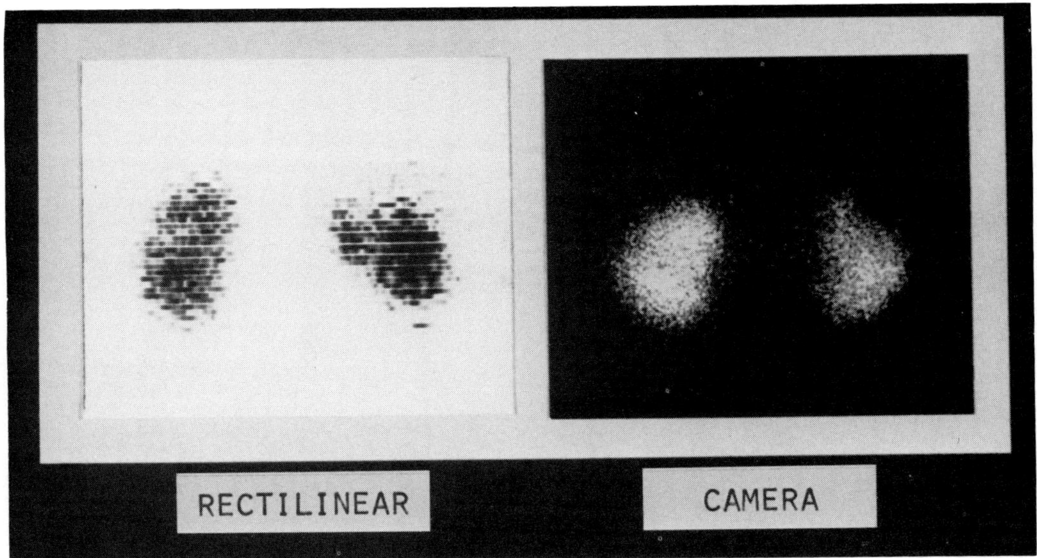

Fig. 5.　Rectilinear scan (left) and scintillation camera study (right) of the same patient. Both show an irregular defect located at the upper pole of the right kidney. This patient had a sudden onset of flank pain and hematuria and was believed to have had an embolus from the left heart to the right kidney with infarction of the upper pole.

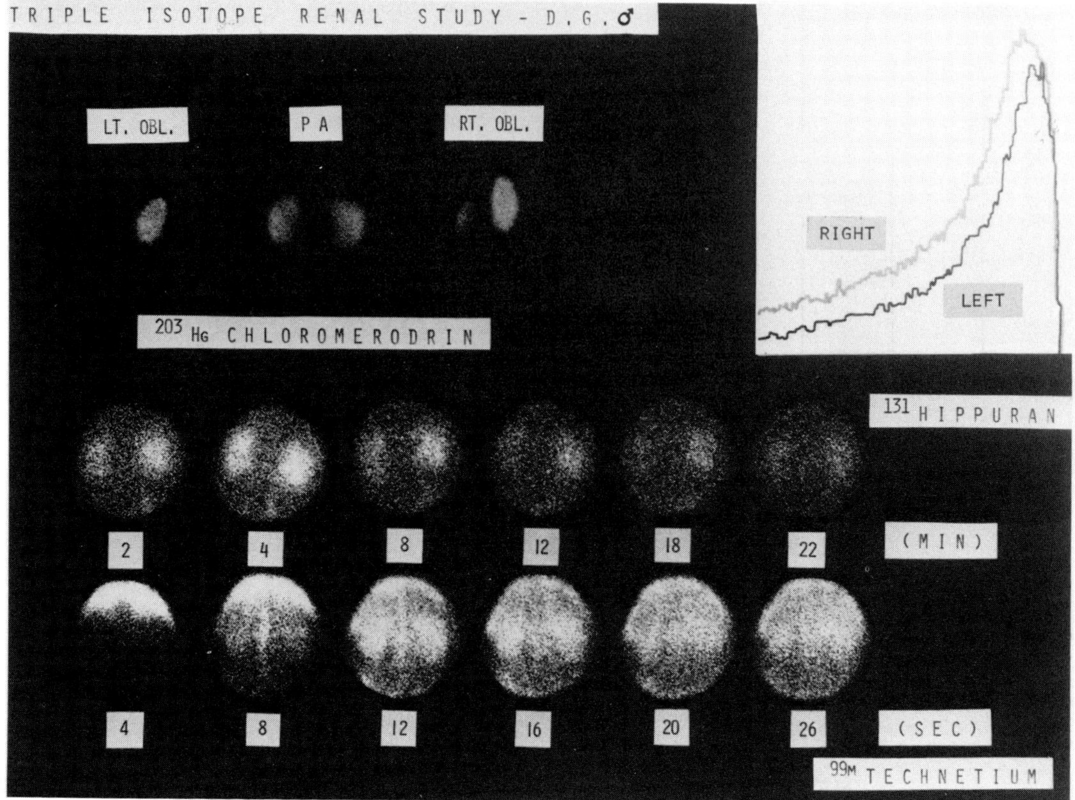

Fig. 6. In this study, the results of three scanning approaches in the same patient are displayed together. The upper left-hand group of images shows the standard renal scan with RMC. Note the left oblique and right oblique projections showing additional aspects of the renal anatomy. In the right-hand upper corner, the renogram is presented and shows a slightly higher amplitude over the right kidney as compared to the left. In reviewing the serial photographs of ROIH passage through the kidneys, it is evident that the right kidney retains activity longer than the left, and that this activity is distributed in a somewhat diffuse fashion throughout the renal parenchyma. It is apparent, therefore, that the slightly elevated renogram curve often seen over the right kidney in standard probe studies may not be due to greater retention in the liver on the right side but may be related to parenchymal or distal obstruction of urinary flow in the right kidney. PTc rapid serial blood flow sequences show a prompt appearance of activity in both kidneys, which is particularly evident in the 12-second frame. The patient was evaluated for hypertension but no significant renal lesions were found in subsequent studies.

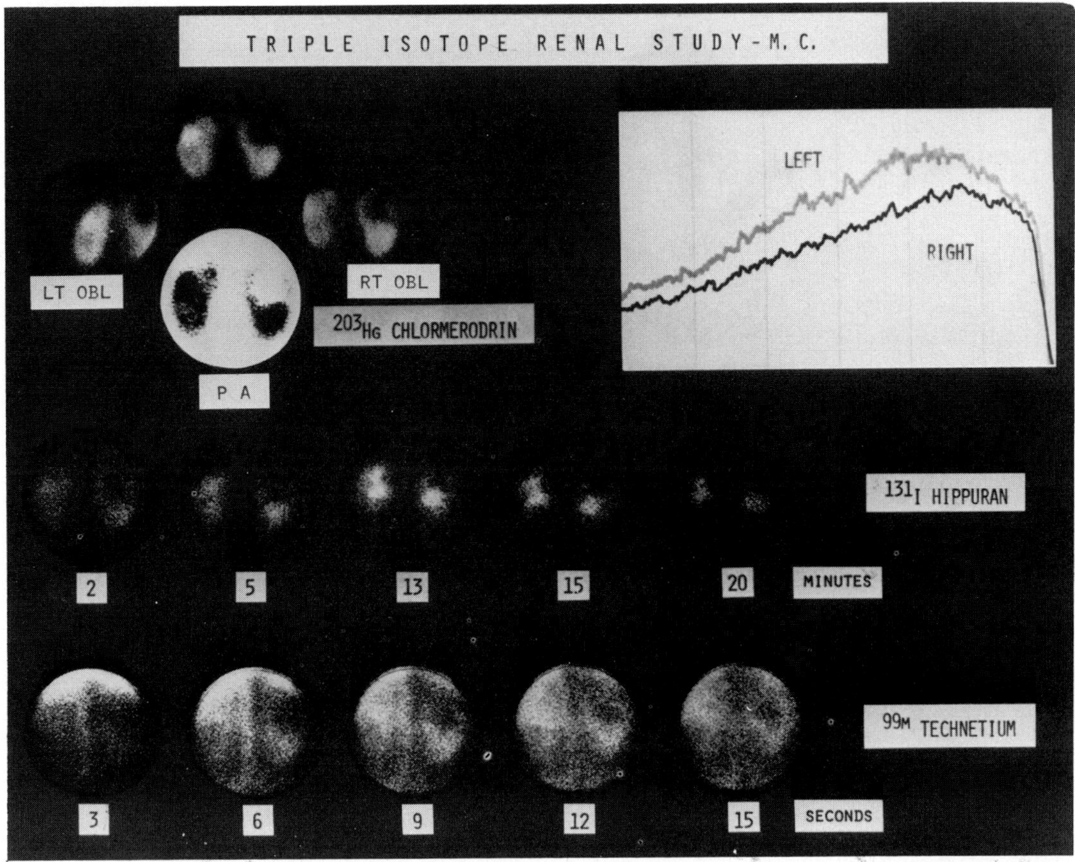

Fig. 7. This is the combined renal study in a patient with obvious polycystic renal disease. This subject is the daughter of a patient with well documented polycystic disease. She was asymptomatic, and the study was performed for screening purposes only. Multiple cysts and irregularities in distribution of activity are evident in the upper left-hand group of photographs, where posterior and right and left oblique projections are presented. The comparable rectilinear study is shown below the posterior projection of the scintillation camera view. In the upper right, the renogram shows a rather slow concentration of activity in the kidneys and a poorly defined and slightly delayed peak. The excretory or downward phase of the curve on both sides is abnormal and indicates retention. The photographs of this ROIH passage through the kidneys show, particularly in the 13- and 15-minute frames, evidence of increased concentration of activity in both kidneys, probably related to upper calyceal obstruction secondary to pressure from adjacent cysts. The renogram and serial ROIH studies suggest that residual renal tissue is functioning normally but that the total amount is probably reduced due to incursion from cysts and that there is secondary obstruction to urinary flow from the multiple intraparenchymal cysts themselves. The rapid serial PTc study shows that there is blood flow in the major functional portions of both kidneys; this is particularly evident in the 9-second frame. The large area in the upper pole of the right kidney devoid of activity corresponds to the well defined cyst seen in the RMC study.

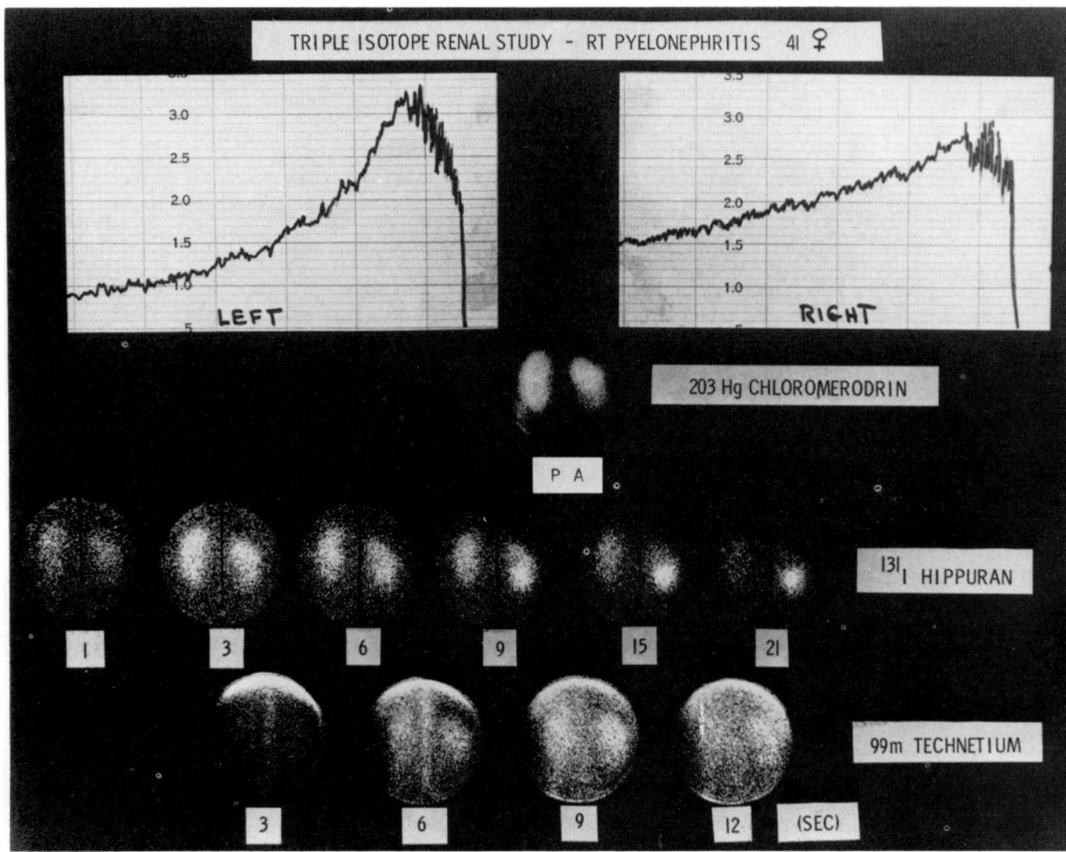

Fig. 8. This patient with chronic pyuria showed x-ray evidence of a duplicated drainage system on the right side. Renograms indicate definite abnormality of function of the right kidney as compared to the left. The RMC scan shows a patchy decrease in activity in the lower pole of the right kidney. Serial ROIH scans clearly define increased concentration and delayed excretion of ROIH in the lower pole of this kidney. This is interpreted as indicating the presence of some functional tissue but poor drainage of the calyceal system in this area of the kidney. The PTc rapid serial studies show essentially normal distribution of flow through both kidneys with only a slight patchy decrease in the inferior pole. The presence of poor drainage, poor tubular concentration of RMC and an abnormal renogram on the right confirm anatomical and functional abnormality of the lower pole of this kidney.

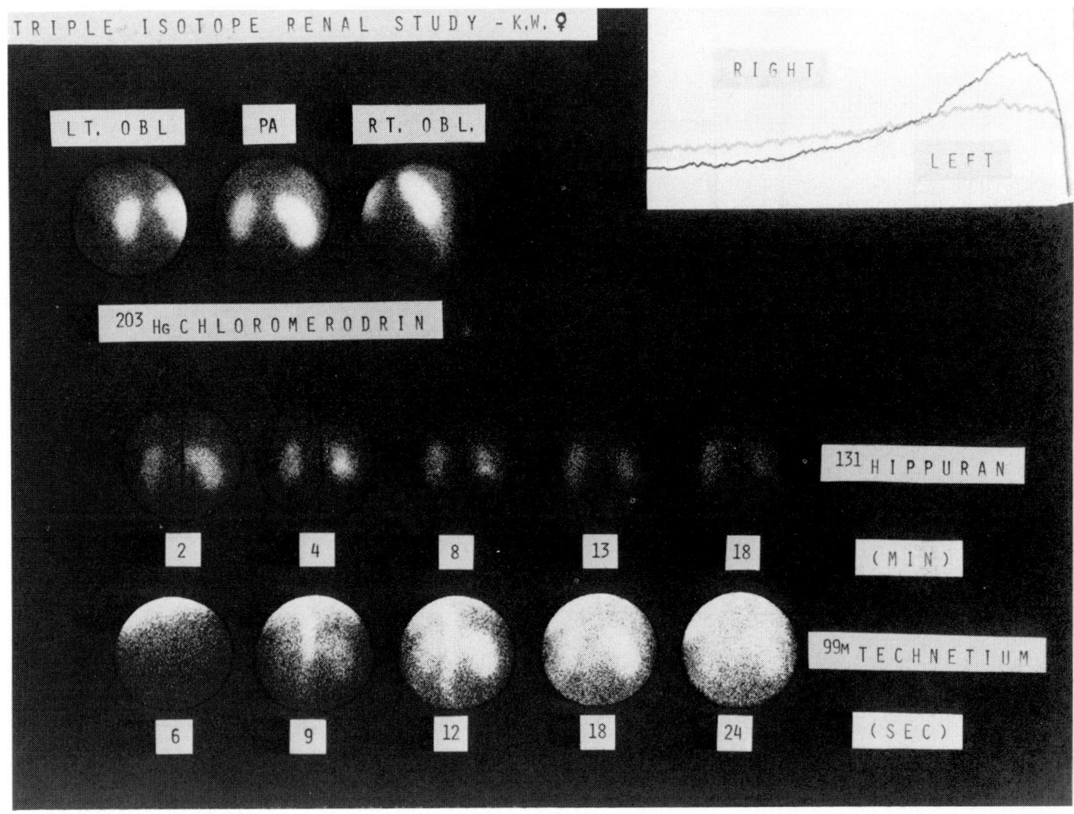

Fig. 9. In this patient screened for unilateral renal disease in the presence of hypertension, the RMC scan clearly shows a discrepancy in the appearance of the right and left kidneys. The right kidney is normal in size and concentration, whereas the left kidney is smaller and shows a striking decrease in total concentration of activity. The renogram shows a normal pattern over the right kidney but an abnormal pattern over the left kidney as characterized by relatively less concentration, poor definition of peak and prolonged retention of activity. Serial ROIH scans also reflect this same phenomenon and show delay in the uptake of activity in the 2-minute frame. Subsequently, a diffuse retention of activity is seen in the 18-minute frame. The PTc rapid serial study, however, shows a striking difference in the flow of blood in the right and left kidneys, with the right kidney filling promptly and a marked delay and relatively lower concentration of activity in the left kidney. The patient was subsequently shown to have an hypoplastic renal artery on the left side.

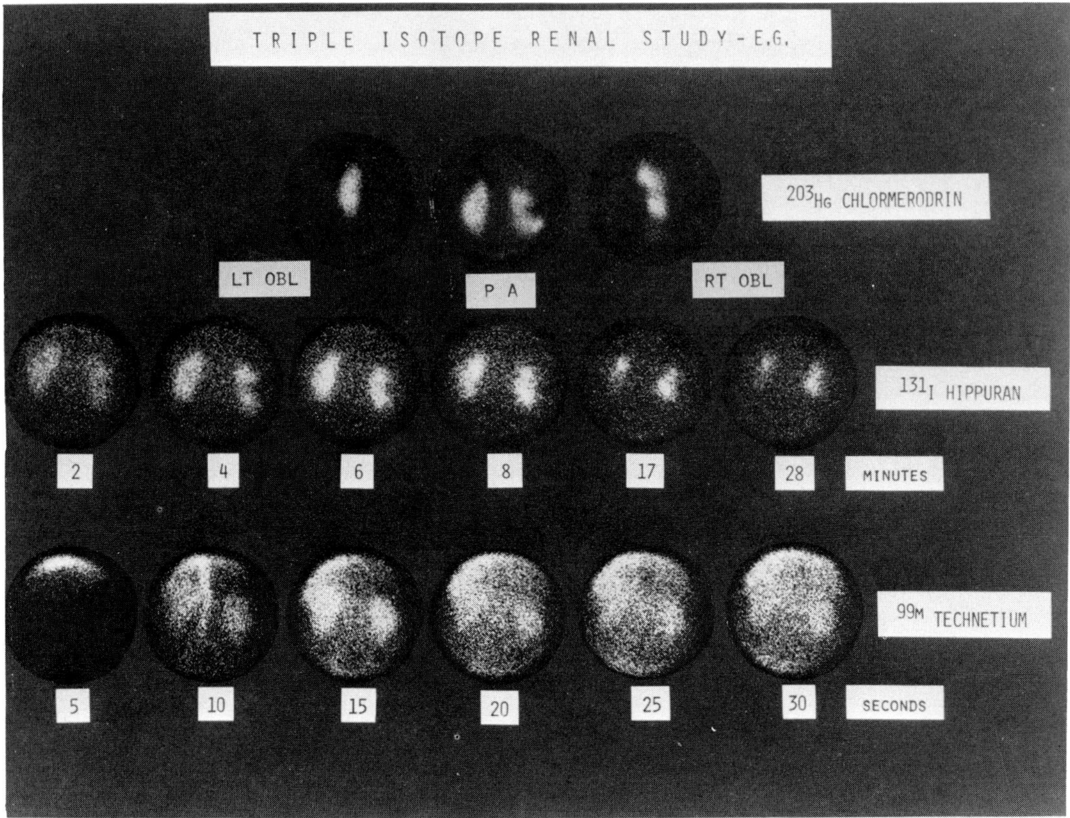

Fig. 10. A middle-aged patient with painless hematuria was shown by intravenous pyelogram to have a mass in the right kidney. The RMC scan shows an obvious defect in the margin of the right kidney as seen in the posterior projection. The left oblique is normal, but the right oblique shows the defect is probably involving the entire thickness of the kidney. The ROIH study shows that this defect in the right kidney did not concentrate and that there was a relative delay in excretion from the right kidney and to a slight extent from the upper pole of the left kidney. The subsequent PTc study clearly shows, especially in the 15-second frame, that the area of defect seen in the RMC posterior projection does in fact fill quite well, with PTc indicating the presence of adequate blood flow in this area. At nephrectomy, a renal carcinoma measuring approximately 4 cm in diameter was observed on bivalve slicing of the kidney. This should be contrasted with the findings in Figure 7, where cystic disease was the underlying pathological lesion.

between vascular (carcinoma) and avascular renal mass can be made (Fig. 10). This differential diagnosis cannot be made by any other technique short of surgery.

REFERENCES

1. Tauxe, W. N., and Hunt, J. C.: Evaluation of renal function by isotope techniques. Med. Clin. N. Amer., *50*:937-955, 1966.
2. Haynie, T. P., Nofal, M. M., Carr, E. A., Jr. and Beierwaltes, W. H.: The use of ^{131}I-labelled contrast media in scintillation scanning of the kidney. J. Lab. Clin. Med., *58*:598-604, 1961.
3. Haynie, T. P., Steward, B. H., Nofal, M. M., Carr, E. A., Jr., and Beierwaltes, W. H.: Renal scintiscans in the diagnosis of renal vascular disease and renal tumors. J. Nucl. Med., *2*:272-281, 1961.
4. Mallard, J. R.: Medical radioisotope visualization (A review of "scanning"). Intern. J. Appl. Radiat., *17*:205-249, 1966.
5. McAfee, J. G., and Wagner, H. N., Jr.: Visualization of renal parenchyma by scintiscanning with [203]Hg-neohydrin. Radiology, *75*:820-821, 1960.
6. Morgan, M. C., Barton, H. L. Erickson, E. E., and Risser, J. R.: Scintiscanning of dog kidneys using diodrast-[131]I. Amer. J. Roentgen., *85*:123-127, 1961.
7. Cassen, B., Curtis, L., and Reed, C.: A sensitive directional gamma-ray detector. Nucleonics, *6*:78-80, 1950.
8. Anger, H. O.: Scintillation camera. Rev. Sci. Instr., *29*:27-33, 1958.
9. Anger, H. O.: Survey of radioisotope cameras. ISA Transactions., *5*:311-334, 1966.
10. Burke, G., Halko, A., and Coe, F. L.: Dynamic clinical studies with radioisotopes and the scintillation camera. I. Sodium iodohippurate-^{131}I renography. J. A. M. A., *197*:15-24, 1966.
11. Gottschalk, A., and Anger, H. O.: Renal scintiphotography with the gamma-ray scintillation camera and [203]Hg-neohydrin. Radiology, *84*:861-867, 1965.
12. Rosenthall, L.: Ortho-iodohippurate-^{131}I kidney scanning in renal failure. Radiology, *87*:298-303, 1966.
13. McAfee, J. G., and Subramanian, G.: Radioactive agents for the delineation of body organs by external imaging devices: A review. ISA Transactions, *5*:349-372, 1966.
14. Taplin, G. V.: The sodium iodohippurate ^{131}I renocystogram: Revised interpretation, termin-

15. Reba, R. C., McAfee, J. G., and Wagner, H. N., Jr.: Radio-mercury-labelled chlormerodrin for in vivo uptake studies and scintillation scanning of unilateral renal lesions associated with hypertension. Medicine, *42*:269, 1962.
16. Beck, R. N.: Radioisotope scanning systems. ISA Transactions, *5*:335-348, 1966.
17. Anderson, E. E., and Wilson, R. E.: Radioisotope renography and radioscintillation scanning in the diagnosis of homograph rejection. Surg. Gynec. Obstet., *122*:1273-1277, 1966.
18. Baum, S., Rabinowitz, P., and Malloy, W. A.: The renal scan as an aid in percutaneous renal biopsy. J. A. M. A., *195*:913-915, 1966.
19. Buse, M. D., Sibrans, D. F., and Buse, J.: Scintillation scanning of kidneys: A pitfall of interpretation in renal insufficiency. Ann. Int. Med., *60*:857-865, 1964.
20. Freeman, L. M., Kay, C. J., and Meng, C. H.: The contribution of renal scanning in the evaluation of renal trauma. Radiology, *86*:1021-1029, 1966.
21. Izenstark, J. L., Burden, J. J., Mardis, H. K., and Varella, R.: Clinical indications for kidney scanning. J. A. M. A., *188*:136-139, 1964.
22. Johnson, P. M.: Renal localization with labelled chlormerodrin. Radiology, *84*:104-107, 1965.
23. Kay, C., Freeman, L., and Avnet, N.: Scintillation scanning in pediatrics. Pediatrics, *37*:794-803, 1966.
24. Kazmin, M. H., Swanson, L. E., and Cockett, A. T. K.: Renal scan: The test of choice in renal trauma. J. Urol., *97*:189-195, 1967.
25. Keller, H. I., Malloy, J. P., and Sauer, G. F.: The renal scan: An aid to renal biopsy. J. A. M. A., *188*:1085-1086, 1964.
26. MacEwan, D. W., and Rosenthall, L.: Assessment of excretory urography and radioisotope renal scanning in diseases of the kidneys. Radiology, *86*:1010-1020, 1966.
27. Morris, J. G., Coorey, G. J., Dick, R., Evans, W. A., Smitanda, N. Pearson, B. B., Loewenthal, J. I., Blackburn, C. R. B., and McCrae, J.: The diagnosis of renal tumors by radioisotope scanning. J. Urol., *97*:40-54, 1967.
28. Meier, D. A., and Beierwaltes, W. H.: Radioisotope renal studies and renal hypertension. J. A. M. A., *198*:1257-1262, 1966.
29. Woodruff, J. H., Jr., Cockett, A. T. K., Cannon, R., and Swanson, L. C.: Radiologic aspects of renal trauma with the emphasis on arteriography and renal isotope scanning. J. Urol., *97*:184-188, 1967.

Chapter 31

Automated Data Processing
in Renal Diseases

HOWARD C. HOPPS, M.D., and ELEMER GABRIELI, M.D.

Automatic Data Processing (ADP) does not make a process *simpler,* it simply speeds it up. In addition, ADP provides for a rigorous consistency in handling data that, otherwise, would be virtually impossible. In turn, this consistency of handling forces a clear and sharp characterization of the data input, the query, and the information output.

Computer technology has advanced beyond biomedical abilities to use it. Apparatus, i.e., hardware, is available in a wide variety of forms to meet virtually any set of technical requirements. Programs, i.e., software, are available to meet most "standard" laboratory needs; and there is no scarcity of programers who, for a price, will design special programs for special purposes.

Sources of basic information on this general aspect of the problem — hardware/software — are listed among the references.

Biomedical scientists have not kept pace with the times and have hardly *begun* to use computers to best advantage. It is true that they are used more and more to accomplish simple data storage/retrieval, to carry out relatively simple accounting-type calculations, and in surveillance systems. But computers have not been used in the area where they could make their greatest contribution, i.e., in converting simple data to complex information and in helping scientists to reach a satisfactory conclusion. It is this aspect of ADP that is emphasized in this chapter and not its use in organizing laboratory work, processing requests, or reporting the results of analyses. Furthermore, the problem is approached in broad terms, concentrating on the design and operation of a *system* rather than getting deeply involved in the detailed characterization of input and the precise manner of processing it.

The system to be considered is presented in its conceptual form in Figure 1, and much of the discussion will relate to this figure. The laboratory determination used for illustrative purposes will be a chemical one, the BUN, although data derived from urinalysis, a clearance study, histopathologic analysis of a renal biopsy, etc. could also have been used.

At the outset, there are two different ways of looking at the laboratory determination (Fig. 1): test-oriented and single patient-oriented. From the *test-oriented viewpoint,* the first consideration is methodology. Without the firm foundation of a specific, sensitive, stable, reproducible test, the superstructure of

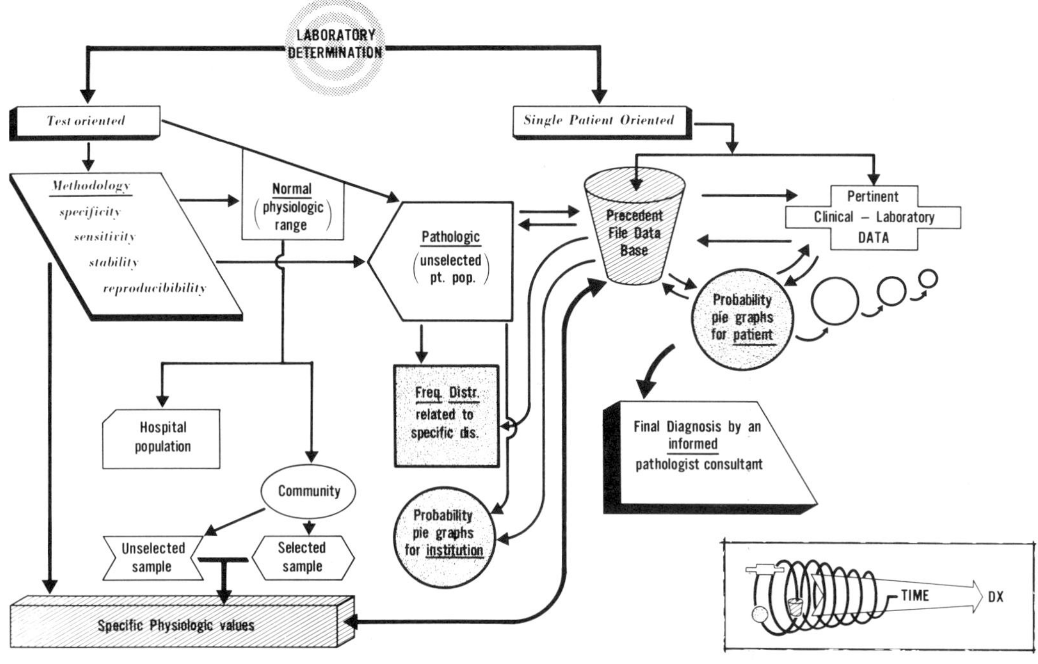

Fig. 1

meaningful interpretation must fall. On the basis of the results derived from proper application of this method, it may be concluded that the test result is within normal limits (a wide physiologic range) or that it is pathologic. Up to this point, the computer is not needed. However, when one steps from the abstract situation, which is the province of general text and reference works into his *own* community and his *own* hospital, then he reaches an area in which it is necessary to develop his *own* particular standards. In a community as a whole (unselected sample), the normal range must be defined. More specific normal ranges may be established in relation to such selected samples as executive groups, occupational groups at high risk for a specific disease, groups of infants who attend a well-baby clinic, the "normal" inmates of an old folks home, etc. A precise characterization of these groups will lead to the collection of *specific* physiologic values which become of special importance when laboratory determinations are viewed from the perspective of the single patient.

The hospital population is, of course, a very biased group, even when one selects those patients who are "normal" with respect to a particular test, and many studies have demonstrated the importance of establishing normal ranges in the context of the particular hospital environment. For example, a recent study

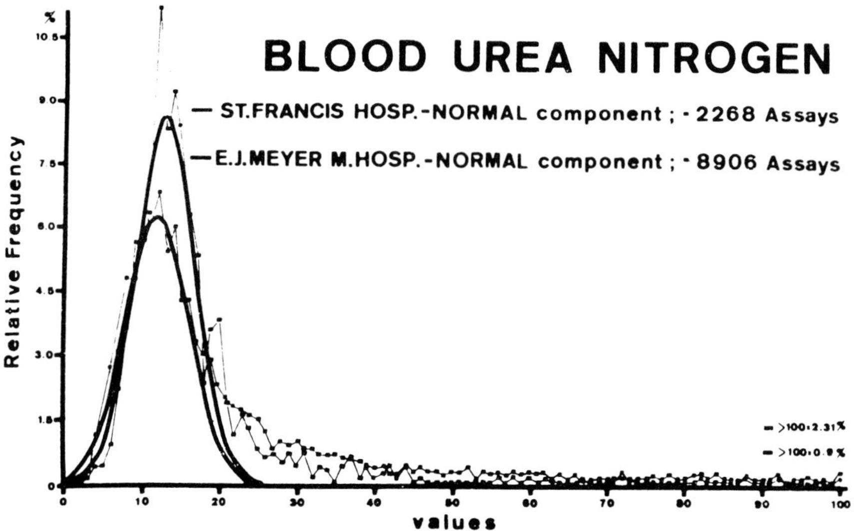

Fig. 2

by one of us (E. G.) shows a significant difference in the distribution of normal BUN values at two hospitals within the same city (Fig. 2).

Turning to pathologic values, ADP can be of even greater help. Adequately characterized input test data coupled with the subsequent input of patient's diagnosis, making certain that *time relationships* are clearly indicated, allows one to develop *for his own institution* a frequency distribution list of test/disease relationships oriented toward *individual diseases.* In our particular illustration, a BUN of 30 mg per 100 ml, the list would include the percentage of cases of pyelonephritis (acute, chronic), obstructive nephropathy, arteriolar nephrosclerosis, glomerulo-nephritis (acute, chronic), G. I. bleeding, toxemia of pregnancy, disseminated lupus erythematosus, amylioidosis, etc., within the hospital experience, which gave this value (actually, a reasonable range *including* this value, e.g., 25 to 40).

Looking at the data a different way,

one could query the computer system for information to provide a probability "pie graph" of disease *diagnosis,* at the particular hospital, based upon the single abnormal laboratory result. This would be quite different from the frequency distribution related to specific diseases. For example, from the aspect of diseases, *per se,* a BUN of 30 mg per 100 ml (group-range of 25 to 40) might characterize 70% of the cases of toxemia of pregnancy in a given hospital. However, when the probability "pie graph" was established for all diseases giving this BUN in the hospital's experience, only 2% of the patients might be found to represent the diagnosis of toxemia pregnancy. In Figure 3 is illustrated a hypothetical probability "pie graph" of diagnoses based upon the BUN determination of 30 (25 to 40), *within the experience of a particular hospital.*

Turning now to the *single patient oriented* view of the laboratory determination, one reaches an area where automated data processing can make its greatest contribution: in helping the physician to arrive at a valid, precise final diagnosis. Looking once again at Figure 1, the most critical aspect of the right half of the figure is the *precedent file data base,* a base which can only be established after much expenditure of time and energy since it must include a great deal of patient data, expressed not only qualitatively, but quantitatively as well. In addition, it must be time-connected to the stage of the disease. Furthermore, all of these data have to be linked, ultimately, to a precise diagnosis. These data (both clinical and laboratory) derived from many patients can, upon proper query, give the information to allow evaluation of a patient under study, in the context of his hospital environment. This may suggest additional pertinent clinical or laboratory data which, in turn, allow a more specific query to the precedent file data base yielding a probability "pie graph" of

greater validity to the patient in question. In this way, a succession of probability "pie graphs" is obtained, each member of the succession taking into consideration the increasing amount of data and drawing on the whole background of experience of the hospital, leading to a more and more precise diagnosis.

Returning to our illustration of a BUN of 30 per 100 ml, with only this information the probability "pie graph" would consider pyelonephritis, arteriolar nephrosclerosis, obstructive nephropathy, etc., all as likely diagnoses. However, if this information were extended to include negative urinalysis and 4+ occult blood in the stool, the probability "pie graph" would change markedly, indicating the most likely diagnosis (by far) to be GI bleeding. This is a rather obvious conclusion, but many conclusions would not be so obvious.

In the lower right hand portion of

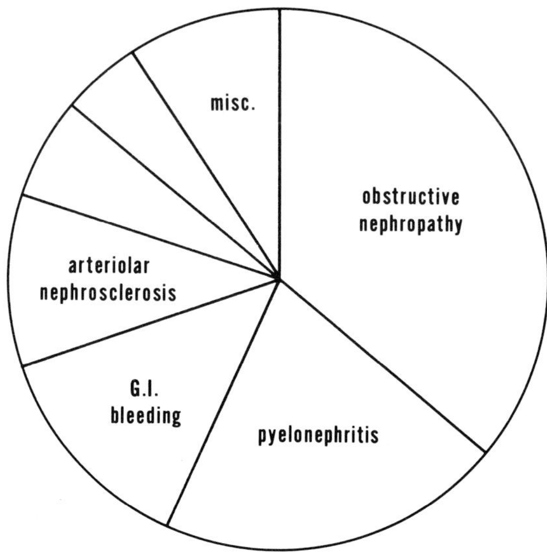

Fig. 3

Figure 1 is an insert which considers the vital importance of time as a "fourth dimension." The positive feed back among pertinent clinical-laboratory data, the precedent file data base, and the probability "pie graphs" for the patient, is greatly augmented by this time factor which provides data on response to specific therapy as well as on the natural progress of the disease.

The authors emphasize that they are *not* advocating machine diagnosis, *per se*, but *are* advocating a computerized system which, operating effectively on well-characterized data, can be of very great assistance to the pathologist and to the clinician, since it would allow recall, on a moment's notice, of the entire experience of the hospital with patients of similar clinical pathologic characteristics.

Clinical laboratory data are *relatively* easy to process because they are sharply characterized both qualitatively and (for the most part) quantitatively. Many new problems are encountered when one attempts to preprocess *histopathologic data* for storage/retrieval/manipulation. The problems inherent in this area are far from solved, and it would be most presumptious to present "the solution" here. However, suggestions are made regarding approaches to this problem. Since these suggestions are to serve primarily as a guide, they are not all-comprehensive although they do attempt to cover the important aspects of the renal *glomerulus* as it might be evaluated in renal biopsy.

Admittedly, it is difficult to characterize precisely each independent variable *qualitatively,* and even more difficult to give a meaningful (semi) *quantitative* value (i.e., measure) for each of these anatomic pathologic changes.

Nevertheless, this *must* be done if the computer input is to be manipulated effectively to yield a truly valuable output.

Not only must *all* pertinent qualitative changes be described — and assigned quantitative values — but the extent of the involvement must be specified, also the location, and also the significant time relationships in terms of duration of the disease or lesion.

EXTENT of involvement must be related to the kidney as a whole, also to the glomeruli. In relation to the *kidney*, per se, the following input terms are suggested:

> all glomeruli (100%), many (99% to 50%), few (49% to 5%), rare (less than 5%)

In relation to the *glomerulus,* per se: diffuse (100%); the major part (99%-50%); the minor part (50%-5%); minimal (less than 5%)

LOCATION could be related to:
Kidney: outer 1/3 of cortex, mid 1/3, inner 1/3, random distribution. *Glomerulus:* hilar, mid portion, peripheral, random distribution.

TIME could be related to the disease in terms of elapsed days, months, or years after the onset, or the process could be considered as: early acute, late acute, sub-acute, sub-chronic, chronic, or healed. (Obviously, the second group of terms is much more subjective than the first and, because of this, less desirable.)

If pertinent, the following terms should also be applied:

> exacerbation
> remission
> inactive
> healing

Many of the *qualitative* factors to be listed can have quantitative values less than normal, or normal, or more than normal, and provisions must be made to indicate this. In order to conserve punch card space, it is suggested that quantitative aspects be related to numbers according to the following scheme:

No. 1 Marked decrease
No. 2 Moderate decrease
No. 3 slight decrease
No. 4 Minimal decrease
No. 5 Within normal range
No. 6 Minimal increase
No. 7 Slight increase
No. 8 Moderate increase
No. 9 Marked increase

Admittedly, these quantitative terms are subjective and, because of this , the user will need to establish his own criteria and equate these with actual figures, figures which may vary considerably from one qualitative factor to another, but which will remain consistent in relation to *the* particular qualitative factor being measured. For example, if one considers "normal" to represent 100%, "marked decrease" may mean less than 10% of the normal (size or quantity); "moderate decrease," from 10% to 50% of the normal; slight decrease, from 50% to 90% of the normal; minimal decrease, from 90% to 99% of the normal. On the positive side, "marked increase" could mean more than 10X; "moderate increase" from 2 to 10X; etc.

The user will need to select and set aside *reference sections* to serve as standards. He will need to refer to these often in order that his criteria do not shift with time. The reference sections will also be very helpful in communicating to others precisely what these particular terms mean.

Qualitative Factors (pertaining to glomeruli), include:

    number (of glomeruli)
    size (of glomeruli)
    cellular (nuclear) density
    exudative infiltration (*cell type)
    fibrosis
    number of epithelial cells
        cytoplasm/nucleus (ratio)
        crescents, caps
    number of endothelial cells,
        cytoplasm/nucleus (ratio)
    number of mesangial cells
        cytoplasm/nucleus (ratio)
    basement membrane
        splitting or duplication
        argyrophilic substance
        PAS positive material
        other
    lobular stalk thickening
    Bowman's membrane (thickness,
        cellularity)
    capillary lumina (amount of space)
    capillary occlusion (*by____)
    Bowman's space (amount)
    *protein ppt., or RBCs, or leukocytes
        in Bowman's space
    karyorrhexis .... (* of what/where)
    karyolysis .... (* of what/where)
    pyknosis .... (* of what/where)
    necrosis (frank) .... (* of what/where)
    fatty changes ...... (* of what/where)
    amyloid .... (* of what/where)
    "hyaline" change ... (* of what/where)
    etc. .... (* of what/where)
    wall/lumen (ratio), afferent arteriole
    wall/lumen ratio, efferent arteriole
    arteriolar hyaline change
    arteriolar "fibrinoid necrosis"
    other ________________________
    other ________________________
    other ________________________

*Three card columns could be allowed for each of the items marked by an asterisk. (The second column would relate to location and extent.) The third column could be utilized as follows:

    1 polymorphonuclear leukocytes
    2 "round cells"
    3 platelets
    4 "cellular"

5 protein ppt.
6 erythrocytes
7 endothelium
8 epithelium
9 basement membrane

*   *   *

Computer technology offers much more to the clinical scientist than just a means to increase his effectiveness in organizing laboratory work, assisting with quality control, and getting out test reports promptly. Computer technology can and should contribute an important dimension to the clinical scientist's intellectual activities, especially in his crucially important role of diagnostician. It will not be easy to achieve this because of the great difficulties inherent in communication between (subjective) man and (objective) machine, but it *can* be accomplished. The crucial factor is selection and characterization of input data so that a comprehensive precedent data file base can be established. This will require a great expenditure of time and effort, and close collaboration between the pathologist and the clinician— but the results will more than repay the cost.

REFERENCES

1. Machine Accountant 1 & C (NAVPERS 10265), published by Bureau of Naval Personnel Navy Training Course, 1964, available from U. S. Printing Office, Wash. - $1.00. (This 165 page manual considers basic principles of automatic data processing, programming, magnetic tape operations, and systems analysis, and will be of particular value to those with limited background in the field of ADP.)
2. Gabrieli, E. R., Pessin, V.: Computer assisted interpretation of laboratory findings. Automation in Analytical Chemistry (MEDIAD), New York, 1966.
3. Gabrieli, E. R., Pessin, V.: The computer's contribution to information content of laboratory data. J.A.M.A., *198*:63-66, 1966.
4. Gabrieli, E. R., Pessin, V., Thorpe, J., and Palmer, R. R. C.: Initial experience with and potential of data processing and computer techniques in a hospital clinical laboratory Am. J. Clin. path., *47*:60-68, 1967.
5. Gabrieli, E. R.: Standardized interpretation of laboratory data. Ann. New York Acad. Sci., Jan. 15-17, 1968 (in press).
6. Gabrieli, E. R.: A practical computer oriented hospital information system. Modern Hospital (in press).
7. Gabrieli, E. R.: Computer oriented documentation of surgical patients. Surg., Gynec., Obst. (in press).
8. Ledley, R. S.: Use of Computers in Biology and Medicine. New York, McGraw-Hill, 1965.
9. Stacy, R. W., Waxman, B. D.: Computers in Biomedical Research. New York, Academic Press, 1965.
10. Sterling, T. E., Pollack, S. V.: Computers and the Life Sciences. New York, Columbia Publishers, 1965.
11. Wilson, I. G., Wilson, M. E.: Information Computers and Systems Design. New York, Wiley Publishers, 1966.

Chapter 32

Percutaneous Renal Biopsy: An Adjunct to the Management of Patients with Renal Disease

ROBERT C. MUEHRCKE, M.D., F.A.C.P.,
and ANIL K. MANDAL, M.B.

INTRODUCTION

Almost simultaneously, PerezAra (17) in 1950 and Iversen and Brun (8) in 1951 reported that percutaneous renal biopsy was a safe and relatively simple clinical procedure. For the past fifteen years, the value of renal biopsy in patients with renal disease has been established as a "routine" procedure. Currently, renal biopsy is the only method of making an exact histological assessment of renal disease during the life of the patient. It is a tremendous aid to the physician in outlining the management and prognosis of patients ill with renal disease. Moreover, tissue specimens "freshly harvest" by renal biopsy can be examined using light, electron and immunofluorescent microsopy and can be analyzed by ultrabiochemical methods.

HISTORICAL REVIEW

As early as 1924, Jungman (9) obtained kidney tissue during an abdominal operation. Later, Castleman and Smithwick (4) reported renal biopsy study of hypertensive patients. They secured renal tissue during lumbar sympathectomy. As far back as 1941, Talbot (21, 22) correlated renal function with renal morphology. Percutaneous renal biopsy was first done by PerezAra (17). Later, Iversen and Brun (8) applied renal biopsy in a systematic study of patients with renal disease. They obtained renal tissue with the patient in a sitting position and used a boring-serrated type needle. However, their yield in obtaining tissue was low (38.2%).

In 1955, Muehrcke *et al.* (13, 15) increased the percent of success (96%) in getting adequate tissue. This was done by use of an exploring needle to find the depth from skin to kidney. The biopsy was taken with Franklin's modification of the Vim-Silverman needle while the patient laid prone on a sand bag. The biopsy site was previously outlined on the patients back by means of measurements obtained from an intravenous pyelogram or a flat film of the abdomen.

Muehrcke and co-workers also were first to use serial renal biopsy studies in clinicopathological correlations of patients with a variety of renal diseases

(14, 15). Currently, Haddad and Mani (6) do percutaneous renal biopsy with the aid of television monitoring and infusion pyelography. Television monitoring permits the operator to visualize the position of the biopsy needle within the opacified kidney. Although the modified Vim-Silverman needle is widely used, plastic disposable biopsy needles are available commercially and their use are gaining in popularity.

INDICATIONS

The indications for doing a renal biopsy are rather broad. A biopsy in indicated for diagnostic purposes in any patient with diffuse renal disease in whom the diagnosis cannot be established by the usual clinical and laboratory methods. The procedure is of particular value to the physician in the differential diagnosis of unsuspected inflammatory and infectious disease of the kidney, of the so-called collagen diseases, of the underlying disease in patients with persistent proteinuria, with the nephrotic syndrome and in patients with unexplained acute oliguric renal failure.

Renal biopsy has been found of equal value in the diagnosis of rare renal disease such as Wegener's granulomatosis, thrombotic thrombocytopenic purpura and Goodpasture disease. Renal biopsy is most helpful in the selection of patients with sudden oliguria for artificial dialysis and in the management of patients with lupus glomerulonephritis who are to be selected for high dosage adrenal corticosteroid treatment. In addition, renal biopsy is of value in patients in whom accurate knowledge as to life expectancy is of particular importance.

CONTRAINDICATIONS

Patients must be evaluated carefully before a renal biopsy is done. Particular contraindications include an uncooperative patient, abnormalities of blood coagulation, a single kidney and terminal chronic renal failure.

Because of the possibility in disseminating infection or spreading tumor cells, renal biopsy should not be done on patients who may have perirenal abscess, renal neoplasm, large cysts or hydro or pyonephrosis. Patients with severe hypertension, malignant hypertension, or toxemia of pregnancy should have their blood pressure lowered before undergoing a kidney biopsy. Moreover, the biopsy should be done with great care and only by an experienced operator. Patients with severe hypertension and patients with toxemia of pregnancy develop complications more frequently than do patients with normal blood pressure.

PRE AND POST RENAL
BIOPSY PRECAUTIONS

To insure the safety of the patient a number of precautions are taken. Prebiopsy studies include examination and culture of urine, timed intravenous pyelogram, clotting, bleeding and prothrombin times and blood urea nitrogen. Patients with uremia due to acute oliguric renal failure should undergo hemodialysis or peritoneal dialysis before a renal biopsy is done. Hypertensive patients should have their blood pressure reduced before renal biopsy.

To insure the safety of the patient after the biopsy is done, a number of precautions must be followed. Firm pressure is applied to the biopsy site by means of the operators hands on a few pads of 4″ x 4″ gauze and later a pressure adhesive tape dressing is applied. The patient remains prone on a sausage-shaped sand bag for thirty minutes. Then the patient is gently transferred to bed and remains flat in bed for one hour, and on bedrest for 24 hours. During this period, the pulse rate, blood pressure and general condition of the patient is frequently observed. The urine is examined for gross and microscopic hematuria and a clear void specimen of urine is obtained for culture. Any complaint of the patient, especially frequency and urgency on micturation or pain at the biopsy site must be carefully assessed.

COMPLICATIONS

In general, the complications of renal biopsy are usually mild and transitory. For example, mild back pain and transient microsopic hematuria are the two most common complications. Transitory gross hematuria and passage of blood clot with clot colic is an infrequent occurrence. In some patients, massive retroperitoneal hematoma with severe shock has occurred (3, 16, 20, 23).

Deaths following renal biopsy were reported in eight incidences in over ten thousand renal biopsy studies.

Elderly patients with severe hypertension and advance arterial disease are more prone to have gross hemorrhage after renal biopsy. Patients with uremia due to chronic renal failure have an increased incidence of hematuria.

TECHNIQUES OF RENAL BIOPSY

The inherent technical difficulties with percutaneous renal biopsy have been overcome by radiological location of the kidney, by confirmation of this location with an exploring needle and by securing a small core of kidney by a relatively atraumatic biopsy needle. The exact biopsy technique is described in detail elsewhere (13).

HANDLING OF RENAL BIOPSY SPECIMENS

In the authors' laboratory, the tissue is routinely fixed in glutaraldehyde for electron microscopic study. A second portion of tissue is fixed in Helly's solution for 3 hours followed by overnight washing in running water. Longer fixation will lead to excessive hardening and brittleness of the tissue. This will not permit the satisfactory cutting of thin sections.

Helly's solution is preferable to buffered formalin solution because it produces less shrinkage of the delicate tubular cells, the glomerular structures and the interstitium. With most staining procedures, material fixed in this solution is generally superior to formalin-fixed specimens. However, frozen sections for lipids stains are not satisfactory following fixation in Helly's solution. When special studies are desired, other methods of fixation are used. These include chilled acetone for alkaline phosphatase; absolute alcohol for glycogen and urates; freeze-drying for various histochemical procedures (10). For ultra-microchemical determinations and in immunofluorescent studies, freezing in liquid nitrogen followed by sectioning in a cryostat is the method of choice (1, 2).

The paraffin-embedded specimen is sectioned at 3-4 micra. This thickness must be strictly adhered to in order to obtain comparable sections and to evaluate accurately and quantatively the glomerular changes, particularly the degree of cellularity and character of the cells. About fifteen to thirty serial sections are usually cut from each biopsy, although at times as many as one hundred sections have been cut. The majority are stained with hematoxylin-eosin. The remaining sections are routinely stained with Alcian Blue-PAS to demonstrate basement membranes, tubular brush borders, and the hyaline granules; periodic acid-silver methenamine to study the basement membranes and tubular droplets; and with Masson trichrome to study connective tissue and fibrin. Oil-Red-O is used on frozen sections to demonstrate lipids (10). In select cases, crystal violet and Congo red stains are used to detect amyloid and Weigert-Van Gieson for evaluation of connective tissue and elastic fibres.

Initially, renal tissue was fixed for electron microscopy studies in buffered 1% osmium tetroxide and embedded in epon (12). Currently, every biopsy specimen is fixes in glutaraldehyde and stained for acid phosphatase using a modification of Gomori's technique (7). After embedding the tissue, it is cut at 0.5 micron and stained with methylene blue-Azure 11 for survey and orientation. These survey sections are also stained with periodic acid-silver methenamine. After the desired structures are identified, sections are cut at 0.025 micron, observed and photographed.

MORPHOLOGICAL ADEQUACY

Kidney specimens obtained with the Vim-Silverman needle usually consist of a cylinder of renal tissue measuring 10 to 15 mm in length and are approximately 2 mm in diameter. Using the aspiration biopsy needle of Iversen and Brun (8), a slightly thicker specimen measuring up to 4 mm diameter is obtained. It is essential that renal cortex is obtained for adequate morphological evaluation; the presence of cortex in the specimen can be determined at the bedside, using a hand lens. This should be done immediately after the biopsy is done.

A second biopsy specimen should be taken if, one hand lens inspection, the first specimen is inadequate. Renal cortex can be readily differentiated from renal medulla because of the lighter color of the cortex and because the glomeruli can be recognized as pinhead-sized structures in formalin fixed specimens. This identification is more difficult in Helly's or Zenker's fixed specimens. Five to ten glomeruli are in general essential to consider a biopsy specimen adequate; however, at times a single glomerulus may be sufficient for an exact diagnosis. By studying multiple serial sections, the maximum number of glomeruli can be examined. This increases the accuracy of the morphological evaluation. When the changes are slight and lack specificity, greater numbers of glomeruli are helpful to the pathologist especially in early stages of renal disorders.

Tissue obtained by renal biopsy will not always permit precise evaluation of focal renal diseases, such as pyelonephritis and arterial or arteriolar nephrosclerosis. In these diseases the pathologist may either over-emphasize or under estimate the severity of renal affliction. In a great majority of diffuse renal diseases, an adequate percutaneous needle biopsy of the kidney reflects the extent and degree of the primary histolotical involvement.

MORPHOLOGICAL ANALYSIS

The renal biopsy requires more careful and detailed morphological study than autopsy material. The pathologist must make a systemic and careful analysis of each of the four major kidney components (glomeruli, tubules, vessels and interstitium). The experienced pathologist should be able to tell the clinician not only the exact renal disease process but the severity of the disease, the acuteness of the disease and the progressiveness of the disease. The pathologist should not cast aside minor histological changes in his evaluation of biopsy material. As the pathologist gains experience in evaluating early changes in various diseases, these minor morphological abnormalities take on new meaning.

A semi-quantitative approach is applied to detailed analytical studies of each major kidney componet and will aid in the correlation of the renal morphology with various clinical and laboratory data. For example, one must systematically study the glomerulus by noting the number of endothelial and epithelial cells, the thickness of the glomerular capillary basement membrane, the narrowing of the capillary lumen, the presence or absence of erythrocytes or leucocytes within the glomerular lumen, glomerular adhesions and other features. An evaluation card listing the numerous detailed abnormalities of renal structures to be quantitatively analyzed is of great value Using this method, clinical and pathological studies have been done in the following diseases; lupus nephritis (14) diabetes mellitus (5) toxemia of pregnancy (18) and the idiopathic nephrotic syndrome (19).

ELECTRON MICROSCOPIC ANALYSIS

Electron microscopic studies of renal tissue is more time consuming and more costly than the study of other organs such as the liver or muscle. In addition, adequacy of renal tissue and random sampling is a much greater problem. In general, due to the extreme thinness of the sections, only a limited portion of a single glomerulus in each section can be examined. A considerable number of sections from a minimum of at least five glomeruli should be studied. However, this number of glomeruli may not have been fixed for electron microscopic study. As usually happens, not a single glomerulus may be found. Initially, a specimen from each end of the biopsy specimen was fixed in glutareldehyde. Currently, the tissue is split longitudinally and fixed. This method usually insures tissue from both cortex and medullae.

To evaluate renal tissue properly by electron microscopy one must study not only several glomeruli but the entire length of the nephron (cortical as well as medullary structures). This includes study of the interstitial tissue and blood vessels. In some studies, as many as forty grids and more than 575 well focused enlarged photographs of a single biopsy specimen were examined. The glomerular, tubular and Bowman's membrane should be quantitatively measured in Angstrom units. Knowledge of the ultra-structure of the glomerulus in health and disease has increased our appreciation of the abnormalities seen by light microscopy. Electron microscopic evaluations of renal tubules must be done with great care. The clinician must have a thorough knowledge of physiological changes occurring in tubules such as those resulting from infusion of various physiological solutions. Currently, electron microscopic studies of the normal renal medullae and papillae are rare. One can distinguish structures such as ascending and descending capillary loops from ascending and descending limbs of Henle only with great difficulty. The medullae is an area of great opportunity for electron microscopic study in health and disease.

ULTRA–BIOCHEMICAL ANALYSIS

The rapid and instantaneous extraction of a core of renal tissue harvests viable cells which can be immediately fixed for ultra-microchemical studies. Bonting and co-workers (1, 2) have applied Lowry's (11) quantitative ultramicrochemical techniques of dissection, weighing and assay of microscopically small fragments of tissue to the study of the nephron. These and similar quantitative biochemical studies are increasing our basic knowledge and understanding of the enzyme topography of the nephron. Changes in quantitative enzyme activity were found to occur in individual units of the nephron long before morphological changes were noted. This information sheds light on the basic adaptive changes in nephrons of diseased kidneys, especially when ultramicrochemical studies are correlated with electron microscopic changes.

IMMUNOPATHOLOGY

The freezing of freshly harvest renal tissue is well adapted for immunopathological study. In our laboratory, a small portion of tissue is transferred onto a saline moistened filter paper within a Petri dish. It can be instantly frozen and cut at 4 micron in a cryostat. Fluorescent-conjugated antihuman immunoglobulins and $Beta_{1C}$ component can stain the tissue.

THE VALUE OF RENAL BIOPSY IN THE CARE OF THE PATIENT

Percutaneous renal biopsy is an extremely valuable, practical adjunct to the physician in his care of the patient afflicted with kidney disease. The procedure should be done only after a careful history is taken, a thorough physical examination is done, and laboratory investigations including tests of renal function and repeated urinalysis is completed.

In the past, renal biopsy studies have modified or changed the initial clinical impression in over 50% of patients investigated with a large variety of renal diseases such as; acute oliguric renal failure, the nephrotic syndrome, persistent proteinuria and other conditions. In an additional 40% of the patients, renal biopsy has confirmed the initial clinical impression. It should be emphasized that in approximately 10% of the patients with renal disease, a definite diagnosis could not be made by either the pathologist or the clinician. In approximately 2% of patients studied by renal biopsy, the morphological diagnosis was incorrectly made by the pathologist.

Once the physician has structural evaluation of the patients's kidney affliction, he can provide a more rational approach to the management of the patient. To provide the maximum aid to physician and patient, this evaluation should include the following: 1) a specific diagnosis; 2) the severity of the disease process; 3) the acuteness of the disease; 4) the activity of the disease process, and 5) the possible reversibility of the disease process.

Renal biopsy has been particularly useful in the histological evaluation of patients with the nephrotic syndrome, in patients with acute oliguric renal failure, in patients with persistent asymptomatic proteinuria, in unsuspected amyloid, in acute intersitial nephritis or in inflammatory disease of the kidneys, in drug induced diseases and in determining exactly the bacteria responsibile for infection. Renal biopsy is also of aid to the physician in patients with widespread vascular disease, such as polyarteritis nodosa, scleroderma, Wegener's granulomatosis, thrombotic thrombocytopenic purpura and Goodpasture's disease.

SUMMARY

For the past fifteen years, the use of renal biopsy has greatly advanced our knowledge of renal disease to the direct benefit of the patient. During this period, renal biopsy has placed clinical nephrology on a firm and more exacting footing.The ability for the investigator to obtain a rapid and instantaneous sampling of renal tissue has increased our knowledge of the kidneys ultrabiochemical, ultrasturctural and immunopathology.

The accurate and faithful correlation of serial quantitative renal biopsy findings using light and electron microscopic and immunopathology with the ever changing clinical course of the patient is an ideal tool to further our understanding of renal disorders.

REFERENCES

1. Bonting, S. L., Pollak, V. E., Muehrcke, R. C., and Kark, R. M.: Quantitative histochemistry of the nephron. Science, *127*:1342, 1958.
2. Bonting, S. L., Pollak, V. E., Muehrcke, R. C., and Kark, R. M.: Quantitative histochemistry of the nephron. II. Alkaline phosphatase activity in man and other species. J. Clin. Invest., *39*:1372-1380, 1960.
3. Brun, C., and Raaschou, F.: Kidney biopsies. Am. J. Med. *24*:676-691, 1958.
4. Castleman, B., and Smithwick, R. H.: The relation of vascular disease to the hypertensive state. Based on a study of renal biopsies from 100 hypertensive patients. J. A. M. A., *121*:1256-1261, 1943.
5. Gellman, D. D., Pirani, C. L., Soothill, J. F., Muehrcke, R. C., and Kark, R. M.: Diabetic nephropathy; a clinical and pathologic study based on renal biopsies. Medicine, Baltimore, *38*:321-367, 1959.
6. Haddad, J. K., and Mani, R. L.: Percutaneous renal biopsy. Arch. Intern. Med., *119*:157-160, 1967.
7. Holt, S. J.: Factors governing the validity of staining methods for enzymes and their bearing upon Gomori acid phosphatase technique. Exp. Cell Res. (Suppl. 7): 1, 1959.
8. Iversen, P. & Brun, C.: Aspiration biopsy of the kidney. Am. J. Med., *11*:324-330, 1951.
9. Jungman, P.: Über chronische streptokokkeninfektionen. Deutsche med. Wchschr., *50*:71, 1924.
10. Lillie, R. D.: Histopathologic technique. Philadelphia, The Blakiston Co.
11. Lowry, O. H.: Quantitative histochemistry of brain, histologic sampling. J. Histochem. Cytochem., *1*:420-428, 1953.
12. Luft, J. H.: Improvements in epoxy resin embedding method. J. Biophys. Biochem. Cytol., *9*:409-414, 1961.
13. Muchrcke, R. C., Kark, R. M. & Pirani, C. L.: Technique of percutaneous renal biopsy in the prone position, J. Urol., *74*:267-277, 1955.
14. Muehrcke, R. C., Kark, R. M., Pirani, C. L., & Pollak, V. E.: Lupus nephritis: A Clinical and pathologic study based on renal biopsies. Medicine, *36*:1-145, 1957.
15. Muehrcke, R. C., Kark, R. M. & Pirani, C. L.: Biopsy of the kidney in the diagnosis and management of renal disease. New Eng. Med., *253*:537-546, 1955.
16. Parrish, A. E., & Howe, J. S.: Needle biopsy as an aid in diagnosis of renal disease. J. Lab. & Clin. Med., *42*:152-157, 1953.
17. PerezAra, A.: La biopsia puntural del rinon no megalico consideraciones generales y aportacion de un nuevo metodo. Bol. Liga Contral el Cancer, *25*:121, 1950.

18. Pollak, V. E., Pirani, C. L., Kark, R. M. Muehrcke, R. C., Freda, V. C. & Nettles, J. B.: Possible glomerular lesion in Toxaemia of pregnancy. Lancet, *2*:59-63, 1956.

19. Rosen, S., Pirani, C. L., Kark, R. M. Muehrcke, R. C. & Pollak, V. E.: Lipoid nephrosis and Idiopathic Membranous glomerulonephritis (Scientific proceedings). The Am. J. Pathology, *44*:14a, 1964.

20. Ross, J. H. & Ross, I. P.: The value of renal biopsy. Lancet, *2*:559-565, 1957.

21. Talbot, J. H.: Medical Progress; Renal function tests. New Eng. J. Med., *226*:197-201, 1942.

22. Talbot, J. H.: Medical Progress; heterogenous renal disorders. Ibid., *226*:228-236, 1942.

23. Zelman, S.: Fatal hemorrhage following needle biopsy in uremia. Report of a case. J.A.M.A., *154*:997-100, 1954.

The Renal Biopsy in Primary Glomerular Disease

ROBERT B. JENNINGS, M.D., and
PETER B. HERDSON, M.B., Ch.B., Ph.D.

Since the percutaneous renal biopsy technique was popularized in the United States by Kark and his associates (1) and Parrish and Howe (2) in 1955, much has been learned about pathological changes which occur in kidneys of living patients suffering from a variety of renal diseases. This information was not available prior to that time, because autopsy studies yielded very little knowledge of the acute stages of non-fatal renal diseases. The recent application to renal biopsies of electron and immunofluorescent microscopy, niether of which were widely used in this context until 1960, has further extended our understanding of the probable pathogenesis of several varieties of renal disease.

Some of the most interesting and significant glomerular diseases are those which can be classified as primary glomerular diseases. These are renal diseases which appear to originate in and chiefly affect glomeruli, even though the renal changes may be part of a more generalized process also occurring elsewhere in the body.

Many different examples of the way in which glomeruli can be altered by disease have been described in preceding papers at this symposium. Suffice it to say that the glomerulus is a relatively simple structure, which can react to disease in only a relatively limited number of morphological changes. These basic types of changes, which are shown in Table 1, can occur in either focal or diffuse forms, involving parts of a few or all glomeruli. Greater precision in description of glomerular lesions has been attempted by the use of the terms 'local' as apposed to 'diffuse' for individual glomerular involvement, and 'focal' as apposed to 'generalized' with reference

TABLE I—TYPES OF GLOMERULAR CHANGE

Endothelium	swelling
	proliferation
	necrosis
Basement membrane	thickening
	deposits
Epithelium	proliferation
	necrosis
Capillaries	thromboses
	inflammatory cells
Infiltrations	amyloid
	hyaline (? nature)

TABLE II
DIFFUSE GLOMERULAR DISEASES

Etiologic Diagnosis	Clinical Diagnosis	Morphologic Diagnosis
Acute post streptococcal glomerulonephritis	Acute glomerulo-nephritis Acute renal failure Other	Proliferative glomerulonephritis Exudative glomerulonephritis Mixed proliferative and exudative glomerulonephritis
?	Toxemia of pregnancy	Endothelial swelling Fibrin deposition
Amyloidosis	Renal failure Nephrotic syndrome	Amyloid deposition
? Soluble antigen-antibody complexes	Nephrotic syndrome	Diffuse membranous glomerular disease
? Virus	Nephrotic syndrome	No glomerular disease (L.M.) Fused foot processes (E.M.)

to the entire kidney (3, 4). However, acceptance of this terminology has been slow, and in the present paper, the term diffuse refers to changes which affect all glomeruli.

Diffuse glomerular diseases have been studied particularly well, because they frequently result in significant functional impairment, thus bringing the patient to the physician. Furthermore, percutaneous renal biopsy is especially useful in this group of glomerular diseases, because the diffuse involvement of glomeruli results in a representative sample of diseased tissue being obtained for study in a high proportion of cases. Information obtained from biopsies of these patients aids in diagnosis, in assessing the effects of treatment, and is an important adjunct to the investigation of the etiology and pathogenesis of these diseases.

In Table 2 are listed most of the important varieties of diffuse glomerular diseases, under the headings of etiologic, clinical and morphological diagnoses. Clearly, etiologic diagnoses are the type that are desired and it is to be hoped that the many question marks under this heading can be removed within the next few years. Also, it is apparent that many of the clinical diagnoses are fairly general. Thus, renal failure and the nephrotic syndrome are not very specific but are simply convenient terms for a set of symptoms and signs manifested by the patient. As might be expected, a variety of morphological changes can be associated with these clinical diagnoses. Although morphological diagnoses can be more specific, difficulties arise in attempting to distinguish mild degrees of these changes, and, at the other end of the spectrum, in distinguishing far-advanced focal from diffuse glomerular diseases.

POST-STREPTOCOCAL GLOMERULONEPHRITIS

This is one of the best studied of the diffuse diseases (5-8). Recent work has established fairly clearly that the disease probably results from the incidental clearing of soluble antigen-antibody complexes from the circulation of the patient (9-13). The antigen has not been identified yet, and until it is, the theory that the disease results from a soluble complex can not be proved. It seems clear, however, that an antigen is present and that it is related somehow to Group A streptococci (14). Gamma-globulin and complement are also parts of the soluble complex, and have been shown by immunofluorescent techniques to be localized focally on the walls of the glomerular capillaries (9, 11-14).

The typical clinical presentation is well known. A patient suddenly develops edema, hypertension and abnormal urine, 7 to 40 days after an infection with a Group A streptococcus. The clinical diagnosis is acute nephritis. The disease develops suddenly and coincidentally with the clearing of the soluble complexes from the circulation, which presumably excite the peculiar and characteristic glomerular inflammatory reaction called acute glomerulonephritis. Oliguria may occur and be so severe that a clinical diagnosis of acute renal failure is made. On the other hand, the disease may be very mild and abnormal urine may be the chief clinical manifestation (5, 7). Renal biopsies of patients with

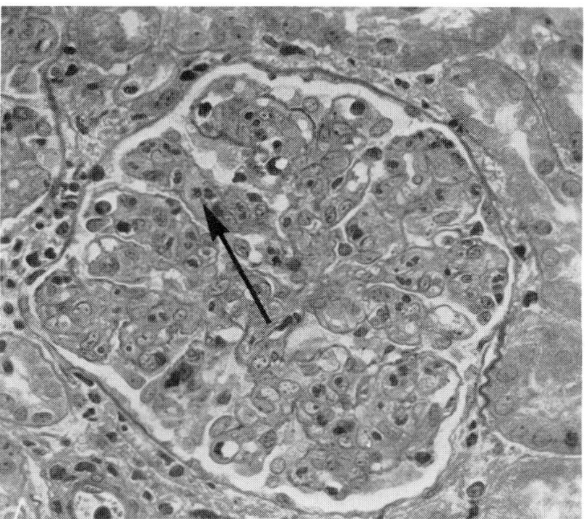

Fig. 1. Section of glomerulus showing increased intracapillary cellularity, lobulation, and about 13 polymorphonuclear neutrophils in the capillary loops. There is a mitotic figure in an endothelial cell (arrow). This glomerulus is typical of moderately severe proliferative glomerulonephritis. From a 5-year-old boy, biopsied six days after the onset of edema, hypertension and abnormal urine. Group A hemolytic streptococci were isolated from his pharynx on admission. He had had a sore throat 2 weeks prior to admission. Heidenhain's connective tissue stain. X 350.

clinical disease will shown diffuse proliferative (Fig. 1) or exudative glomerulonephritis (Fig. 2), or often a mixture of the two. Electron microscopy of tissue obtained within the first 40 days after onset of renal symptoms reveals characteristic electron-dense deposits ("humps") on the epithelial aspect of the glomerular capillary basement membrane (6) (Fig. 3). The intracapillary hypercellularity is confirmed, and basement membrane-like material is seen between many of these cells. In addition, electrondense material frequently is present irregularly between endothelium and basement membrane, and within the basement membrane, especially in patients with marked histological changes. Immunofluorescent microscopy

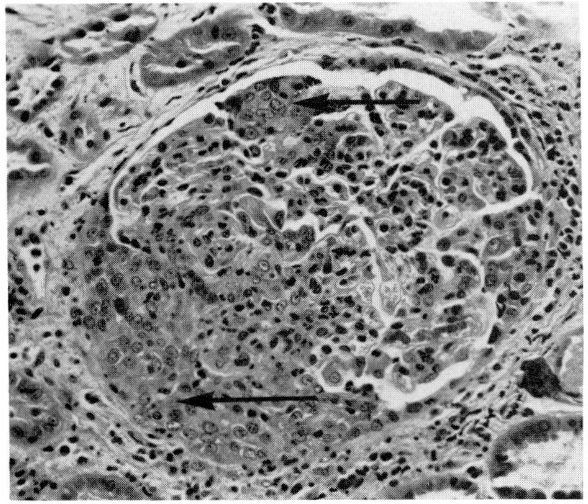

Fig. 2. Section of glomerulus showing increased cellularity due to the presence of increased numbers of polymorphonuclear neutrophils within the capillary loops, and crescents at the arrows. There is no proliferation of endothelial cells. This patient developed clinical acute nephritis with oliguria, azotemia, and hypertension about one week after being treated with 300,000 units of procaine penicillin for severe acute pharyngitis. The ASO titer rose after admission, showing the patient had had a recent infection with a group A streptococcus. The serum complement was depressed to 23 units. Biopsy was performed 30 days after the onset and two days before the patient died in acute renal failure. This diseased glomerulus is representative, showing acute inflammation, and the name exudative is applied because of the abundant granulocytes and the crescents. Crescents have been shown to be a response of the epithelial cells in Bowman's space to exudation of fibrin (7). Hematoxylin and eosin stain. X 276. (Reprinted with permission from J. Clin. Invest. (5).)

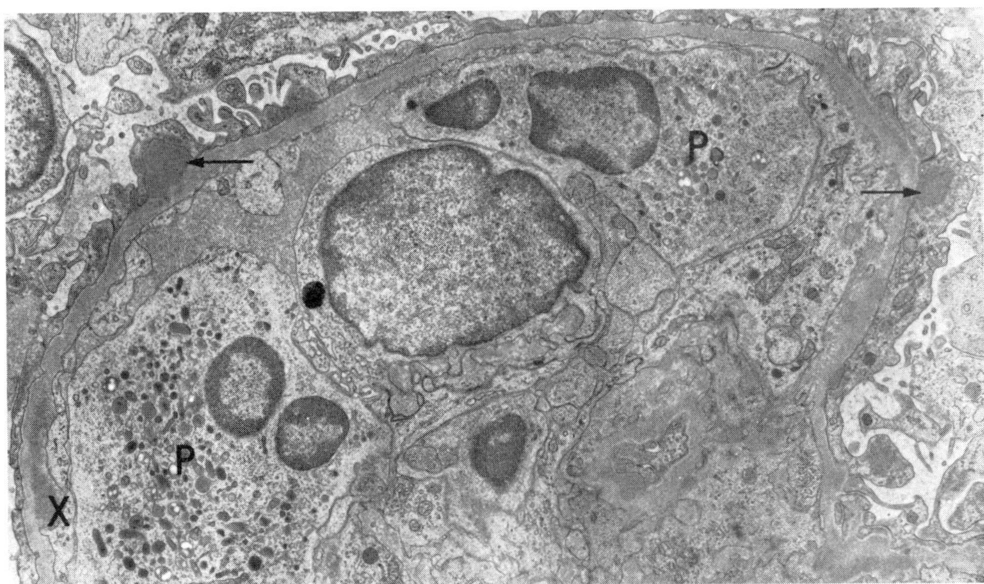

Fig. 3. Electron micrograph of part of a glomerular capillary loop from the same patient as Figure 1. The capillary lumen is virtually occluded by at least three inflammatory cells including two polymorphonuclear leucocytes (P). Electrondense material is noted between the basement membrane at X. Two "humps" (arrows) are present. Sub-epithelial deposits of this particular type are characteristically seen in post-streptococcal acute diffuse glomerulonephritis up to 40 days after the onset of symptoms. Deposits of identical morphology may occur in other diseases believed to be associated with antigen-antibody complexes, including secondary syphilis (16). X 4000.

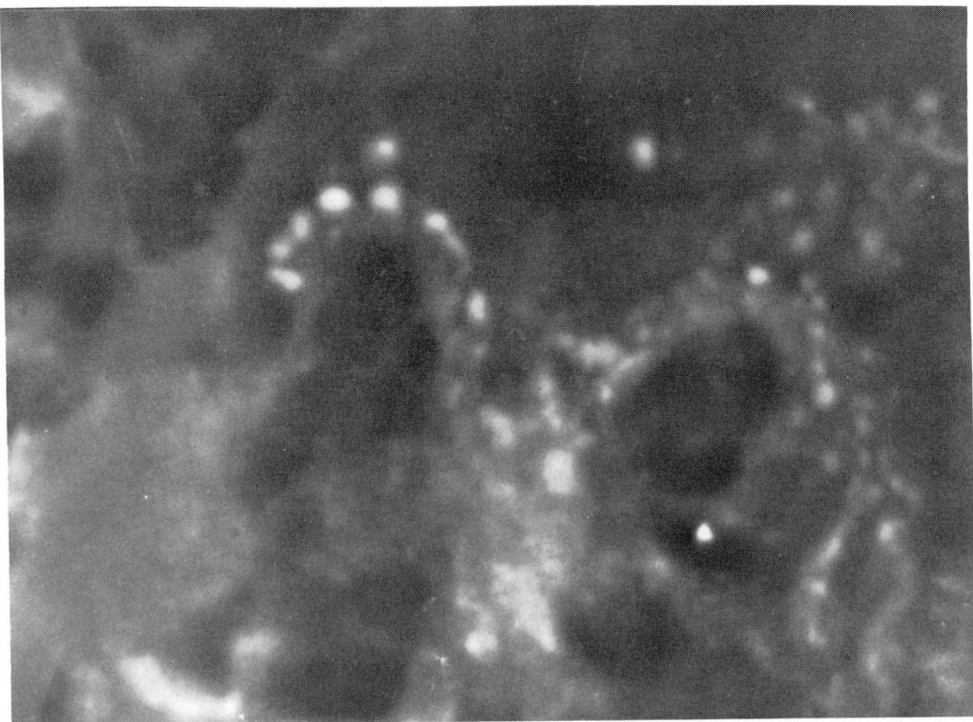

Fig. 4. Glomerulus obtained 23 days after the onset from a 20-year-old white female with acute diffuse proliferative poststreptococcal glomerulonephritis. Fluorescence for gamma globulin is present along the basement membranes in a discrete granular pattern. This distribution of gamma globulin was found during the acute phase of post-streptococcal clinical acute glomerulonephritis of all histologic types. Complement had the same distribution as gamma globulin. Both gamma globulin and complement decreased in quantity and finally disappeared in patients with healed acute glomerulonephritis. Preliminary studies of gamma globulin distribution in glomeruli of patients whose acute attack failed to heal has shown gamma globulin is still present a year or more after the acute attack (17).

of such tissue shows a fairly characteristic distribution of gamma-globulin and complement (Fig. 4).

Histologic evidence of hypercellularity often still is present when the nephritis has healed clinically, as defined by the patient being free of signs and symptoms, and having urine which has returned to normal. However, our experience suggests that the proliferative lesions eventually disappear in such patients (7). On the other hand, there is fairly good evidence that some patients develop persistent disease after an acute attack of post-streptococcal glomerulonephritis. If this is true, then these patients should develop granular contracted kidneys and should show chronic diffuse proliferative glomerulonephritis some 5 to 25 years after the onset (7). This concept is still under investigation.

TOXEMIA OF PREGNANCY

This is a reversible lesion which electron microscopy has shown to be characterized chiefly by swelling of the endothelium of the glomerular capillaries (18-20). Fibrin often is present and may be etiologically related to the glomerular response (21). The disease is included here because it is one of the diffuse

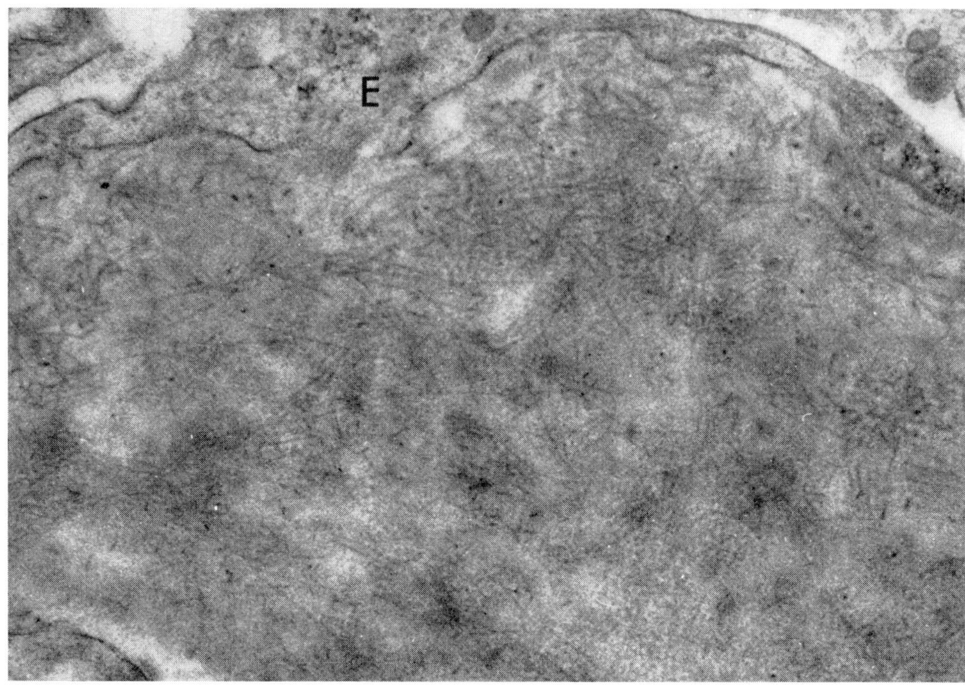

Fig. 5. Electron micrograph of a segment of glomerular capillary basement membrane infiltrated and thickened by amyloid. Typical amyloid fibrils are readily distinguished, E, epithelial cytoplasm. X 52,000.

glomerular lesions, and because toxemia and post-streptococcal acute glomerulonephritis are the only diffuse glomerular diseases in which there is fairly precise information concerning their time of onset. The time of onset of all the other conditions listed in Table 2 is completely unknown.

AMYLOIDOSIS

This is an uncommon alteration. It has fairly characteristic histological and fluorescent staining reactions and a specific electron microscopic appearance (22) (Fig. 5). The proteinuria associated with glomerular involvement by amyloid is often so extensive as to lead to the nephrotic syndrome (23, 24). During the 11 years that the Northwestern University group has been doing biopsies,

several cases of completely unexpected primary amyloidosis have been discovered.

DIFFUSE MEMBRANOUS GLOMERULAR DISEASE

This disease is manifest clinically by proteinuria with or without the nephrotic syndrome. The incidence of the pathological changes which are involved is unknown, because they are detected only if proteinuria or edema lead to clinical investigation including renal biopsy. The morphological renal abnormalities associated with this disease are found occasionally at autopsy in patients dying of renal failure. Other names which have been applied to this type of glomerular alternation are diffuse membranous glomerulonephritis (25-28),

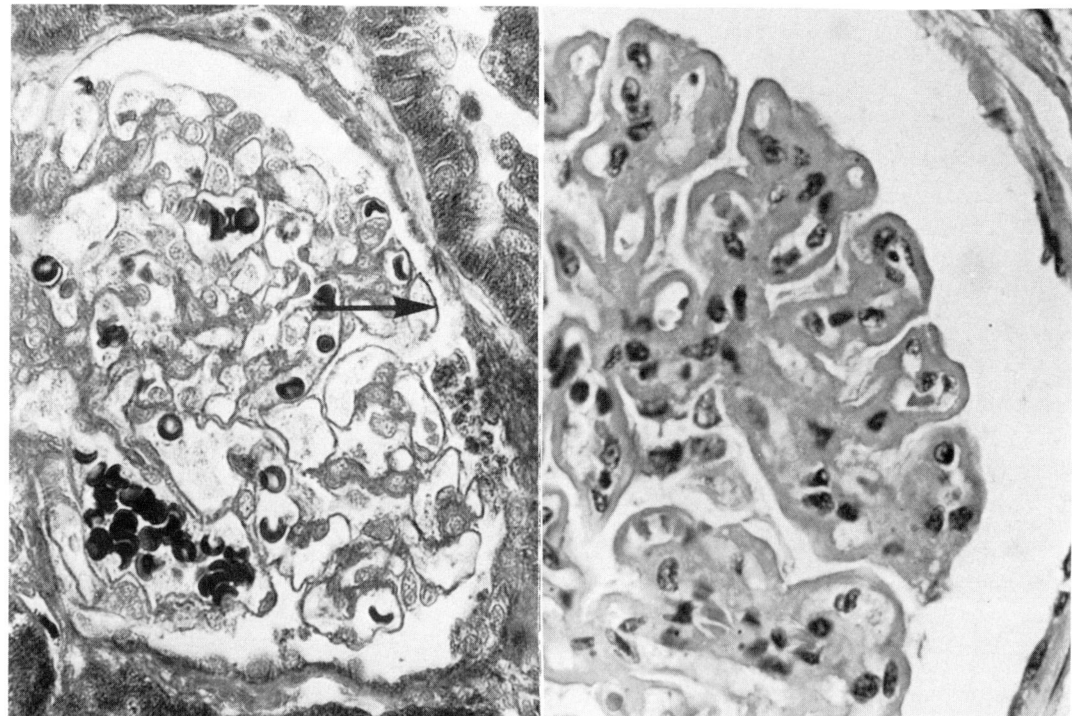

Fig. 6a. Section of a glomerulus from a 22-year-old patient with the nephrotic syndrome of 15 months' duration. The walls of the capillary loops are not thickened and a "red line" can not be positively identified, but there is a suggestion of a red deposit on the loop marked by the arrow. Electron microscopy revealed mild membranous glomerular disease. Immunofluorescence staining was not done. Heidenhain's connective tissue stain. X 850.

Fig. 6b. Severe membranous glomerular disease, in a 36-year-old Negro female who lived 28 months after the onset of the nephrotic syndrome. She died in chronic renal failure. This section is of a representative glomerulus obtained at autopsy. When the first biopsy was obtained three weeks after the onset of proteinuira, basement membrane thickening was no more severe than that noted in Figure 6a. Hematoxylin and eosin. X 840.

glomerulonephrosis (29), and recently, membranous nephrosis (30). The authors shifted from the eponym membranous glomerulonephritis (25) to membranous glomerular change or disease in 1962 because there was no proof that this "disease" had an inflammatory origin as implied by the name glomerulonephritis.

Diffuse membranous glomerular disease is characterized by thickening of the walls of the peripheral capillary loops of all glomeruli (25). The thickening ranges from slight (Fig. 6a), to very marked (Fig. 6b). The lesion was first identified by light microscopy by Bell (26) and later by Allen (27) but subsequent work with electron microscopy, immunofluorescence, and the study of thin sections by light microscopy has made the diagnostic criteria more precise. It seems clear that the thickening is due to the presence of a sub-epithelial layer of dense material (usually called "deposits"), which is attached to or is a part of the basement membrane (Fig. 7) (28-32). The deposits are usually more electron-dense than the basement membrane but occasionally may show a vacuolated appearance. Study of fresh tissue by the immunofluorescent techni-

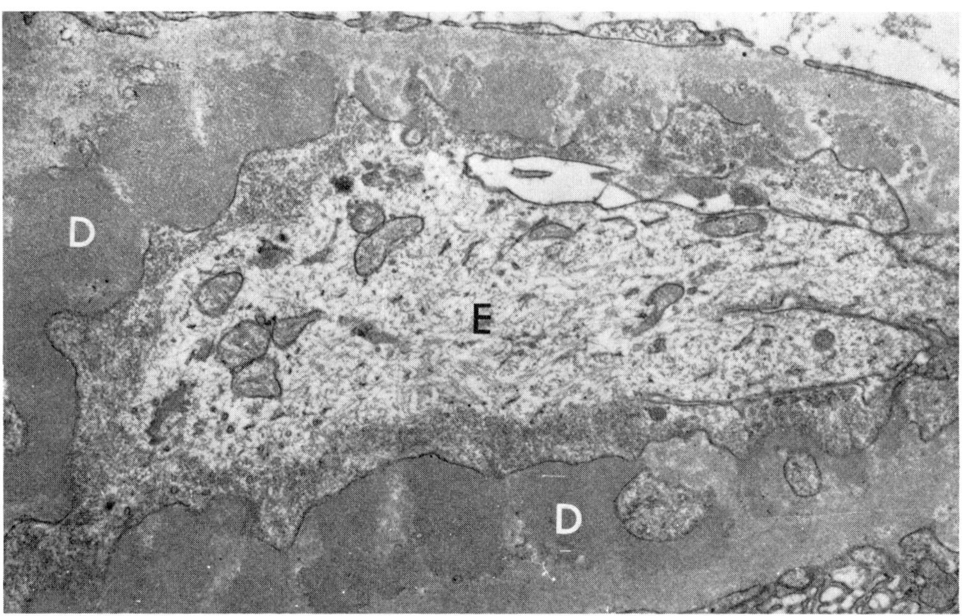

Fig. 7. Electron micrograph of part of a glomerulus from a case of typical diffuse membranous glomerular disease. Thick subepithelial electron-dense deposits (D) are seen along the basement membrane, and electron-dense granular material is present in neighboring epithelial cytoplasm. E, epithelial cytoplasm, X 16,000.

que shows that the deposits contain gamma-globulin (Fig. 8) and βIC globulins complement (12, 13, 33). Examination of thin sections stained by Heidenhain's modification of Mallory's connective tissue reveals that the inner portion of the thickened glomerular capillary wall is blue and the outer part deep red (Fig. 9). When we first identified this differential staining in 1957 we called this change "red line disease" (25). Later work has established that the "red line" is probably the deposit seen on electron microscopy. The deposit can also be seen in 0.5 μ sections of kidney fixed in osmium tetroxide, embedded in Epon and stained with toluidine blue (34). Here the material stains more deeply blue than the basement membrane itself (Fig. 10).

The objective diagnosis of diffuse membranous glomerular disease is rela-tively easy in the classic case, where there is obvious thickening of the walls of peripheral capillary loops, the "red line" is present in thin sections, gamma-globulin and complement are found along the basement membrane by immunofluorescence, and electron microscopy shows characteristic subepithelial deposits. Mallory's connective tissue stain colors the deposits violet against a green background and the PAS-methanamine stain shows spikes of silver-positive material in the basement membrane (35).

However, there are patients with diffuse membranous glomerular disease in whom the glomeruli do not show objective thickening of the basement membrane by routine techniques of light microscopy. Frequently, a "red line" can be detected in this group, but it is very thin, and difficult to resolve (Fig. 6a).

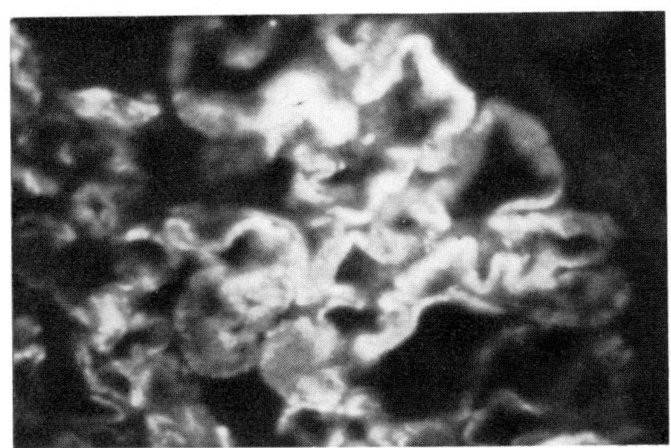

Fig. 8. Glomerulus showing typical irregular generally linear fluorescence for gamma globulin along the basement membranes of the peripheral capillary loops in a 39-year-old Puerto Rican male with membranous glomerular disease. Complement had the same distribution as gamma globulin and is not illustrated. Proteinuria was present for two years prior to time of biopsy. Edema was intermittant and minimal. The patient has not responded to steroid therapy. Electron microscopy showed a pattern similar to Figure 7.

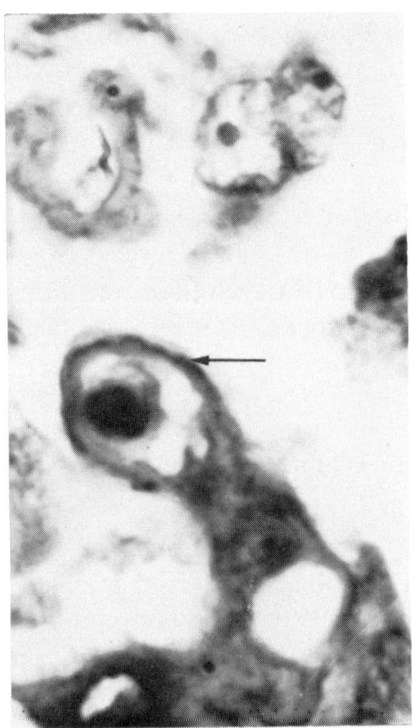

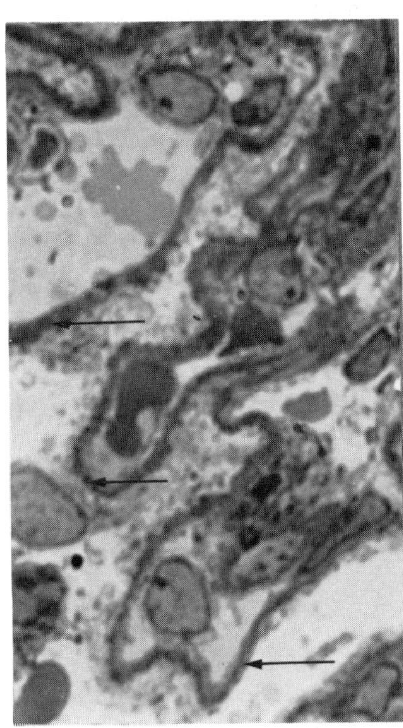

Fig. 9. Glomerular capillary loop from a patient with moderate membranous glomerular disease, showing marked thickening of the wall chiefly due to a red-staining layer, which appears black in the photomicrograph (arrow). It was in this 56-year-old man who was suffering from the nephrotic syndrome associated with renal vein thrombosis, that the red line was first seen by Dr. Martin P. Hutt and R. B. J. Heidenhain's connective tissue stain. X 2,400.

Fig. 10. Mild membranous change in the kidney of a 47-year-old Caucasian male with a history of proteinuria of two years' duration. The nephrotic syndrome had not been clinically apparent, but proteinuria averaged 1 to 2 mg per 24 hours. The serum cholesterol was 464 mg per 100 ml. This high power view is of parts of three glomerular capillaries in a 1μ section embedded in Epon. The section was stained with toluidine blue and shows the deposit which was stained deep blue in a subepithelial position (arrows). The structure equivalent to the lamina densa appears light gray and is adjacent to the lumen of the capillary. Toluidine blue. X 2,000.

This is because the thickness of the deposit in such instances is close to or less than the resolving power of the light microscope. Moreover, the intensity of the azocarmine stain may vary from patient to patient depending on the chemical character and density of the deposit. Biopsies from patients with these lesser degrees of diffuse membranous glomerular disease usually show positive immunofluorescence and always show sub-epithelial deposits by electron microscopy. This type of diffuse membranous change was not diagnosed by light microscopy until correlative studies with electron microscopy enabled us to establish appropriate criteria. It seems probable that kidney tissue of some patients with the nephrotic syndrome, classified in the earlier literature on renal biopsy as "no glomerular disease by light microscopy," "nil disease," "lipoid nephrosis," and "glomerular epithelial cell disease," really had diffuse membranous glomerular change which was not detected.

The etiology of diffuse membranous glomerular disease has not been established. A lesion that is very similar has been induced in rabbits by creating a situation in which soluble antigen-antibody complexes are continuously present (9, 10). The presence of gamma-globulin and complement in the complexes and in the glomerular capillary membranes in these experimental animals, as in man, lends support to the idea that the disease in man results from a kind of antigen-antibody reaction. However, a similar lesion also can be induced by injecting homologous or heterologous soluble material from renal cortex in Freund's adjuvant, in which case a direct rather than an incidental antigen-antibody reaction may be occurring in the glomeruli (36-39). The

hypothesis that the continuous clearance of soluble complexes may cause the disease in man is attractive. The fact that similar glomerular changes develop in some patients after administration of drugs like Tridione (40) suggests that such chemicals may somehow be related to the antigenic response.

Whether or not diffuse membranous glomerular disease has a single etiology remains to be seen. It seems more likely that multiple mechanisms may be involved (40-42). The observations and criteria for diagnosis presented here have allowed us to identify 50 patients with these glomerular changes. None has responded well to steroid therapy, and their course, with few exceptions, has been one of relentless significant proteinuria with variable degrees of edema. About one-third of them are now dead, almost always as a result of either renal failure or infection.

NO GLOMERULAR DISEASE BY LIGHT MICROSCOPY

The last diffuse glomerular alteration which will be considered is often called "lipoid nephrosis." The glomeruli do not show any lesion by light microscopy, but electron microscopy reveals widespread fusion of epithelial foot-processes, together with microvillation of epithelial cytoplasm (25, 43) (Fig. 11). There usually are no deposits of gamma-globulin or complement in such glomeruli (12, 33). The lesion is reversible, and responds well to steroids. Virus infection has been suggested as a possible etiology of this disease.

Some investigators would include diabetic renal disease amongst diffuse glomerular diseases. Our decision not to do so is arbitrary and is based on the belief that the thickening of peripheral

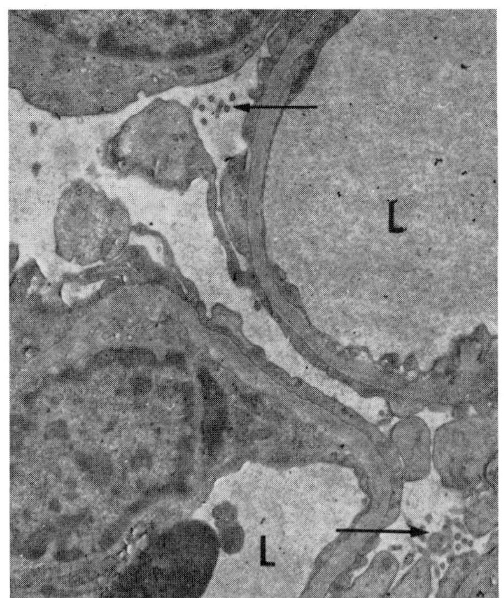

Fig. 11. Electron micrograph of portion of a glomerulus from a patient with the nephrotic syndrome, whose biopsy showed "no disease by light microscopy." There is widespread fusion of epithelial cell foot processes, and microvillation of epithelial cytoplasm is present (arrows). L, capillary lumen. X 4,000.

capillary loops and occasional nodular glomerular lesions seen in diabetes mellitus may be associated more with extension of the arteriolar disease which is always present in these patients (26) than with primary glomerular disease.

Finally, brief reference should be made to focal glomerulitis which is considered in section B of this chapter. In our series of more than 1000 renal biopsies, this is one of the most common diagnoses (44). A small proportion of cases of focal glomerulitis are associated with diseases such as systemic lupus nephropathy (4), Henoch-Schönlein purpura (44, 45), so-called Goodpasture's syndrome (46) and subacute bacterial endocarditis (47), but in the vast majority, there is meagre knowledge of the etiology or pathogenesis of the glomerular changes. In the present context of

diffuse glomerular diseases, it is of importance to realize that repeated sporadic involvement of glomeruli by focal glomerulitis may result eventually in disease affecting all glomeruli. The chief clue that the renal disease may have originated focally lies in the fact that the glomerular lesions are almost always of different ages. However, once the kidney is diffusely involved, one can only guess that the alterations began focally.

REFERENCES

1. Kark, R. M., Muehrcke, R. C., Pirani, C. L., and Pollak, V. E.: The clinical value of renal biopsy. Ann. Int. Med., *43*:807-847, 1955.
2. Parrish, A. E., and Howe, J. A.: Kidney biopsy. A review of one hundred successful needle biopsies. Arch. Int. Med., *96*:712-716, 1955.
3. Heptinstall, R. H., and Joekes, A. M.: Focal glomerulonephritis. A study based on renal biopsies. Quart. J. Med., *28*:329-346, 1959.
4. Muehrcke, R. C., Kark, R. M., Pirani, C. L., and Pollak, V. E.: Lupus nephritis: A clinical and pathologic study based on renal biopsies. Medicine, *36*:1-145, 1957.
5. Jennings, R. B., and Earle, D. P.: Post-streptococcal glomerulonephritis: Histopathologic and clinical studies of the acute, subsiding acute and early chronic latent phases. J. Clin. Invest., *40*:1525-1595, 1961.
6. Herdson, P. B., Jennings, R. B., and Earle, D. P.: Glomerular fine structure in post-streptococcal acute glomerulonephritis. Arch. Path., *81*:117-128, 1966.
7. Jennings, R. B., and Earle, D. P.: Glomerulonephritis. In, Becker, E. L. (ed.): Structural Basis of Renal Disease. New York, Hoeber Inc., 1967.
8. McCluskey, R. T., and Baldwin, D. S. Natural history of acute glomerulonephritis. Am. J. Med., *35*:213-230, 1963.
9. Dixon, F. J.: The role of antigen-antibody complexes in disease. Harvey Lect., *58*:21-52, 1962-63.
10. Dixon, F. J.: The pathogenesis of immunologically induced nephritis. Proc. 3rd Int. Congr. Nephrol., Washington 1966, Vol. 2; pp. 97-112, Basel/New York, Karger, 1967.
11. Michael, A. F., Jr., Drummond, K. N., Good, R. A., and Vernier, R. L.: Acute poststreptococcal glomerulonephritis: Immune deposit disease. J. Clin. Invest., *45*:237-248, 1966.

12. McCluskey, R. T., Vassalli, P., Gallo, G., and Baldwin, D. S.: An immunofluorescent study of pathogenic mechanisms in glomerular diseases. New Eng. J. Med., *274*:695-701, 1966.

13. Earle, D. P., and Jennings, R. B.: Glomerulonephritis. Proc. 3rd Int. Congr. Nephrol., Washington 1966, Vol. 3, pp. 51-68, Karger, Basel/New York, 1967.

14. Seegal, B. C., Andres, G. A., Hsu, K. C., and Zabriskie, J. B.: Studies on the pathogenesis of acute and progressive glomerulonephritis in man by immunofluorescein and immunoferritin techniques. Fed. Proc., *24*:100-108, 1965.

15. Vassalli, P., and McCluskey, R. T.: The coagulation process and glomerular disease. Am. J. Med., *39*:179-183, 1965.

16. Falls, W. F., Jr., Ford, K. L., Ashworth, C. T., and Carter, N. W. The nephrotic syndrome in secondary syphilis. Report of a case with renal biopsy findings. Ann. Int. Med., *63*:1047-1058, 1965.

17. Potter, E. L., Earle, D. P., Humair, L., Gallo, G., Jennings, R. B., and Herdson, P. B.: Immunofluorescent and morphologic studies of chronic latent, healing and healed post-streptococcal glomerulonephritis. In preparation.

18. Pirani, C. L., Pollak, V. E., Lannigan, R., and Folli, G.: The renal glomerular lesions of pre-eclampsia: Electron microscope studies. Am. J. Obstet. Gynec., *87*:1047-1070, 1963.

19. Spargo, B., McCartney, C. P., and Winemiller, R.: Glomerular capillary endotheliosis in toxemia of pregnancy. Arch. Path., *68*:593-599, 1959.

20. Mautner, W., Churg, J., Grishman, E., and Dachs, S.: Preeclamptic nephropathy. An electron microscopic study. Lab. Invest., *11*:518-530, 1962.

21. Vassalli, P., Morris, R. H., and McCluskey, R. T., The pathogenic role of fibrin deposition in toxemia of pregnancy. J. Exper. Med., *118*:467-478.

22. Bergstrand, A., and Bucht, H.: Electron microscopy of renal glomerular amyloidosis. In Ciba Foundation Symposium on "Clinical and Pathological Significance of Renal Biopsy," Ed. by G. E. W. Wolstenholme and M. P. Cameron, Boston, Little Brown & Co., 1962, pp. 51-65.

23. Lindsay, S.: Primary systemic amyloidosis with nephrosis. Am. J. Med., *4*:765-772, 1948.

24. Lindeman, R. D., Scheer, R. L., and Raisz, L. G.: Renal amyloidosis. Ann. Int. Med., *54*:883-898, 1961.

25. Earle, D. P., Jennings, R. B., and Bernik, M.: A consideration of the histopathologic basis for the nephrotic syndrome. Prog. in Cardiovascular Dis., *4*:148-169, 1961.

26. Bell, E. T.: Renal Diseases, Ed. 2. Philadelphia, Lea & Febiger, pp. 448, 1950.

27. Allen, A. C.: The clinicopathologic meaning of the nephrotic syndrome. Am. J. Med., *18*:277-314, 1955.

28. Habib, R., Michielsen, P., deMontera, E., Hinglass, N., Galle, P., and Hamburger, J.: Clinical microscopic and electron microscopic data in the nephrotic syndrome of unknown origin. In, Ciba Foundation Symposium on "Clinical and Pathological Significance of Renal Biopsy." Ed. by G. E. W. Wolstenholme and M. P. Cameron. Boston, Little Brown & Co., 1962, pp. 70-92.

29. Kimmelstiel, P., Kim. O. J., and Beres, J.: Studies on renal biopsy specimens, with the aid of the electron microscope. II. Glomerulonephritis and glomerulonephrosis. Am. J. Clin. Path., *38*:280-296, 1962.

30. Churg, J., Grishman, E., Goldstein, M. H., Yunis, S. L., and Porush, J. G.: Idiopathic nephrotic syndrome in adults. A study and classification based on renal biopsies. New Eng. J. Med., *272*:165-174, 1965.

31. Movat, H. Z., and McGregor, D. D.: The fine structure of the glomerulus in membranous glomerulonephritis (lipoid nephrosis) in adults. Am. J. Clin. Path., *32*:109-127, 1959.

32. Spargo, B., and Arnold, J. D.: Glomerular extrinsic membranous deposit with the nephrotic syndrome. Ann. N. Y. Acad. Sci., *86*:1043-1063, 1960.

33. Drummond, K. N., Michael, A. F., Good, R. A., and Vernier, R. L.: The nephrotic syndrome of childhood: Immunologic, clinical, and pathologic correlations. J. Clin. Invest., *45*:620-630, 1966.

34. Trump, B. F.: Electron microscopic studies of human renal disease. Observations of normal visceral glomerular epithelium and its modification in disease. Lab. Invest., *11*:753-781, 1962.

35. Jones, D. B.: Nephrotic glomerulonephritis. Am. J. Path., *33*:313-330, 1957.

36. Blozis, G. G., Spargo, B., and Rowley, D. A.: Glomerular basement membrane changes with the nephrotic syndrome produced in the rat by homologous kidney and hemophilus pertussis vaccine. Am. J. Path., *40*:153-165, 1962.

37. Heymann, W.: Further studies in experimental autoimmune renal disease of rats. In, renal Metabolism and Epidemiology of Some Renal Diseases. Proceedings of the 15th Annual Conference on the Kidney, Ed. by J. Metcoff. New York, National Kidney Foundation. pp. 217-221, 1964.

38. Okuda, R., Kaplan, M. H., Cuppage, F. E., and Heymann, W.: Deposition of autologous gamma globulin in kidneys of rats with nephrotic renal disease of various etiologies. J. Lab. Clin. Med., *66*:204-215, 1965.

39. Heymann, W.: Experimental analogies of human nephropathies. Proc. 3rd Int. Congr. Nephrol. Washington 1966, Vol. 2; pp. 164-177, Basel/New York, Karger, 1967.

40. Barnett, H. L., Simons, D. J., and Wells, R. E., Jr.: Nephrotic syndrome occurring during tridione therapy. Am. J. Med., *4*:760-764, 1948.

41. Pollak, V. E., Kark, R. M., Pirani, C. L., Shafter, H. E., and Muehrcke, R. C.: Renal vein thrombosis and the nephrotic syndrome. Am. J. Med., *21*:496-520, 1956.
42. Panner, B.: Nephrotic syndrome in renal vein thrombosis. Arch. Path., *76*:303-317, 1963.
43. Farquhar, M. G., Vernier, R. L., and Good, R. A.: Studies on familial nephrosis II. Glomerular changes observed with the electron microscope. Am. J. Path., *33*:791-818, 1957.
44. Earle, D. P., and Jennings, R. B.: Focal glomerular lesions. Trans. Am. Clin. & Climatol. Ass'n., *72*:24-37, 1960.
45. Vernier, R. L., Farquhar, M. G., Brunson, J. G., and Good, R. A.: Chronic renal disease in children. Am. J. Dis. Child., *96*:306-343, 1958.
46. Duncan, D. A., Drummond, K. N., Michael, A. F., and Vernier, F. L.: Pulmonary hemorrhage and glomerulonephritis. Report of six cases and study of the renal lesion by the fluorescent antibody technique and electron microscopy. Ann. Int. Med., *62*:920-938, 1965.
47. Bell, E. T. Glomerular lesions associated with endocarditis. Am. J. Path., *8*:639-664, 1932.

The Renal Biopsy of Focal Glomerular Disease

ROBERT H. HEPTINSTALL, M.D.

The renal biopsy has opened up a completely new era of renal pathology, for whereas the pathologist at one time was dependent almost entirely on material obtained at autopsy or surgery, he is now confronted with tissue from the early stage of disease or from conditions which do not ultimately prove fatal. It is obvious in such circumstances that new pictures are constantly being encountered, whose interpretation is difficult, and because of our ignorance, frequently frustrating. One of the interesting outcomes of the early years of the renal biopsy is the recognition of various forms of focal glomerulonephritis, and this account is devoted mainly to this subject.

FOCAL GLOMERULONEPHRITIS

Focal glomerulonephritis is a glomerulonephritis in which only a certain number of glomeruli show lesions, the others being normal. It is of interest that those glomeruli having lesions frequently show an involvement of only a portion of the tuft, a change that will be referred to as a local lesion. In general, it can be said that focal glomerulonephritis can occur as a manifestation of well recognized entities such as systemic lupus erythematosus, polyarteritis nodosa, subacute bacterial endocarditis, or Schönlein-Henoch syndrome, or it may occur outside these diseases with a variety of clinical pictures.

FOCAL GLOMERULONEPHRITIS AS PART OF SYSTEMIC DISEASE

Systemic lupus erythematosus in its early stages affects the glomeruli in a focal way and the affected glomeruli show a predominantly local involvement, this consisting of one or two adjacent lobules showing necrotizing or proliferative changes. In the later stages, most of the glomeruli show involvement, but the tendency to localized involvement of individual glomeruli is often apparent.

Polyarteritis in the classical Kussmaul and Maier (6) form shows no glomerular change apart from those of ischemia, but in what is often referred to as the microscopic form (2), the glomeruli are involved. The changes here are essentially focal and even in advanced cases it is quite frequent to see a significant number of glomeruli not showing involvement. The glomerular lesion is almost invariably a necrotizing change affecting usually only part of the tuft which is rendered eosinophilic and structureless. A proliferative change may be seen in the affected part of the tuft and the epithelium lining Bowman's capsule is frequently excited to produce crescents.

Subacute bacterial endocarditis has long been recognized to produce a focal glomerulonephritis and the appearance is no different from that of focal glomerulonephritis not appearing as part of a systemic disease; this will be described later. The way in which the lesion is produced in endocarditis is not known but the two main possibilities are that it is embolic, or that it represents some immunologic mechanism.

Schönlein-Henoch purpura has long been known to give rise to a form of nephritis. Up to the time of the renal biopsy, the only picture recognized was that of a florid proliferative glomerulonephritis accompanied by extensive crescent formation in the patients with a rapidly progressing azotemic course. However, the more usual renal manifestation is much milder with complete recovery occurring as a rule. This form has been shown to have a renal picture of a mild focal glomerulonephritis of the type to be described.

FOCAL GLOMERULONEPHRITIS OCCURRING OUTSIDE SYSTEMIC DISEASE

The great majority of cases diagnosed as focal glomerulonephritis on biopsy do not present clinically with these various systemic illnesses. Their presentation is varied: some are first seen with a nephrotic syndrome with no distinguishing clinical features: others have recurrent attacks of hematuria: others may have hemoptysis and an abnormal urine noted on urinalysis, while some have urinary abnormalities or other symptoms or signs referable to the kidney; skin rashes and joint pains have been noted to occur in a good proportion of patients (3). The prognosis in most of these non-specific cases is good, the exception being the group with hemoptysis which frequently develop a rapidly progressive glomerulonephritis with death in uremia. In these cases, the renal pathology changes drastically over a relatively short time from a focal glomerulonephritis to a widespread florid glomerulonephritis with extensive crescent formation (1, 4, 7).

The pathology of focal glomerulonephritis not associated with systemic disease consists of a certain number of the glomeruli showing changes that are usually localized to one or two lobules of the tuft, although sometimes the tuft is diffusely involved. The usual localized change consists of an increase in cell nuclei often accompanied by necrosis, although one may occur without the other. There is sometimes proliferation of adjacent epithelium lining Bowman's capsule, and adhesions may form. In some cases, the localized area is solid and hyaline and this appears to be a later lesion as judged by a study of sequential biopsies. It is of interest that necroses have not been seen in our cases accompanied by a nephrotic syndrome (3). The tubules are frequently unaffected but focal loss may be found. Lymphocytes and plasma cells may be seen in the interstitium, and increased fibrosis is present in those with tubular loss. The changes in arteries are not impressive.

DISCUSSION

Apart from those forms accompanying systemic disease very little has been written about focal glomerulonephritis. This is almost certainly because it is either an early manifestation of disease, or because it represents a mild illness, with the result that it was never encountered in an autopsy service. Its recognition is largely a result of the extended use of the renal biopsy. It should not be diagnosed with abandon and certain of the pitfalls in diagnosis should be discussed.

In the first place, it is essential that some of the glomeruli should be normal, and this obvious fact should always be borne in mind. This is important in the differential diagnosis from resolving acute diffuse glomerulonephritis. In the latter condition, there is a widespread proliferative lesion in all glomeruli; during resolution the number of cells decreases at a more or less even rate in all glomeruli but persistence of increased numbers of cells in the mesangium may be seen for several months. In certain cases of acute diffuse glomerulonephritis it is found that some glomeruli show one or two lobules to be more severely affected, such as having greater numbers of nuclei than others. It is reasonable to assume that such glomeruli might resolve more slowly than others so that an appearance resembling a focal glomerulonephritis could be produced. The contrast between these more severely affected glomeruli and the others, would become accentuated during resolution, but the presence of mesangial hypercellularity would still be present in those less severely affected initially. There is still uncertainty, however, regarding the antecedent picture in the kidney of those cases in which partial solidification of an occasional glomerulus is seen on biopsy. It is conceivable that some of these might be the end result of what originally was a diffuse process, the affected glomeruli representing those that were irreparably damaged during the acute phase. For this reason, it seems best to include under the diagnosis of focal glomerulonephritis only those cases showing proliferative lesions, with or without necrosis.

Proliferative changes in both the tuft and in the cells lining Bowman's capsule may be seen around the periphery of infarcts. This change could be confused with focal glomerulonephritis if such an area were to be sampled by the biopsy needle. It is of interest that this is a likely cause of the glomerular lesions of subacute bacterial endocarditis where infarcts of the kidney are commonly encountered.

In cases of chronic pyelonephritis with hypertension, it is not infrequent to see what has been referred to as alterative glomerulitis (5). This consists of certain glomeruli showing localized nuclear proliferation with pyknosis of some of the nuclei and sometimes being associated with necrosis. Loss of surrounding tubules and other stigmata of chronic pyelonephritis should help to exclude this lesion.

In malignant hypertension, the glomeruli may show necrosis of part of the tuft with an occasional cellular increase. The necrosis in this case is usually in continuity with a necrotic arteriole and other vascular changes of severe hypertension will be seen.

In many renal biopsies, it is frequent to find scattered completely hyalinized glomeruli and the question invariably arises as to how this is to be interpreted. This is often impossible to determine especially in the older age group where aging and ischemic changes are present.

In a young person, hyalinized glomeruli are more likely to be of significance, but even here their presence in small numbers should not be taken as indicative of old glomerulonephritis, nor should focal glomerulonephritis be diagnosed on this basis.

COURSE OF FOCAL GLOMERULONEPHRITIS

In general, it has been our experience that the prognosis in focal glomerulonephritis not associated with systemic disease has been good. In sequential biopsies, it has been obseved that healing of the localized glomerular lesions takes place with the production of localized scars. The exception is the group of cases associated with hemoptysis, a condition referred to by many as Goodpasture's syndrome, in which an apparently benign-looking focal glomerulonephritis has changed into a widespread florid glomerulonephritis with rapid death from renal failure. Some of the cases associated with recurrent hematuria may, after many years, develop permanent renal impairment but the proportion behaving in this way is not great.

Of course the progress is quite different in focal glomerulonephritis occurring as a manifestation of polyarteritis or systemic lupus.

ETIOLOGY

Little can be said of the etiology but the varied circumstances under which it is encountered make it unlikely that there is any common etiologic factor.

REFERENCES

1. Benoit, F. L., Rulon, D. B., Theil, G. B., Doolan, P. D., and Watten, R. H.: Goodpasture's syndrome: A clinicopathologic entity. Amer. J. Med., *37*:424, 1964.
2. Davson, J., Ball, J., and Platt, R.: The kidney in in periarteritis nodosa. Quart. J. Med., *17*:175, 1948.
3. Heptinstall, R. H., and Joekes, A. M.: Focal glomerulonephritis. In, Wolstenholme, G. E. W., and Cameron, M. P. (Eds.): Ciba Foundation Symposium of Renal Biopsy. Boston, Little, Brown, 1961. P. 194.
4. Johnson, J. R., and McGovern, V. J. Goodpasture's syndrome and Wegener's granulomatosis. Aust. Ann. Med., *11*:250, 1962.
5. Kimmelstiel, P., and Wilson, C.: Inflammatory lesions in the glomeruli in pyelonephritis in relation to hypertension and renal insufficiency. Amer. J. Path., *12*:99,1936.
6. Kussmaul, A., and Maier, R.: Ueber eine bisher nicht beschriebene eigenthümliche Arterienerkrankung (Periarteritis nodosa), die mit Morbus Brightii und rapid fortschreitender allgemeiner Muskellähmung einhergeht. Deutsch. Arch. Klin. Med., *1*:484, 1866.
7. Rusby, N. L., and Wilson, C.: Lung purpura with nephritis. Quart. J. Med., *29*:501, 1960.

Chapter 34

Functional Correlates of the Juxtaglomerular Apparatus

JOHN P. CAPELLI, M.D., GONZALO E. APONTE, M.D., and LAURENCE G. WESSON, JR., M.D.

INTRODUCTION

Although the renin-angiotensin system had its inception some 70 years ago by Tigerstedt and Bergman (1), the physiologic role of this complex humoral system in body homeostasis still remains to be established. Through the intervening years of investigative effort, the areas of physiologic importance can be broadly categorized into three:

1) Volume homeostasis-the direct and specific stimulation of aldosterone by angiotensin (2, 3, 4) leading to sodium and water retention and in this manner indirectly aiding in volume control (5) and blood pressure homeostasis;

2) Intrarenal Regulatory Hormone-under this category, there are generally two leading concepts:

   (a) Autoregulation of renal blood flow (Thurau)
   (b) Maintenance of glomerulo-tubular balance-through a direct regulatory influence on proximal tubular sodium reabsorption (Leyssac).

3) Extra-renal sites of renin synthesis and function-this being an ex-tremely new area, the knowledge is no more than fragmentary. However, certain facts seem to be clear:

   (a) Interaction with catechol-amines-angiotensin facilitating the release of adrenal medullary catecholamines (6).
   (b) Multiorgan sites of synthesis and probable function, e.g. mouse submaxillary gland (7, 8) and human uterus (9).

Of these many areas of investigative interest, major efforts have been directed toward two, i.e., control of renin release and a direct renal tubular action of angiotensin. In this chapter are discussed investigations of the role of the macula densa in renin synthesis and/or release, and the effects of the biological effector of this system, angiotensin, upon renal tubular function. The studies were conducted in rats combining histochemical techniques, to localize metabolic changes, with biochemical (quantitative) determination of whole tissue. Although the kidney was the primary organ of interest, parallel responses were studies in the salivary and adrenal glands since both are sodium-responsive organs.

THE JUXTAGLOMERULAR COMPLEX

Angiotensin II, an octapeptide with pressor activity ten fold that of norepinephrine, is formed by the action of renin on a plasma substrate found in the alpha$_2$ globulin fraction. Renin is an enzyme located within the juxtaglomerular complex of the nephron; it has no known pharmacologic action which is not mediated by angiotensin. There appears to be little doubt that renin is stored within the granular component of the epithelioid cells in the afferent arteriole. However, the question remaining unsettled concerns the site of renin synthesis, since more recent studies have localized renin to the macula densa as well as the granular cells of the afferent arteriole (10).

The studies conducted with electron microscopy have indicated an unusually intimate relationship with the cells of the macula densa and those of the afferent arteriole (11, 12). There is a reduced cytoplasmic/nuclear ratio in the macula densa cells with a rearrangement of the subcellular structures, i.e., the Golgi apparatus and endoplasmic reticulum, at the basal side of the cell. The basement membrane separating the macula densa cells and the granular cells of the afferent arteriole lacks continuity and appears fragmented. Of further significance, the presence of intercytoplasmic bridges, and possibly channels, between the two cell types have strengthened the potential for functional interplay.

From the functional standpoint, the possibility for interaction was first suggested by the histochemical studies of Hess, Pearse, Fisher and Gross (13, 14, 15, 16). Basically, these investigators showed that with renal artery stenosis or adrenalectomy, increases in the key enzyme of the monophosphate shunt pathway, glucose-6-phosphate dehydrogenase (G-6-PD), occurred in the macula densa concomitantly with increases in juxtaglomerular granularity. From these studies, the suggestion emerged that this enzyme may be implicated in certain aspects of sodium metabolism. However, biochemical confirmation of this relationship remained to be proven and was carried out in the authors' investigations.

THE EFFECTS OF ELECTROLYTE IMBALANCE ON RENAL RENIN AND G-6-PD

Following two weeks of sodium deprivation, increases of G-6-PD activity are observed throughout the cortical nephrons. In addition, marked increases of enzyme activity occur in the macula densa. In the adrenal gland, the zona glomerulosa demonstrates increases in activity as well. Quantitatively, the mean G-6-PD content with sodium deficiency was 9.5 uM/gm dry wt/min (E.U.) while the control groups had a mean value of 4.4 E.U. (Fig. 1). The mean juxtaglomerular index was similarly significantly increased over the control groups. The renal content showed a five-fold rise, 13.8 units per gm dry wt (R. U.) over normal controls (2.6 R. U.). (17).

Conversely, when animals are subjected to sodium loading by dietary manipulations and DCA, a marked reduction in enzyme activity is observed both histochemically and quantitatively (Fig. 2). Renal renin content is similarly reduced to negligible amounts.

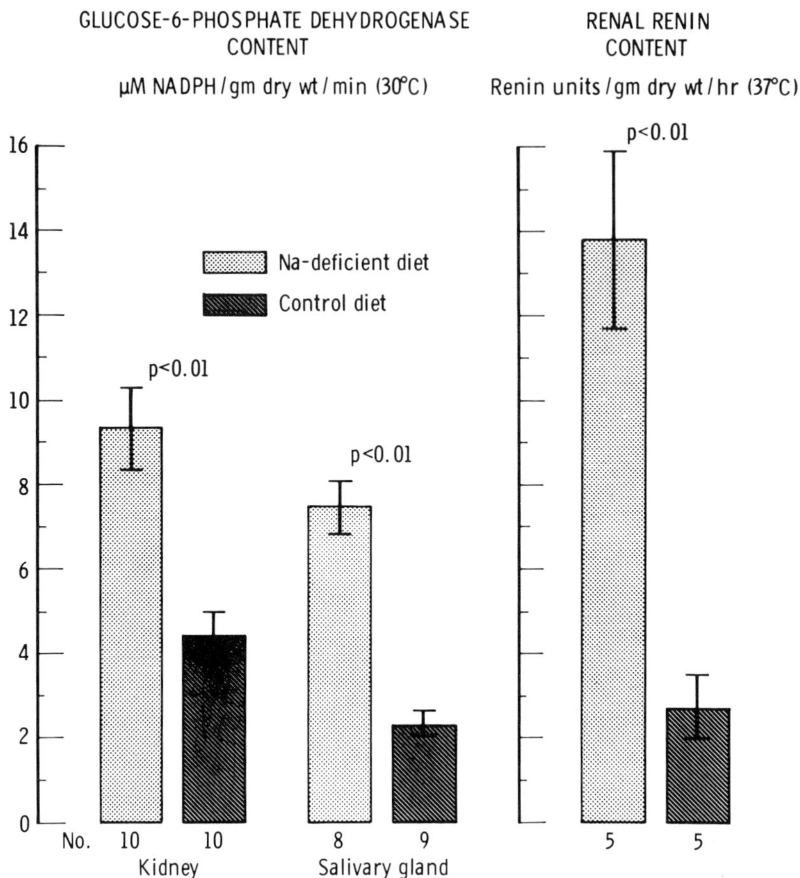

Fig. 1. Quantitative glucose-6-phosphate dehydrogenase levels for kidney and salivary gland and renal renin content after 2 weeks of sodium deprivation. Values are expressed as mean ± S.D.

THE EFFECTS OF VASOACTIVE AGENTS AND MERALLURIDE ON RENAL REININ AND G-6-PD

In sodium-loaded rats, marked reduction of enzyme activity throughout the nephron, including the macula densa, permits any changes increasing enzyme activity induced by exogenous agents readily observable. Intraperitoneal injections of synthetic angiotensin II (1.5 mg/kg) induced considerable return of enzyme activity in the proximal convoluted tubule and the ascending limb of Henle (Fig. 2). Salivary gland ducts and zona glomerulosa also show increased enzyme activity. The mean renal G-6-PD content was 5.2 E. U. in the angiotensin treated groups and 2.1 E. U. in the control groups. Macula densa enzyme activity remained low in both groups and renal renin content assessed both quantitatively and by juxtaglomerular counting was negligible (18).

In animals under similar positive sodium balance, the administration of exogenous bradykinin failed to induce any significant changes from the control group.

However, the administration of meralluride to salt loaded animals induced considerable return of enzyme activity in the kidney and salivary gland (Fig. 3). Of

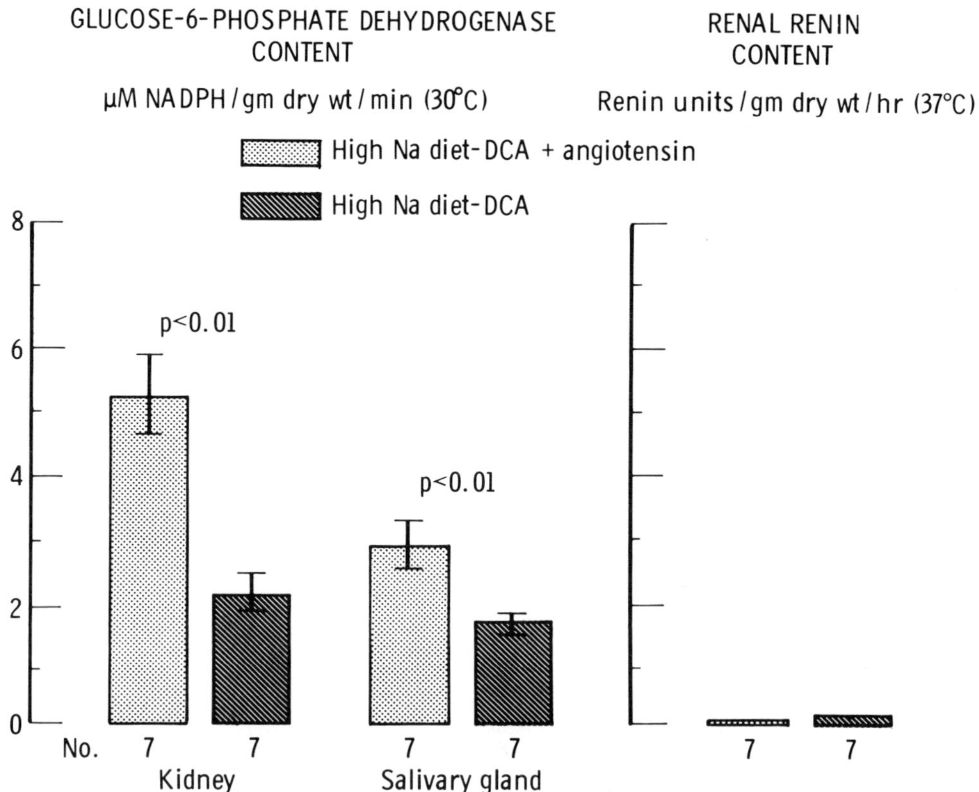

Fig. 2. Response of renal renin and renal and salivary gland glucose-6-phosphate dehydrogenase after angiotensin administration to the salt loaded rat. (Reproduced by permission of *Laboratory Investigation.)*

particular significance is that the pattern of histochemical staining is similar to angiotensin treated animals, i.e., the proximal convoluted tubules, the ascending limb of Henle, and the salivary gland excretory ducts. The zona glomerulosa show no changes. Renal salivary gland G-6-PD content averaged 8.0 E. U. and 3.6 E. U., respectively for this group, a significant increase over control values. The renal renin content remained negligible in each group.

THE FUNCTIONAL SIGNIFICANCE OF G-6-PD

This particular enzyme is the key component of the hexose monophos-phate shunt pathway. The monophosphate shunt is not a high energy yielding system, however it can function in two possible roles. First, it can provide reduced NADP which is a necessary element for the interaction of the glycolytic pathway with the Krebs cycle. In this way, amino acids can be synthesized and energy made available for protein (and possibly renin) synthesis. Alternatively, the monophosphate shunt may act by providing dihydroxyacetone phosphate to the glycolytic cycle. This in turn, by means of triose isomerase and alpha-glycerophosphate dehydrogenase could provide essential components to the glycolytic cycle, a high energy yield system which could be used in

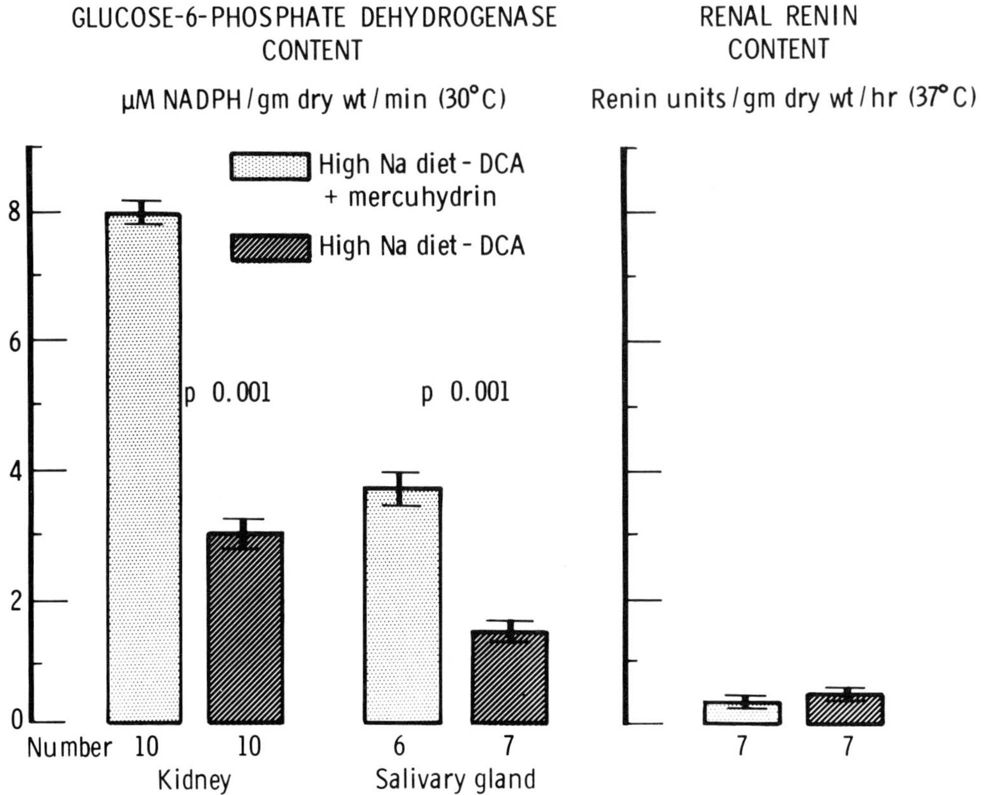

Fig. 3. Response of renal renin and renal and salivary gland glucose-6-phosphate dehydrogenase after meralluride administration to the salt loaded rat.

synthesizing renin. Hess and Pearse (19) have demonstrated high activity of alpha-glycerophosphate dehydrogenase in the granular cells of the afferent arteriole.

The macula densa appears to contain significant quantities of this enzyme which in turn is influenced by changes in sodium balance. The macula densa by its anatomic localization is in a position to sample tubular fluid just prior to its entry into the distal convoluted tubule, the site of potassium and acid secretion. The major remaining tubular fluid cation at this point is sodium, since potassium and calcium are probably all removed proximally. The results obtained in these studies suggest that those factors leading to reductions of sodium load to the macula densa provide a stimulus for increasing its activity, as evidenced by increased G-6-PD activity; concomitant increases in juxtaglomerular granularity and renal renin content occur. Although earlier studies led to the conclusion that changes in mean arterial pressure in the afferent arteriole affected renin release (5), several recent experiments have shown that even with persistent reductions in mean arterial pressure, increasing the delivery of distal sodium load will blunt the release of renin (20).

THE EFFECT OF ANGIOTENSIN ON THE RENAL TUBULE

The results of our studies indicate that angiotensin II has the capacity to alter the metabolic properties of proximal convoluted tubule and the ascending limb of Henle. The failure of a similar peptide, bradykinin, to induce similar changes suggests that the effect of angiotensin II may eventually be discovered to be a specific one. How angiotensin actually induces enzyme activity is unknown. It may represent a direct action, *e.g.* the result of inhibition of the aerobic metabolism with compensatory activation of the anaerobic pathways of metabolism, or an indirect action mediated through changes in glomerular filtration or peritubular vascular pressures. These suggestions are highly speculative, and the results obtained in no way substantiate any conclusions.

The similarity of enzymatic activity induced by meralluride was striking. Renal functional data (21) as well as histochemical observations (22) suggest that the mercurial diuretics exert their action on the proximal portion of the nephron. The similar histochemical patterns of activity between angiotensin II and meralluride gives added significance to the specific intranephron effect of angiotensin.

The intrarenal function of the renin-angiotensin system has centered around two possibilities: a hemodynamic-autoregulatory function, and a specific tubular action. However, because of the complex interrelations of renal blood flow, glomerular filtration rate, and separate compartmental tubular functions of the nephron, a clear separation as to site of action of this agent is not possible by the usual renal function tests.

The observations obtained from our study support a tubular action of angiotensin although autoregulation of blood flow or glomerular filtration cannot be disproven. Peters (23) demonstrated a tubular inhibitory effect of sodium reabsorption with a consequent dose-dependent natriuresis and diuresis in a normal rat during isotonic saline diuresis; GFR remained unchanged during angiotensin administration, while p-aminohippurate clearance declined markedly. During diuresis, angiotensin II was estimated to be 15,000 to 30,000 times more potent, on a molar basis, than hydrochlorothiazide. Langford (24) also demonstrated a dose-dependent sodium diuresis resulting from angiotensin II infusion. Further, when angiotensin was infused with a mercurial diuretic no augmentation of a diuresis with either one alone occurred, suggesting a similar site of action for each.

Studies in man relating to electrolyte excretion under the influence of angiotensin II infusions have failed thus far to clearly separate hemodynamic from tubular effects. Although angiotensin II is usually antinatriuretic in normal man (25, 26), an effect which may be attributed in whole or in part to marked reductions in GFR, natriuresis is observed in patients following severe salt depletion (27), with moderate degrees of diastolic hypertension (28), and in patients with cirrhosis and ascites (29). Louis and Doyle (27) clearly demonstrated that the antinatriuretic response to angiotensin in normal subjects will become natriuretic and diuretic following severe sodium depletion. The diuresis occurred with no detected changes in creatinine clearance. This seemingly paradoxical effect of angiotensin on electrolyte excretion has been explained two ways: a) the renal vascula-

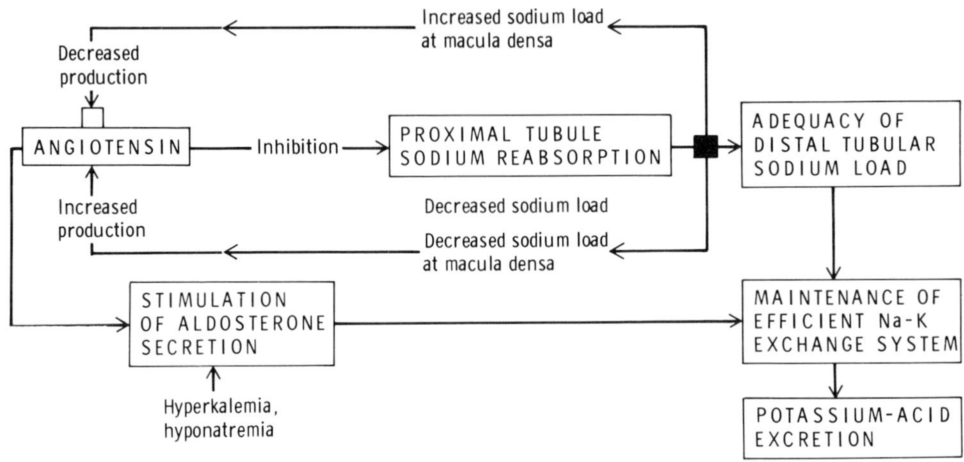

Fig. 4. Tubulo-tubular control of Na-K balance-A physiologic role of the renin-angiotensin system. The macula densa occupies a central role responding to reductions in tubular fluid sodium load affecting increased renin-angiotensin production which in turn reduces proximal sodium reabsorption increasing the distal tubular sodium load providing adequate substrate for ionic exchange and K-H secretion. Increasing sodium loads withdraw the stimulus to the macula densa. The stimulation of aldosterone by angiotensin acts to complement the system.

ture fails to respond to angiotensin with vasoconstriction as in the control state (30); or b) tachyphylaxis of the renal vasculature secondary to high levels of endogenous angiotensin II pre-exists (26, 31). In either event, the unresponsive renal vasculature would permit a direct tubular effect of angiotensin II to be detected. Thus, although these clearance studies do not provide clear evidence for a direct tubular effect, they are wholly compatible with one.

A direct, experimental test for a tubular and more specifically, a proximal tubular effect for angiotensin II are the studies of Leyssac (32). It was initially shown by Leyssac, Lassen and Thaysen that sodium "transport" was inhibited by angiotensin II in isolated renal tissue (33). In a later series of studies, Leyssac (32) demonstrated a significant prolongation of the proximal tubular occlusion (collapse) time following angio-

tensin II infusion in the rat. Prolongation of proximal tubule collapase time is interpreted as measuring inhibition of sodium and water reabsorption in this segment. More direct evidence for this effect is the micropuncture studies of Gertz (34) who, using the split droplet technic, observed an approximately 30% inhibition of sodium reabsorption in the proximal tubule following angiotensin II instillation. Our findings indicate an effect of angiotensin II on the proximal tubule and also on the ascending limb of Henle, but they cannot determine whether sodium reabsorption is inhibited at these sites.

The final aspect of an intranephron effect of the renin-angiotensin system is its physiological significance (Fig. 4). If angiotensin does, in some way, inhibit sodium transport in the proximal convoluted tubule, or in the loop of Henle, a very real question then becomes the survival value of the system. Others have suggested a general role in the maintenance of glomerulotubular balance (32). However, on comparing the effects of the renin-angiotensin system on sodium balance with the effects on aldosterone secretion, and the relationship of the latter to potassium balance, a different role seems possible. The most important defense of the vertebrate body against potassium (and acid) intoxication is renal tubular secretion of potassium by an ion exchange system in the distal segment. The renin-angiotensin system, as an intrarenal hormone can assure efficiency of this defense by maintaining adequate delivery of sodium substrate to distal potassium exchange regions of each nephron by inhibition of sodium reabsorption in the proximal segment. At the same time, angiotensin enhances utilization of substrate sodium through stimulation of aldosterone secretion. When sodium delivery to the distal tubule is adequate or in excess, the macula densa senses this chemical change and renin release is inhibited. This would give the juxtaglomerular apparatus a primary intrarenal role for the *tubulo-tubular* control of sodium-potassium transport by a negative feedback system responsive to sodium load at the macula densa.

THE RENIN-ANGIOTENSIN SYSTEM IN PATHOLOGICAL STATES

The etiologic role of the renin-angiotensin systems in the production of experimental and human hypertension has attracted a great deal of enthusiasm. Clamping one renal artery in rats regularly produces an increased renin content in the ischemic kidney with or without a corresponding rise is systemic arterial pressure (35). If the kidney is then removed and the contralateral kidney made ischemic, hypertension will persist, but in the absence of elevated blood renin levels (35). When both adrenals are removed and the rats are not given saline, renal and blood renin concentrations increase markedly, yet the systemic blood pressure remains low (35). Conversly, salt loading and DCA administration elevate systemic blood pressure followed by the disappearance of renin from the kidney and blood (35). Thus, there may be increases in renal and plasma renin without increase in blood pressure, hypertension with or without increased renin secretion, and finally even hypertension in the virtual absence of renin.

Studies of renin activity in various forms of hypertension in humans have failed to demonstrate significant elevations except in the accelerated or "malignant" form of the disease (36, 37). These results have been the authors' observations as well (Fig. 5). The demonstration of significant elevations of plasma renin activity in malignant hypertension has been a rather consistent finding in the majority of instances. Furthermore, the vascular damage characteristically seen in this entity may be a direct effect of the liberated humoral agents acting at the vascular (cellular) level. Masson and co-workers have demonstrated intense vasculitis following the administration of renin to salt loaded animals (38).

Renal artery stenosis undoubtedly can lead to sustained diastolic hypertension. However, demonstration of elevated peripheral plasma renin activity in this condition has not been a consistent observation (36, 37). Although renal vein renin activity may be more helpful (39), unless simultaneous measurement of renal blood flow is determined, con-

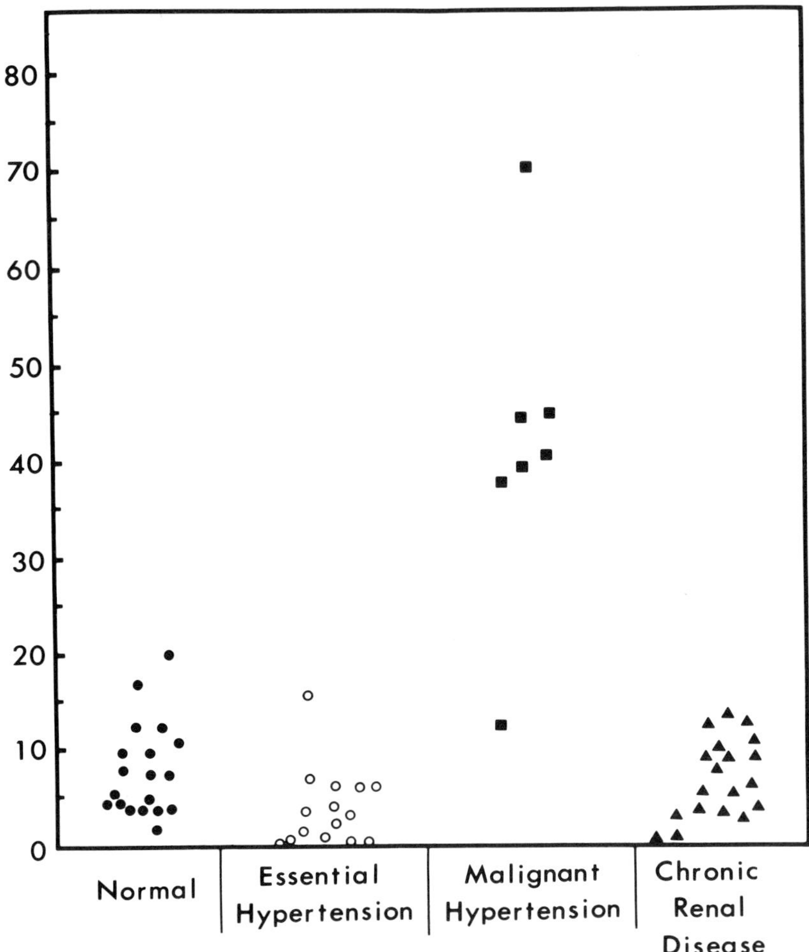

Fig. 5. Plasma renin activity in various forms of hypertensive disease. (Chronic renal disease include all forms of chronic parenchymal disease with blood urea nitrogen levels greater than 75 mg per 100 ml.)

clusions as to the actual increase or decrease in the rate of renin production cannot be drawn. Such studies have yet to be performed. Thus although renin would appear to be the responsible factor in the production of hypertension on a renovascular basis, the evidence to date fails to warrant that conclusion.

Plasma renin activity is usually elevated in cirrhosis with ascites, nephrosis and certain instances of congestive heart failure (36, 37). The significance of these observations in unknown, and what role the renin-angiotensin system may contribute to the edematous state, particularly through its action on aldosterone, remains to be defined.

Untreated Addison's Disease will invariably lead to marked elevations of plasma renin activity. With correction of the electrolyte derangement, return to normal values occurs, again indicating the responsiveness and activity of this system to sodium balance (36).

Toxemia of pregnancy has currently become of interest in the area of neuroendocrine hypertension, particularly since the recent demonstration that the human uterus and chorion is capable of renin synthesis (9, 40). Nevertheless, studies of plasma renin activity in toxemia of pregnancy, have generally demonstrated values lower than that seen in normal pregnancy yet still higher than that observed in the normal, non-pregnant female. Again, as with essential hypertension, undefined factors enhancing vascular "responsiveness" to normal or mild elevations in plasma renin activity may be occurring in the pregnant woman who develops the syndrome.

Reduced or absent plasma renin activity takes on significance in the patient with primary aldosteronism (41). This finding in the patient with hypertension, who fails to show a significant (3-5 fold) rise in plasma renin activity following sodium deprivation, is an extremely important diagnostic clue for primary aldosteronism. Presently, this is probably the foremost diagnostic tool that measurement of plasma renin activity can offer.

Thus, it becomes quite clear that despite many years of study, both in the physiologic and pathologic areas, the role of the renin-angiotensin system remains elusive.

BIBLIOGRAPHY

1. Tigerstedt, R., and Bergmen, P. G.: Niere and Kreislauf. Skand. Arch. Physiol., 8:223, 1898.
2. Laragh, J. H., Angers, M., Kelly, W. G., and Lieberman, S.: Hypotensive agents and pressor substances. The effect of epinephrine, norepinephrine, angiotensin II and others on the secretory rate of aldosterone in man. J. A. M. S., 174:234, 1960.
3. Mulrow, P. J., Ganong, W. F., Cera, G., and Kuljian, A.: Nature of aldosterone stimulating factor in dog kidneys. J. Clin. Invest., 41:505, 1962.
4. Kaplan, N.: The biosynthesis of adrenal steroids: Effects of Angiotensin II, Adrenocorticotropin, and potassium. J. Clin. Invest., 44:2029, 1965.
5. Tobian, L.: Physiology of the juxtaglomerular cells. Ann. Int. Med., 52:395, 1965.
6. Peach, M. J., Cline, W. H., and Watts, D. T.: Release of adrenal catecholamines by angiotensin II. Circulation Res., 19:571, 1966.
7. Bing. J., and Faarup, P.: Location of renin (or a renin-like substance) in the submaxillary glands of albino mice. Acta Path. Microbiol. Scand., 64:203, 1965.
8. Trautschold, I., Werle, E., Schmal, A., and Hendrikoff, N. G.: Die hormonelle beeinflussung des isorenin-spiegels der submandibularisdruse der seisser maus and zur lokalisierung des enzyme in der druse. Z. Physiol. Chem., 344:232, 1966.
9. Capelli, J. P., Wesson, L. G., Jr., Aponte, G. E., Faraldo, C., and Jaffe, E.: Characterization and source of a renin-like enzyme in anephric humans. J. Clin. Endocr. 28:221, 1968.
10. Warren, B., Johnson, A. G., and Hoobler, S. W.: Characterization of the renin-antirenin system. J. Exper. Med., 123:1109, 1966.
11. Oberling, Ch., and Hat, P. Y.: Etude de l'appareil juxtaglomerulaire due rat au microscope electronique. Ann. Anat. Path., 5:441, 1960.
12. Hartroft, P. M., and Newmark, L. W.: Electron Microscopy of renal juxtaglomerular cells. Anat. Rec., 139:185, 1961.
13. Hess, R., and Pearse, A. G. E.: The significance of renal glucose-6-phosphate dehydrogenase in experimental hypertension in the rat. Brit. J. Exp. Path., 40:243, 1959.
14. Fisher, E. R.: Correlation of juxtaglomerular granulation, pressor activity and enzymes of the macula densa in experimental hypertension. Lab. Invest., 10:707, 1961.
15. Gross, F., and Hess, R.: Histochemical changes in kidneys and in salivary glands of rats with experimental hypertension. Proc. Exp. Biol. Med. 104:509, 1960.
16. Hess, R., and Regoli, D.: Correlation of enzymatic activity of the juxtaglomerular complex with renin content in renal hypertensive rats. Brit. J. Exp. Path., 45:666, 1964.
17. Capelli, J. P., Wesson, L. G., Jr., and Aponte, G. E.: The effect of sodium on renal renin and on glucose-6-phosphate dehydrogenase in the kidneys, salivary glands and adrenal glands. Nephron, 5:106, 1968.
18. Capelli, J. P., Wesson, L. G., Jr., and Aponte, G. E.: The effect of sodium and angiotensin on renal renin and renal, adrenal and salivary gland glucose-6-phosphate dehydrogenase. Evidence for

a proximal tubular effect of angiotensin. Lab. Invest., *16*:925, 1967.

19. Hess, R., and Pearse, A. G. E.: Mitochondrial a-glycerophosphate dehydrogenase activity of juxtaglomerular cells in experimental hypertension and adrenal insufficiency. Proc. Soc. Exp. Biol. Med., *106*:895, 1961.

20. Vander, A. J.: Control of renin release. Physiol. Rev., *47*:359, 1967.

21. Wesson, L. G., Jr.: Physiology of the kidney. In, Alken, C. C., Dix, V. W., Weyrauch, H. M., and Wildbolz, E. (eds.): Encyclopedia of Urology. II Berlin. Springer-Verlag, 1965. pp. 147-154.

22. Cafruny, E. J.: Histochemical demonstration of mercury in renal cells. Biochem. Pharm., *9-10*:15, 1962.

23. Peters, G.: Renal tubular effect of val$_5$-angiotensin II amide in rats. Proc. Soc. Exp. Biol. Med., *112*:771, 1963.

24. Langford, H. G.: Tubular action of angiotensin. Canad. M. A. J., *90*:332, 1964.

25. Biron, P., Chretien, M., Koiew, E., and Genest, J.: Effects of angiotensin infusions on aldosterone and electrolyte excretion in normal subjects and patients with hypertension and adrenocortical disorders. Brit. Med. J., *1*:1569, 1962.

26. Peart, W. S.: Hypertension and the Kidney. II. Experimental basis of renal hypertension. Brit. Med. J., *2*:5164, 1959.

27. Louis, W. J., and Doyle, A. E.: The effects of aldosterone and angiotensin on renal function. Clin. Sci., *30*:179, 1966.

28. Brown, J. J., and Peart, W. S.: The effect of angiotensin on urine flow and electrolyte excretion in hypertensive patients. Clin. Sci., *22*:1, 1962.

29. Laragh, J. H., Cannon, P. J., Bentzel, C. J., Sicinski, A. M., and Meltzer, J. I.: Angiotensin II, norepinephrine, and renal transport of electrolytes and water in normal man and in cirrhosis with ascites. J. Clin. Invest., *42*:1179, 1963.

30. Peart, W. S., and Brown, J. J.: Effect of angio-tensin (hypertensin or angiotensin) on urine flow and electrolyte excretion in hypertensive patients. Lancet., *1*:28, 1961.

31. Louis, W. J., and Doyle, A. E.: The effects of varying doses of angiotensin on renal function and blood pressure in man and dogs. Clin. Sci., *29*:489, 1965.

32. Leyssac, P. P.: The regulation of proximal tubular reabsorption in mammalian kidney. Acta Physiol. Scand., *70* (Suppl): 291, 1966.

33. Leyssac, P. P., Lasser, U. V., and Thaysen, J. H.: Inhibition of sodium transport in isolated renal tissue by angiotensin. Biochem. Biophys. Acta., *48*:602, 1961.

34. Gertz, K. H.: Direct measurements of the transtubular flux of electrolytes in the intact rat kidney. Proc. XXII Congr. Int. Union Physiol. Sci. Leiden, *1* (Supple. 3): 370, 1962.

35. Gross, F., Schaechtelin, G., Brunner, H., and Peters, G.: The role of the renin-angiotensin system in blood pressure regulation and kidney. Canad. M. A. J., *90*:258, 1963.

36. Brown, J. J., Davies, P. L., Lever, A. F., and Robertson, J. I. S.: Variations in plasma renin concentration in several physiological and pathological states. Canad. M. A. J., *90*:201, 1964.

37. Brown, J. J., Lever, A. F., and Robertson, J. I. S.: Plasma renin concentration in human hypertension. Amer. Heart J., *74*:413, 1967.

38. Masson, G. M. C., Mikush, A., and Yasuda, H.: Experimental vascular disease elicited by aldosterone and renin. Endo., *71*:505, 1962.

39. Kirkendall, W. M., Fitz, A. E., and Lawrence, M. S.,: Renal Hypertension. Diagnosis and Surgical Treatment. New Eng. J. Med., *276*:479, 1967.

40. Symonds, E. M., Stanley, M. A. and Skinner, S. L.: Production of renin by in vitro cultures of human chorion and uterine muscle. Nature *217*:1152, 1968.

41. Conn, J. W., Cohen, E. L., and Rovner, D. R.: Suppression of plasma renin activity in primary aldosteronism. J. A. M. A., *190*:213, 1964.

Chapter 35

Clinicopathological Correlations in the Nephrotic Syndrome

MARVIN FORLAND, M.D., and BENJAMIN H. SPARGO, M.D.

In an introduction to his monograph on *Bright's Disease* written in 1948, the distinguished American physician Henry A. Christian noted, ". . . structure has been decreasing in clinical importance as in recent years pathological physiology increasingly has become a dominant concern in medicine" (4). Within a very few years, the development of techniques for percutaneous renal biopsy by Iversen and Brun (12), Kark and Muehrcke (13), and others was to abruptly bring about renewed opportunity for emphasis on clinicopathological correlations in renal disease. The introduction of electron microscopy has been an additional key factor leading to a more fundamental understanding of renal disease which has been of nosological and diagnostic interest to the physician and consequently of prognostic and therapeutic importance to his patient.

The usefulness of renal biopsy coupled with careful clinical follow-up

TABLE I—THE NEPHROTIC SYNDROME
UNIVERSITY OF CHICAGO RENAL BIOPSY SERIES

	Total Series	Adult	Pediatric (Below 15 yrs.)
1. Idiopathic Nephrotic Syndrome			
A. Lipid Nephrosis	25	8	17
B. Glomerular Membranous Change	19	19	
2. Chronic Glomerulonephritis	26	17	9
3. Systemic Lupus Erythematosus	14	13	1
4. Diabetic Glomerulosclerosis	8	8	
5. Amyloidosis	8	8	
6. Miscellaneous			
A. Congenital Nephrosis	1		1
B. Anaphylactoid Purpura	1	1	
C. Periarteritis Nodosa	1	1	
D. Focal Glomerulonephritis	1	1	
TOTAL	104	76	28

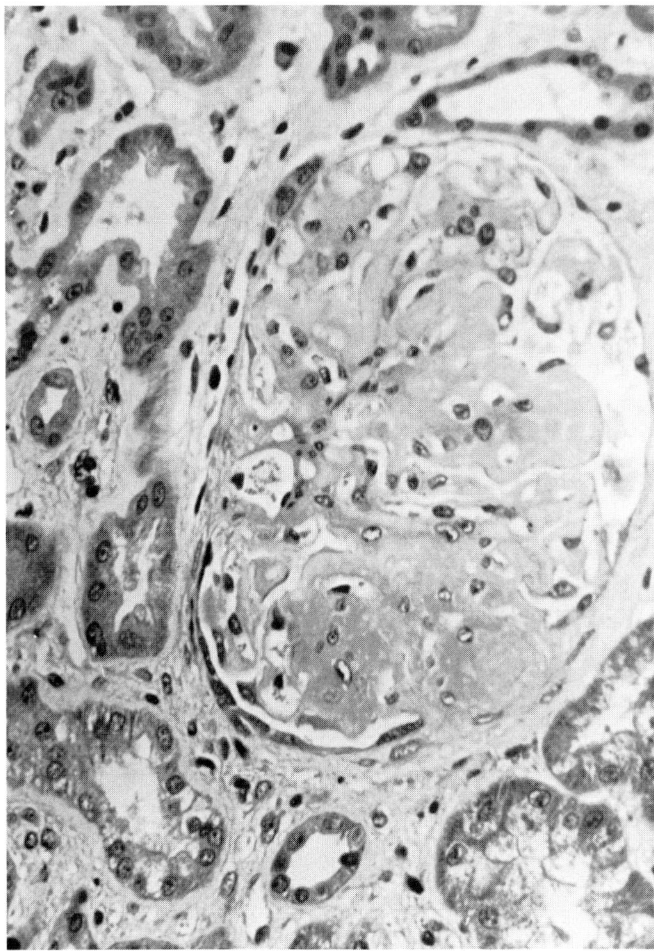

Fig. 1. Amyloid nephrosis. The decreased glomerular cellularity is related to accumulations of the amyloid resulting in irregular lobular distortion and mild glomerular ischemia. Tubular changes are secondary to the glomerular damage. H & E, 450X

has been particularly significant in the study of patients presenting with the nephrotic syndrome. While the clinical features of edema, proteinuria, hypoalbuminemia and hypercholesterolemia have defined this as a clinical syndrome for more than half a century (20), debate concerning its pathological correlations has raged for a similar period of time. Points of contention have concerned whether this was the characteristic picture of a distinct pathological lesion, and if so, was this lesion primarily a glomerular or tubular abnormality, and finally, was this indeed a uniquely renal disease or was the kidney merely partici-

pating in a systemic metabolic abnormality.

The current status of some of these questions will be considered by reviewing the clinicopathological correlations in 104 patients with a clinical diagnosis of nephrotic syndrome who had renal biopsies performed at the University of Chicago Hospitals over the past twelve years (Table 1). All biopsies have been examined by light microscopy and over 95% of patients have had a portion of renal biopsy studied by electron microscopy.

The occurrence of the clinical picture of nephrosis in the course of systemic

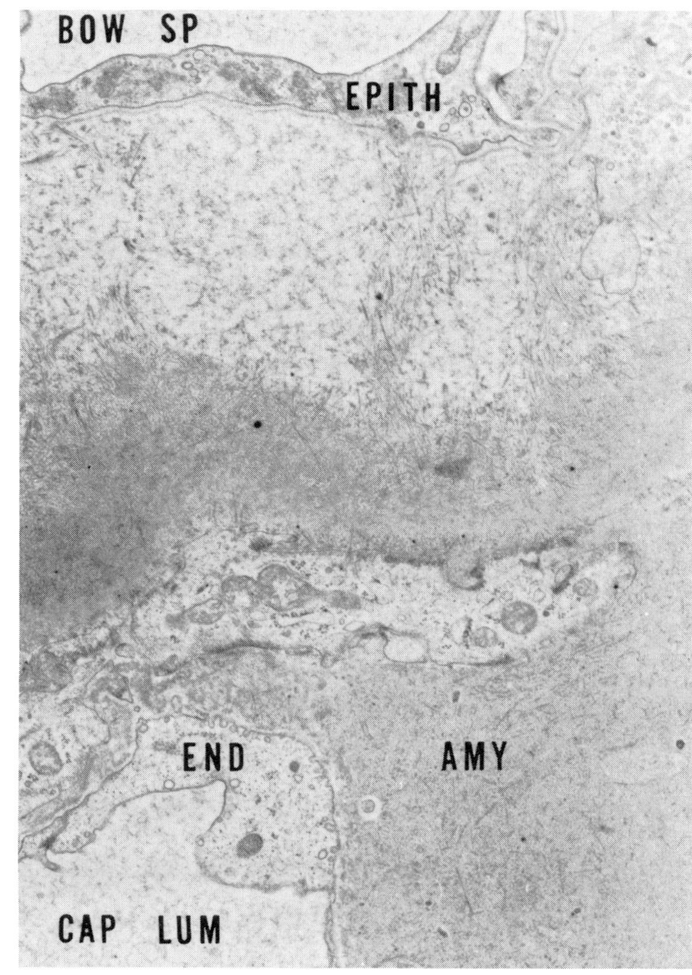

Fig. 2. The amyloid deposits extend from the displaced endothelium through the basement membrane, which can no longer be identified, and elevate the epithelial cells. A prominent ultrastructural characteristic of amyloid is the coarse fibrillar material. This can be most clearly shown away from the denser matrix. 13,800X

ABBREVIATIONS FOR ALL ILLUSTRATIONS

AMY = Amyloid
B M = basement membrane
BOW SP = Bowman's space
CAP LUM = capillary lumen
EPITH = epithelium
END = endothelium
MES = mesangium
RBC = red blood cell

disease and earlier described renal diseases such as glomerulonephritis was appreciated as early as 1913 by Munk who pointed out what was then a frequent but not exclusive relationship of nephrosis to syphilis (21). This is clearly demonstrated in our series in which 60 of 104 cases, or 58%, have been associated with other distinct clinical diagnoses. A few pertinent examples will be cited.

A 40-year-old Negro male was admitted with a four-year history of intermittent edema, treated with mercurial diuretics over the previous eight months. Clinical and laboratory findings indicated a diagnosis of nephrotic syndrome. A renal biopsy established the presence of amyloidosis (Fig. 1, 2). Combined diuretic therapy led to a 55 pound weight loss during five weeks of hospitalization. Diuretic treatment has been continued in the outpatient department and the patient has been able to work during the past 18 months despite a slowly rising BUN. Renal biopsy made possible the rapid establishment of a diagnosis and, in the absence of evidence for an underlying disease, therapy has been directed at maintaining the patient relatively free of edema. Eight of our 76 adult patients were found to have renal

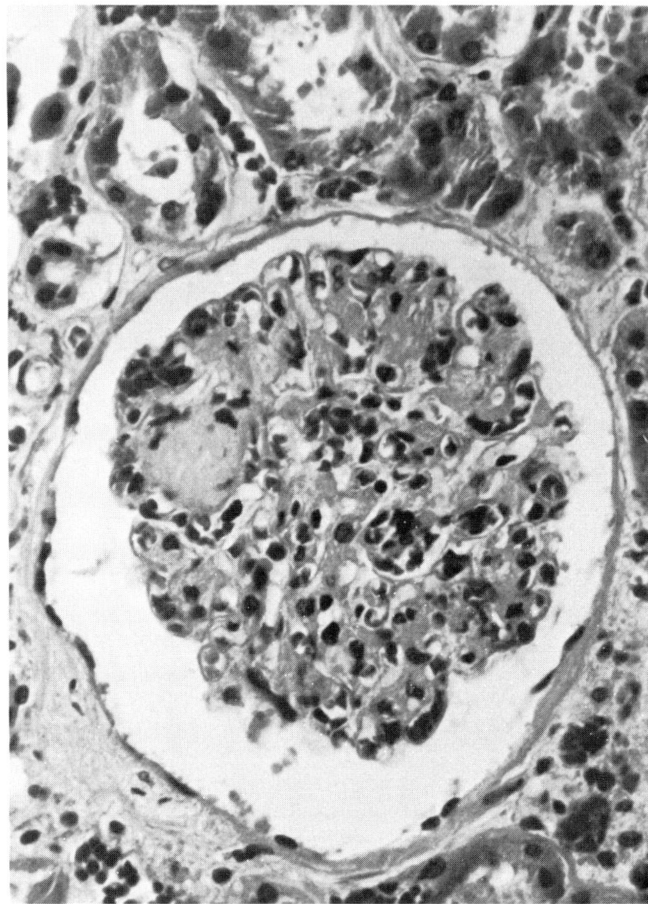

Fig. 3. Nodular diabetic glomerulosclerosis. The conspicuous nodular cellular lesion is wreathed by dilated capillaries. Residual mesangial nuclei are present along the periphery of the nodule. H & E, 450X

amyloidosis. Other series have reported a 3 to 12% incidence (17). Two of our patients had multiple myeloma, with this diagnosis also made by renal biopsy in one. A third had long-standing regional enteritis. Primary amyloidosis has been considered the diagnosis in the remaining five. Seven of the eight have expired with a mean survival of 20.3 months following the onset of symptoms. This is similar to a 17.6 month survival in a recent review of reported cases (17). As in other series, the majority of our patients were males and the age of onset was usually over 40, with a mean of 56.2 years in our group. Corticosteroid

therapy has not been useful and is generally considered contraindicated because of potentially harmful side effects.

A second example of systemic disease responsible for nephrotic syndrome is illustrated by a 46-year-old Negro woman hospitalized for evaluation of hematemesis. A history of recent congestive heart failure and labile hypertension was elicited. A diagnosis of diabetes mellitus had been made two months earlier. Laboratory and clinical findings of the nephrotic syndrome were present. A renal biopsy taken four months later, when blood pressure was

Fig. 4. Diabetic glomerulosclerosis with thickening of the lamina densa of the basement membrane in addition to the irregular accumulation of dense basement membrane-like material extending through the lobular stalk distorting the mesangial cells. 11,000X

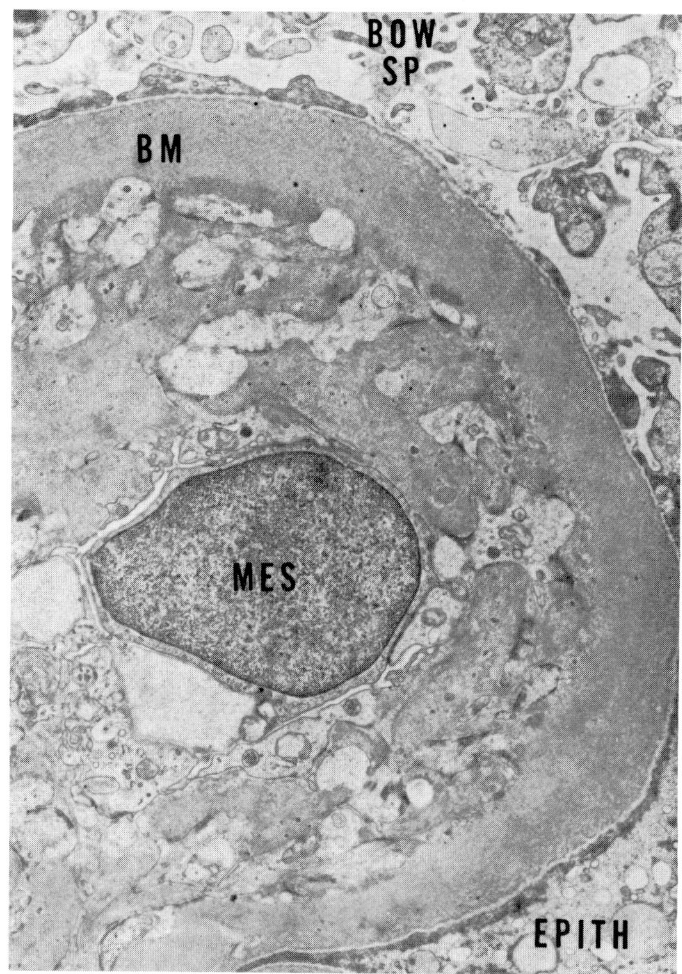

satisfactorily controlled, indicated a diagnosis of diabetic glomerulosclerosis (Fig. 3, 4).

The finding of renal lesions characteristic of diabetes mellitus soon after the clinical appearance of the abnormality in carbohydrate metabolism, or even prior to its clinical presentation, has now been frequently reported (1, 6, 16). These observations have been cited as evidence for a more basic metabolic abnormality in diabetes mellitus which may progress as a vascular or renal lesion or make its initial appearance with hyperglycemia and glycosuria. A second patient in our group of eight also had a

diagnosis of diabetes mellitus and nephrotic syndrome due to diabetic glomerulosclerosis made on the same hospital admission. While it has been observed that the degree of proteinuria, renal failure and hypertension correlates more closely with the diffuse lesion (9) than the classic Kimmelstiel-Wilson nodular lesion (14), all eight of our patients had clearcut nodular lesions as well as diffuse basement membrane changes.

A particularly useful clarification made possible by study of renal biopsies with electron microscopy has occurred in idiopathic nephrotic syndrome. Electron microscopy has revealed that char-

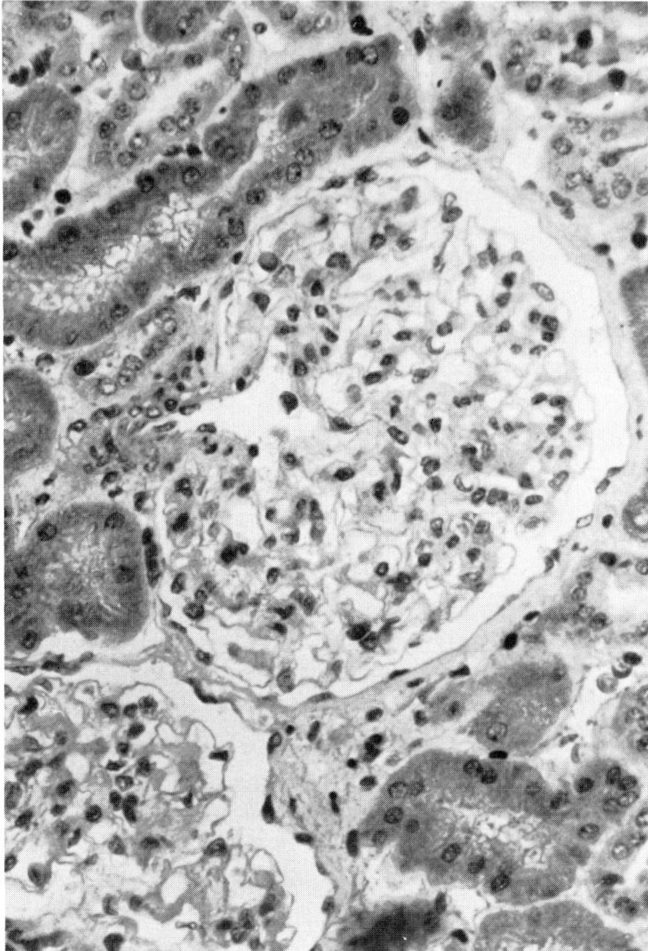

Fig. 5. Lipid nephrosis. This is often referred to as "nil" disease because a lesion can not be discerned by light microscopy. H & E, 450X

TABLE II
IDIOPATHIC NEPHROTIC SYNDROME

	Lipid Nephrosis	*Glomerular Membranous Change*
Light Microscopy	no lesion ("nil")	"Membranous glomerulonephritis"
Electron Microscopy	foot process fusion	membranous change
Age of Onset	majority children	almost exclusively adults
Immunofluorescence	usually negative	stain for IgG and Beta$_{1c}$ C′
Proteinuria	"selective"	heavier weight globulins
Steroid Response	$> 60\%$ remission	infrequent
Prognosis	$< 10\%$ mortality	50% mortality

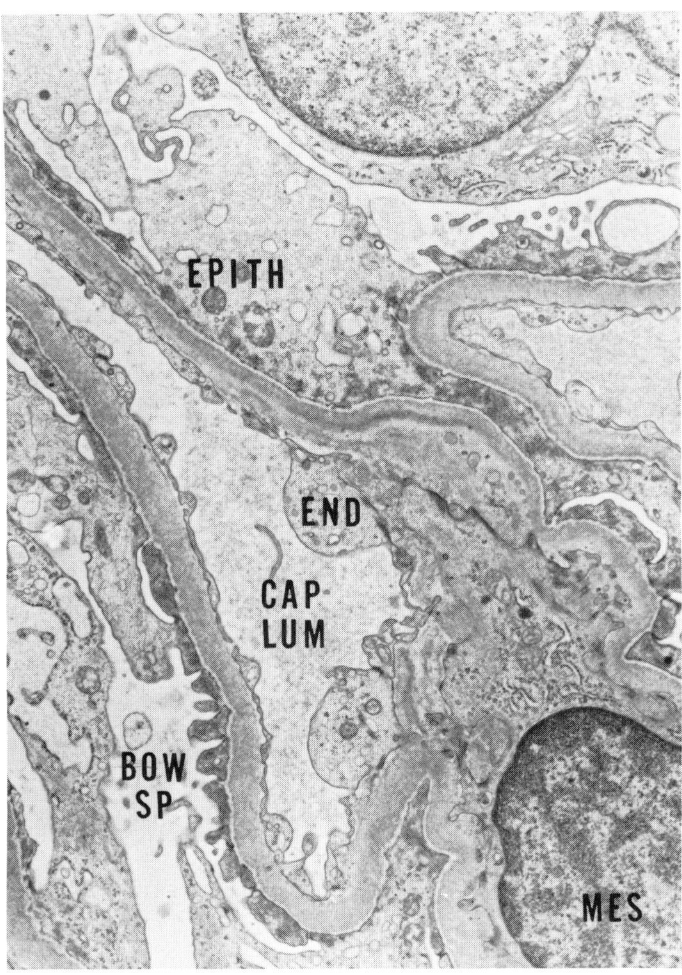

Fig. 6. Large areas of fused foot processes cover the entire outer surface of the basement membrane in the absence of other ultrastructural changes. 11,000X

acteristic changes are present in the glomerular capillary wall in all such patients and form the basis for division into two categories which have important clinical distinctions (Table II). The predominantly childhood form of idiopathis nephrotic syndrome, or lipid nephrosis, is frequently associated with a normal-appearing glomerulus by light microscopy, the "nil" lesion (Fig. 5). As first reported by Farquhar, Vernier and Good in 1957 (8), ultrastructural study reveals fusion or smudging of the epithelial cell foot processes (Fig. 6). Whether the epithelial cell is the primary site of damage or reacts to submicroscopic alterations in the basement membrane remains speculative. This lesion is reversible with clinical remission.

The second form, seen almost exclusively in adults, was termed membranous glomerulonephritis by Bell in 1950 (2) (Fig. 7). The technical restrictions of light microscopy led this careful observer to equate capillary wall thickening with basement membrane thickening and hence both lipid nephrosis and the membranous lesion were included in this grouping. On electron microscopy, the lesion is characterized by marked variation in basement membrane thickness and staining properties, as well as

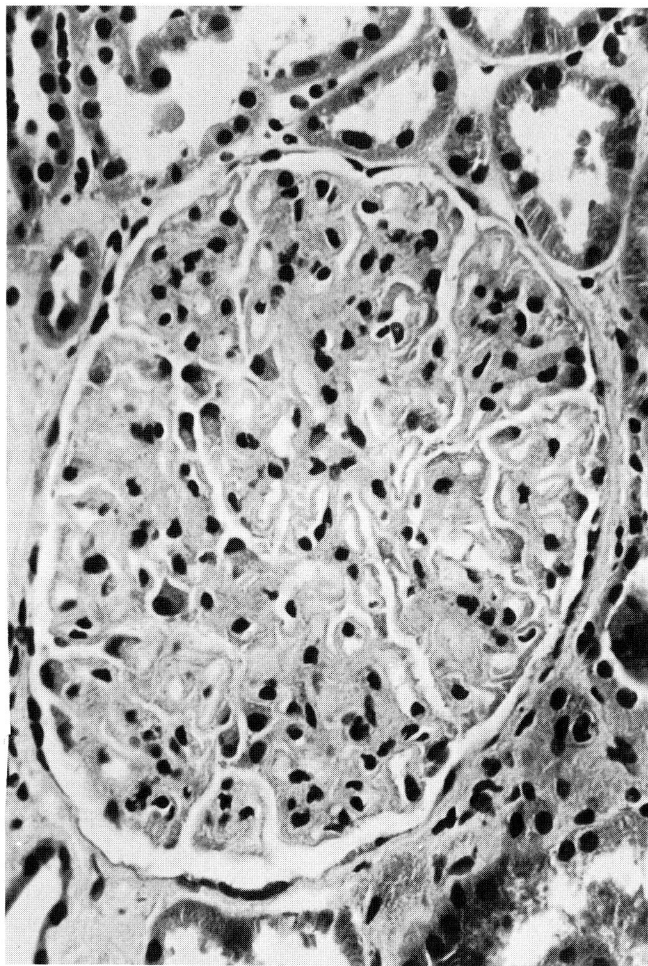

Fig. 7. Membranous glomerular change with the idiopathic nephrotic syndrome has a diffuse glomerular capillary thickening without evidence of inflammation. H & E, 450X

what are thought to be proteinaceous deposits between the membrane and epithelial cell. Foot process fusion is also often present (Fig. 8, 8a). This lesion shows neither inflammatory change nor does it appear related to streptococcal infection and consequently the term glomerulonephritis has received strong criticism (5). Our preference has been to call this idiopathic nephrotic syndrome with glomerular membranous change.

The difference in age of onset is evident in the group of 44 patients with idiopathic nephrotic syndrome which comprises 42% of our series. Of the 25 with lipid nephrosis, 17 or 68% were below age 15. In contrast, all 19 patients with glomerular membranous change were age 15 or above and the mean age of onset for this group was 41 years, with a range of age 15 to 72.

Two additional means of differentiating between these two groups have been suggested in recent years. Again using renal biopsy material and immunofluorescent techniques, several groups have reported the glomerular membranous lesion stains positively for the immunoproteins IgG and the $beta_{1c}$-globulin component of complement (15, 18). In contrast, such staining is usually not seen in lipid nephrosis (7).

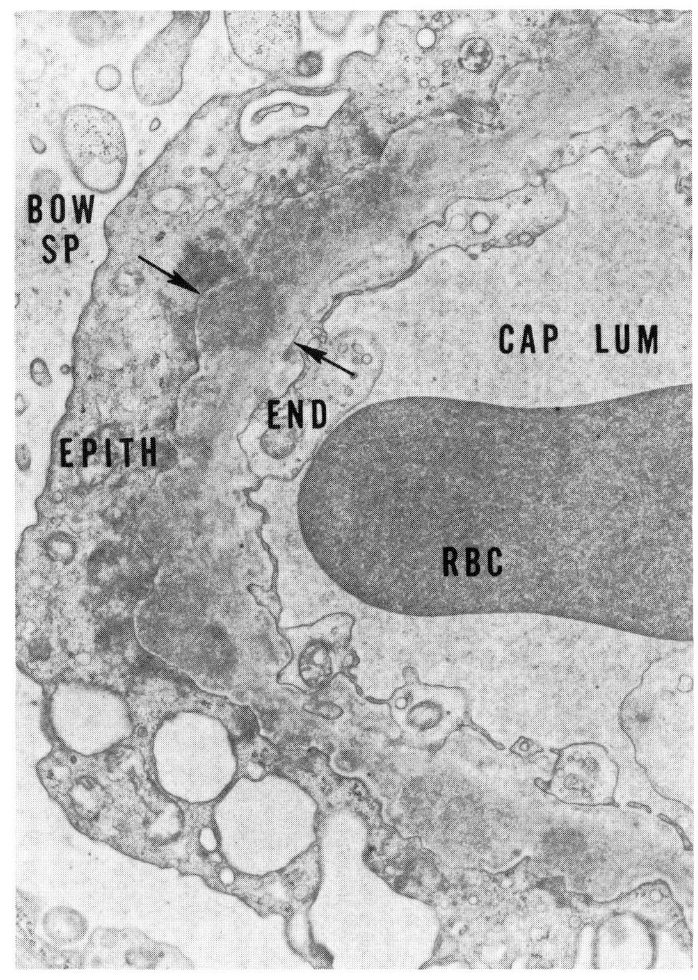

Fig. 8. The most prominent alteration is the irregularity and widening of the basement membrane with osmophilic material distorting the epithelial cell margin. Secondary changes in the glomerular epithelial cell include foot process fusion and microvillus formation. Only minor changes can be shown in the endothelial cells, 16,000X

Vernier has suggested the positive staining lesions probably represent immune complexes and may be the factor responsible for the renal damage (28). The absence of immunoproteins in the lesions of lipid nephrosis suggests a different etiology or pathogenesis.

The second differential technique is based on the pattern of urinary protein excretion according to molecular size (26). The milder structural lesions have been characterized by a "selective" proteinuria, with loss of albumin and smaller globulins such as transferrin (molecular weight 88,000). With more severe histologic damage, and particularly basement membrane thickening, loss of higher weight globulins, such as IgG (molecular weight 155,000) becomes more prominent. Simplifications in procedures for such determinations including Sephadex column chromatography (10) and commercially available immunoplates now have been reported (3).

The importance of distinguishing between these two forms of idiopathic nephrotic syndrome is apparent upon examining their therapeutic response and prognosis. With the introduction of effective antibiotic therapy and later corticosteroids, the mortality rate at five

Fig. 8a. Other stages of the membranous lesion may have more prominent basement membrane widening with areas of both decreased and increased density. This progressive sclerosis may be associated with a decreased cellularity. 16,000X

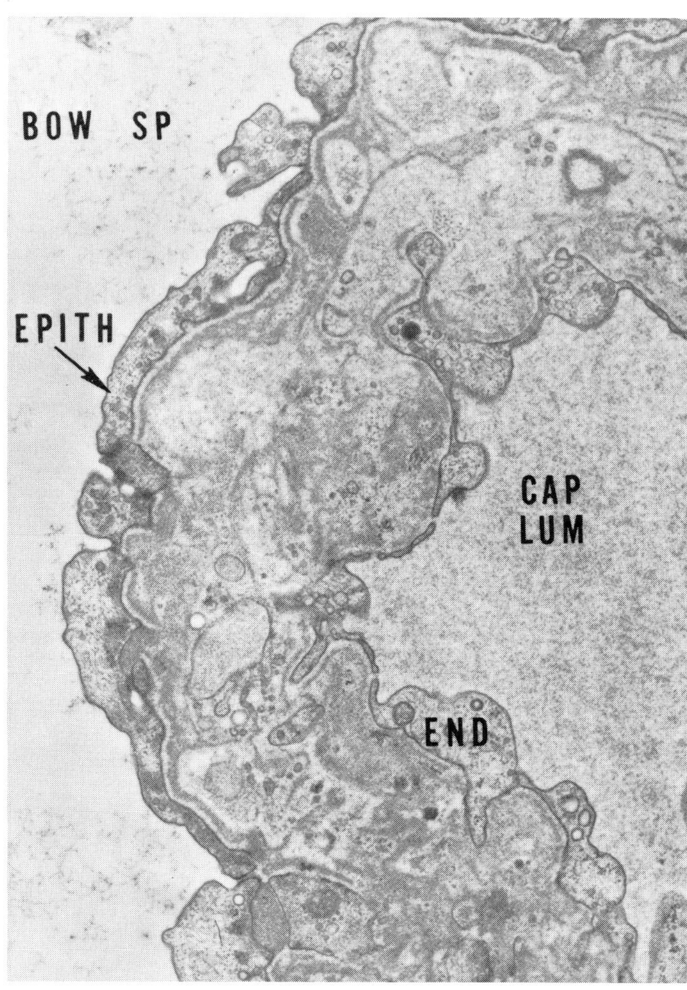

years with lipid nephrosis has fallen from approximately 50 to 60% to less than 10%. From a spontaneous remission rate of about 20%, we now see remissions in greater than 60% and relatively few patients need be burdened by massive edema (25). Of our eight adult patients, one has expired due to Hodgkin's Disease. Seven have had remissions or are well-controlled on corticosteroids. Comparable favorable results have been reported by Rosen *et al.* (23) and Hardwicke and associates (11).

By contrast, in our group of nineteen patients with glomerular membranous change, nine have expired with a mean survival of six years following the onset of symptoms. Eight of the deaths appeared to be directly related to the renal disease. One patient has been lost to follow-up and nine are surviving. Progressive renal insufficiency with hypertension and intercurrent infection have been the principal causes of death. In our experience, corticosteroid therapy, in high or low dosage, has rarely appeared to favorably influence the clinical or morphological picture. Improvement occurred concurrent with corticosteroid therapy in several patients, but deterioration was equally frequent and remissions have been observed to occur without

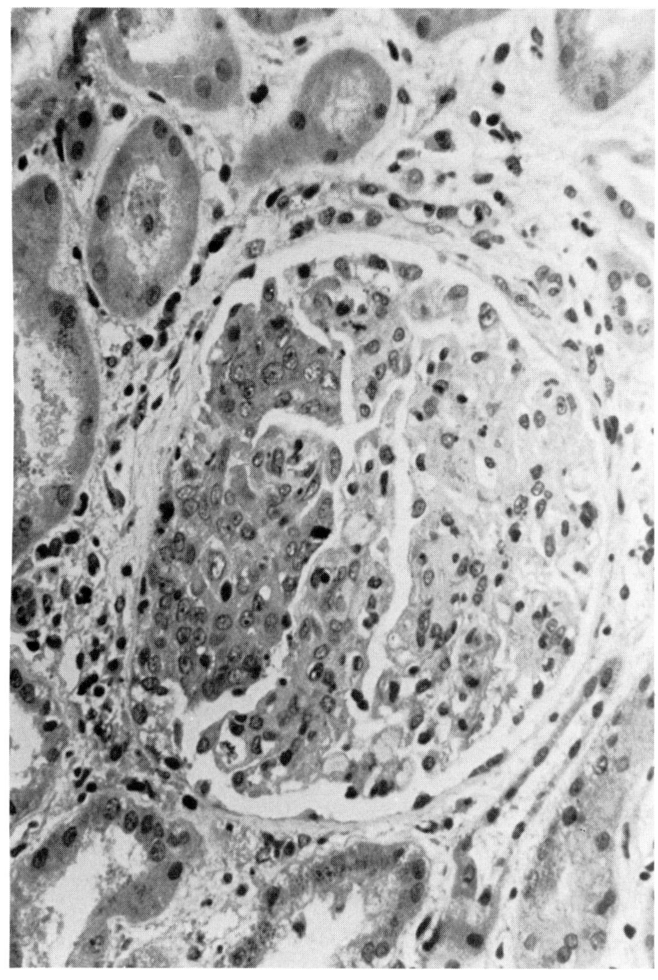

Fig. 9. Lupus glomerulonephritis. Irregular glomerular inflammatory changes involve both intra- and extra-capillary cells with frequent areas of focal necrosis. H & E, 450X

corticosteroid therapy. Two of nine survivors are now in complete remission and four have mild, asymptomatic proteinuria. Three require intermittent diuretic therapy. One patient, a 59-year-old male, has had a gradual fall in urea clearance to 20 ml/minute despite prednisone therapy, but he remains asymptomatic. Because of the wide variation in the course of the disease, prognosis must be offered with caution in these patients. Recent trials of immunosuppressive therapy for this lesion have been stimulated by the previously described finding of immunoglobulins on fluorescent microscopy, but data is inadequate for

evaluation of the efficacy of such therapy at this time (19).

Mention should be made of the nephrotic syndrome in systemic lupus erythematosus (SLE). Fourteen such cases comprise almost a quarter of the group associated with other primary diseases. Renal involvement is generally present in more than half the patients presenting with SLE and may vary from a local and focal glomerulitis, to a diffuse glomerular involvement associated with tubular and interstitial changes, or a basement membrane lesion which in our experience is morphologically indistinguishable from the membranous change lesion in

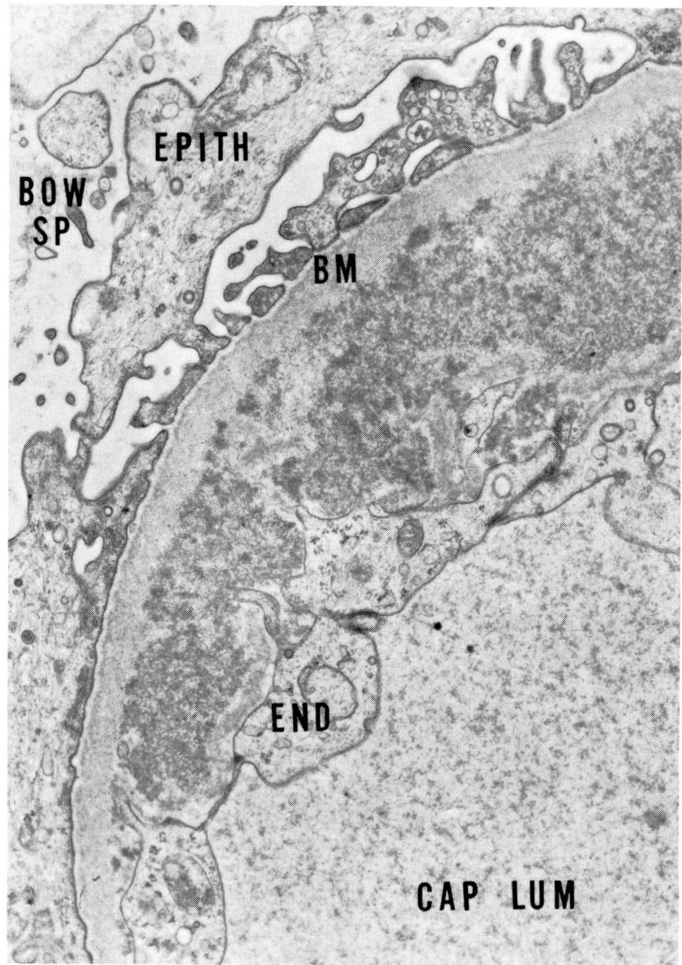

Fig. 10. Wire-loop lesions characteristically have ultrastructural alterations including subendothelial osmophillic deposits. These may accumulate in the mesangial areas and be related to the inflammatory response. Extension through the basement membrane occurs with the progression of the lesion. 16,000X

All tissues for electron microscopy were fixed in Collidine-buffered Osmium, dehydrated in graded alcohols, cleared in propylene oxide, embedded in Epon, stained with lead hydroxide and uranyl acetate.

the adult form of the idiopathic nephrotic syndrome (27).

Other series have indicated a 15% incidence of nephrotic syndrome in patients with SLE (24). Eleven of our fourteen cases with the clinical syndrome in association with this disease had severe proliferative lesions fitting the lupus glomerulonephritis categorization of Pollak and associates (22) (Fig. 9, 10). Our approach has been to utilize high-dose corticosteroid therapy in these patients who usually have other serious manifestations of systemic disease. Three patients have had the membranous lesion. Additional clinical and laboratory confirmation of SLE is necessary to establish the diagnosis with the finding of such a lesion on biopsy. Our impression has been that this group is relatively stable and less often develops clinical nephrotic syndrome or rapid progression.

With further opportunity for careful serial study of biopsies in the evaluation of the natural history and therapeutic response of renal lesions, and the development of a uniform nomemclature which is now "in committee," the second fifteen years of renal biopsy should prove as rewarding as the first.

BILIOGRAPHY

1. Arnold, J. D., Tarlov, A. R., Spargo, B., and Brewer, G. J.: Subclinical Diabetes Mellitus in patients presenting with clinical chronic "glomerulonephritis." Trans. Assoc. Am. Physicians, *71:*189-195, 1958.
2. Bell, E. T.: Renal Disease, 2nd ed. Philadelphia, Lea and Febiger, 1950.
3. Cameron, J. S., and Blandford G.: The simple assessment of selectivity in heavy proteinuria. Lancet, *ii:*242-247, 1966.
4. Christian, H. A.: Bright's Disease. Oxford, Oxford Univ. Pres, 1948.
5. Churg, J., Grishman, E., Goldstein, M. H., Yunis, S. L., and Porush, J. G.: Idiopathic nephrotic syndrome in adults: A study and classification based on renal biopsies. New Engl. J. Med., *272:*165-174, 1965.
6. Daysog, A., Jr., Dobson, H. L., and Brennan, J. C.: Renal glomerular and vascular lesions in prediabetics and in diabetes mellitus: a study based on renal biopsies. Ann. Int. Med., *54:*672-684, 1961.
7. Drummond, K. N., Michael, A. F., Good, R. A., and Vernier, R. L.: The nephrotic syndrome of childhood: immunologic, clinical, and pathologic correlations. J. Clin. Invest., *45:*620-630, 1966.
8. Farquhar, M. G., Vernier, R. L., and Good, R. A.: Electron microscope study of the glomerulus in nephrosis, glomerulonephritis, and lupus erythematosus. J. Exper. Med., *106:*649-660, 1957.
9. Gellman, D. D., Pirani, C. L., Soothill, J. F., Muehrcke, R. C., and Kark, R. M.: Diabetic nephropathy: A clinical and pathologic study based on renal biopsies. Medicine, *38:*321-367, 1959.
10. Hardwicke, J.: Estimation of renal permeability to protein on Sephadex G 200. Clin. Chim. Acta, *12:*89-96, 1965.
11. Hardwicke, J., Blainey, J. D., Brewer, D. B., and Soothill, J. F.: The nephrotic syndrome. Proc. 3rd Int. Congr. Nephrol., Washington 1966, Vol. 3, 69-82, Basel/New York, Karger.
12. Iversen, P., and Brun, C.: Aspiration biopsy of the kidney. Amer. J. Med., *11:*324-330, 1951.
13. Kark, R. M., and Muehrcke, R. C.: Biopsy of kidney in prone position. Lancet, *i:*1047-1049, 1954.
14. Kimmelstiel, P., and Wilson, C.: Intercapillary lesions in the glomeruli of the kidney. Am. J. Path., *12:*83-98, 1936.
15. Lange, K., Treser, G., Sagel, I., Ty, A., and Wasserman, E.: Routine immunohistology in renal diseases. Ann. Int. Med., *64:*25-40, 1966.
16. Linnér, E., Svanborg, A., and Zelander, T.: Retinal and renal lesions of diabetic type, without obvious disturbances in glucose metabolism, in a patient with family history of diabetes. Am. J. Med., *39:*298-304, 1965.
17. Maxwell, M. H., Adams, D. A., and Goldman, R.: Corticosteroid therapy of amyloid nephrotic syndrome. Ann. Int. Med., *60:*539-555, 1964.
18. McCluskey, R. T., Vassalli, P., Gallo, G., and Baldwin, D. S.: An immunofluorescent study of pathogenic mechanisms in glomerular diseases. New Engl. J. Med., *274:*696-701, 1966.
19. Michael, A. F., Vernier, R. I., Drummond, K. N., Levitt, J. I., Herdman, R. C., Fish, A. J., and Good, R. A.: Immunosuppressive therapy of chronic renal disease. New Engl. J. Med., *276:*817-828, 1967.
20. Müller, F.: Morbus Brightii. Verhandl. Deut. Pathol. Ges., *9:*64-99, 1905.
21. Munk, F.: Klinische Diagnostik der degenerativen Nierenerkrankungen. Zeit. Klin. Med., *78:*1-52, 1913.
22. Pollak, V. E., Pirani, C. L., and Schwartz, F. D.: The natural history of the renal manifestations of Systemic Lupus Erythematosus. J. Lab. Clin. Med., *63:*537-550, 1964.
23. Rosen, S., Pirani, C. L., Kark, R. M., Muehrcke, R. C., and Pollak, V. E.: "Lipoid Nephrosis" and Idiopathic Membranous Glomerulonephritis. Am. J. Path., *44:*14a, 1964.
24. Rothfield, N. F., McCluskey, R. T., and Baldwin, D. S.: Renal disease in Systemic Lupus Erythematosus. New Engl. J. Med., *269:*537-544, 1963.
25. Saxena, K. M., and Crawford, J. D.: The treatment of nephrosis. New Engl. J. Med., *272:*522-526, 1965.
26. Squire, J. R., Hardwicke, J., and Soothill, J. F.: Proteinuria. *In*, Black, D.A.K. (ed.): Renal Disease. Philadelphia, F. A. Davis Company, 1962, pp. 213-232.
27. Spargo, B. H., and Forland, M.: The differential diagnosis of glomerular ultrastructural lesions. Proc. 3rd. Int. Congr. Nephrol. Washington 1966, Vol. 2, 33-44. Basel/New York, Karger, 1967.
28. Vernier, R. L., Tinglof, B., Urizar, R., Litman, N., and Smith, F. G., Jr.: Immunofluorescence studies in renal disease. Proc. 3rd Int. Congr. Nephrol., Washington 1966, Vol. 3, 83-94, Basel/New York, Karger, 1967.

Chapter 36

Drug-Induced Nephropathy

GEOFFREY KENT, M.D., PH.D., R. C. MUEHRCKE, M.D. and F. I. VOLINI, M.D.

The kidney, with its rich blood supply and highly specialized excretory function, is especially vulnerable to the adverse effects of drugs. Nephropathy induced by drugs may result from a variety of mechanisms and produce clinical manifestations. These may range from mild and reversible glomerular and tubular lesions to severe and irreversible chronic renal failure.

This presentation is not intended to review exhaustively the subject of drug-induced renal disease but rather to highlight a clinicopathological correlation of manifestations commonly encountered in the practice of medicine. The drugs to be discussed will be arbitrarily grouped according to their presumed site of action with particular reference to the tubules, interstitium, glomeruli and blood vessels (Fig. 1 and 2).

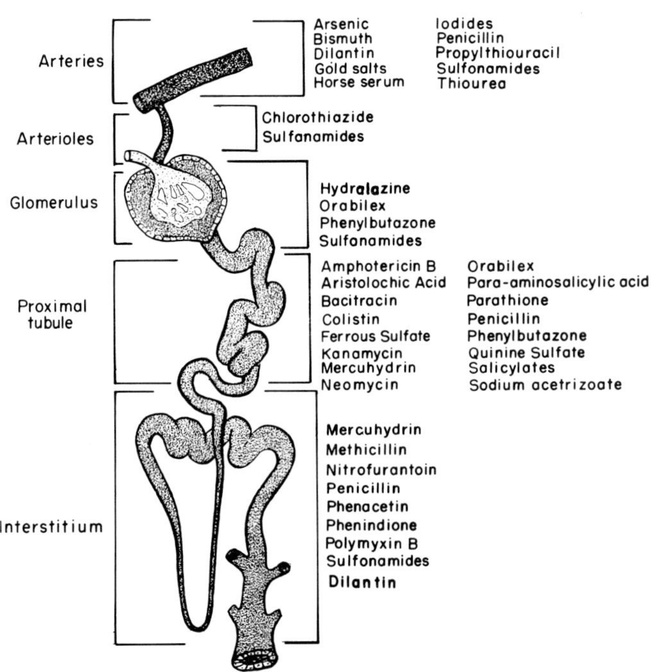

Fig. 1.   Morphologic site of drug induced nephropathy.

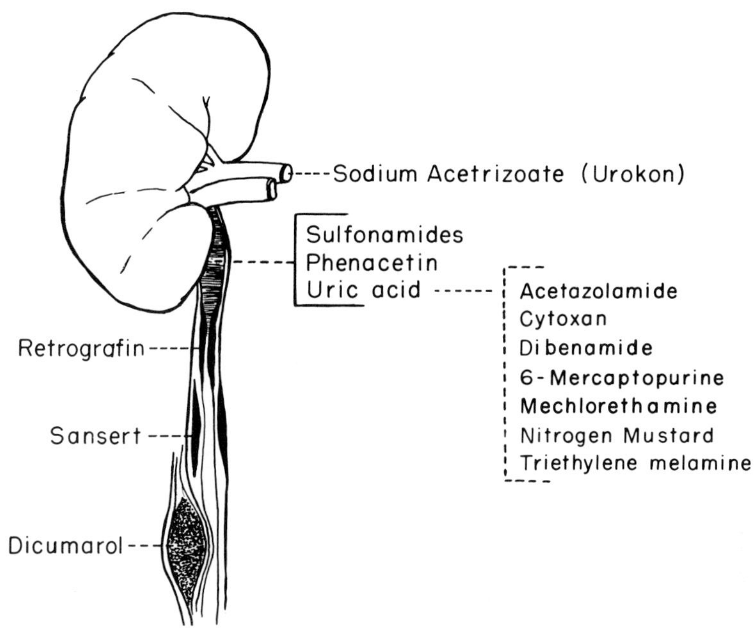

Fig. 2. Gross morphologic site of drug induced acute renal failure.

MECHANISMS

The precise mode of action by which drugs exert adverse renal effects remains poorly understood and in many instances is difficult to determine. The mechanisms to be considered either singly or in combination include direct nephrotoxic effects, immune phenomena, mechanical effects, metabolic effects and secondary effects such as hemolysis.

Direct nephrotoxicity akin to such poisons as inorganic mercurials (1) or carbon tetrachloride (2) is best exemplified by certain antibiotics (Fig. 1). The toxic effects are dose and time related and characteristically should be reproducible in animals. As these substances undergo progressive concentration within the tubular lumen, they reach toxic levels and damage the tubular epithelial cells. A similar concentrating mechanism may be operative in producing lesions of the renomedullary

interstitium (counter-current multiplier system) as seen following the prolonged use of analgesic agents.

In the main, immune or hypersensitivity reactions involve the endothelial surfaces and walls of arteries, arterioles and glomerular capillaries. The lesion produced may be in the form of vasculitis, polyarteritis nodosa, glomerulonephritis, and "foot-process disease" of the glomerular capillary epithelium. An additional morphological site for hypersensitivity reactions may be the renal interstitium which displays an acute interstitial nephritis characterized by infiltrates of plasma cells, small lymphocytes and eosinophils. This type of interstitial nephritis was first described by Councilman in 1898 (Fig. 3).

Mechanical obstruction due to drug action may result from the presence of the drug as insoluble crystals, as for example crystallization of sulfonamides, or it may be the result of a secondary

Volume III　JULY and SEPTEMBER, 1898　Nos. 4 and 5

THE JOURNAL

OF

EXPERIMENTAL MEDICINE

ACUTE INTERSTITIAL NEPHRITIS.

By W. T. COUNCILMAN, M. D.

(From the Sears Pathological Laboratory of Harvard University.)

PLATES XXXVII and XXXVIII.

DEFINITION.—An acute inflammation of the kidney characterized by cellular and fluid exudation in the interstitial tissue, accompanied by, but not dependent on, degeneration of the epithelium; the exudation is not purulent in character, and the lesions may be both diffuse and focal.

Fig. 3. From original paper by Councilman on acute interstitial nephritis.

effect of drugs. Such an example is the precipitation of uric acid following the use of cytoxan (4), or the development of periureteral fibrosis following the use of Sansert (5). Metabolic effects of drugs on the kidney are best exemplified by potassium deficiency which results from the chronic use of cathartics and oral diuretic agents (6 and 7).

DRUG–INDUCED RENAL TUBULAR DAMAGE

The direct nephrotoxicity of drugs on renal tubules may give rise to clinical features ranging from mild tubular dysfunction to acute renal failure. The morphologic features likewise vary from hardly discernible ultrastructural changes to severe tubular necrosis. Approximately 20% of 284 patients with acute oliguric renal failure seen by one of us (RCM) had drug or chemical-induced disease. While the relationship of the patient's symptoms to drug dosage may often be doubtful, severe damage, when present, may usually be correlated with underlying renal disease or excessive drug dosage. The drugs belonging to this category include the antibiotics such as neomycin (8 and 9), kanamycin (10) and colistin methanesulfonate (11) as well as such agents as aristolochic acid (4) and degraded tetracycline (epiahydrotetracycline and anhydrotetracycline) (12-14). A number of brief patient illustrations may serve best to emphasize the clinicopathological features of drug-induced nephropahty.

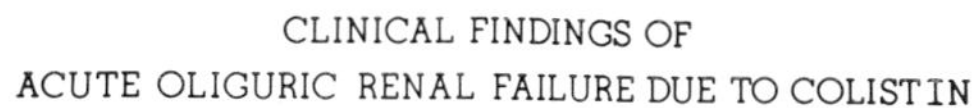
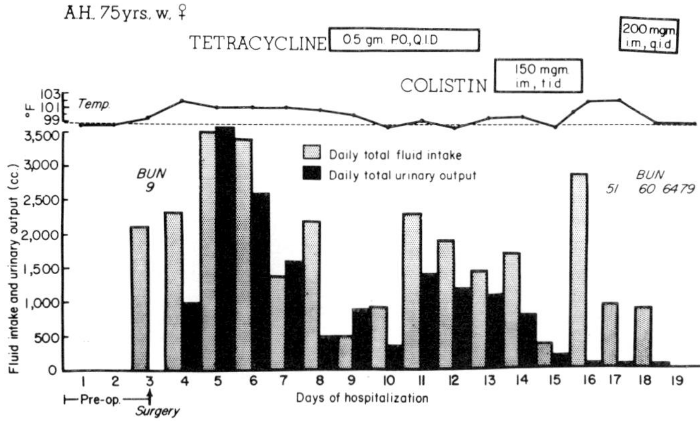

Fig. 4.

Case 1. Acute Oliguric Renal Failure Due to Colistin Methanesulfonate

A. H., a 75-year-old female, was admitted to the hospital because of a fracture to the neck of the femur. Urinalysis and blood urea nitrogen (BUN) were normal. On the 3rd hospital day prosthetic replacement of the femoral head was performed (Fig. 4). Because of mild pyuria, collistin methanesulfonate was give intramuscularly in doses of 6.3 mg/Kg/day. She promptly developed oliguria, moderate azotemia and later total anuria. Hemodialysis was done on the sixth day but she expired shortly thereafter. Autopsy revealed extensive renal tubular necrosis (Fig. 5).

Case II. Polyuria Due to Aristolochic Acid

A. W., a 57-year-old male underwent surgery for carcinoma of the rectum. Three years later, he developed metastatic lesions in bone and pelvic soft tissue associated with severe back pain. He was given a total of 1069 milligrams aristolochic acid intravenously over 42

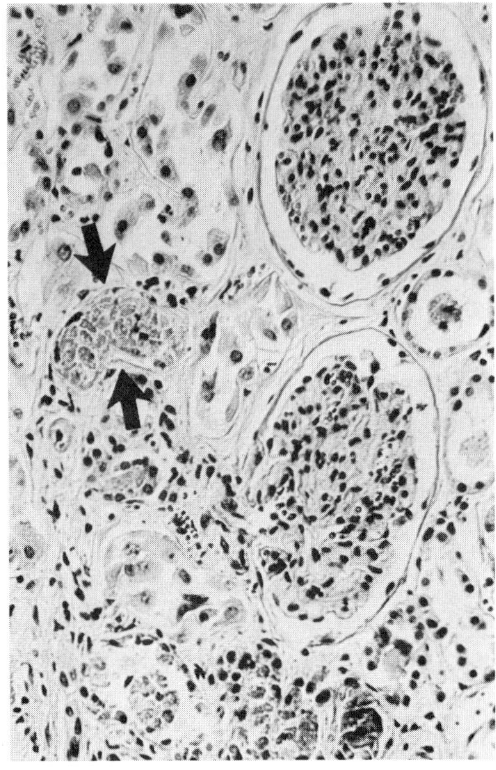
Fig. 5. Autopsy finding in patient treated with colistin methanesulfonate. The photograph shows tubular necrosis (arrows). Hematoxylin and Eosin. X 210.

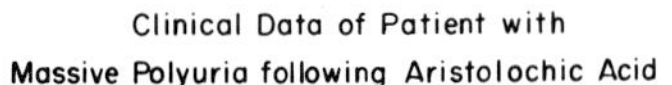

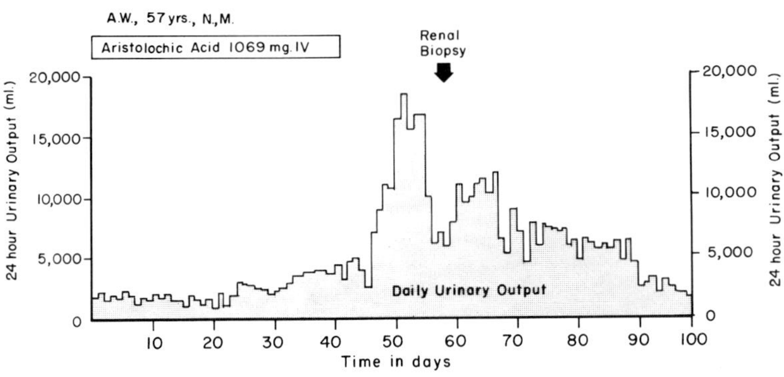

Fig. 6.

days (Fig. 6). Following discontinuance of aristolochic acid therapy, he developed polyuria. The urinary output continued to rise to a peak of 18 liters and was unaffected by administration of pitressin or chlorothiazide. Renal biopsy at this time showed only few changes consisting of dilatation of tubules and flattening of the lining epithelium. Fluid and electrolyte balance was maintained by oral and I. V. fluid supplements. The polyuria subsided gradually over the next three weeks and further observations revealed no evidence of permanent renal damage.

Case III. Fanconi Syndrone Due to Degraded Tetracycline

M. K., a 44-year-old physician's wife developed a flu-like syndrome with fever while on a trip abroad. Her husband gave her tetracycline capsules which were outdated (2-1/2 years old). She continued to be febrile and was hospitalized. Admission urinalysis was normal. One day later, she was found to have 2+ glucosuria and 1+ proteinuria. Chromatography of urine revealed a large excess of amino acids. The concentration of blood urea nitrogen was normal. The fever subsided within two days, and urinalysis was normal three weeks later.

Comment

These case histories illustrate the occurrence of acute oliguric renal failure with acute tubular necrosis and transient tubular dysfunction in the form of polyuria or the Fanconi syndrome (Table 1). Colistin has been shown to produce proximal renal tubular necrosis in rats (15). The mechanism of drug toxicity in this instance may be related to its ability to disrupt certain cell membranes (16) by acting as a cationic detergent. The action may resemble that of amphotericin B, a fungicide also known to disrupt cell membranes (17) and to produce the Fanconi syndrome (18).

TABLE I
DRUG-INDUCED FANCONI SYNDROME

Amphotericin B (18)
Degraded Tetracycline (13)
Degraded Oxytetracycline (40)
Bismuth Compounds (39)

The effect of colistin on renal function in man is unpredictable. Patients
with and without renal disease have
received the drug without significant
changes in urinary output, BUN or urinalysis. Although transient azotemia or
further increases in a previously elevated
BUN have been reported, almost all such
patients have returned to pre-treatment
BUN levels once medication was discontinued. When patients on treatment with
colistin develop acute oliguric renal
failure, one may suspect either that the
drug was given in doses greater than the
recommended upper limit of 5 mg per
Kg per day or that some degree to renal
insufficiency pre-existed (11).

DRUG–INDUCED DAMAGE TO THE RENAL INTERSTITIUM

The most important example for this
group is chronic interstitial nephritis
associated with analgesic (phenacetin)
abuse (19). The outstanding clinical features are emotional disturbances,
anemia, peptic ulcers and azotemia.
These are reflected pathologically in
interstitial fibrosis and papillary necrosis
(20). The patient may experience renal
colic when necrotic papillae are passed.
Grossly, the necrotic papillae are brown
due to the deposition of lipofuscin. By
contrast with the papillary necrosis seen
in diabetic or obstructive uropathy,
baterial infection does not play a role
and evidence of suppuration is lacking.
Neutrophilic infiltrates are not a feature
at the line of demarcation between the
necrotic papillae and the adjacent viable
tissue.

In addition to this non-bacterial type
of papillary necrosis, the interstitial
space of the medulla is widened due to
an increase of both mucopolysaccharides
and collagen (Fig. 7). The blood supply

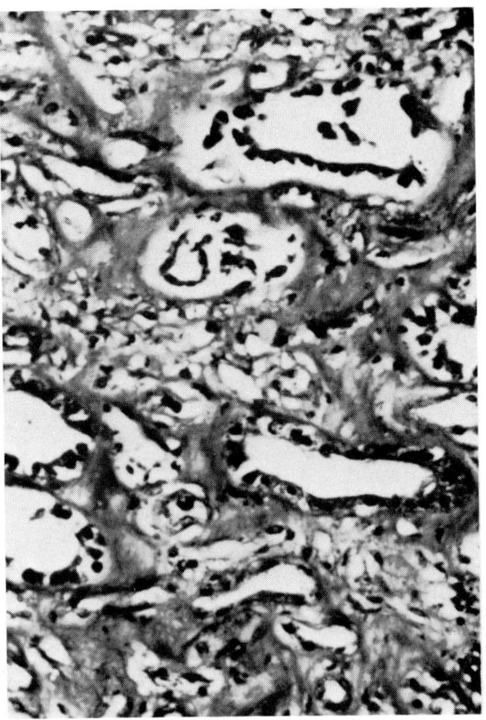

Fig. 7. Renal medulla in patient with analgesic abuse showing widening of interstitial space and scanty blood supply. X 400.

is scanty. Presumably, a metabolite of
the analgesic agent or possibly a contaminant reaches the interstitium at a
high concentration, causing the primary
injury. The increase in interstitial tissue
then results in secondary tubular atrophy, obliteration of peritubular capillaries and finally papillary necrosis.
Some patients may not be seen until
they have developed terminal uremia,
while in other patients papillary necrosis
may be an early feature and discovered
in the urine following an attack of
ureteral colic. The features are illustrated
by the following case histories.

*Case IV. Analgesic-induced
interstitial Nephritis*

L. G., a 42-year-old physician ingested
3 kg. of phenacetin contained in APC
tablets during a five-year period for relief

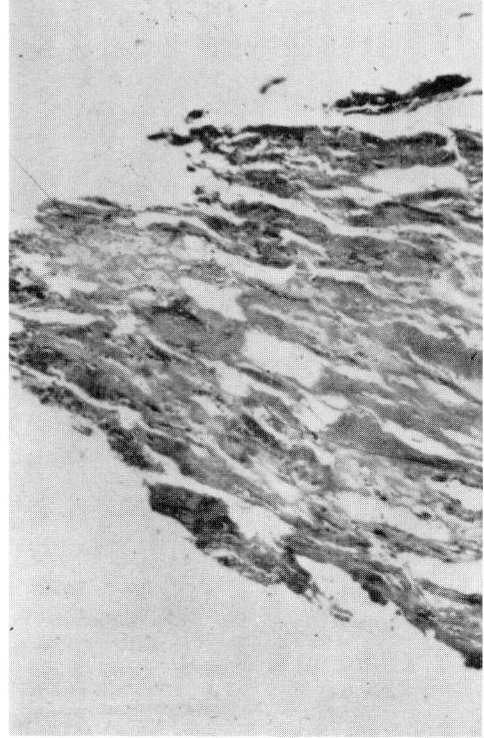

Fig. 8. Necrotic renal papilla passed following ureteric colic. The patient had taken large quantities of phenacetin-containing tablets. X80.

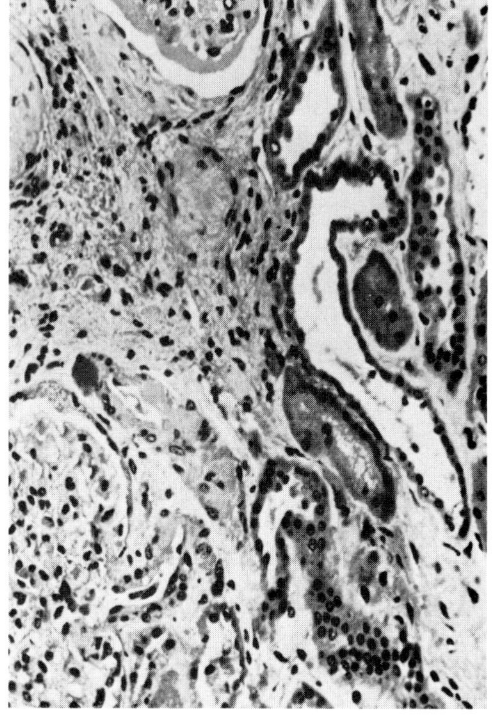

Fig. 9. Renal biopsy from same patient. The photograph shows interstitial fibrosis and a round cell infiltrate. X 210.

of sinus headaches. He was admitted to hospital for ureteral colic associated with the passage of material which proved to be necrotic renal papilla (Fig. 8). Renal biopsy revealed interstitial nephritis (Fig.9). He improved after withdrawal of the phenacetin containing analgesic tablets.

Case V. Analgesic-induced interstitial Nephritis with Uremia

D. M., a 57-year-old female was admitted to hospital with uremia and a history of having taken 14 APC tablets daily for headaches over the past 40 years. She had hypertension for two years previously. She developed uremic frost and died with a BUN of 310 mg

per 100 ml. At autopsy, both kidneys were diminished in size. Their surfaces were granular and on section revealed papillary necrosis. Microscopically, chronic interstitial nephritis was in the foreground, and the necrotic papillae showed the features described above.

DRUG-INDUCED RENAL GLOMERULAR AND VASCULAR DISEASE

The effect of drugs on blood vessels is usually considered to be the result of hypersensitivity or immune reactions. In this category are included drugs that result in the nephrotic syndrome (21-25), although the mechanisms lead-

TABLE II—DRUG-INDUCED NEPHROTIC SYNDROME

Bismuth Tartrate (33)	Phenindione (Hedulin) (37)
d-Pencicillamine (25)	Phenylbutazone (41)
Gold Salts (34)	Probenacid (38)
Mercuhydrin (24)	Smallpox Vaccination
Mercurous Chloride (Caromel) (35)	Thallium Salts
Paramethadione (Paradione) (21)	Tolbutamide (Orinase) (23)
Perchlorate (36)	Trimethadione (Tridione) (22)

ing to this clinical syndrome may be less apparent and the role of blood vessel disease may only be recognized by electron microscopic study. Other conditions belonging to this group are hypersensitivity angiitis and acute glomerulonephritis. Hypersensitivity angiitis is typically seen following the use of sulfa drugs or the thiazides (26). Acute proliferative glomerulonephritis has been observed following administration of such agents as dextran (27), Sulfonamides (28), orabilex (29) and hydralazine (29), while the nephrotic syndrome has occurred following the use of tridione (21), paradione (22), orinase (23), mercuhydrin (24), d-penicillamine (25) and trichlorethylene (Table II). The following case histories may illustrate the pertienent clinicopathological features.

Case VI. TTp-like Syndrome Produced by Phenylbutazone

H. B., a 44-year-old female complained of intermittent pain and swelling of the joints for the past five years. Because her wrists and hands became involved, she was given phenylbutazone. Following a total dose of 600 mg she developed chills, fever, vomiting, oliguria, Coombs-positive hemolytic anemia and thrombocytopenic purpura. This case was reported in detail elsewhere (30). The BUN was 74 mg per 100 ml.

Renal biopsy study revealed dilated glomerular capillaries containing eosinophilic hyaline thrombi (Fig. 10). She developed anuria which persisted for three weeks. During this time, peritoneal dialysis was used repeatedly; however, she developed pneumonia and expired. The condition was interpreted as thrombotic thrombocytopenic purpura with intravascular coagulation.

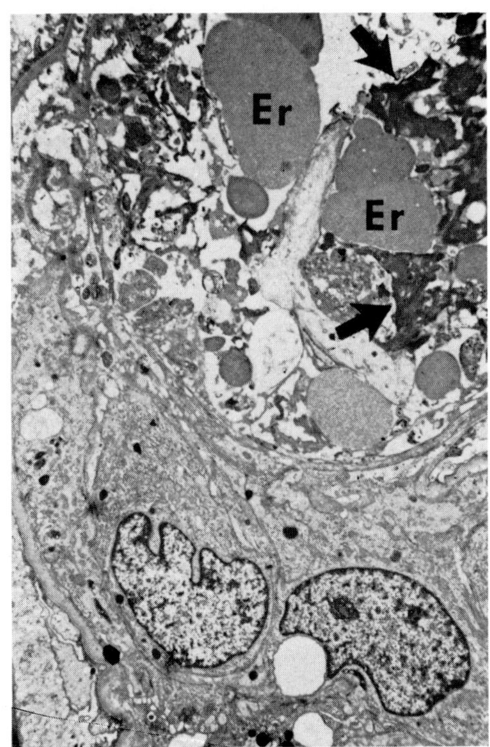

Fig. 10. Thrombus within lumen of glomerular capillary. Note fibrin (arrows) about erythrocyte (Er). X 4200.

Case VII. Hypersensitivity Angiitis following the use of Sulfa Drugs

J. S., a 23-year-old male was admitted to the hospital with fever and pyuria. Urine cultures revealed 10 million E. coli/cc. Four grams of Gantrisin were given daily. The patient developed a skin rash, eosinophilia and acute oliguria. The previously normal blood pressure rose to 190/100 and the blood urea nitrogen to 176 mg per 100 ml. Oliguria progressed to anuria. Peritoneal dialysis were performed over the next four days resulting in a decline of the blood urea nitrogen to 88 mg per 100 ml. Hypertension and anuria, however, persisted and the patient expired on the 14th hospital day. Autopsy revealed acute fibrinoid necrosis of the wall of small caliber vessels together with an intense leukocytic infiltrate which permeated into perivascular tissues (Fig. 11).

Case VIII. Acute Glomerulonephritis following Administration of Dextran

A 40-year-old female patient had an iron deficiency anemia due to a bleeding peptic ulcer and was given iron-dextran intramuscularly with good response. She was given 500 ml of 6% dextran and over the next few days developed fever, backache and pain around the iron-dextran injection sites. Biopsy of this region revealed an allergic type of inflammation with vasculitis. Nine days after the febrile reaction, the patient developed massive proteinuria with numerous hyaline and red cell casts in the urine sediment. Renal biopsy study revealed proliferative glomerulonephritis (Fig. 12). Following administration of prednisone, the fever subsided and the proteinuria diminished. This case was studied at the Research and Education Hospital of the University of Illinois in conjunction with Dr. V. Pollack and will

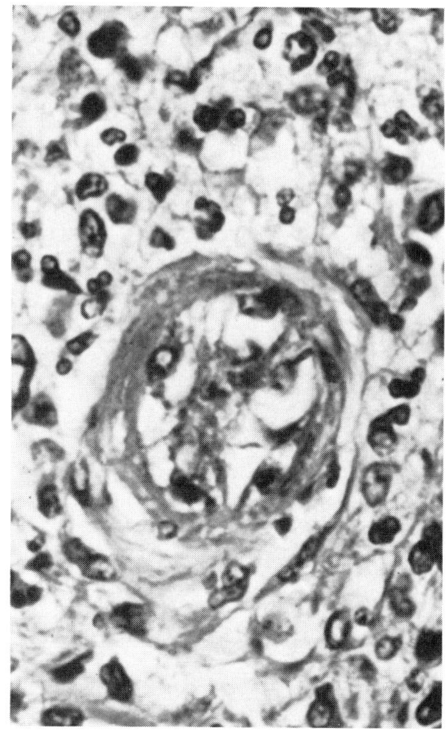

Fig. 11. Hypersensitivity angiitis following sulfa therapy. Small caliber vessel with fibrinoid necrosis surrounded by leukocytic infiltrate. X 525.

be reported in detail elsewhere.

Large molecular weight Dextran is known to be a potent antigen, and it is probable that the patient was sensitized through the previous administration of iron dextran. Low-molecular-weight dextran produces acute renal failure due to nephron occlusion as a result of increased urinary viscosity (31) or swelling of tubular cells (32).

Case IX. Nephrotic Syndrome due to Mercuhydrin

K. F., a 67-year-old female was admitted to hospital in acute pulmonary edema. She had been hypertensive for the past 11 years. On admission, she was given digoxin and mercuhydrin. Admission urinalysis was normal and the blood

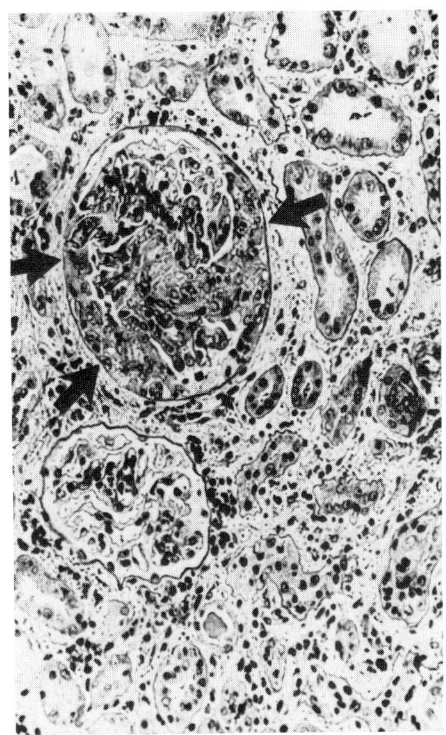

Fig. 12. Proliferative glomerulonephritis following Dextran therapy. Arrows point to crescent formation. X 150.

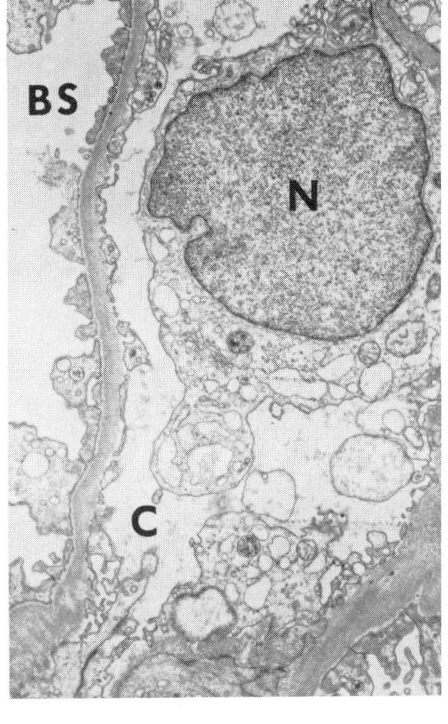

Fig. 13. Electron micrograph of patient with nephrotic syndrome following d-penicillamine. Note fusion of foot processes (C=capillary; BS=Bowman's space). X 6000.

urea concentration was 28 mg per 100 ml. Following a second injection of mercuhydrin, she developed fever, 2+ proteinuria and a macular skin rash. On the 4th day, edema of the face and arms appeared and proteinuria became more abundant. The BUN was 28 mg per 100 ml. The serum cholesterol was 480 mg per 100 ml. The 24-hour urinary output diminished to 300 ml. She was treated conservatively and after two weeks the proteinuria diminished and the edema subsided.

Case X. Nephrotic Syndrome following d-Penicillamine

M. W., a 32-year-old female was found to have hepatolenticular degeneration (Wilson's Disease) with severe ataxia, intention tremor, and Kayser-Fleischer rings. She was given d-penicillamine, and because a severe skin rash developed the drug was withdrawn. Months later, the neurologic signs were found to be more advanced and another course of d-penicillamine was instituted. The blood urea nitrogen was 12 mg per 100 ml and routine urinalysis was normal. After three days on d-penicillamine, the patient developed 4+ proteinuria. Hyaline and granular casts and doubly refractile lipid bodies were found in the urinary sediment. The blood cholesterol was 435 mg per 100 ml. The 24-hour urine protein was 5 gms. Serum albumin was 2.0 gm per 100 ml, PSP excretion was 35% in 15 minutes, and the 24-hour endogenous creatinine clearance was 71 ml per min. Moderate edema of the face was noted. Electron microscopic study of a renal biopsy specimen revealed fusion of epithelial cell foot processes (Fig. 13). She was given adrenocortical steroids (prednisone) which resulted in a decrease in proteinuria and edema. Three months later urinalysis revealed a trace of protein and a normal urinary sediment.

Discussion

The foregoing illustrates the great variety of reactions displayed by the kidney in response to drug injury. The physician's awareness of the potential hazards of therapeutic agents and of the clinical manifestations encountered will make for judicious employment of these agents and reduce both incidence and severity of adverse reactions. However, the exact mechanism of drug induced renal disorders is often difficult to ascertain in the individual patient, and before one can implicate the adverse action of drugs it is necessary to consider other disease processes.

The major difficulty in identifying drug reactions stems from the variability in response between different individuals. The lack of uniform response is due largely to inherent biochemical differences between recipients of the drug (42). The transformation of drugs may require a series of enzymatic reactions, the activity of which is regulated by genes (42-44). An altered inactivation of the drug or an inability to maintain critical cellular metabolites in the presence of the drug may be one mechanism by which toxic levels are reached. Impairment of renal function may further exaggerate toxicity by interfering with the elimination of the drug or its metabolites and by increasing the patient's cellular susceptibility to the drug. Patients with disturbed renal function thus have an increased predisposition to the nephrotoxic action of drugs, particularly those excreted by the kidneys.

The lack of uniform patient response to drugs is even more pronounced in the case of immune reactions. Like immune responses to protein antigens, those induced by drugs are associated with an induction period, the production of immune globulins, and the appearance of allergic phenomena (anaphylaxis, serum sickness, cutaneous reactions, delayed hypersensitivity). However, by contrast with reactions to proteins, the incidence of sensitization to drugs is low, the antibody response is difficult to demonstrate, readministration may fail to produce hypersensitivity, and allergic manifestations may be localized to a single organ or even a single cell type. The reason for the low degree of drug immunogenicity lies in the requirement of simple chemicals to react with proteins before becoming antigenic (45-47). Aside from the drug itself, moreover, the reactant may be a derivative of the drug or even a contaminant. The manner in which the combination with protein occurs may also play a role; thus covalent coupling seems important in the reactivity of a compound and its capability to be immunogenic (46, 47). Genetic differences which play a role in drug toxicity may further influence the degradation and antigenicity of drugs, thereby increasing the variability in response (48, 49).

The differences noted between the response of individuals to drugs and macromolecules apply not only to the induction of immune responses but also to their recognition. Thus, the drug alone may not combine effectively with antibody because of a difference in antigenic determinant or lack of sufficient combining sites. Where the drug cannot be demonstrated to react with protein, a contaminant or a metabolic intermediate of the drug may well carry out the required conjugation. In penicillin hypersensitivity (50, 51), for example, there is evidence for antibody formation to a number of penicillin derivatives, but not to penicillin alone or to derivatives not bound covalently by protein.

Because of the difficulty in demonstrating antibodies, the toxic or allergic nature of an injury is gauged by indirect criteria. For some compounds, such as bichloride of mercury or some of the antibiotics, potential toxicity is well established. Vascular reactions, by contrast, such as glomerulonephritis and angiitis, are presumed to be allergic in origin. Immune reactions are likely to be present also where an induction period, eosinophilia or cutaneous reactions are displayed or where renal biopsy studies demonstrate the presence of small lymphocytes, plasma cells, and eosinophils. Renal tubular syndromes, such as the Fanconi syndrome, are generally considered the result of drug toxicity. Recently, however, the Fanconi syndrome has also been described in conjuction with immunologic disorders, such as systemic lupus erythematosus or other hypergammaglobulinemias, suggesting that the syndrome may on occasion have an immunologic basis.

CONCLUDING REMARKS

Nephrotoxic and hypersensitivity reactions are the foremost complications in drug-induced nephropathy. They produce a great variety of clinical manifestations ranging from mild renal tubular syndromes to irreversible renal failure. Optimal patient care requires familiarity with the potential hazards of therapeutic agents and early recognition of adverse effects. Caution in the administration of certain drugs is particularly indicated in the presence of underlying renal disease.

REFERENCES

1. Freeman, R. B., Maher, J. F., Schreiner, G. E., and Mostofi, F. K.: Renal tubular necrosis due to nephrotoxicity of organic mercurial diuretics. Ann. Int. Med., *57*:34, 1962.
2. Shreiner, G. E., and Maher, J. F.: Toxic nephropathy. Am. J. Med., *38*:409, 1965.
3. Murphy, F. D., Kuzma, J. F., Polley, T. Z., and Grill, J.: Clinicopathological studies of renal damage due to sulfonamide compounds. Arch. Int. Med., *73*:433, 1944.
4. Muehrcke, R. C., Rosen, S., Thiele, K. G., Pirani, C. L., and Kark, R. M.: Drug-induced renal disease. Ann. Int. Med., *64*:1181, 1966.
5. Schwartz, F. D., and Dunea, G.: Progression of retroperitoneal fibrosis despite cessation of treatment with methysergide. Lancet, *1*:955, 1966.
6. Relman, H. S., and Schwartz, W. B.: The nephropathy of potassium depletion; a clinical and pathological entity. New Engl. J. Med., *255*:195, 1956.
7. Muehrcke, R. C., and McMillan, J. C.: The relationship of chronic pyelonephritis to chronic potassium deficiency. Ann. Int. Med., *59*:427, 1963.
8. MacLean, L. D.: Renal failure following the administration of intraperitoneal neomycin. Minnesota Med., *40*:557, 1957.
9. Emmerson, B. T., and Pryse-Davies, J.: Studies of the nephrotoxic effects of neomycin. Austral. Ann. Med., *13*:149, 1964.
10. Kleeman, C. R., and Maxwell, M. H.: The nephrotoxicity of antibiotics: A review. In, Quinn, E. L., Kass, E. H., (eds): Biology of Pyelonephritis. Boston, Little, Brown and Co., 1960.
11. Elwood, C. M., Lucas, G. D., and Muehrcke, R. C.: Acute renal failure associated with sodium colistimethate treatment. Arch. Int. Med., *118*:326, 1966.
12. Gross, J. M.: Fanconi syndrome (adult type) developing secondary to the ingestion of outdated tetracycline. Ann. Int. Med., *58*:523, 1963.
13. Frimpter, G. W., Trimpanelli, A. E., Eisenmenger, W. J., Stern, H. S., and Ehrlich, L. I.: Reversible Fanconi syndrome cause by degraded tetracycline. J.A.M.A., *185*:111, 1963.
14. Shils, M. E.: Renal disease and the metabolic effects of tetracycline. Ann. Int. Med., *58*:389, 1963.

15. Jawetz, E.: Polymyxin, Colistin and Polymyxin E. Lancet, *1*:922, 1963.

16. Feingold, D. S.: Antimicrobiol. chemotherapeutic agents: The nature of their action and selective toxicity. New Engl. J. Med., *269*:900, 1963.

17. Weissmann, G., Pras, M., and Hirschorn, R.: A common mechanism for the fungicidal and nephrotoxic effect of amphotericin-B. J. Clin. Invest., *45*:1084, 1966.

18. Wertlake, P. T., Butler, W. T., Hill, G. J., and Utz, J. P.: Nephrotoxic tubular damage and calcium deposition following amphotericin-B therapy. Am. J. Path., *43*:449, 1963.

19. Zollinger, H. V.: Chronische Interstitielle Nephritis bei Abusus von Phenacetinhaltigen Analgetica. Schweiz. Med. Wschr., *85*:746, 1955.

20. Harvald, B., Valdorf-Hansen, F., and Nielsen, A.: Effect on the kidney of drugs containing phenacetin. Lancet, *1*:333, 1960.

21. Wren, J. C., and Nutt, R. L.: Nephrotic syndrome occurring during paramethadion therapy; report of case with clinical remission. J.A.M.A., *153*:918, 1953.

22. Barnett, H. L., Simons, D. J., and Wells, R. E.: Nephrotic syndrome occurring during Tridione therapy. Am. J. Med., *4*:760, 1948.

23. Schnall, C., and Wiener, J. S.: Nephrosis occurring during tolbutamide administration. J.A.M.A., *167*:214, 1958.

24. Munck, O., and Nissen, N. I.: Development of nephrotic syndrome during treatment with mercurial diuretics. Acta Med. Scand., *153*:307, 1956.

25. Adams, D. A., Goldman, R., Maxwell, M. H., and Latta, H.: Nephrotic syndrome associated with penicillamine therapy of Wilson's Disease. Am. J. Med., *36*:330, 1964.

26. Kjellbo, H., Stakeberg, H., and Mellgren, J.: Possibly thiazide-induced renal necrotizing vasculitis. Lancet, *1*:1034, 1965.

27. Thiele, K. G., Muehrcke, R. C., and Berning, H.: Wierenerkrankungen durch Medikamente. Dent. Med. Wschr., *36*:1632, 1967.

28. Lehr, D.: Clinical toxicity of sulfonamides. Ann. N. Y. Acad. Sci., *69*:417, 1957.

29. Stetter, J. G., Maher, J. F., and Schreiner, G. E.: Acute renal failure following cholecystography. J. Am. Med. Assoc., *184*:102, 1963.

30. Dunea, G., Muehrcke, R. C., Nakamoto, S., and Schwartz, F. D.: Thrombotic thrombocytopenic purpura with acute anuric renal failure. Am. J. Med., *41*:1000, 1966.

31. Mailloux, L., Swartz, D. C., Capizzi, R., Kim, K. E., Onesti, G., Ramirez, O., and Brest, A. N.: Acute renal failure after administration of low-molecular-weight dextran.

32. Morgan, T. O., Little, J. M., and Evans, W. A.: Renal failure associated with low-molecular-weight dextran infusion. Brit. Med. J., *2*:737, 1966.

33. Karelitz, S., Freeman, A. D.: Hepatitis and nephrosis due to soluble bismuth. Ped., *8*:772, 1951.

34. Gregorie, F., MacMendier, C., and Lambert, P.: Syndrome nephrotique apres traitement aux seis door. J. Urol., *62*:140, 1956.

35. Troen, P., Kaufman, S. H., and Katz, K. H.: Mercuric bichloride poisoning. New Engl. J. Med., *244*:459, 1951.

36. Lee, R. E., Verner, R. L., and Ulstrom, R. A.: The Nephrotic syndrome or a complication of perchlorate treatment of thyrotoxicosis. New Engl. J. Med., *264*:1221, 1961.

37. Baker, S. B. de C., and Williams, R. T.: Acute interstitial nephritis due to drug sensitivity. Brit. Med. J., *1*:1655, 1963.

38. Ferris, T. F., Morgan, W. S., and Levitin, H.: Nephrotic syndrome caused by probenacid. New Engl. J. Med., *265*:381, 1961.

39. Czerwinski, A. W., and Ginn, H. E.: Bismuth nephrotoxicity. Am. J. Med., *37*:969, 1964.

40. Castell, D. O., and Sparks, H. A.: Nephrogenic diabetes insipidus due to demethylclortetracycline hydrochloride. J.A.M.A., *193*:237, 1965.

41. Scheitlin, W., and Jeanneret, P.: Uber akuto nierinschadgengen unter phenylbutazonherapie. Schweiz. med Wschr., *87*:881, 1957.

42. Motulsky, A. G.: Pharmacogenetics. In, Progress in Med. Gen., *3*:49, 1964. New York, Grune & Stratton, Inc., N. Y.

43. Remmer, H., and Merker, H. J.: Drung-induced changes in the liver endoplasmic reticulum: Association with drug metabolizing enzymes. Science, *142*:1657, 1963.

44. Remmer, H.: Drugs as activators of drug enzymes. Proceed. I. Intern. Pharm. Meet., *6*:235, 1962.

45. Parker, C. W.: The biochemical basis of an allergic drug response. Ann. N. Y. Acad. Sci., *123*:55, 1965.

46. Eisen, H. N.: Hypersensitivity to simple chemicals. In, Lawrence, H. S. (ed.): Cellular and Humoral Aspects of the Hypersensitive States. New York, Hoeber, 1959.

47. Gell, P. G. H., Harington, C. R., and Rivers, R. P.: The antigenic function of simple chemical compounds: Production of Precipitins in Rabbits. Brit. J. Exp. Path., *27*:267, 1946.

48. Chase, M. W.: Models for hypersensitivity studies. In, Lawrence, H. S. (ed.): Cellular and Humoral Aspects of the Hypersensitive States.

49. Arquilla, E. R., and Finn, J.: Genetic differences in antibody production to determinant groups on insulin. Sci., *142*:400, 1963.

50. Parker, C. W., Shipiro, J., Kern, M., and Eisen, H. N.: Hypersensitivity to penicillenic acid derivatives in human beings with penicillin allergy. J. Exp. Med., *115*:821, 1962.

51. Parker, C. W.: Editorial: Penicillin allergy. Am. J. Med., *34*:747, 1963.

Chapter 37

Acute Renal Failure: Correlative Clinical-Pathological Study

ROBERT C. MUEHRCKE, M.D.

Introduction

Acute oliguric renal failure was first recognized by physicians at least one hundred years ago. (1) Like many other clinical disorders, it remained dormant in medical literature except for a sporadic report in the English literature by such pathologists as Councilman (2) and Kimmelstiel (3) or in the German literature by Colmers (4) and Minami. (5) However, it was not until World War II that Eric Bywaters permanently established it as a clinical syndrome. (6, 7, 8)

Today, acute oliguric renal failure is a well substantiated clinical syndrome occurring in an adult with previously healthy kidneys and characterized by sudden decrease below 400 ml (less than 17 ml per hr) in daily urinary output delivered to the urinary bladder. Acute renal failure can occur in patients with renal disease as well as in those receiving a renal transplant. Acute oliguric renal failure is associated with progressive and fatal clinical and biochemical manifestations. In some patients, acute renal failure may not be associated with oliguria but with a "high urinary output" (non-oliguric) (9). In time, both conditions can be reversible either spontaneously by diuresis or by proper and effective management. On the other hand, acute renal failure can be irreversible and produce a progressive deterioration in the clinical and biochemical status of the patient leading to death.

The reversibility of acute renal failure depends on several important conditions. The most important is early diagnosis with differentiation from chronic "end-stage" renal disease, renal circulatory failure (pre-renal) and obstructive uropathy (post-renal). It can also occur superimposed on chronic renal disease. Once an exact diagnosis is made, prompt and adequate intensive management must follow. An all important factor in the outcome of the patient with acute renal failure is the pathophysiological process especially the specific site and severity of renal damage. There are few clinical disorders that demand from the physician his scientific knowledge, his practical skill and clinical common sense as does the syndrome of acute renal failure. The gravity of the disorder and its complete and dramatic reversibility greatly taxes the physicians' ability and yet he may experience tremendous gratification once the patient recovers.

Acute oliguric renal failure as known today was a by-product of military and civilian casualty medicine from World War I and II. It has long been known to result from shock. (10) Although shock was effectively treated, progressive and fatal renal insufficiency contributed significantly to the final outcome of the battle casualty. During World War I, studies made on combat and civilian casualties with shock revealed the frequent occurrence of renal involvement with progressive azotemia and death. (5) In 1939, Jeghers and Bakst reviewed acute renal failure under the term extra-renal azotemia (11) These reports attracted little attention or interest from the medical profession.

During the war years 1939-1945, Bywaters and colleagues (6, 7, 8) aroused considerable attention and stimulated the military physicians' interest in acute oliguric renal failure. During the 1940 bombardment of London, they studied air raid casualties injured by fallen masonry or heavy material. Their patients recovered from shock but sustained crushing and compressed muscle injuries. Renal insufficiency followed and in many it was fatal. They designated this disorder the "crush syndrome." At autopsy, they found acute necrosis of renal tubules and blanched necrotic muscle. Bywater's original and accurate drawings of abnormal renal morphological findings are most impressive and should be reviewed by those interested in this disorder. (7)

Differential Diagnosis

The physician must make a prompt differentiation of sudden oliguria or anuria due to acute renal failure from that of chronic "end-stage" renal failure. Patients with acute renal failure may not display the typical course in which there is an onset stage or oliguria may not be striking. For further differentiation, it seems important to subdivide acute oliguric renal failure into three distinct clinical groups. These are acute parenchymal disease, acute renal circulatory failure (pre-renal) and obstructive uropathy (Post-renal).

Prompt and accurate differential diagnosis is very important for two reasons. First, acute circulatory failure if not corrected may progress to parenchymal lesions. Secondly, hasty and poorly considered managment using fluid and electrolytes may be extremely hazardous if parenchymal abnormalities are present. The pre-renal disorders include renal circulatory insufficiency due to a variety of causes; acute myocardial infarction, dehydration and electrolyte and acid-base deficiencies such as hyponatremia, hypopotassemia and acidosis.

PRE-RENAL FAILURE

Acute renal circulatory failure or pre-renal failure is a term applied to patients with acute oliguria or anuria. It implies two clinical conditions: one, impairment of circulation to the kidney with resultant oliguria and, two, renal parenchymal damage has not yet occurred. Acute renal circulatory failure results from renal ischemia. The clinical course of acute renal circulatory failure is short and usually reversible. If untreated, acute renal circulatory failure may progress to varying degrees of renal parenchymal damage such as acute tubular necrosis; for example, severe and prolonged ischemia may result in bilateral renal cortical necrosis. The urine then has a low osmolarity and increased sodium concentration.

POST-RENAL FAILURE

The complexity and distance from the

renal pelvis to the urinary bladder predisposes the ureter to a variety of pathological conditions leading to obstructive uropathy. The diagnosis of obstructive causes of acute renal failure is very imporant as its management is completely different than when the parenchyma is primarily involved. In the past, acute oliguric renal failure owing to mechanical obstructive uropathy was referred to as "surgical anuria" and the only treatment was surgical intervention with the objective to relieve the obstruction. Mechanical obstruction of the ureter and subsequent acute anuria usually presents diagnostic difficulties and not conceptual problems.

The diagnosis of obstructive uropathy must be made as quickly as possible so as to relieve the obstructive process before irreversible parenchymal damage occurs. Some patients will have no symptoms related to ureteral obstruction, although, the foremost diagnostic clue is usually a sudden and complete anuria. Total anuria over 24 hours is rare in acute tubular necrosis but it can occur if the necrosis is extensive, severe and diffuse such as in arsine-induced anuria. Total anuria can occur in severe acute glomerular afflictions and in diffuse necrotizing vasculitis. These glomerular diseases include acute post-streptococcal glomerulonephritis, hypersensitivity glomerulonephritis lupus glomerulonephritis, acute thrombotic thrombocytopenic purpura and bilateral renal cortical necrosis. Erythrocyte casts and subsequent absolute anuria that develops in a patient receiving sulfonamides usually indicates an underlying renal vasculitis.

RUPTURED URINARY BLADDER

Absolute anuria can be erroneously diagnosed if the urinary bladder was ruptured and the urine is diverted into the peritoneal cavity. A penetrating injury or blunt trauma in the lower abdomen can result in perforation of the bladder. Extravasation of urine into the peritoneal cavity may produce findings of acute renal failure and, later, peritonitis. This occurs in approximately 60 per cent of the patients with bladder rupture.

Urine trapped inside the peritoneal cavity approaches the osmolarity and chemical composition of the blood. For example, the initial urinary potassium concentration is greater than that in the vascular space and would cross the peritoneal membrane into the blood. The overall effects of this "auto-dialysis" would result in a relative blood loss of sodium and chloride but a gain in blood urea nitrogen and serum potassium.

Clinical Features of Acute Oliguric Renal Failure

Acute oliguric renal failure is an omnibus syndrome that is an acute result of innumerable causes steming from involvement of the major and minor renal arteries, the renal veins, the glomeruli, the renal interstitium the renal tubules and from obstructive uropathy. The primary illness precipitating acute renal failure can greatly modify the natural history of the disorder. Thus, the clinical course and prognosis of patients with acute oliguric renal failure may be extremely variable.

Today, the most common underlying pathological abnormality of acute oliguric renal failure has been attributed to

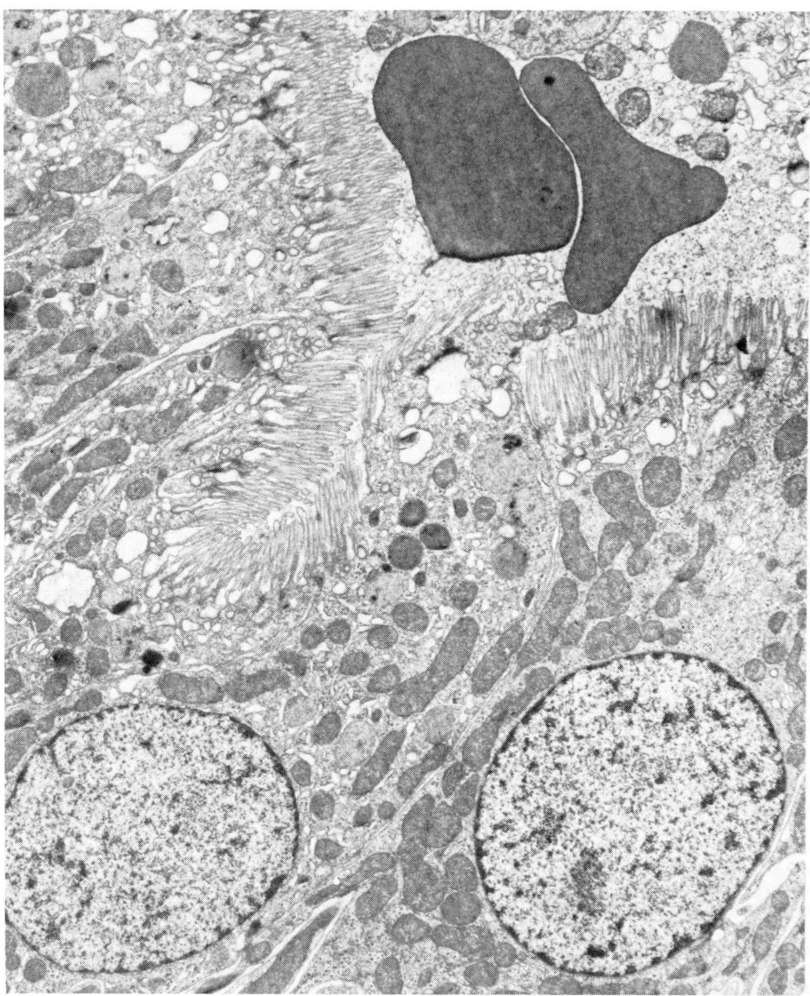

Fig. 1. Electron-micro-photograph from patient with acute oliguric renal failure due to unknown causes. A 54-year-old housewife developed oliguria and weakness. Her blood urea nitrogen was 114 mg per 100 ml. She was given mannitol intravenously without a diuresis. A clinical diagnosis was made of acute oliguric renal failure due to "acute tubular necrosis." A renal biopsy was done on the fourth day of oliguria. The tubules appeared normal by light microscope. The renal tissue was studied by electron microscopy and was found normal. Note the proteinaceous material in the tubular lumen (L). Normal cellular constituents are seen. There is interstitial edema (IE). The tubular basement membrane (BM) is laminated. X9,720.

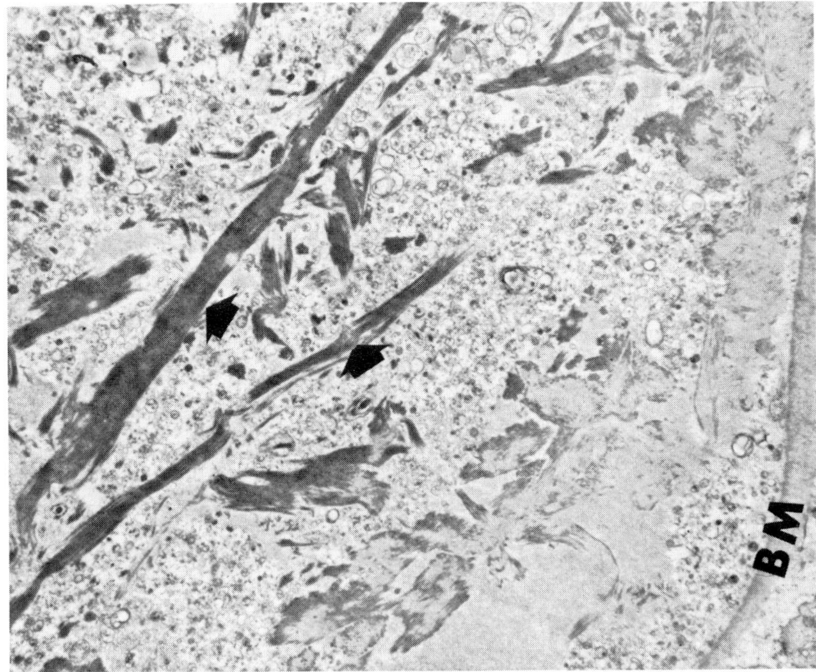

Fig. 2. Electron-micro-photograph of severe acute tubular necrosis. A 44-year-old housewife with metastatic adenocarcinoma of the breast was given aristolochic acid intravenously. She developed acute oliguria. A renal biopsy was taken on the 9th day. Severe acute tubular necrosis was found extending down to the tubular basement membrane (BM). Strands of fibrinoid material (F) were noted in the necrotic cellular debris. X2,100.

"acute tubular necrosis." Although electron microscopic studies of renal tissue obtained early in oliguria revealed normal or minimal tubular changes the term "acute tubular necrosis" will be used in relation to the wide spectrum of these tubular abnormalities. This spectrum of tubular changes extends from morphologically normal tubules by electron microscopy (Fig. 1) to severe tubular necrosis with dissolution of the tubular basement membrane (Fig. 2).

When acute oliguric renal failure owing to "acute tubular necrosis" is uncomplicated by high catabolic conditions such as infection or fever or by surgical trauma or associated injuries, the clinical course and natural history with its biochemical abnormalities and clinical complications are quite predictable. With proper treatment, the patient has an excellent chance of survival and recovery may be relatively complete.

STAGES OF ACUTE OLIGURIC RENAL FAILURE

The course of the illness may be short or long and the disorder mild or severe. In general, the clinical course of patients with acute oliguric renal failure follows similar basic stages regardless of difference in etiology or pathogenesis. The clinical course was divided by Bull, Joekes and Lowe (12) into five distinct stages. These stages were more precisely adapted for clinical use by Loughbridge *et al.* (13) and were related to patients with uncomplicated "acute tubular necrosis" (Fig. 3). The first is the onset

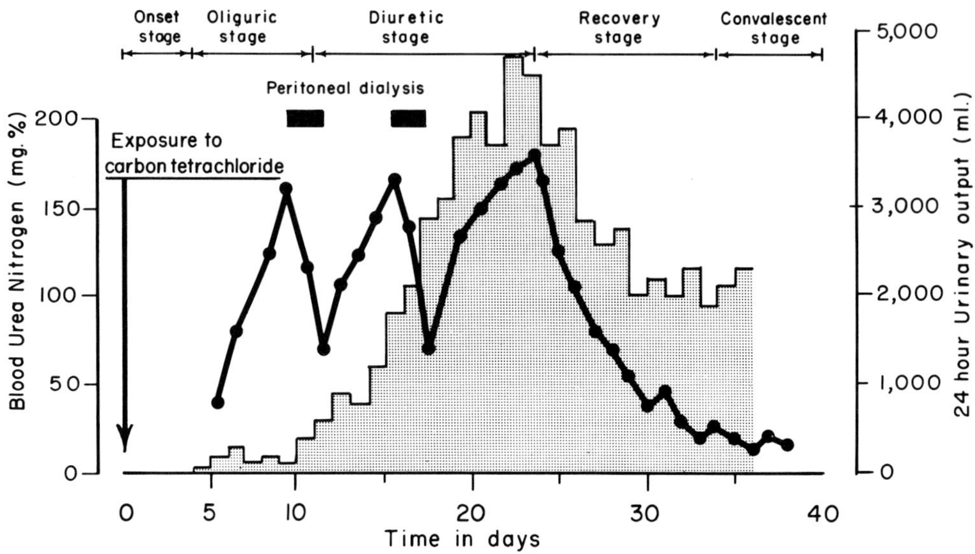

Fig. 3. Five stages of acute oliguric renal failure are illustrated in this clinical chart. The onset stage extends from the exposure to the precipitating factor to the occurrence of oliguria. The oliguric stage starts from the first day the 24-hour urinary output is below 400 ml to the onset of diuresis. The diuretic stage starts from the first day the urinary output increases over 400 ml to the point when the blood urea starts to fall. The recovery stage starts from the first day the blood urea nitrogen starts to fall until it returns to normal or is stabilized at a new level. The convalescent stage follows and ends when the patient returns to work.

stage followed by the oliguric-anuric stage. Following oliguria is the early diuretic stage. Then the late diuretic or recovery stage. During this phase, the recovery of renal function and tubular healing takes place. Finally, the convalescent stage in which the patient is rehabilitated and returned to productivity and usefulness as a member of society. Although the course of acute renal failure can often be forecast initially as related to the type of the precipitating disorder, in at least 25 to 30 per cent of the cases no exact diagnosis can be made.

ACUTE NON-OLIGURIC (HIGH OUTPUT) RENAL FAILURE

Although oliguria or anuria are the classical clinical features of most patients with acute renal failure, some patients with acute renal failure will have neither oliguria or anuria but will have a normal or a high urinary output. The frequency with which this occurs is not known as many patients with non-oliguria will go unrecognized. It is possible that acute non-oliguric renal failure occurs in a similar, if not a greater incidence, as does acute oliguric renal failure. Moreover, patients with acute non-oliguric renal failure often do well without dialysis and are not referred to renal dialysis centers should they be diagnosed by their physicians.

Acute renal failure without oliguria or anuria can result from the same numerous causes that produce oliguria. This type of acute renal failure was emphasized by Graber and Sevitt (9) in patients who develop a high urinary ouput associated with a rapid increasing blood urea nitrogen and an impaired creatinine clearance. In this condition, the kidneys have an inability to excrete a large urea load.

Acute non-oliguric renal failure can be induced by nephrotoxic drugs and chemicals, eclampsia, burns, shock and hemorrhage. Why the same nephrotoxic agent produces severe oliguria in one patient and massive urinary output in others is not known.

COMPLICATIONS

In general, the ability of the patient to recovery depends on the primary illness and associated complications. For example, in patients with uncomplicated acute renal failure due to medical or obstetrical causes the mortality is approximately 25 per cent. On the other hand, when acute renal failure is complicated by infection and trauma both surgical and accidental, the mortality was over 70 per cent.

The overall mortality of patients with acute oliguric renal failure reported by several renal dialysis centers varies from 34 per cent to 65 per cent. In an extensive analysis of 1,354 patients, the overall mortality was 42 per cent. (14) The mortality in the group aged above 51 years is approximately 58 per cent and similar in both sexes. The mortality below 50 years is approximately 31 per cent with twice as many men as women.

This sex difference in mortality rate is due to the large group of obstetrical patients who have a better prognosis. When they are excluded the sex ratio below 50 years is quite similar. From this analysis, the mortality of acute oliguric renal failure is greatly dependent upon the following factors: the nature and severity of the primary illness, the precipitating factors producing acute renal failure, the site and severity of the renal lesion, the clinical condition of the patient on arrival at a renal dialysis center and, finally, the effectiveness of the medical team in utilizing adequate facilities and knowledge in the management of the patient.

THE CAUSES OF DEATH

Death from acute renal failure affects men at the peak of their greatest economic benefit to their family and community. Women are usually affected at the height of child bearing or at the time of greatest need in "raising their faimly." Prior to our present knowledge and recognition of the ill effects of water and electrolyte abnormalities, the principal cause of death in patients with acute renal failure was pulmonary edema, uremia, acidosis and potassium intoxication.

The chief cause of death in patients with acute oliguric renal failure is equally divided between infections and the primary illness. Each are approximately one-third of all causes. Should infection produce acute oliguric renal failure then this infection is included as the primary illness. In patients with acute renal failure due to acute glomerulonephritis, the cause of death due to infection was similar to the group of patients with "acute tubular necrosis."

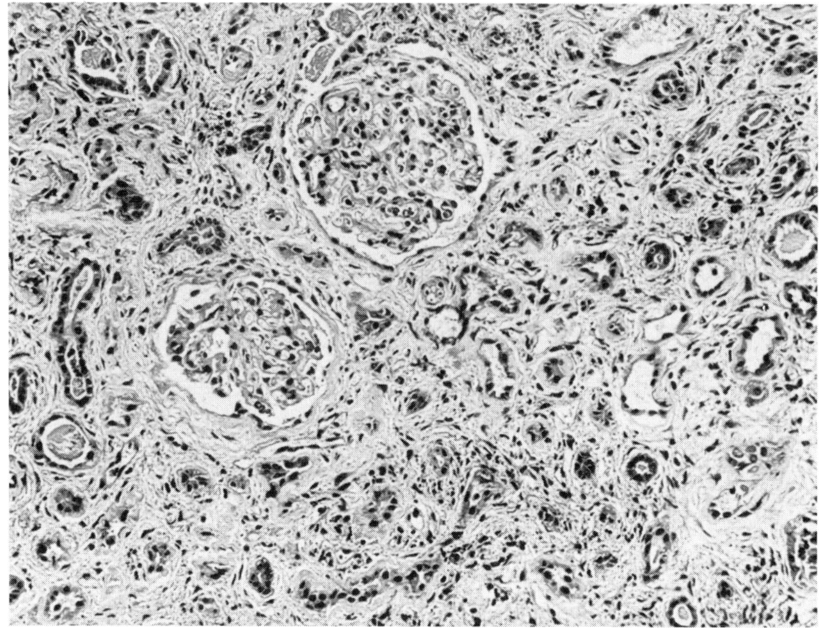

Fig. 4.   Diffuse interstitial fibrosis due to prolonged auria. A renal biopsy
was taken 5½ months after onset of severe and prolonged (37 days of)
anuria. Diffuse interstitial fibrosis is noted. The tubules have undergone
repair. There is thickening of the proximal and distal tubular basement
membrane. H & E X 175.

The biochemical abnormalities, mainly uremia and hyperkalemia, account for approximately 10 per cent each. Hemorrhage and administration of excessive fluids and excessive sodium chloride produces approximately 5 per cent of the deaths each. Digitalis toxicity, unexplained shock and unknown causes are equal at 3 per cent each.

OTHER COMPLICATIONS

The vast knowledge on the pathophysiology of acute renal failure has greatly lead to sound therapeutic principles. The application of this knowledge in the management of patients ill with acute renal failure has greatly reduced complications and morbidity due to uremia or due to abnormalities in fluid and electrolytes. However, extra-renal complications occur and constitute the largest percentage of the morbidity and mortality of patients with acute renal failure. These complications include: neurological, gastrointestinal, cardiovascular, hemorrhagic tendency, anemia and nutritional.

PERSISTENT PATHOPHYSIOLOGICAL ABNORMALITIES

Impairment in renal function and structure may persist following the patient's recovery from acute renal failure. Impairment in renal function may revert to normal in time or it may persist. In general, only a rare patient has progressed to chronic renal failure. (15) Structural abnormalities such as severe tubular necrosis may require as long as six to eight months before healing is complete by ultrastructural studies. Focal or diffuse interstitial fibrosis as a sequelae to acute renal failure is a common morphological finding. (Fig. 4)

URINE AND URINARY SEDIMENT

Urinalysis remains as much an art today as it did centuries ago when first introduced by the Persians. Physicians ritually use urinalysis as an aid in the diagnosis and the management of patients with renal disease. Clinicopathological correlations made of urinalysis with the vivid and dynamic morphology of renal biopsy is transforming the "art" of urinalysis into a "science." However, in acute oliguric renal failure, there is no specific abnormality to differentiate it from other renal disease. The findings in the urinary sediment do not reflect the extent of renal damage or the nature of the renal lesion. Moreover, urinalysis is of no value to the physician in making a prognosis during oliguria.

The gross appearance of the urine gives the physician a clue as to hematuria, hemoglobinuria, myoglobinuria and increased bilirubinuria. Gross hematuria occurs with renal infarction such as a renal artery occlusion and renal cortical necrosis (Table 1). Hematuria must be distinguished from hemoglobinuria. In states of intravascular hemolysis, free hemoglobin within the glomerular capillaries is excreted when the serum level of hemoglobin exceeds 135 mg per 100 ml. This excretory rate depends on the plasma haptoglobin level.

TABLE I–CAUSES OF HEMATURIA
IN THE PRESENCE OF ACUTE
OLIGURIC RENAL FAILURE

I. *Vascular Disease*
   a. Renal Artery Occlusion
   b. Renal infarction
   c. Acute Renal Cortical Necrosis
   d. Polyarteritis Nodosa
   e. Hypersensitivity Angiitis
   f. Necrotizing Vasculitis
   g. Scleroderma
   h. Malignant Nephrosclerosis
   i. Renal Vein Thrombosis

II. *Tubular Disease*
   a. Acute Tubular Necrosis

III. *Glomerular Disease*
   a. Acute Post-streptococcal Glomerulonephritis
   b. Hypersensitivity Glomerulonephritis
   c. Lupus Glomerulonephritis
   d. Thrombotic Thrombocytopenic Purpura
   e. Hemolytic Uremic Syndrome

IV. *Interstitial Disease*
   a. Hypersensitivity Interstitial Nephritis
   b. Granulomatous Interstitial Nephritis
   c. Lymphomatous Interstitial Nephritis
   d. Acute Bacterial Pyelonephritis
   e. Leptospirosis Interstitial Nephritis

V. *Pelvic Ureteral Disease*
   a. Ureteral Calculi
   b. Ureteral Tumor
   c. Crystallization (Uric Acid or Sulfonamides)

RENAL BIOPSY

Percutaneous renal biopsy is a valuable clinical adjunct to the physician in the management of patients with acute oliguric renal failure. It is a relatively safe and painless procedure. Renal biopsy should be done after all other clinical and laboratory investigations fail to differentiate or clarify the underlying renal disorder. Renal biopsy will provide morphological information on which the physician can base his managment and prognosis.

Caution should be taken not to obtain a biopsy from patients who received heparin while undergoing hemodialysis, in patients with thrombocytopenia, those in a clinical state of uremia or in patients about to die. To insure the safety of the patient clotting and bleeding times, prothrombin time and platelet counts should be done. The

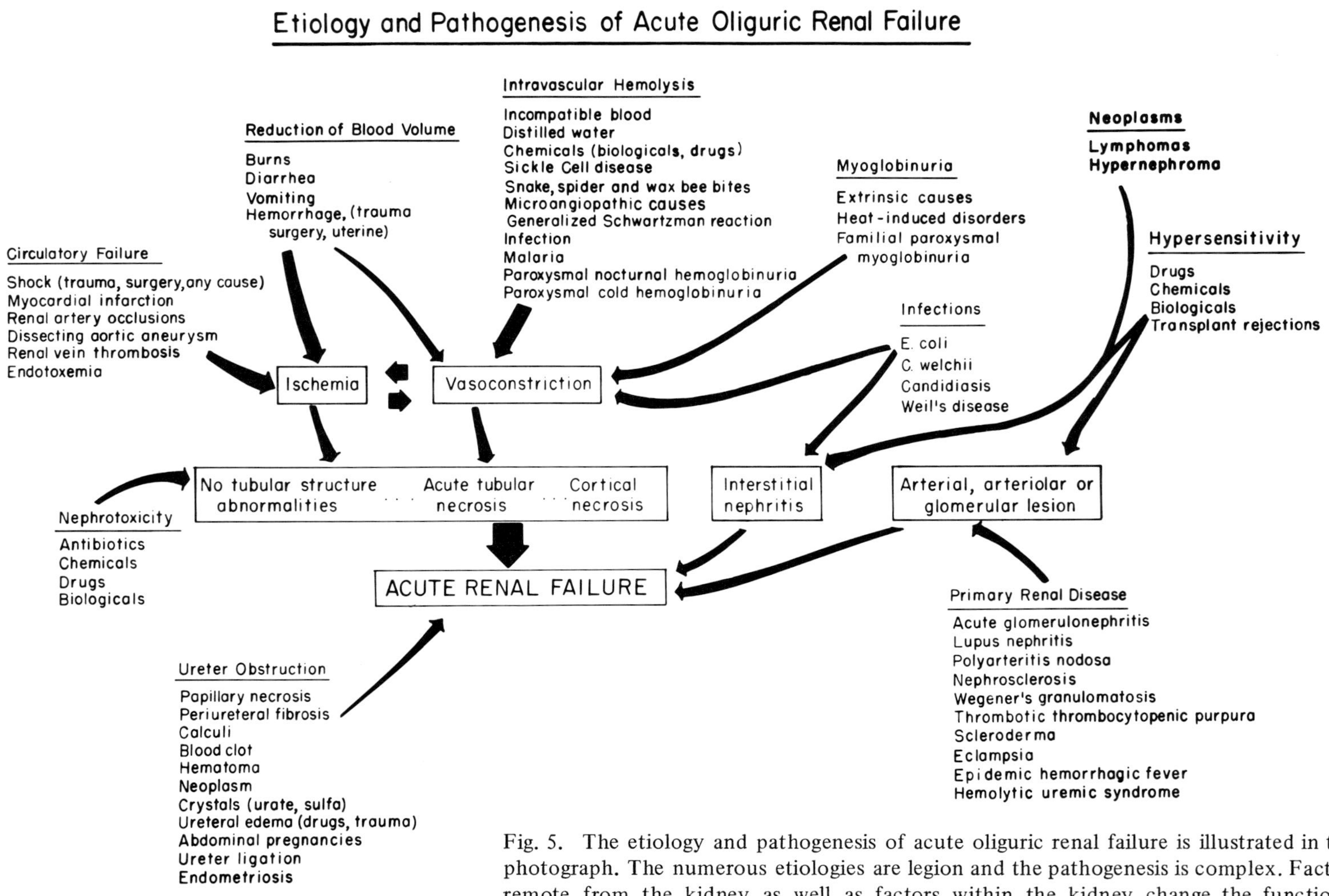

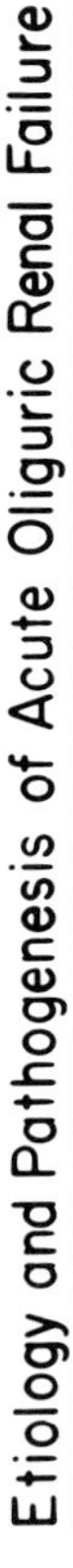

Fig. 5. The etiology and pathogenesis of acute oliguric renal failure is illustrated in this photograph. The numerous etiologies are legion and the pathogenesis is complex. Factors remote from the kidney as well as factors within the kidney change the functional environment and may damage the parenchymal. (Permission of C. B. Mosby and Company, from Acute Renal Failure: Diagnosis and Management, By Robert C. Muehrcke.)

author has found it necessary to improve the clinical fitness of the patient by dialysis before doing a renal biopsy. The renal biopsy is done either the same day dialysis is completed or the very next day.

The patient with acute oliguric renal failure is a poor risk. It must also be stressed that there is a much greater risk in doing a renal biopsy in patients with severely elevated blood pressure than in a normotensive individual. When severely elevated blood pressure was present, the author has either reduced the blood pressure prior to taking the renal biopsy or has taken an "open biopsy."

THE ETILOGY AND PATHOGENESIS OF "ACUTE TUBULAR NECROSIS"

Acute renal failure results from numerous etiological conditions. Their frequency varies from one country to another as well as in different age groups. Precipitating factors are legion and include shock, endotoxins, ischemia, infection, hemolytic crisis, nephrotoxins, acute hypersensitivity reactions, intrinsic renal disease, renal vascular damage and numerous other causes (Fig. 5).

Insults to the body far remote from the kidney may reduce the renal blood flow to such low levels that little or no urine is formed. These etiological factors disturb renal function, damage the kidney and result in acute renal failure. In view of the etiological uncertainties for acute renal failure, a number of terms were offered to describe this condition. They include traumatic edema, traumatic anuria, (7) post-traumatic anuria, hemoglobinuric nephrosis, (16) anoxic nephrosis, ischemic nephrosis, crush syndrome, (17) compression syndrome,

(8) lower nephron nephrosis, (18) traumatic shock, (19) shock kidney and acute tubular necrosis. (12)

In approximately 30 per cent of all patients, the etiology for acute oliguria is unknown. In other patients, the etiology is specific and, in some, the etiology is multiple. Therefore, not only single mechanisms but combinations of mechanisms may explain the pathophysiology of "acute renal failure."

Excluding primary parenchymal disease of the glomeruli, interstitium, arteries and arterioles the pathogenesis of acute renal failure can be discussed from two major aspects. These were emphasized by Oliver (20) as ischemia and nephrotoxicity. Oliver studied the morphological lesions produced by these two salient groups and found that in "severely damaged kidneys" not all nephrons were affected and in some kidneys "only occasional ones." He interpreted this finding as the effect of patchy renal vasoconstriction and ischemia. In addition, Oliver found that ischemia (tubulorrhexis) produced complete disruption of the tubular epithelium with basement membrane fragmentation. With nephrotoxins, he found tubular necrosis without basement membrane changes (nephrotoxic). Oliver believed this finding was a major factor in the pathogenesis of acute renal failure.

ISCHEMIA

Renal ischemia due to reduction of the renal blood flow is the most common factor responsible for acute renal failure. It is present when acute tubular necrosis occurs in association with severe circulatory failure. The concept of renal ischemia has been accepted without critical review and was first made by Foy in 1943. (21) The exact pathogenesis involving renal ischemia is a complex mechanism and is confused by experimental data. If ischemia was the sole factor in producing "acute tubular necrosis," one would expect to find distal tubular necrosis as frequently as proximal necrosis. This is not the case.

There are few observations available on renal circulation during acute renal failure. The renal blood flow using radioactive Krypton (22) has been reported as normal in dogs with oliguria. Other investigators using a flowmeter in the renal vein and taking direct measurements found a decrease in renal blood flow with acute renal failure. To measure renal blood flow Bull and colleagues (12) used the direct Fick principle and PAH for determination. They found renal blood flow during oliguria reduced in two patients to 3 and 5 per cent of normal. They did not take into consideration that low A-V differences of PAH made this particular technique inaccurate. Moreover, their observations not only lack controls but no comparison was made to healthy individuals. This data is scanty and if available may shed light on this problem. The prolonged reduction in effective circulating blood volume with prolonged vasoconstriction is sufficient to result in renal ischemia. When ischemia is intense, prolonged renal damage usually occurs. This damage can vary from mild tubular abnormalities to diffuse complete renal cortical necrosis. Brun and Munk (22, 23) studied patients with acute renal failure during oliguria due to acute tubular necrosis. They found that renal blood flow frequently exceeded the levels considered necessary to produce irreversible tubular lesions. Although ischemia is necessary in initiating the sequence, it is not the only factor causing tubular necrosis.

NEPHROTOXINS

The kidney has several characteristics in its structure and function that makes it vulnerable to nephrotoxins such as chemicals, drugs and biological products. These characteristics are explained as follows. The kidneys comprise 0.4 per cent of the body in weight and they have a high oxygen consumption. The kidneys receive approximately 20 to 25 per cent of the cardiac output. The kidneys have the largest surface area of endothelial cells in comparison to any other organ. In addition, the kidneys are second to the liver in the most complex metabolism of any organ. They have an extremely vascular renal medulla with its reta mirabile that functions in a counter current multiplier system. This complex mechanism results in hypertonicity of the renal interstitium with concentration of nephrotoxic chemicals and drugs.

Nephrotoxic chemicals have exerted their adverse effects on the kidney through one or a combination of pathopharmacological mechanisms. One example of such a mechanism is the direct nephrotoxicity that results from the direct effect on the tubular epithelial cells which concentrates the protoplasmic poison. Secondly, is the progressive concentration of the filtered nephrotoxic agent within the lumen of the nephron. Some nephrotoxins penetrate the cell and interact with cellular constituents to poison the cell. For example, a nephrotoxin such as mercuhydrin interacts with enzyme systems both within the glycolytic cycle and Krebs cycle. The resulting structural change can vary from no apparent morphological abnormalities through the range of tubular necrosis to diffuse renal cortical necrosis.

Drug-induced Acute Oliguric Renal Failure

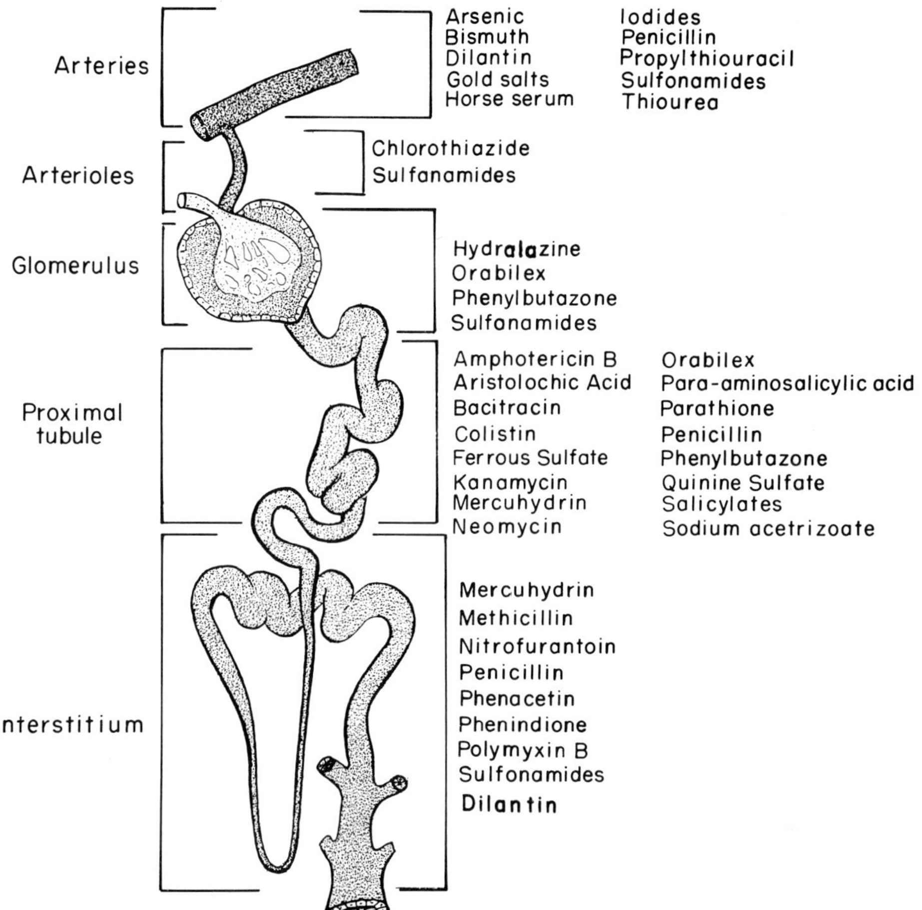

Fig. 6. The morphological site involved by drugs that induce acute oliguric renal failure. The arteries, glomeruli and interstitium are involved with hypersensitivity reactions. The tubules are sites of nephrotoxic reactions. (Permission of C. B. Mosby and Company, from Acute Renal Failure: Diagnosis and Management, by Robert C. Muehrcke.)

Other nephrotoxins such as sulfonamides produce their adverse patho-pharmacological effects through a hypersensitivity reaction. The morphological site is usually the large endothelial surface of the glomerular capillaries, arterioles and arteries. Last but not least, the forgotten renal interstitium is a frequently involved site of hypersensitivity reactions (Fig. 6) (Table II).

TABLE II–ACUTE OLIGURIC RENAL FAILURE DUE TO DRUG-INDUCED ACUTE INTERSTITIAL NEPHRITIS

1. Dilantin
2. Mercuhydrin
3. Methicillin
4. Nitrofurantoin
5. Penicillin
6. Phenacetin
7. Phenindione
8. Polymyxin B
9. Sulfonamide

PATHOLOGY OF ACUTE OLIGURIC RENAL FAILURE

Fifteen years ago, much of the morphological knowledge associated with acute renal failure was based on innumerable case reports describing the classical morbid anatomy. Since 1952, freshly harvested tissue obtained by serial renal biopsy has provided a dynamic and vivid cinematographic image of the exact structural lesions of acute renal failure. In addition, serial electron microscopic studies have further clarified this dynamic morphology. The complex clinical, biochemical, and renal functional abnormalities of acute renal failure can be attributed to a wide range of renal structural findings.

Numerous morphological findings must be considered. They vary from apparently normal and mild findings to severe and progressive irreversible damage. In addition, these findings involve all four anatomical segments of the kidney; the interstitium, the tubules, the glomeruli, and the vasculature. In the past, emphasis was placed on each of these segments either singularly or in combination as to the specific site producing acute renal failure. It is very likely that many of these morphological changes are of an accessory nature that accompanies acute renal failure but do not produce the syndrome.

"ACUTE TUBULAR NECROSIS"

Morphological findings of tubular necrosis were first described in 1917 by Hackradt (10) and later by Minami. (5) Although tubular necrosis was not commonly recognized it was in 1942 that the lesion was fully established by Bywaters. (6, 7, 8) He described the lesion in patients with "traumatic anuria" as an involvement of the distal convoluted tubules and the ascending limb of Henle's loop. Bywaters emphasized the intense catarrh of the proximal tubular epithelium. He observed that the most severe damage occurred primarily in small areas of Henle's loop and secondary in convoluted tubules. He also emphasized the findings of metaplasia in the parietal epithelial cells of Bowman's capsule with cuboidal cell formation adjacent to the tubular entrance. In addition, Bywaters associated interstitial cellular infiltrates and interstitial fibrosis with tubule repair. These observations received support by renal biopsy studies in the author's laboratory.

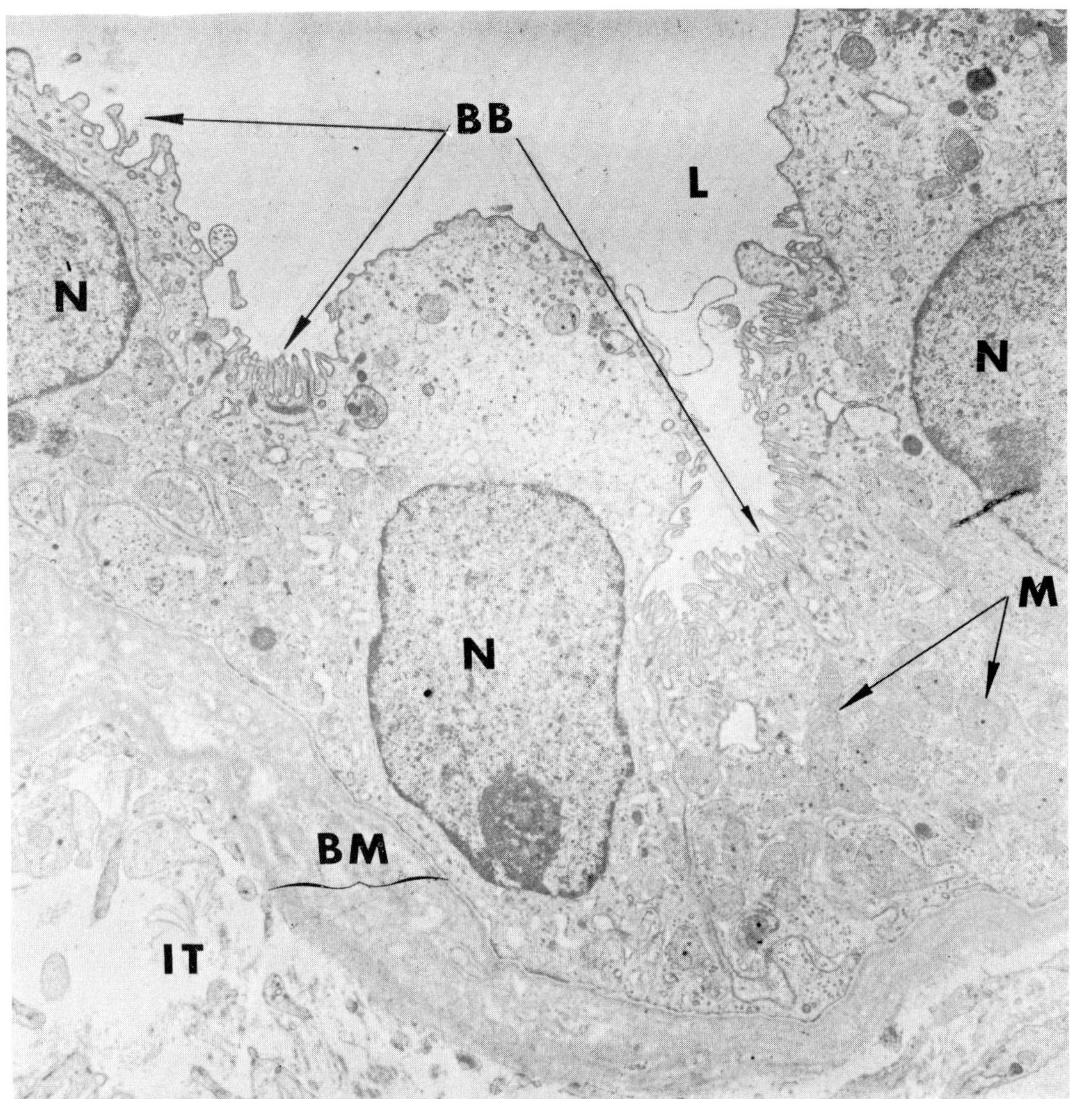

Fig. 7. Tubular regeneration following tubular necrosis: A proximal tubular epithelial cell is seen approximately 6 months after prolonged anuria induced by arsine. The brush border (BB) is low, sparse and protrude into the tubular lumen (L). The necleus (N) is large and occupies much of the cell. The mitochrondria (M) appear normal The tubular basement membrane (BM) is markedly thickened. The interstitial tissue (IT) is edematous and contains collagen bundles. (X 7,728)

HISTOLOGIC EVOLUTION OF REPAIR IN "ACUTE TUBULAR NECROSIS"

Primary electron microscopic abnormalities are not seen to the same degree in all tubules. (24) The degree of tubular abnormalities depends on the severity of the initial insult. In such studies, one must also consider the time relationship after onset of acute renal failure to the time morphological study was made. However, the author has observed some tubules completely damaged and tubules in an adjacent nephron spared. Uncomplicated tubular necrosis undergoes a rapid repair and tubular lesions of mild necrosis may heal within days after the initial insult. This may explain why necrotic lesions are not found if a renal biopsy is taken too late in the course of acute renal failure.

Serial renal biopsy study using the elctron microscope revealed that tubular necrosis and tubular regeneration are extensive. In some patients, it may be impossible to differentiate specific tubules as proximal, distal or collecting.

In severe "acute tubular necrosis," only remanents of the basement membrane may be seen in the epithelial cell debris (Fig. 2). When tubular necrosis is less severe cortical tubules can be identified. The proximal tubules may lose much of their brush border. In repair, the epithelial cells have a simplified structure and mitosis is frequently seen. The epithelial cells are low, cuboidal and contain an enlarged round to oval shaped nucleus. The mitochondria appear increased in numbers and have prominent cristae. Many months are required for epithelial cells of the cortical tubules to heal significantly for a possible differentiation of cell type (Fig. 7). The histological evolution of acute tubular necrosis is diagrammed in Figure 8.

ACUTE BILATERAL RENAL CORTICAL NECROSIS

In 1896, Juhel-Renoy (25) first described bilateral renal cortical necrosis at autopsy of a 16-year-old girl. She developed anuria on the ninth day after

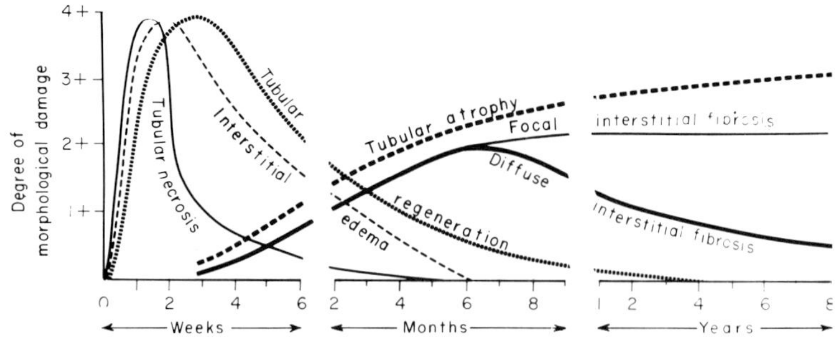

Fig. 8. Histological evolution of acute tubular necrosis. Acute tubular necrosis is rapidly followed by tubular repair. Tubular regeneration occurs over months. Interstitial edema accompanies tubular damage. Should oliguria be prolonged interstitial fibrosis occurs. Diffuse interstitial fibrosis may persist and in time lead to a focal interstitial fibrosis. (Permission of C. B. Mosby and Company, from Acute Renal Failure: Diagnosis and Management, by Robert C. Muehrcke.)

developing scarlet fever and died on the fifteenth day. Ten years later, Bradford and Lawrence (26) described renal cortical ncerosis associated with pregrancy. Since then numerous monograms have been written on this subject. The most well known discussion is that by Sheehan and Moore (27) and that by Duff and Murray. (28)

In general, bilateral renal cortical necrosis involves both kidneys in relatively the same severity. It is a fulminant ischemic necrosis of the cortex involving glomeruli and tubules. On a single occasion, the disease afflicted only one kidney. The opposite kidney had renal artery stenosis. Renal cortical necrosis can be suspected clinically but the diagnosis can only be made by renal biopsy study or by post mortem examination.

GLOMERULAR DISEASE

In the past, acute oliguric renal failure as a result of glomerular abnormalities was considered rare. More recently, acute oliguric renal failure has resulted from a number of diseases involving the glomeruli. These include acute post-streptococcal glomerulonephritis, lupus glomerulonephritis, glomerulonephritis due to polyarteritis nodosa, drug-induced hypersensitivity glomeruloncphritis and necrotizing glomerulonephritis due to Wegener's granulomatosis. In addition, thrombotic thrombocytopenic purpura has produced acute renal failure due to glomerular lesions.

The prominent clinical features of glomerular disease are hematuria and a rapidly decreasing urinary output ending in absolute anuria. There may be some degree of periorbital edema and hypertension. The urine is grossly bloodly and contains erythrocyte casts and large quantities of proteinuria. Unlike the fixed urinary specific gravity of "acute tubular necrosis," the urinary specific gravity is usually high, e.g., 1,025. In "acute tubular necrosis," the urinary sodium is above 30 mEq per L while in acute glomerulonephritis the urinary sodium concentration during oliguria is usually below 30 mEq per L. Life should be sustained using repeated dialysis until a morphological evaluation of the kidney is made. This provides a precise histological diagnosis on which the physician can base his treatment and prognosis. In some patients with acute oliguric renal failure due to glomerular disease, the use of adrenocortical steroids may be beneficial in resolving the glomerular abnormalities, otherwise the prognosis is usually very poor and recovery is nil.

ACUTE INTERSITIAL NEPHRITIS

The earliest description of interstitial involvement was reported by Biermer (29) in 1860. He studied a patient with absolute anuria of ten days duration. At autopsy, he found acute interstitial nephritis. Subsequently, Councilman (2) in 1898, and forty years later, Kimmelstiel (3) related acute hematogenous interstitial nephritis to acute renal failure.

The first outstanding morphological study of acute interstitial nephritis was that of Councilman. (2) He described the disease as an acute inflammation of the kidney characterized by interstitial cellular infiltrates and interstitial edema. In the majority of his patients, lymphocytes, eosinophils, plasma cells and histocytes infiltrated the interstitium.

Kimmelstiel (3) observed acute hematogenous interstitial nephritis in association with hemolytic reactions following blood transfusions and in the hepatorenal syndrome. Kimmelstiel described the renal morphology in patients with anuria as a "cellular infiltration, interstitial edema, hematin casts within the tubular lumen, tubular dilatation and epithelial cell regeneration." He pointed out that these changes could be present simultaneously or any one of these processes could be absent. He differentiated acute hematogenous interstitial nephritis from the lymphogenic ascending type of interstitial nephritis. Kimmelstiel regarded it as an allergic hyperergic response to either foreign proteins or protein breakdown products. Moreover, they pointed out that the renal intersititium was an area where hypersensitivity reactions can occur. Time has proved his postulate.

Neither Councilman or Kimmelstiel attributed acute interstitial nephritis to a direct bacterial invasion of the interstitium. They based this on finding a diffuse lesion and not a focal interstitial lesion. However, Munk (23) believed that the interstitial lesion was not a primary kidney disease but a general cellular exudation caused by bacterial or viral infection of the interstitium such as complicating streptococcal infections or smallpox.

SUMMARY

Acute oliguric renal failure is an omnibus clinical syndrome resulting in acute clinical and biochemical manifestations. This syndrome is precipitated from innumerable causes steming from renal artery involvement, the renal veins, glomeruli, interstitium, renal tubules and from obstructive uropathy. Its etiology is legion and its pathogenesis is complex. Through serial clinicopathological studies of patients with acute renal failure, the histological evaluation of renal abnormalities continues to clarify the syndrome.

REFERENCES

1. Cumin, W.: Cases of severe burns with dissection and remarks. *Edinburgh M & S J., 19*:337, 1823.
2. Councilman, W. T.: Acute interstitial nephritis. *J. Exp. Med., 3*:393, 1898.
3. Kimmelstiel, P.: Acute hematogenous interstitial nephritis. *Am. J. Path., 14*:737, 1938.
4. Colmers, Dr.: Ueber die durch das Erdbeden in Messina am verursachten Verletzungen. *Arch f. klin. Chir., XC*:701, 1909.
5. Minami, S.: Über Nierenveränderungen Nach Verschüttung. *Virchows Arch. Path. Anat., 245*:247, 1923.
6. Bywaters, E. G. L., and Beall, D.: Crush injuries with impairment of renal function. *Brit. Med. J., 1*:427, 1941.
7. Bywaters, E. G. L., and Dible, J. H.: The renal lesion in traumatic anuria. *J. Path. Bact., 54*:110, 1942.
8. Bywaters, E. G. L.: Ischemic necrosis crushing injury, traumatic edema, the crush syndrome, traumatic anuria, compression syndrome: A type of injury seen in air raid casualities following burial beneath debris. *J.A.M.A., 124*:1103, 1944.
9. Graber, I. G., and Sevitt, S.: Renal function in burned patients and its relationship to morphological changes. *J. Clin. Path., 12*:25, 1959.
10. Hackradt, A.: Über Acute Tödliche Vasomotorische Nephrosen Nach Verschüttung (Munchen). Worishofen, Wagner, 1917.
11. Jeghers, H., and Bakst, H. J.: The syndrome of extrarenal azotemia. *Ann. Int. Med., 11*:1861, 1938.
12. Bull, G. M., Joekes, A. M., and Lowe, K. G.: Renal function studies in acute tubular necrosis. *Clin. Sc., 9*:379, 1950.
13. Loughbridge, L. W., Milne, M. D., Shackman, R., and Wootton, I.D.P.: Clinical Course of Uncomplicated Acute Tubular Necrosis. *Lancet, 1*:351, 1960.
14. Lunding, M., Steiness, I., and Thaysen, J. H.: Acute renal failure due to tubular necrosis: Immediate prognosis and complication. *Acta. Med. Scand., 176*:103, 1964.
15. Muehrcke, R. C., Rosen, S., Pirani, C. L., and Kark, R. M.: Renal lesions in patients recovering from acute renal failure. *J. Lab. Clin. Med., 64*:888, 1964.
16. Mallory, T. B.: Hemoglobinuric nephrosis in traumatic shock. *Am. J. Clin. Path., 17*:427, 1947.

17. Dunn, J. S., Gillespie, M., and Niven, J. S. F.: Renal lesions in two cases of crush syndrome. *Lancet, 2*:549, 1941.

18. Lucke, B.: Lower nephron nephrosis. The renal lesions of the crush syndrome of burns, transfusions and other conditions affecting the lower segments of the nephrons. *Military Surgeon, 99*:371, 1946.

19. Husfeldt, E., and Bjering, T.: Renal lesions from traumatic shock. *Acta. Med. Scand., 91*:279, 1937.

20. Oliver, J., MacDowell, M., and Tracy, A.: The pathogenesis of acute renal failure associated with traumatic and toxic injury. Renal ischemia, nephrotoxic damage and the ischemic episode. *J. Clin. Invest., 30*:1307, 1951.

21. Foy, H., Altmann, A., Barnes, H. D., and Kondi, A.: Anuria with special reference to renal failure in blackwater fever, incompatible transfusions and crush injuries. *Trans. Roy. Soc. Trop. Med., and Hyg., 36*:197, 1943.

22. Brun, C., Crone, C., Davidsen, H. G., Fabricius, J., Tybjaerg Hansen, A., Lassen, N. A., and Munck, O.: Renal blood flow in anuric human subject determined by use of radioactive Krypton 85. *Proc. Soc., Exper. Biol. & Med., 89*:687, 1955.

23. Munk., O.: *Renal Correlations in Acute Renal Failure.* Oxford, Blackwell Scientific Publications, 1958.

24. Dalgaard, O. Z., and Pedersen, K. J.: Renal tubular degeneration: Electron microscopy in ischemic anuria. *Lancet, 2*:484, 1959.

25. Juhel-Renoy, E.: De l'anuric Precoce Scarlatinense. *Arch. Gen. Med., 17*:385, 1886.

26. Bradford, J. R., and Lawrence, T. W. P.: Endoarteritis of the renal arteries causing necrosis of the entire cortex of both kidneys. *J. Path. & Bact., 5*:195, 1898.

27. Sheehan, H. L., and Moore, H. C.: *Renal Cortical Necrosis and the Kidney of Concealed Accidental Hemorrhage.* American Lecture Series. Springfield, Thomas, 1953.

28. Duff, G. L., and Murray, E. G. D.: Bilateral cortical necrosis of the kidneys. *Am. J. Med. Sc., 201*:428, 1941.

29. Biermer, quoted in Councilman, W. T.: Acute interstitial nephritis. *J. Exp. Med., 3*:393, 1898.

Chapter 38

Laboratory Tests as a Guide to Therapy by Acute Dialysis

FRANCESCO del GRECO, M.D., and NORMAN M. SIMON, M.D.

The role of the laboratory in acute dialysis may be best appreciated by a brief outline of the clinical problems of acute renal failure and acute drug intoxication for which therapy by dialysis may be indicated. In acute renal failure, the clinician must initially determine whether the condition is due to remediable or irremediable causes (9, 12). Remediable causes imply prerenal and postrenal mechanisms which are amenable to correction by simple medical or surgical intervention, and in which the structural integrity of the kidney is preserved. Irremediable causes include a host of disorders causing structural renal changes which are not directly amenable to therapy. Briefly, prerenal mechanisms which may lead to acute renal failure include hypotension and shock of diverse etiology, fluid and electrolyte depletion, congestive heart failure, and renal arterial obstruction. Postrenal mechanisms are included under the category of urinary tract obstruction secondary to stricture, stone, clot, tumors and prostatic hypertrophy. Next, if the renal failure is due to intrinsic renal damage rather than to prerenal or postrenal mechanisms, an attempt must be made to determine nature, pathogenesis, and extent of renal injury so that appropriate management may be planned. In cases of acute drug poisoning the clinician should make every effort to identify the drug and dosage. If the patient is critically ill when first seen, therapy by dialysis may assume priority over detailed diagnostic studies.

The purpose of the chapter is to consider the role of the laboratory in acute renal failure and acute drug poisoning. Our experience is based on observations in 160 consecutive patients with acute renal failure and 70 patients with acute barbiturate poisoning.

ROLE OF THE LABORATORY

The laboratory offers an array of procedures that may be useful in guiding dialysis therapy. A perusal of the procedures listed in Table 1 will give an idea of the diversity of tests currently available. It should be emphasized at this point that a fundamental premise to the correct interpretation of laboratory data, is a careful history and thorough physical examination. Essential initial laboratory studies include urinalysis, blood count, urea nitrogen and sugar, plasma creatinine, bicarbonate, sodium and potassium, urine and blood culture, chest x-ray, and electrocardiogram. If

TABLE I—LABORATORY PROCEDURES
THAT MAY BE USEFUL IN ACUTE RENAL FAILURE AND ACUTE DIALYSIS

1. Urinalysis:
   specific gravity, protein, sugar, ketones,
   sediment (cells, casts, crystals, bacteria)

2. Hematologic Studies:
   a. CBC, reticulocyte count, platelet count
   b. Coagulation tests
   c. G-6-P-D assay

3. Blood and Urine Chemistries:
   a. Blood urea nitrogen and creatinine, and osmolality ratio
   b. Urine sodium concentration
   c. Serum Na, K, CO_2, pH, Ca, P, amylase, FBS

4. Blood and Urine Electrophoresis: protein, hemoglobin, myoglobin

5. Serologic Studies:
   a. Serologic test for syphilis
   b. LE cells, anti-nuclear antibodies
   c. Anti-streptococcal antibodies
   d. RBC antibodies
   e. Serum conplement

6. Toxicologic Analysis of Blood & Urine

7. Bacteriology:
   throat, blood, skin, urine, and stool cultures

8. X-ray and Isotope Studies:
   a. Chest film
   b. KUB
   c. IVP, drip infusion nephrotomography
   d. Aortography
   e. Venography
   f. Cystography and retrograde pyelography
   g. Isotope
   h. Renal scan

9. Electrocardiogram:
   contour (infarction, pericarditis, electrolyte disturbance) and arrhythmia

10. Bladder and Ureteral Catheterization

11. Tissue Biopsy—Kidney, Skin, Muscle, Lung:
    a. Light microscopy
    b. Immunofluorescent studies
    c. Electron microscopy

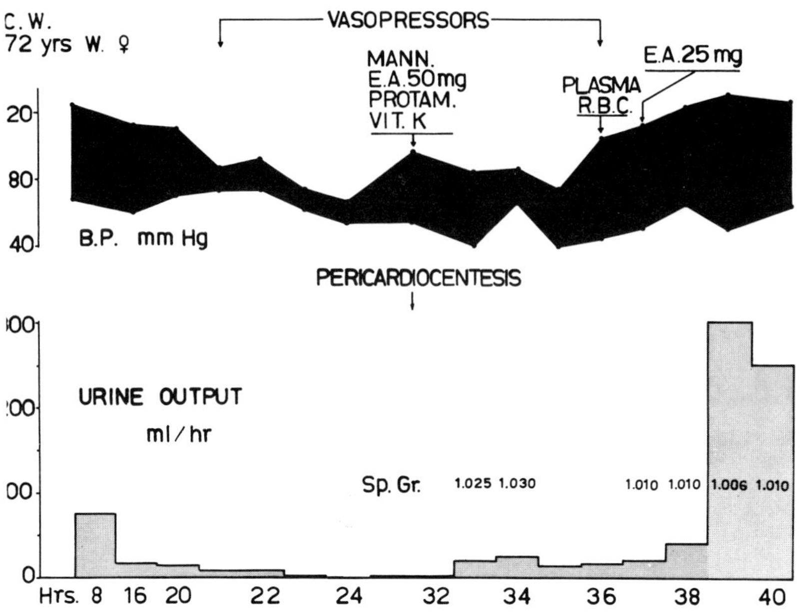

Fig. 1. Blood pressure and urine output in a patient with pericardial tamponade (Case 1).

acute drug intoxication is suspected, appropriate samples of blood, gastric content and urine should be obtained as soon as possible. On the basis of the clinical findings and initial laboratory results, it is usually possible to formulate judgement as to whether the patient can be managed by conservative means alone, or whether dialysis should be undertaken without delay.

Pertinent points relating to the role of the laboratory in acute renal failure and acute poisoning are delineated by clinical examples described below.

1. Value of Laboratory in Determining Underlying Pathophysiology

The abrupt onset of oliguria is always a dramatic event which should lead to the immediate application of appropriate tests. Among these, urinalysis, urine specific gravity and urine and plasma osmolality (7, 16) are of the utmost

value. This point is illustrated by the following case:

Case 1. A 72-year-old female entered the hospital with a history of recurrent thrombophlebitis and clinical features suggestive of pulmonary embolization. She was treated with combined heparin-coumarin anticoagulant therapy for 2 weeks and was progressing satisfactorily until she went into shock from pericardial tamponade. A progressive fall in urine output was noted as tamponade developed until the patient became markedly oliguric (Fig. 1). There was a slight increase in urine output as the patient was vigorously treated with vasopressor infusions, intravenous mannitol, ethacrynic acid, 50 mg, protamine, vitamin K and pericardiocentesis. Urine specific gravity at this time ranged from 1.025 to 1.030. Cautious volume expansion with plasma and packed red cells was then carried out with stabilization of the circulation and restoration of normal blood pressure, following which a repeat infusion of ethacrynic acid in smaller dosage, 25 mg, resulted in prompt, marked and sustained diuresis.

Comment: The high specific gravity of the urine at a time when the patient was markedly oliguric, indicated preservation of tubular concentrating ability and suggested that the renal failure was caused by a prerenal mechanism (i.e., hypovolemia and shock) rather than by intrinsic renal damage. Accordingly, administration of fluids was carried out to restore blood volume and normal blood pressure.

The value of simultaneous measurement of urine and plasma osmolality in the early stage of acute renal failure has been recently documented (7). In this study, the urine to plasma osmolality ratio was 1.0 in acute tubular necrosis, but in excess of 1.3 in prerenal failure. Another laboratory procedure of value in acute oliguric renal failure is the determination of urinary sodium. If a prerenal or postrenal mechanism has precipitated renal failure, the concentration of urinary sodium will be very low, usually less than 20 mEq per liter. In contrast, if tubular necrosis is the underlying mechanism, urinary sodium concentration usually will exceed 30 mEq per liter (17). Measurement of urea excretion in acute renal failure is of limited clinical value (3).

2. Value of Laboratory in Establishing Diagnosis

Acute renal failure may be caused by a wide range of disorders which can be diagnosed by judicious use of laboratory procedures and critical review of clinical findings. Cases 2, 3 and 4 illustrate this point clearly.

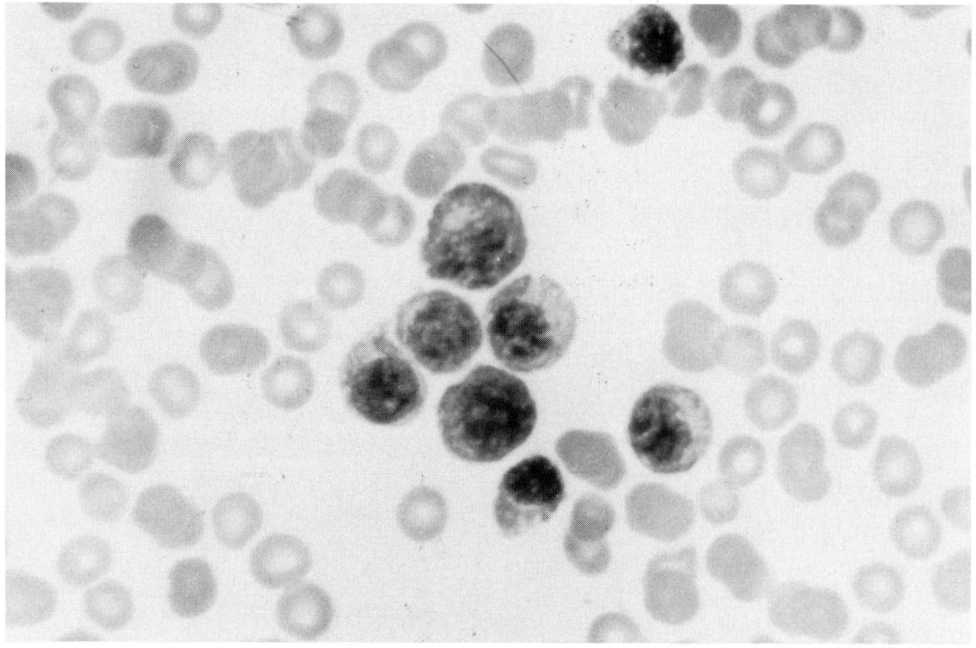

Fig. 2.   Peripheral blood smear in a patient with plasma cell myeloma and acute renal failure (Case 2).

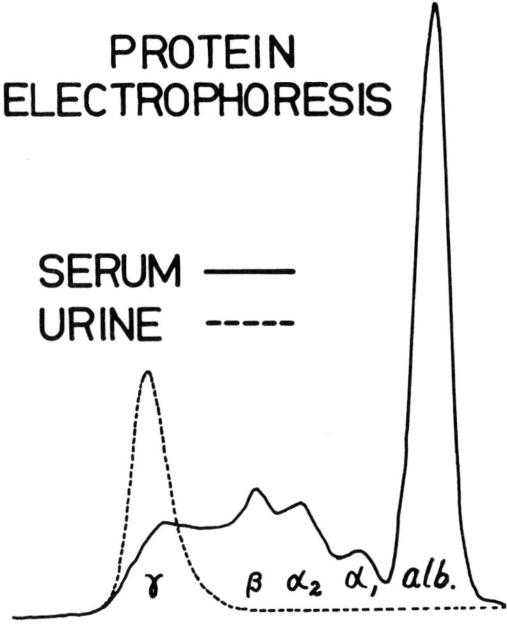

Fig. 3. Serum and urine electrophoretic patterns in a patient with plasma cell myeloma and acute renal failure (Case 2).

Case 2. A 41-year-old white male was admitted with rapidly progressive renal failure, and a history of low back pain for nearly 6 months. Recent work-up at another hospital including intravenous and retrograde pyelograms, and renal arteriography failed to establish a diagnosis. A rapid increase in blood urea nitrogen from 50 to 123 mg per 100 ml was noted. On admission, diagnosis of plasma cell myeloma and leukemia was suggested by the hemogram, which revealed a white blood cell count of 43,100 with 40% plasma cells and rouleaux formation (Fig. 2)

The diagnosis was confirmed by demonstration of Bence-Jones protein in the urine and of plasma cells of varying maturity in the bone marrow. The serum and urine electrophoretic patterns, shown in Figure 3, revealed the abnormal protein to be present in the urine but not in the blood.

Comment: In this case, routine blood smear and blood count on admission pointed toward the diagnosis which was supported by appropriate chemical and hematological studies.

Case 3. A 21-year-old Negro male was admitted to the hospital with nausea and abdominal pain after a drinking binge and was found to be markedly oliguric. Bleeding from the gums and melena were also noted. Massive intravascular hemolysis with hemoglobinemia was present. Striking abnormalities (Fig. 4) were found in the peripheral blood smear, indicating red cell fragmentation and thrombocytopenia. Additional hematological studies, including bone marrow examination and investigation of clotting mechanism were then performed and diagnosis of thrombotic thrombocytopenic purpura was made. Treatment with urokinase, heparin, and corticosteroids was instituted. With the aid of hemodialysis, the patient made a remarkable recovery.

Comment: In this case, careful examination of the blood smear obtained on admission revealed unusual morpho-

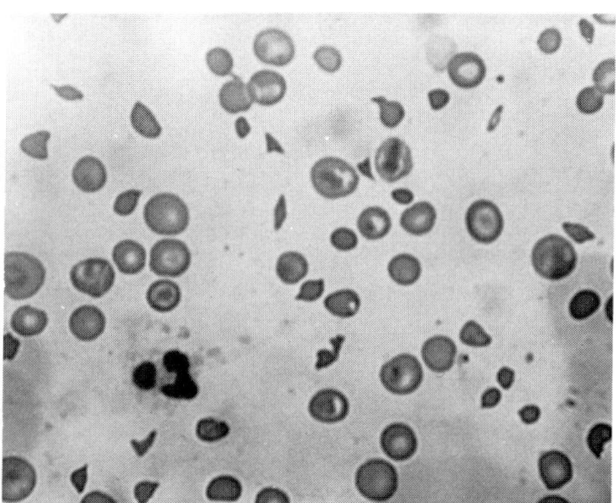

Fig. 4. Peripheral blood smear in a patient with thrombotic thrombocytopenic purpura and acute renal failure (Case 3).

logical abnormalities of the red cells and prompted more extensive and detailed laboratory studies leading to the diagnosis of an unusual cause of acute renal failure.

Case 4. A 56-year-old white male was admitted with acute renal failure of 4 days duration. He had been hospitalized elsewhere 11 days previously with recurrent melena and hematemesis for bleeding peptic ulcer and had been given two units of whole blood without untoward reactions. A third unit, given on the 7th hospital day, was followed by chills, fever, hemoglobinuria, and oliguria. Past history revealed that ten years previously he had been given blood transfusions for bleeding peptic ulcer. He remained oliguric for several weeks and required frequent hemodialysis to control uremia and acidosis. The mechanism of the transfusion reaction which had precipitated acute renal failure was worked out by serologic studies (Table 2), after appropriate blood samples from the three donors had been secured from the referring hospital. The indirect Coombs test was positive with red cells from the third donor but not with those from the first two donors. Typing showed the patient to be group O, Rh negative, and Kell negative. The anti-Kell antibody titer in the patient's serum was 1:16.

Comment: The serologic studies carried out after the patient's admission to our hospital showed that acute renal failure had been precipitated by the rare phenomenon of Kell incompatibility (6), and were essential to the safe conduct of the repeated hemodialyses that were required to control uremia.

At times, it is not possible to establish definitive diagnosis in the early stage of acute renal failure and therapy by

TABLE 2—SEROLOGIC STUDIES IN A PATIENT WITH KELL INCOMPATIBILITY
(Case 4)

Test:	Blood Donor	
	1st & 2nd	*3rd*
Saline Cross Match	negat.	negat.
Indirect Coombs	negat.	posit.
Kell Factor	negat.	posit.
Patient's blood group O-, cde/cde, k/k		

dialysis must be undertaken to control uremia and hyperkalemia. This often is the case in patients with renal failure precipitated by trauma or extensive surgery.

The persistence of prolonged oliguria despite careful medical and dialysis therapy poses the problem of diagnosis in a different perspective. The following case illustrates this point and documents the value of laboratory studies.

Case 5. A 36-year-old Negress was transferred from another hospital with acute oliguric renal failure, developing after abruptio placentae in the 30th week of her 12th pregnancy. The patient had been transfused with 4 units of whole blood without reactions. On admission to our hospital, she was severely uremic and markedly lethargic. However, with a combined program of conservative management and repeated hemodialyses she improved rapidly and felt very well. She remained oliguric with urine output below 150 ml per day for one month. A variety of laboratory studies including renal arteriography and retrograde pyelography, suggested that the patient had intrinsic renal disease. Accordingly, renal biopsy was carried out to establish the definitive diagnosis. The biopsy (Fig. 5) showed extensive renal

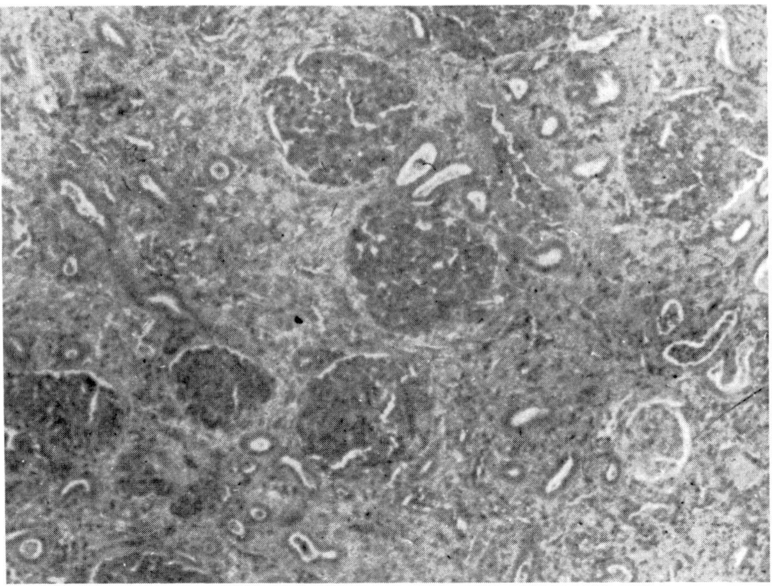

Fig. 5. Renal biopsy in a patient with acute renal failure (Case 5). Findings demonstrate extensive renal cortical necrosis.

cortical necrosis with no evidence of regenerating process.

Comment: Owing to the prolonged period of severe oliguria, renal biopsy was performed to determine the nature and severity of organic renal damage. The question was whether the patient had a potentially reversible lesion, such as acute tubular necrosis, or whether she had sustained irreparable renal damage. The demonstration by biopsy of renal cortical necrosis indicated that recovery was impossible and that the patient's life could be maintained only by periodic dialysis or by renal transplantation.

3. Value of Laboratory in Determining Need and Frequency of Dialysis

In acute renal failure, or in acute drug poisoning, the physician is often faced with the question of deciding when to undertake and how frequently to employ dialysis (12, 15). The laboratory plays a major role in both types of decisions. For example, in acute barbiturate poisoning knowledge of blood levels of barbiturate is particularly critical since the decision must be made whether conservative management or dialysis should be employed, as illustrated by the following case.

Case 6. A 23-year-old white male was admitted in deep coma 11 hours after ingestion of approximately 10 gm of phenobarbital. The blood barbiturate level was 25 mg per 100 ml at this time. Initially, the patient was treated with gastric lavage, respiratory assistance and intravenous fluids. However, despite these measures on the evening of admission, the patient developed severe respiratory distress and fever up to 103° F rectally, at which time tracheostomy was carried out and peritoneal dialysis instituted. Twelve hours later his condition had deteriorated with hypotension, oliguria and generalized edema, and blood barbiturate level was 22 mg per 100 ml. This high level of barbiturate remaining in the blood despite peritoneal dialysis, combined with deteriorating clinical condition prompted the decision to undertake hemodialysis. After the initial 3½ hours of hemodialysis, response to pain and patellar reflexes were noted, the blood pressure stabilized within normal levels and respiratory distress decreased. Hemodialysis was continued for 9 hours, after which all superficial and deep tendon reflexes returned and blood barbiturate level decreased to 17 mg per 100 ml. Subsequently, the patient made an uneventful recovery and was fully awake nearly three days after termination of hemodialysis.

Comment: The finding of an elevated blood level of barbiturate despite seemingly adequate conservative management and peritoneal dialysis, along with the clinical findings indicating deterioration was critical to the decision to undertake hemodialysis. Our experience in the past several years has confirmed the wisdom of serial measurements of blood barbiturate levels to assess more objectively the effectiveness of conservative therapy and to determine the need for dialysis.

Experimental and clinical studies have led to the development of a variety of procedures for identifying and quantitating a large number of drugs (11). Methods of analysis of many drugs have made possible evaluation of the dialysance (i.e., the ability of dialysis in effecting removal from the blood stream).

Until recently, the application of dialysis to the treatment of acute renal failure was based on biochemical criteria (9) which included blood urea nitrogen in excess of 150 mg per 100 ml, carbon dioxide content lower than 12 mEq per liter, and serum potassium above 7.0 mEq per liter.

With the advent of prophylactic dialysis (15), these criteria have been modified and dialysis is started somewhat earlier in the course of acute renal failure. Further, in an attempt to control uremia more effectively, to lessen the "catabolic" rate and to maintain the patient in better general condition, dialysis is carried out more frequently regardless of the levels of blood urea nitrogen, serum bicarbonate and potassium. Nevertheless, the results of laboratory studies are not to be overlooked, for valuable information as to the catabolic rate in acute renal failure can be obtained. For practical purposes, the rates of change of blood urea nitrogen and serum potassium can be taken as indices of the catabolic rate (1, 2, 8, 13). As shown in Table 3, in uncomplicated acute renal failure blood urea nitrogen

TABLE 3—ESTIMATE OF ENDOGENOUS CATABOLISM
IN ACUTE RENAL FAILURE

Acute Renal Failure	Tissue Catabolic Rate	BUN mg/100 ml		K mEq/L	Number of Dialyses
		Range	Δ/Day	Range	
Uncomplicated	Low	8 → 96	10.3	3.9 → 5.7	2
Complicated	High	35 → 300	44.9	4.2 → 9.3	4

Δ Increment per day

increases slowly during the oliguric phase and hyperkalemia is not a serious problem. By contrast, in renal failure complicated by trauma or extensive surgery, blood urea nitrogen and serum potassium tend to increase rapidly. So that, in the former instance, dialysis may be needed on one or two occasions, while in the latter dialysis may have to be employed more frequently, even at intervals of 48 hours. At this point, it should be mentioned that in cases of complicated renal failure such as those associated with burns, major surgery and massive fluid and electrolyte deficits, frequent laboratory measurements of hematocrit, blood volume, and composition of drainage fluids are as essential as determining the levels of blood urea nitrogen and serum electrolytes.

Finally, mention should be made of the electrocardiogram in acute renal failure and in course of dialysis. Electrolyte disturbances distort the electrocardiogram to varying degree (4, 14), and patterns attributable to abnormal serum levels of potassium and calcium have long been recognized. Dialysis can produce very rapid and perhaps dangerous serum electrolyte changes. Thus, while correction of hyperkalemia and hypocalcemia by dialysis may be associated with a normal electrocardiographic pattern (Fig. 6), development of arrhythmias in course of dialysis may also be expected. This is especially true in patients with underlying heart disease treated with digitalis, quinidine or procaine amide. In such instances, the electrocardiogram should be monitored throughout dialysis

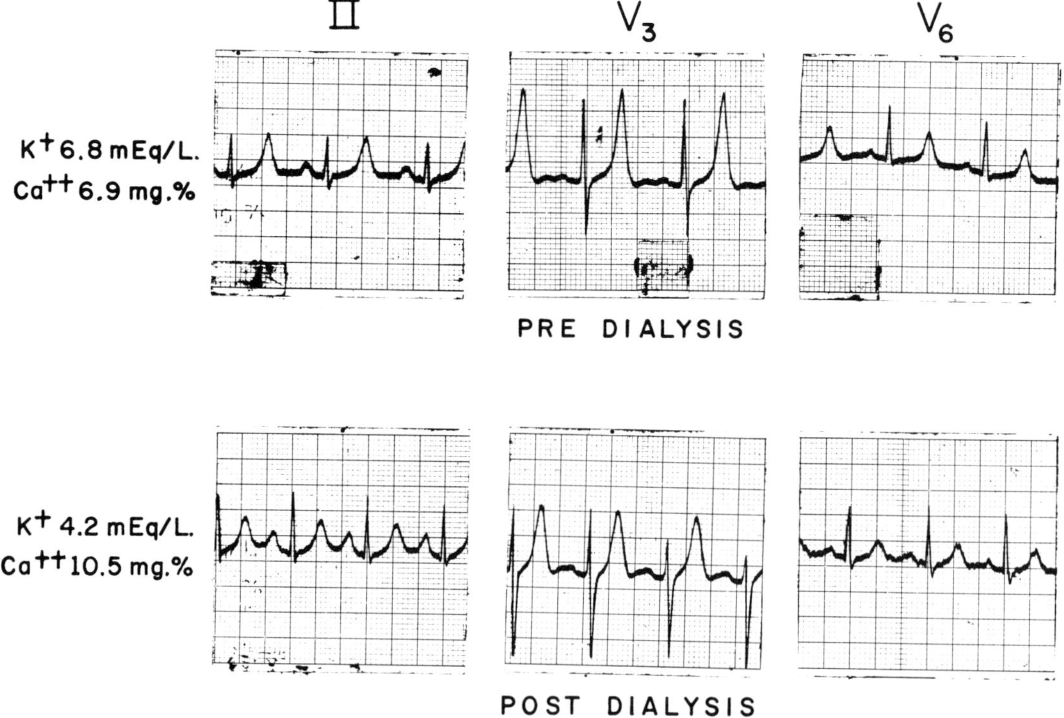

Fig. 6. Electrocardiographic tracings (Lead II) in a patient with acute renal failure demonstrating predialysis distortion caused by hyperkalemia and hypocalcemia and correction produced by dialysis.

so that arrhythmias may be detected at onset and appropriate measures applied. In our experience we have found that this approach contributes greatly to the safe conduct of dialysis.

SUMMARY

The laboratory plays a critically useful role in the management of patients with acute renal failure and acute poisoning. The laboratory procedures include a wide range of tests which permit a rational approach to the problems of diagnosis, conservative management and dialysis.

ACKNOWLEDGMENTS

We wish to thank the personnel of the Dialysis Unit, Passavant Memorial Hospital, and all the fellows and residents who in the past eight years have shared our experience in studying so many patients with acute renal failure and barbiturate poisoning. Drs. P. Herdson and J. Sherrick, Department of Pathology, and Dr. H. Kwan, Department of Medicine, have been most helpful in studying certain of the patients referred to us. The secretarial assistance of Mrs. L. Van Stone is greatly appreciated.

REFERENCES

1. Blagg, C. R., and Parsons, F. M.: The use of norethandrolone in acute renal failure from obstetric causes. Lancet, *2*:577-581, 1960.
2. Blondeel, N. J., Goodman, S., Simon, N. M., and del Greco, F.: The production of urea nitrogen and creatinine in chronic azotemia and the effect of hemodialysis. Proc. Soc. Exp. Biol. Med., *122*:156-161, 1966.
3. Chisholm, G. D., Charlton, C. A. C., and Orr, W. McN.: Urine-urea/blood-urea ratios in renal failure. Lancet, *1*:20-23, 1966.
4. del Greco, F., and Grumer, H.: Electrolyte and electrocardiographic changes in the course of hemodialysis. Am. J. Cardiol., *9*:43-50, 1962.
5. del Greco, F., Arieff, A. J., and Simon, N. M.: Acute barbiturate and glutethimide intoxication. Quart. Bull. N. U. Med. School, *36*:306-315, 1962.
6. del Greco, F., and Kurtides, E.: Kell incompatibility with acute renal failure. Arch. Int. Med., *112*:727-730, 1963.
7. Eliahou, H. E., and Bata, A.: The diagnosis of acute renal failure. Nephron, *2*:287-295, 1965.
8. Giordano, C.: Use of exogenous and endogenous urea for protein synthesis in normal and uremic subjects. J. Lab. Clin. Med., *62*:231-246, 1963.
9. Kolff, W. J.: Acute renal failure: Causes and treatment. Med. Clin. North America. Philadelphia & London, W. B. Saunders Co., 1955, pp. 1041-1071.
10. Maher, J. F., Schreiner, G. E., and Waters, T. J.: Successful intermittent hemodialysis, longest reported maintenance of life in true oliguria (181 Days). Trans. Amer. Soc. Artif. Int. Organs, *6*:123-133, 1960.
11. Maher, J. F., and Schreiner, G. E.: The dialysis of poisons and drugs. Trans. Amer. Soc. Artif. Int. Organs, *13*:369-393, 1967.
12. Merrill, J. P.: The Treatment of Renal Failure, 2nd Ed. New York & London, Grune & Stratton, 1965, pp. 255-259.
13. McCracken, B. H., Pearl, M. A., and Carvajal, E.: Dietary protein and renal failure, New Eng. J. Med., *272*:1050-1054, 1965.
14. Rubin, A. L., Lubash, G. D., Cohen, B. D., Brailousky, D., Braveman, W. S., and Luckey, E. H.: Electrocardiographic changes during hemodialysis with the artifical kidney. Circulation, *19*:552-556, 1959.
15. Teschan, P. E., Baxter, C. R., O'Brien, T. F., Freyhof, J. N., and Hall, W. H.: Prophylactic hemodialysis in the treatment of acute renal failure. Ann. Int. Med., *53*:992-1004, 1950.
16. Ward, E. E., Richards, P., and Wrong, O. M.: Urine concentration after acute renal failure. Nephron, *3*:289-294, 1966.
17. Waugh, W. H.: Functional types of acute renal failure and their early diagnosis. Arch. Int. Med., *103*:686-689, 1959.

Chapter 39

Laboratory Tests for the Management of Patients Undergoing Chronic Dialysis

ERVIN A. GOMBOS, M.D.

INTRODUCTION

By definition, uremia is a syndrome complex, both clinical and biochemical, stemming from renal functional impairment resulting in retention of by-products of metabolism. These, in turn, create alone, or in concert, secondary biochemical derangements and affect practically all functions of the organism.

The uremic syndrome is known to be manifest clinically by generalised weakness, gastrointestinal, hematological, dermatological, cardiovascular and neurological manifestations. The latter may appear in form of sensory and motoric disturbances. Prior to the development of chronic intermittent hemodialysis, patients reaching endstage renal disease became progressively and severely debilitated and died of uremia without exception. Depending on the type of underlying renal disease and success of the conservative management, the terminal event could sometimes be delayed for weeks or months. With the advent of chronic dialysis, however, the natural course of chronic renal disease was altered, albeit for a relatively small patient population.

Methods

Table I indicates one type of dialysate in use. Table II and III indicates some biochemical values obtained prior and after hemodialysis utilising single pass warm dialysate in a parallel flow pumpless system.

The rate of removal of any substance during hemodialysis is affected by usual factors influencing dialysance of this substance, e.g., blood flow through the dialyser, rate of fluid flux across the cellophane membrane, and dialysate temperature and flow rate; all independently and in concert, affect blood levels during dialysis.

Discussion of all the principles of dialytic therapy, the systems presently in use and their relative merits can be found in literature (1, 2, 3).

TABLE I—COMPOSITION
OF THE DIALYSATE BATH

Ion	mEq / Liter
Calcium	2.5
Magnesium	1.5
Potassium	2.0
Acetate	33
Sodium	126
Chloride	105
Dextrose	200 mg. per 100 ml

TABLE 2—PRE-DIALYSIS AND POST-DIALYSIS VALUES OF SOME BLOOD CHEMISTRIES*

	Serum Urea Nitrogen mg/100 ml Dialysis		Serum Creatinine mg/100 ml Dialysis		Serum Na mEq/L Dialysis		Serum K mEq/L Dialysis		Serum Ca mEq/L Dialysis		Serum P mg/100 ml Dialysis		HCO_3 mEq/L Dialysis		Serum Mg mEq/L Dialysis		Uric Acid mg/100 ml Dialysis	
	Pre	Post	Pre	Post	Pre	Post	Pre	Post	Pre	Post	Pre	Post	Pre	Post	Pre	Post	Pre	Post
	78.21	21.83	14.70	4.13	140	136	3.51	3.20	4.33	4.72	4.91	2.95	23.1	24.0	2.92	2.40	8.14	3.88
S.D.	18.11	12.03	2.13	1.01	3	2	1.21	1.31	1.02	1.83	1.01	1.26	2.1	1.21	1.70	0.81	2.23	1.01

*Values represent means of 20 consecutive 12 hour dialyses in 18 patients on diet containing 60 gm protein/day.

TABLE 3—ACID BASE VALUES PRIOR AND POST CHRONIC DIALYSIS

Ph		PCO_2 mm Hg		HCO_3 mEq/L		Buffer Base mEq/L Blood	
Pre	Post	Pre	Post	Pre	Post	Pre	Post
7.31	7.39	40.1	39.2	21.7	25.0	27.4	30.9

*Values represent means of 3 consecutive determinations in 5 patients.

LABORATORY TESTS FOR EVALUATION OF PATIENTS UNDERGOING CHRONIC HEMODIALYSIS

Blood or serum urea nitrogen is the most valuable single laboratory test reflecting the degree of uremia and the biochemical correction as accomplished by dialysis. It is well established that blood urea levels reflect the total urea distribution space (usually total body water) and are affected by dietary nitrogen intake, endogenous protein catabolism and the rate of urea synthesis. Blood in the gastrointestial tract may contribute to the rise in BUN. Evidence is accumulating that indicates that at a dietary, high quality protein intake of 0.78 gm per kg, nitrogen balance is accomplished and that there is reutilisation in the uremic of urea N in protein anabolism.

CREATININE

Creatinine, an anhydride of creatine, is principally formed from creatine phosphate present in muscle tissue. Creatinine values are thus affected by muscular mass, and muscle wasting would tend to exaggerate creatinine levels. In chronic renal failure with high blood levels of creatinine, the ratio of creatinine to blood urea nitrogen is usually well maintained. In patients undergoing chronic hemodialysis, this ratio, normally 1:10, is upset. Because of its free diffusion during dialysis, urea appears to dialyse at a faster rate than creatinine. It is therefore conceivable that larger molecules moving slowly through the cellophane are dialysed at rates more congruent with creatinine.

It is therefore probable that serum creatinine levels reflect the degree of biochemical improvement to a greater degree than urea levels alone.

SERUM ELECTROLYTES

Serum sodium levels prior to dialysis usually are in the normal range, and are affected between dialysis primarily by the sodium and water intake of patients. Since most patients undergoing chronic intermittent dialysis have no substantial urine output, any intake of fluid in excess of the output and insensible loss will reflect itself in serum sodium levels. Excessive and undesirable intake of fluid may depress serum sodium levels and only agressive fluid removal during dialysis will correct its concentrations. Occasionally, a patient, still capable of significant urine output in spite of almost total nephron loss will appear hyponatremic because of a sodium wasting pattern of output. These losses are further enhanced by the osmotic diuresis and dietary salt restrictions occasionally imposed upon them. In this small patient population, augmented sodium intake between and during dialysis aids in restoring serum sodium levels toward normal. The total body sodium content equally affects total circulating blood volume. Increased sodium space correlates well with expanded circulating blood volume and hypertension. To aid in removal of water, hyponatremic dialysate can be utilized for better control of hypertension. Post-dialytic concentrations of sodium shift readily toward equilibration with the dialysate concentration. Hypernatremia in chronic dialysis is rare and is seen only in severely dehydrated patients. If mild (140 to 145 mEq per L), only the laboratory findings would indicate its presence. If severe (> 145 mEq per L), clinical signs could appear indicating hypervolemia, hypertension, confusion and other electrolyte disturbances.

SERUM POTASSIUM

Serum potassium concentration prior to dialysis tends to be normal or slightly elevated. Low serum values are extremely rare, and when present indicate severe total body potassium depletion. High values, if not due to error introduced by haemolysis, are found during periods of dietary indiscretions, severe uncontrolled acidosis, catabolic states (e.g., during infection) or during severe dehydration associated with hyperkalemia. Usually, potassium concentrations in the dialysate are kept low (0 to 2.0 mEq per L). This is applicable to the majority of patients. Occasionally, normal concentrations (4.0 mEq per L) are necessary, e.g., in digitalized patients. However, in digitalized patients dialysate with concentrations of 2.0 mEq per L are administered without any untoward effects.

CHLORIDES

Serum chloride is usually in the normal range but may be high or low. When abnormally low, they are usually congruent with the clinical history of the interval between dialysis. Vomiting is not uncommon, especially during the early months of chronic dialysis. Later, it may still occur during periods of postdialytic dysequilibrium syndrome.

ACID-BASE BALANCE

Blood pH before dialysis tends to be acid (7.19 to 7.30). During dialysis significant correction is accomplished and over correction (pH 7.48) is not uncommon. Serum bicarbonate levels are usually low (21.7 mEq per L) prior to

dialysis and augmented after. Correction is readily accomplished utilizing either sodium bicarbonate or acetate. The respiratory alkalosis regularly observed after dialysis has not been adequately explained. The tendency of the chronic uremic to replenish buffering capacity during equilibration against sodium acetate containing dialysate could possibly be due to absorption of bicarbonate at the skeletal crystal—extracellular fluid interface.

CALCIUM PHOSPHATE

Long standing renal insufficiency is found to be associated frequently with hyperfunction of the parathyroid glands, and renal osteodystrophy may be present in patients with chronic renal disease or develop while undergoing chronic intermittent hemodialysis. Abnormalities can be found on x-ray surveys of bone, and spontaneous fractures of ribs and other bones have been reported. Total serum calcium levels tend to be low prior to dialysis with complete correction after 6–12 hours. On occasion, especially in geographic areas where tap water calcium levels are high and no de-ionisation of the water is carried out, periods of transient dialysis induced hypercalcemia are common. Inorganic phosphate, always high prior to dialysis, tends to diminish during dialysis. No good correlation is known to exist between manifest bone disease and serum calcium or serum inorganic phosphate levels. No specific laboratory test other than radiological evidence of bone disease is available as an absolute indication of its existence. On the other hand, patients with significant bone disease tend to have high alkaline phosphatase activity which is unaffected by the dialytic procedure. Elevated activity of alkaline phosphatase has been observed in about 50% of patients undergoing chronic dialysis and in all of these patients manifest bone disease was present. Occasionally osteodystrophy may be present in absence of high alkaline phosphatase activity.

Magnesium

Hypermagnesemia is of frequent occurence in chronic renal failure. The significance of high plasma and red blood cell magnesium levels is still debated but evidence is accumulating that implicates magnesium, at least in part, in neuropathy. All patients undergoing chronic hemodialysis have elevated serum magnesium levels prior to dialysis. Depending on the magnesium content of dialysate, a drop in serum levels can be expected. The water content of magnesium varies depending on geographical areas and this has necessitated deionisation procedures which aleviate the problem. In our experience, symptoms have not been attributed to elevated levels of serum magnesium.

Carbohydrate Metabolism

Carbohydrate metabolism is deranged in chronic uremia. The syndrome of "Azotemic Pseudiabethes" consists of an abnormal glucose tolerance curve and is clinically manifest by an apparent improvement of fasting hyperglycemia and glycosuria in diabetics with renal insufficiency. In addition, there is an increased sensitivity to hypoglycemic agents. The present evidence suggests a generalized reduction in cellular glucose uptake leading to reduced liver glycogen and decreased cellular utilization. It has been proposed that the defect is a function of diminished phosphorylation manifest primarily in the liver whose demands for ATP for the detoxification of nitrogen are maximal. Others suggest as the cause a peripheral insensitivity to endogenous insulin.

Seventy per cent of our patients undergoing chronic intermittent hemodialysis have had high fasting concentrations of blood glucose. Utilizing a slightly elevated glucose content in our dialysate (200mg per 100 ml) no significant hyperglycemia has been observed during or after dialysis. Since methods other than high glucose gradient are available for removal of fluid from the patient undergoing dialysis, it is likely that dialysate-glucose concentrations in excess of normal range are not indicated.

Lipemia

Elevated plasma lipids have been observed in chronic uremia. Elevation of fasting plasma triglycerides (TG) (normal > 150 mg per 100 ml) has been frequently noted in well controlled uremic patients undergoing chronic hemodialysis. Fasting TG concentrations in dialysed patients are higher than in the undialysed group and it is concluded that this elevation may result from a combination of increased endogenous TG synthesis and defective TG removal.

Amino Acids

In chronic uremia, rigid dietary protein restriction is indicated as part of the conservative management. Evidence is accumulating that indicates that end-stage uremics are low on both dietary essential amino acids (valine, isoleucine and tryptophan) and dietary non-essential amino acids (tyrosine and alanine). Improved food intake and dialysis result in partial or total correction of several of these deficiencies (alanine, valine, isoleucine) while tyrosine and tryptophan deficiencies persist. It appears that dialysis aggravates threonine and cystidine deficiency. It is as yet not known what the long term effects of these metabolic changes are. A severely restricted protein intake in association with vigorous hemodialysis is most likely to result in serious nutritional deficiencies.

COMMENTS

The goal of chronic intermittent hemodialysis is improvement, preferably complete correction of biochemical abnormalities of uremia. In completely anuric patients, this involved 20 to 30 hours of dialysis time per week. Dietary protein restriction would shorten dialysis time but would increase the nutritional deficiencies inherent in the dialytic form of therapy. The question has been raised if the goal of dialysis is normal chemistries or only significant rehabilitation. The two are not synonymous. Most patients do not feel the difference between the post-dialytic serum urea nitrogen values of 15 or 50. On the other hand, the long term effects of "underdialysis" are yet to be seen.

BIBLIOGRAPHY

1. Doyle, D. E.: Extracorporeal Hemodialysis Therapy in Blood Chemistry Disorders. Springfield, Thomas, 1962.
2. Hampers, C. L., Soeldner, S., Doak, P. B., and Merrill, J. P.: Effect of chronic renal failure and hemodialysis on carbohydrate metabolism. J. Clin. Invest., *45:*1719-1731, 1966.
3. Henderson, L. W., Rodriguez, B., and Bluemle, L. W., Jr.: Factors influencing blood pH changes during extracorporeal dialysis in patients with chronic renal failure. Trans. Amer. Soc. Artif. Intern. Organs, *12:*193-199, 1966.
4. Hendler, E. D., Eglin, J. M., Jr., Hendler, R. G., Cummings, J. W., Vietzke, B. F., Hinckley, B. I., and Gombos, E. A.: Chronic intermittent hemodialysis: Clinical considerations. Med. Ann. of D. C., *36:*335-340, 1967.
5. Hutchings, R. H., Hegstrom, R. M., and Scribner, B. H.: Glucose intolerance in patients on long-term intermittent dialysis. Ann. Int. Med., *65:*275-285, 1966.
6. Maher, J. F., Freeman, R. B., and Schreiner, G. F.: Hemodialysis for chronic renal failure, II, Biochemical and clinical aspects: Ann. Int. Med., *62:*535-550, 1965.
7. Ogden, D. A., and Holmes, J. H.: Changes in total and ultrafilterable plasma calcium and magnesium during hemodialysis. Trans. Amer. Soc. Artif. Inter. Organs, *12:*200-204, 1966.
8. Schreiner, G. E., and Maher, J. F.: Uremia. Springfield, Thomas, 1961.
9. Transactions of the American Society for Artificial Internal Organs, Vol. I-XIII
10. Westervelt, F. B., Jr., and Schreiner, G. E.: The carbohydrate intolerance of uremic patients. Ann. Int. Med., *57:*266-276, 1962.
11. Young, G. A., and Parsons, F. M.: Amino nitrogen loss during hemodialysis, its dietary significance and replacement. Clin. Sci., *31:*299-307, 1966.

Chapter 40

The Clinical Pathology of Renal Homotransplantation

ROBERT CADE, M.D., and ALEJANDRO DE QUESADA, M.D.

In human renal transplantation, initial technical success is usually achieved; survival of the allograft, however, requires control of graft rejection. If the best possible function is to be obtained, early recognition of rejection is imperative. Precise diagnosis, however, is equally important, for intensive use of immune suppressive agents may cause death from bone marrow depression or infection when given to stop rejection which is not occurring.

Allograft rejection may be manifest, clinically. by fever, pain and tenderness around the graft, and swelling of the graft (8, 14). Hypertension, edema, malaise and arthralgia have also been reported as manifestations of rejection (8, 14, 16, 17). Perhaps the most frequently used criterion for rejection has been a decrease in function manifest by oliguria (14), rising BUN or serum creatinine (8, 14, 16), falling creatinine clearance (17), and decreased urinary sodium (15).

Jackson (10) and Kountz (12) have stressed the utility of renal blood flow or PAH clearance in early detection of rejection. Serial examination of the urinary sediment for lymphocytes has also proven useful (5, 8, 11), for an increase in urinary lymphocytes is apparently an early and sensitive sign of rejection.

As rejection is an immunologic phenomenon, measurement of serum hemolytic complement activity (9) and of the components of complement (3) have also been studied and reported to be useful when rejection is suspected.

Serial determinations have been made of the various parameters in ten patients who received cadaver transplants at the University of Florida; the data accumulated is the source of material for this report.

When examining rejection episodes in our patients, two rather clear patterns emerge. One, occurring during the first month after transplantation, has been termed "early rejection"; The other, occurring in the remote post-transplant period, has been called "late rejection."

Methods and Materials

All transplants were done utilizing cadaver kidneys; matching of ABO blood groups was the only criterion for selection of donors. Although several of the allografts functioned immediately, evidence of significant ischemic damage, assessed by tubular function, or biopsy, or both, was present in all cases. All recipients

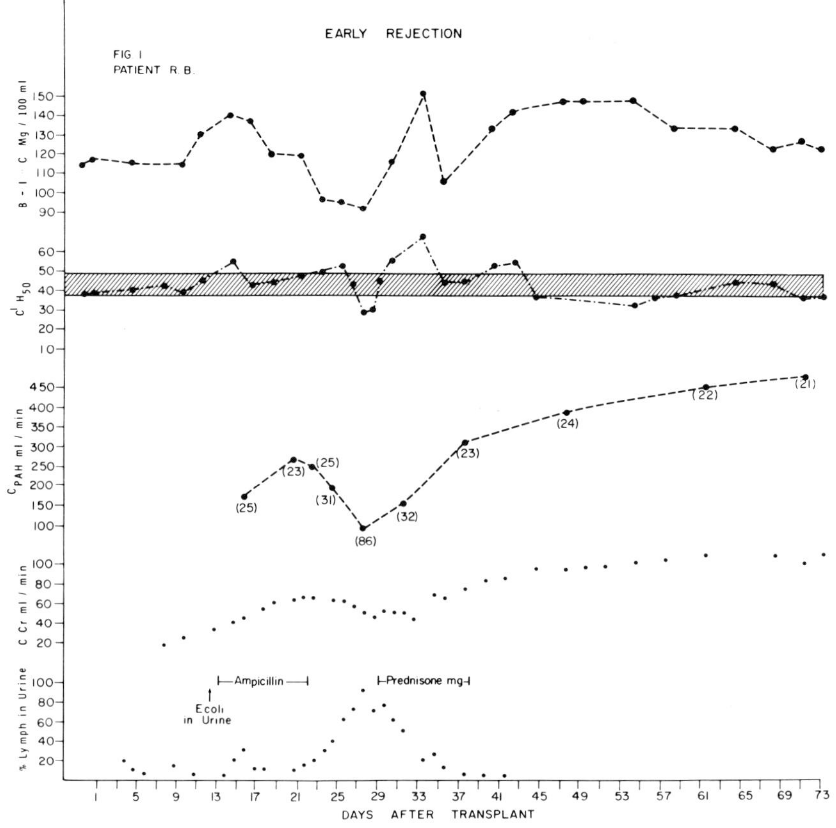

Fig 1.   (N) = Ratio Ccr/C_{PAH}

Prednisone dose 200 mg/day for three days then rapidly decreased to 50 mg/day.

were given Imuran from the time of transplantation. Several also received adrenal corticosteroids beginning at the time of transplantation. This practice was abandoned, however, to facilitate wound healing, and steroids were then given only when rejection became apparent.

In the early-post transplant period, daily 24-hour creatinine clearances were performed (13). An Addis count and differential cell count on the urinary sediment were also done each day. Whole serum hemolytic complement activity (9) and B-1-C concentration (3) were determined at least three times each week. PAH clearances, using stan-dard techniques (13), were performed at frequent intervals.

In the remote post-transplant period, all studies were performed but with decreased frequency.

Results

In Figure 1 are illustrated the characteristics of early rejection. The concentration of B-1-C and hemolytic complement activity of serum expressed in $C'H_{50}$ units are shown at the top of the figure; renal plasma flow and creatinine clearance are shown in the center; and at the bottom is given the percentage of lymphocytes among white cells in the

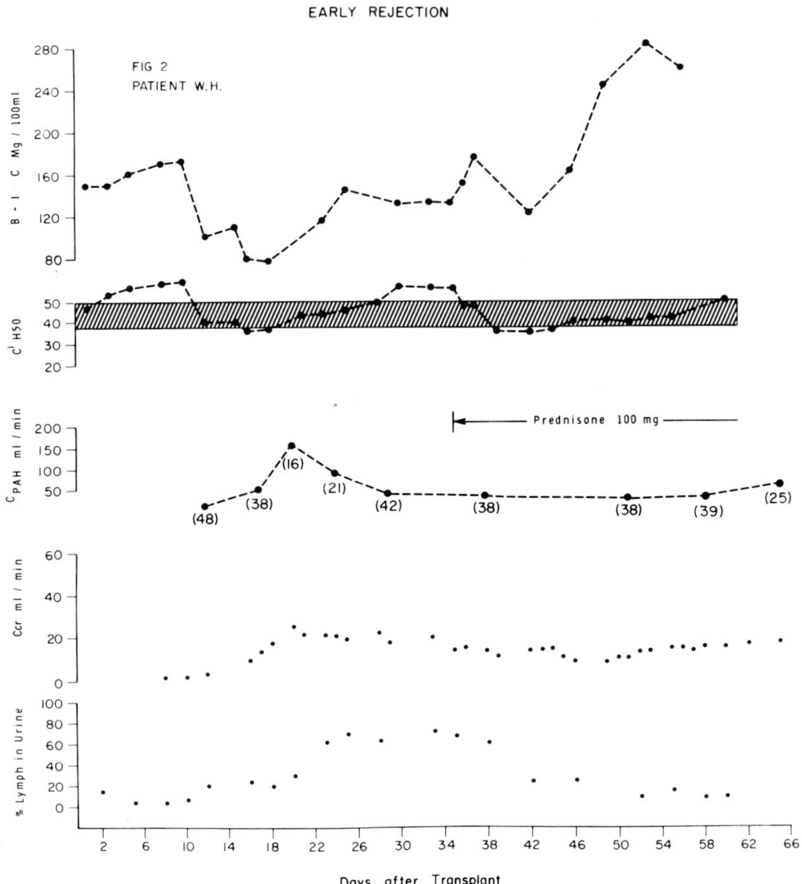

Fig 2.   (N) = Ratio Ccr/C_{PAH}

urinary sediment. In parentheses, under the PAH clearance points, are the calculated creatinine / PAH clearance ratios.

At day 12, there was an increase in urinary lymphocytes. Both B-1-C and $C'H_{50}$ were also increased at that time, probably as a result of the urinary tract infection which became apparent the next day. The total lymphocyte excretion continued to increase although for several days the percentage of lymphocytes went down since large numbers of granulocytes were excreted as a result of the infection. As the infection subsided and granulocyte excretion fell, the percentage as well as total number of lymphocytes excreted, increased sharply. As the kidney continued to recover from the ischemic damage suffered at transplantation, both creatinine and PAH clearance improved progressively until day 21 when creatinine clearance was 63 and PAH clearance 275 ml per minute. On day 22, PAH clearance was 250 ml per minute and by day 25 was only 180. Creatinine clearance during this time varied between 60 and 63 ml per minute. Serum B-1-C concentration fell abruptly to 95 mg per 100 ml of serum on day 22 while serum hemolytic complement activity remained in a normal range until day 26. Between days 22 and

28, both PAH and creatinine clearances fell progressively. The decrease in PAH clearance was proportionately much greater and began earlier then the decrement in creatinine clearance so that the clearance ratio rose very sharply from 0.16 on day 21 to 0.86 on day 28. Prednisone, 250 mg daily, was started on day 29; by day 31 both $C'H_{50}$ and B-1-C had returned to the normal ranges, the percentage of lymphocytes in the urine was falling and PAH clearance had increased. Improvement was continuous and by day 70 creatinine clearance was 100 and PAH clearance 475 ml per minute.

Figure 2 shows a second example of early rejection. As the kidney recovered from acute tubular necrosis, both creatinine and PAH clearances increased rapidly and the clearance ratio fell. On day 12, however, the percentage of lymphocytes in the urine increased and both B-1-C concentration and $C'H_{50}$ fell sharply. Function continued to improve, however, and on day 20 creatinine clearance was 24 and PAH clearance 152 ml per minute. Both creatinine and PAH clearances then began to fall; again the decrease in PAH clearance began earlier and was proportionately greater than the fall in creatinine clearance. The percentage of lymphocytes in the urine continued to increase. On day 26, the patient became febrile and on day 28 signs of acute prostatitis became apparent. In retrospect, this probably began on day 21 when the patient began to complain of distal urethral pain. The rise in B-1-C and $C'H_{50}$ which occurred at that time was probably a reflection of prostatic infection. Antibiotics were started on day 29 and Prednisone on day 35. After steroid therapy was started, lymphocytes in the urine decreased, and function became stable and then slowly

improved. There was an initial sharp rise in the concentration of B-1-C and then both B-1-C and $C'H_{50}$ fell to low levels before returning to a normal range. These changes in $C'H_{50}$ and B-1-C, an initial increase when steroids are started with a secondary fall as production of complement is depressed, appear to be characteristics of supression of rejection with steroids as they have occurred in all the rejections we have treated.

An example of late rejection is shown in Figure 3. This rejection began about two months after transplant when the patient was taking 40 mg of Prednisone and 150 mg of Imuran each day. Creatinine clearance was still improving slowly, $C'H_{50}$ was stable and in a normal range, and blood pressure was moderately elevated. The blood pressures shown in this figure are the maximal and minimal pressures for each day; the temperature shown is the highest recorded for the day. On day 2 of this sequence, the patient became febrile and complained of pain and fullness in the area of the graft. A diagnosis of rejection was made on the basis of clinical findings and a large dose of Prednisone started. On day 4, however, it was apparent the fever and symptoms were due to a large pelvic and perinephric abscess which was promptly drained. Clinically, marked improvement occurred immediately. Complement activity which had increased with the infection remained elevated, however, and the septic temperature curve continued in spite of antibiotics and steroids until day 10 when loculations in the abscess tract were broken and a large volume of purulent material drained. Immediately after this procedure, her blood pressure fell sharply and remained down for almost six hours. Urine flow decreased abruptly and creatinine clearance for that day was greatly reduced

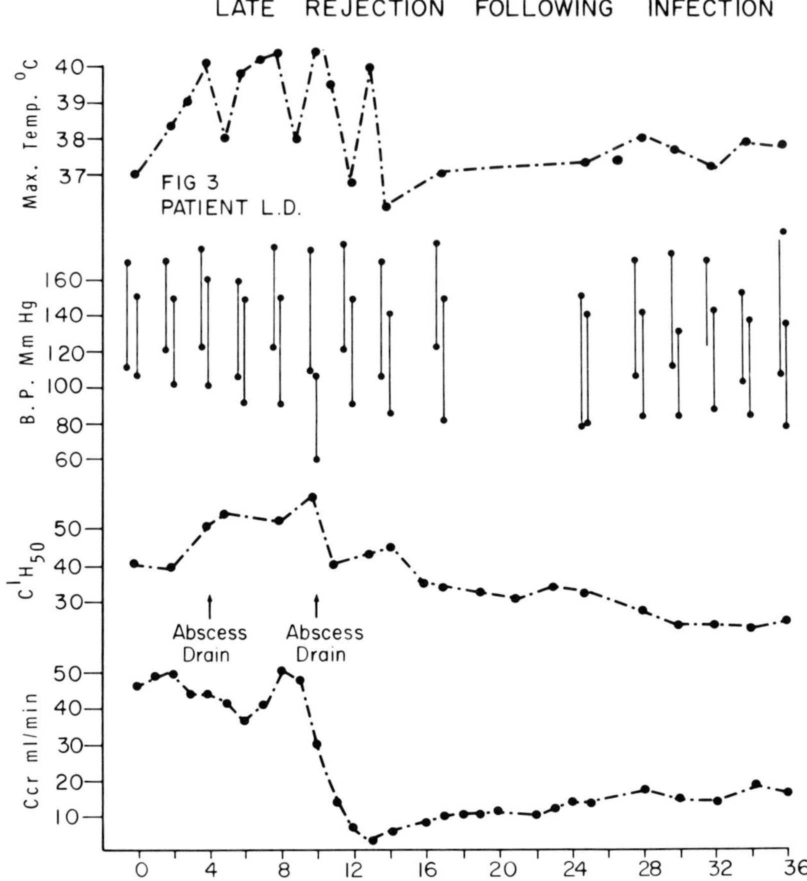

Fig. 3. Blood pressure values are highest and lowest readings for each day, all taken with patient supine.

and continued to fall. $C'H_{50}$ fell to a normal range after good drainage was established and she became afebrile. On day 16, $C'H_{50}$ fell below normal and remained low until her death 20 days later of a cerebral hemorrhage. Creatinine clearance, which was 5 ml per minute on day 13, improved very slowly and reached a peak of 19 ml per minute just before her death. Autopsy showed not only classic evidence of rejection, but also findings of a generalized Shwartzman reaction (18).

It seems likely that in this patient increased production of complement due to infection more than compensated for the increased consumption occurring with rejection so that $C'H_{50}$ was normal or high until the infection was controlled. In retrospect, it seems likely that the marked fall in creatinine clearance immediately after the second surgical drainage of the abscess was due to a Shwartzman reaction rather than rejection (18).

In Figure 4 are given pertinent data from a late rejection which began about five months after transplant. With prostatitis there was a rise in both $C'H_{50}$ and B-1-C. When rejection began both fell to depressed levels before any change in function occurred; function then fell

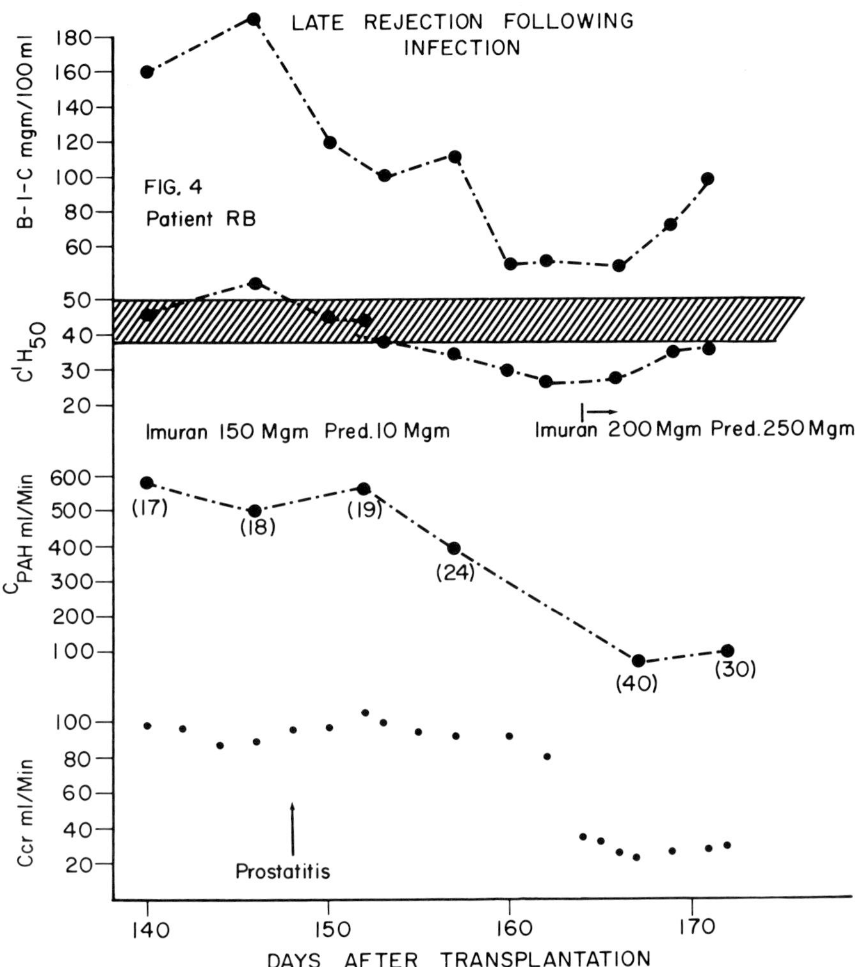

Fig 4. (N) = Ratio Ccr/C_{PAH}
Antibiotic treatment of prostatitis was begun on day 156.

rapidly until large doses of adreno-cortical steroids were given; then stabilized and slowly increased. The sequence of events, infection with a rise in serum complement activity followed by rejection is the same as that shown in Figure 3.

In Figure 5 are shown data which, initially, were thought to indicate a late rejection. Because no evidence of infection could be found, and because no change in either B-1-C or $C'H_{50}$ occur-red, treatment for rejection was not started. When hydrochlorothiazide, which had been given for mild steroid induced hypertension was discontinued, function improved progressively.

Discussion

Attempted rejection of allografts from non-related cadaver donors in such a constant occurrence during the first month after transplant that it should be anticipated. When steroids are not given

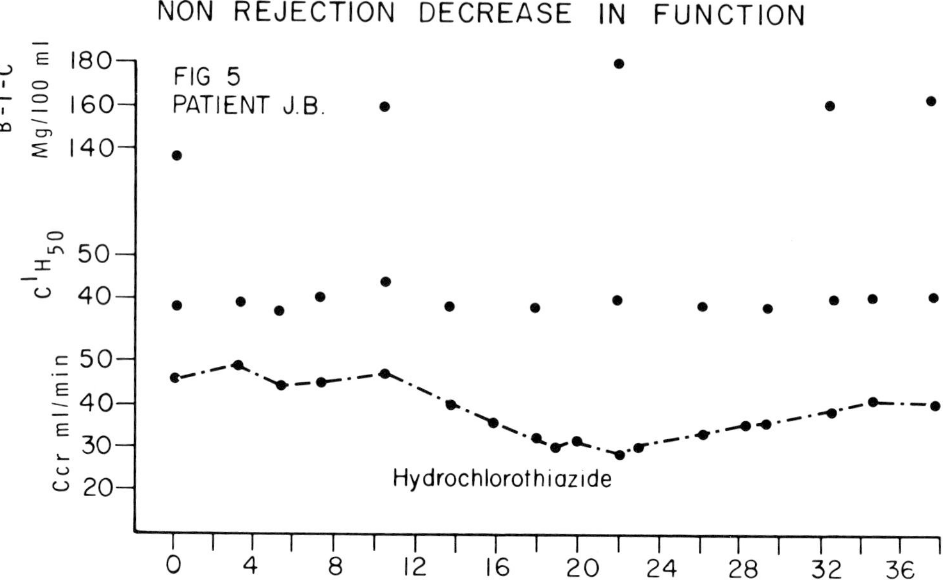

Fig. 5. Hydrochlorothiazide was discontinued on day 22.

as initial immune suppression so that wound healing can proceed normally, a very constant sequence of events occurs.

Renal function improves progressively from the time of transplantation. Between the tenth and fourteenth day B-1-C and $C'H_{50}$ both fall, the decline in B-1-C usually preceding the fall in $C'H_{50}$. At this time, lymphocytes in the urine increase in number. Although these findings surely indicate rejection is occurring, function as assessed by PAH and creatinine clearance continues to improve as the kidney is rapidly recovering from acute ischemic damage. Between the third and fourth week, however, reparative and destructive processes reach a balance and function decreases; the decline in PAH clearance almost always precedes the fall in creatinine clearance.

With concomitant infection, or with the inflammation associated with rejection, an acute phase response with a rise in $C'H_{50}$ and B-1-C may occur (2, 6)

which masks the increased utilization of complement by the rejection. When steroids are started and the inflammatory response with its resultant stimulation of complement is suppressed, serum complement activity and B-1-C concentration abruptly fall and remain low until the rejection is controlled.

Late rejection, in our experience, has always followed infection. Five episodes of late rejection in males have followed exacerbation of chronic prostatitis. The sequence of events has been a rise in $C'H_{50}$ and B-1-C associated with the infection. Both B-1-C and $C'H_{50}$ then fall when rejection starts; as in early rejection B-1-C is apparently a more sensitive index than is $C'H_{50}$. The change in PAH clearance in late rejection, as in early rejection, also began before and is of greater magnitude than the change in creatinine clearance.

While fever in our patients has frequently occurred during rejections, it has not been present in the absence of significant infection. In several instances of early rejection, significant decrease in function occurred with decreased complement and elevated urinary lymphocytes although temperature remained normal. Tenderness around the renal transplant has been a fairly constant occurrence in early rejection and probably reflects perirenal inflammation; in late rejection, when the kidney in encased by fibrous tissue it has not occurred.

BIBLIOGRAPHY

1. Austen, K. F., and Russell, P. S.: Detection of renal allograft rejection in man by demonstration of a reduction in the serum concentration of the second component of complement. Ann. N. Y. Acad. of Sci. Seventh International Transplantation Conference, *129:*657-672, 1966.
2. Boltax, A. J., and Fischell, E. E.: Serologic tests for inflammation. Serum complement, C reactive protein, and erythrocyte sedimentation rate in myocardial infarction. Am. J. Med., *20:*418, 1956.
3. Fahey, J. L., and McKehley, E. M.: Quantitative determination of serum immunoglobulins in antibody agar plates. J. of Immunol., *94:*85, 1965.
4. Gewurz, H., Clark, D. A., Finstad, J., Kelly, W. D., Varco, R. L., Good, R. A., and Gabrielson, A. F.: Role of the complement system in graft rejection in experimental animals and in man. Ann. N. Y. Acad. Sci. Seventh International Transplantation Conference, *129:*673-713, 1966.
5. Goodwin, W. E., Kaufman, J. J., Mims, M. M., Turner, D. R., Glassock, R., Goldman, R., and Maxwell, M. M.: Human renal homotransplantation I. Clinical experiences with six cases of renal transplantation. J. Urol., *89:*13, 1963.
6. Guiney, E. J., Austen, K. F., and Russell, P. S.: Measurement of serum complement during homograft rejection in man and rat. Proc. Soc. Exper. Biol. and Med., *115:*1113, 1964.
7. Gunn, W. C.: The variation in the amount of complement in the blood in some acute infectious diseases and its relation to the clinical features. J. Path., *19:*155, 1914-15.
8. Hume, D. M., Magee, J. H., Kauffman, H. M., Rittenbury, M. S., and Prout, G. R.: Renal homotransplantation in man in modified recipients. Ann. Surg., *158:*608-644, 1963.
9. Kabat, E. A., and Mayer, M. M.: Assay of Complement in Experimental Immunochemistry, 2nd ed. Springfield, Thomas, p. 135-153, 1961.
10. Jackson, B. T., and Mannick, J. A.: Serial blood flow in first set renal homotransplants undergoing rejection. Surg. Gynec. Obst., *119:*1265-1270 1964.
11. Kountz, S. L., Williams, M. A., and Williams, P. L., Kapros, C., and Dempster, W. J.: Mechanism of rejection of homotransplanted kidneys. Nature (London), *199:*257-260, 1963.
12. Kountz, S. L., Knudsen, D. F., and Cohn, R.: The pathophysiology of renal allotransplant rejection. International Congress of Nephrology, Abstracts p. 225, Sept., 1966.
13. Levin, D. M., and Cade, J. R.: Effect of dietary sodium intake on renal function in patients with renal disease. Ann. Int. Med., *62:*231-245, 1965.
14. Murray, J. E., Merrill, J. P., Harrison, J. H., Wilson, K. E., and Damin, G. J.: Prolonged survival of human-kidney homografts by immunosuppressive drug therapy. New Eng. J. Med., *268:*1315-1323, 1963.
15. Ogden, D. A., and Holmes, J. H.: Urinary solute excretion as an index of renal homograft rejection. Ann. Int. Med., *64:*806-816, 1966.
16. Starzl, T. E., Marchioro, T. L., and Waddell, W. R.: The reversal of rejection in human renal homografts with subsequent development of homograft tolerance. Surg. Gynec. Obst., *117:*385-395, 1963.
17. Starzl, T. E., Machioro, Porter, K. A., Moore, C. A., Rifhind, D. and Waddell, W. R.: Renal homotransplantation: late function and complications. Ann. Int. Med., *61:*470-497, 1964.
18. Thomas, L., and Good, R. A.: Studies on the generalized Shwartzman reaction. J. Exp. Med., *96:*605-623, 1952.
19. Vaughn, J. H., Boyles, T. B., and Favour, C. B.: The response of serum gamma globulin level and complement titer to adrenocorticotrophic hormone (ACTH) therapy in lupus erythematosus disseminaters. J. Lab. Clin. Med., *37:*698.

Chapter 41

Clinical Significance of the Renal Pressor System

FRANCESCO DEL GRECO, M.D., and NORMAN M. SIMON, M.D.

The demonstration by arteriography and differential function studies of renal arterial obstructive lesions in patients with hypertension does not always imply a cause and effect relationship. Indeed, obstructive lesions of the renal arteries have been found in a significant series of normotensive subjects (11, 13). Among the major criteria proposed for establishing the diagnosis of renovascular hypertension, the finding of increased levels of renin or renin activity in the blood should provide the most important evidence (13). However, despite the recent development of improved methods of assay, it is yet to be unequivocally demonstrated that the measurement of renin does provide the ultimate evidence for or against the diagnosis of renovascular hypertension (23). Several series of cases have been published in the past few years and the results have been variable (10).

At this point, it should be emphasized that the renal pressor system is not only concerned with the regulation of blood pressure but also with other important physiological functions. There is now abundant evidence that the renin-angiotensin system is also concerned with the regulation of sodium metabo-lism, aldosterone secretion and, possibly, with the regulation of the intrarenal circulation and tubular function (2, 6, 7, 9, 24, 30). It is therefore apparent that an understanding of the role of the renal pressor system in hypertension must take into account all of the various factors which influence the blood levels of renin and angiotensin.

The purpose of this presentation is to describe: 1) the relationship between sodium balance and renin activity in normotensive subjects and in patients with benign essential hypertension; 2) the results of studies performed to assess the significance of renin activity in hypertensive patients with renovascular lesions, or with kidneys unequal in size and shape.

MATERIAL AND METHODS

Normotensive Controls

Seventeen healthy men and women, 2 Negroes and 15 whites, aged from 20 to 58 years were utilized to determine the effects of changes in body posture and quiet ambulation on the level of renin activity in the peripheral venous blood while on *ad libitum* sodium intake, and while on reduced sodium intake alone and in combination with diuretic therapy.

Before the study, each subject was maintained on *ad libitum* sodium intake for at least three days. On the morning of the fourth day, 20 ml of clotted or slightly heparinized venous blood were obtained in the early morning after overnight fast and half hour of recumbency in a quiet room, and again after 4 hours of ambulation. Each subject was then placed on a diet containing 10 mEq sodium and 60 to 80 mEq of potassium, and blood samples for the measurement of renin activity were again collected 4 days later while recumbent and after 4 hours of ambulation. Administration of hydrochlorothiazide, 50 mg t.i.d. for 4 days, was then begun and on the morning of the fifth day blood samples were collected under conditions similar to those mentioned above. With each collection of blood with the patient supine, samples of heparinized blood were also withdrawn for the determination of plasma sodium, potassium and creatinine. Body weight was measured daily, and urinary sodium, potassium and creatinine were determined in aliquots of 24 hours urine collections made during *ad libitum* sodium intake and on the fourth day of each of the two experimental periods.

Patients with Essential Hypertension.

Thirteen patients, aged 19 to 62 years, were studied. Four were Negroes and 9 white. In each case, detailed diagnostic studies failed to reveal a cause of the hypertension. Supine diastolic blood pressure with the patients on *ad libitum* sodium intake and after 3 days of hospitalization ranged from 90 to 135 mm Hg, and endogenous creatinine clearance ranged from 52 to 171 ml per minute. The studies concerning renin activity were carried out in a manner similar to those described above for normotensive subjects. In 2 patients, the studies were repeated on two separate occasions from six to thirteen months apart.

Patients with Renovascular Hypertension.

Twenty-five patients, one Negro and 24 white, were included in this study. Each case was subjected to at least two or more of the following procedures: timed intravenous pyelography, differential renal function (29), I^{131} labelled hippurate renography, renal arteriography, and the angiotensin infusion test (18). Peripheral blood samples for the measurement of renin activity were obtained in every case on two or more separate occasions with the patients recumbent on *ad libitum* sodium intake and off diuretic therapy for at least 5 days. Samples of renal venous blood were also obtained in 19 patients either by retrograde catheterization or at the time of surgery. In addition, in 7 patients the effect of sodium depletion and ambulation on peripheral blood renin activity was studied according to the protocol used for normotensive controls.

On the basis of the results of surgery and of the other diagnostic studies, the patients were divided into the following groups:

1. *Renovascular Hypertension Cured or Improved by Surgery.* Seven were included (Table 2). Renal surgery, i.e., arterioplasty or nephrectomy, on the involved kidney was followed by a significant decrease or return of blood pressure to normal from 6 to 20 months, postoperatively.

2. *Renovascular Hypertension Un-*

improved by Surgery. This group included 4 patients (Table 3) in whom nephrectomy or arterioplasty failed to have any beneficial effect.

3. *Presumptive Renovascular Hypertension.* This group includes 14 patients (Table 4). In 10 patients, no operation was performed due to advanced age, poor general condition, or mildness of the hypertensive process. In 4 patients, surgery was performed and was followed by significant decreases in blood pressure. However, since the postoperative follow-up period included from 2 weeks to 2 months only, the diagnosis of renovascular hypertension is still considered presumptive at this time.

Patients with Kidneys Unequal in Size.

Eight patients (Table 6) were found to have kidneys unequal in size by intravenous pyelography, although renal arteriography was normal in all. Six patients were hypertensive and 2 normotensive. Three patients had unilateral hydronephrosis, one unilateral blunting of the calyces suggestive of pyelonephritis, one nephrosclerosis by renal biopsy of the smaller kidney, while the other 3 patients had no apparent cause of unilateral kidney contraction. One of the patients with unilateral hydronephrosis (W.W., Table 6) was subjected to ureteroplasty and was cured of her hypertension. R. A. was determined in peripheral venous blood in all 8 patients, and in renal venous blood in 7.

Measurement of Renin Activity.

Renin activity (R.A.) was estimated from the angiotensin II released by incubation of plasma or serum, according to the procedure described by Pickens *et al.* (25, 26). The angiotensin II formed during incubation was mea-

sured by its pressor effect in anesthetized ganglion-blocked rats. In each rat several injections of angiotensin II* standards were given to ensure that sensitivity was constant. Subsequently, injections of the unknown samples and standards were given in alternating sequence. Each unknown was assayed at least three times in each of two or three different rats. R. A. was expressed in nanograms (ng) of angiotensin II produced by 10 ml of plasma after 4 hours of incubation.

RESULTS

Normal Controls. The results are listed in Table 1 and illustrated in Figure 1.

On *ad libitum* sodium intake, R. A. of peripheral venous blood averaged 21.5± 2.2 S.E. ng/10 ml during recumbency, and 46.8± 4.2 S.E. ng/10 ml after 4 hours of ambulation. Following sodium restriction, R. A. increased to an average of 67.8± 7.3 S.E. ng/10 ml during recumbency, and to an average of 115± 9.2 S.E. ng/10 ml after 4 hours of ambulation. Both these means were significantly higher ($p < 0.001$) than during *ad libitum* sodium intake. The administration of hydrocholorothiazide produced a further significant increase in R.A., which averaged 406± 62.2 S.E. ng/10 ml during recumbency and 816± 123 S.E. ng/10 ml after ambulation.

Urinary sodium excretion decreased to an average of 12.1 mEq/24 hours after 4 days of sodium restriction, and to an average of 10.8 mEq/24 hours on the fourth day of hydrochlorothiazide administration. The decrease in sodium

---

*Prepared from angiotensin II (Hypertensin, Ciba) standardized against a known concentration of angiotensin research standard A (asp-val-angiotensin II), kindly supplied by Division of Biological Standards, Medical Research Council, London, England.

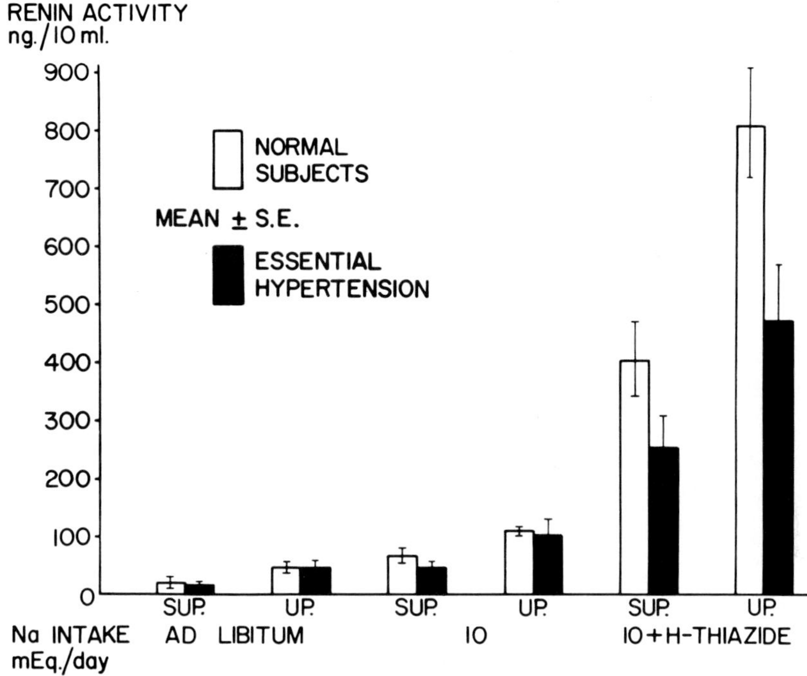

Fig. 1. Renin activity in healthy subjects and patients with essential hypertension supine (Sup.) and upright (Up.) after four hours of ambulation, receiving *ad libitum* and reduced sodium intake.

excretion closely corresponded with an increase in the level of R. A., both during recumbency and after ambulation. Plasma sodium and potassium which averaged 142.6± S.E. 0.8 mEq per liter and 4.6± S.E. 0.07 mEq per liter, respectively, during *ad libitum* sodium intake, either did not change or decreased slightly after sodium restriction and diuretic administration.

Essential Hypertension.

The results are summarized in Table I and illustrated in Figure 1. On *ad libitum* sodium intake, R. A. averaged 17.7± S.E. 2.7 ng/10 ml during recumbency, and 46± S.E. 5.4 ng/10 ml after ambulation. These values did not differ from those of normal subjects. With sodium restriction and administration of hydrochlorothiazide, R. A. increased in 8 patients to levels comparable to those found in normal subjects. However, in 5 patients, 3 of whom were Negroes, R. A. increased much less. In 3 patients, urinary aldosterone excretion ranged from 11.0 to 24.0 μg per 24 hours (normal range: 5 to 32) during unrestricted sodium intake.

Urinary sodium excretion corresponded with the intake of sodium in most patients, and the highest levels of R. A. were found in those excreting less than 20 mEq per 24 hours. Plasma sodium and potassium averaged 141.4 ± S.E. 0.8 mEq per liter and 4.1 ± S.E. 0.2 mEq per liter, respectively, during *ad libitum* sodium intake. With sodium restriction and diuretic administration, the changes were similar to those noted in normal subjects.

TABLE 1—EFFECT OF DIETARY SODIUM RESTRICTION AND DIURETIC ADMINISTRATION ON RENIN ACTIVITY

	Sodium Intake											
	Ad Libitum				*10 mEq/day*				10 mEq/day + Hydrochlorothiazide			
	B. Wt. *kg*	*B.P.* *mm Hg.* *Sup.*	*R.A. ng/10 ml* *Sup.*	*Up.*	*B. Wt.* *kg*	*B.P.* *mm Hg.* *Sup.*	*R.A. ng/10 ml* *Sup.*	*Up.*	*B. Wt.* *kg*	*B.P.* *mm Hg.* *Sup.*	*R.A. ng/10 ml* *Sup.*	*Up.*
Normal Controls												
Mean	70.9	113/72	21.5	46.8	69.3	107/68	67.8	115.3	65.5	108/68	406.0	816.0
±S.E.	3.2		2.2	4.2	0.3		7.3	9.2	0.5		62.2	121.8
Essential Hypertensives												
Mean	71.2	165/108	17.7	46.4	69.6	138/95	44.9	106.2	67.7	134/92	262.3	473.0
±S.E.	2.1		2.7	5.4	0.2		10.2	27.8	0.3		54.2	112.5

B. Wt., body weight.   R.A., renin activity.   Sup., supine.   Up., upright.

TABLE 2—RENIN ACTIVITY IN PATIENTS WITH RENOVASCULAR HYPERTENSION CURED OR IMPROVED BY SURGERY

Pat.,Age/Sex	B.P. mm Hg.	Fundi (K-W)	Renal Arteriogram	R.A. ng/10 ml Renal Vein Involv. Side	Uninv. Side	Differ-ence	Periphe-ral Vein	Surgery	Follow-up B.P. mm Hg.	R.A.† ng/10 ml
P.A.,40/M	190/112	0	Lt. main Art. stenosis	344*			75, 224*	Lt. nephrectomy	6 mos. 160/102	19
P.N.,33/F	204/114	0	Rt. main branch occlusion				46, 176*	Rt. nephrectomy	10 mos. 110/70	20
A.L.,60/M	176/94	I	Rt. main Art. stenosis				12	Rt. nephrectomy	2 yrs. 132/76	36
J.B.,72/M	220/124	II	Lt. main Art. stenosis	1226*			19, 83*	Lt. arterioplasty	6 mos. 150/80	20
R.T.,28/M	198/120	I	Rt. main Art. occlusion	8901*	1133*	7768*	1264,1870*	Rt. arterioplasty	2 yrs. 168/108	
D.W.,46/F	186/109	0	Lt. main Art. stenosis	870*	360*	510*	25, 340*	Lt. nephrectomy	1 yr., 120/80 10 mos.	28
M.B.,46/F	192/100	0	Rt. main Art. stenosis	23,127*	21,48*	2,79*	60	Rt. arterioplasty	1 yr., 120/72 5 mos.	15

R.A., renin activity
*Specimen obtained at surgery
†Peripheral venous blood

TABLE 3—RENIN ACTIVITY IN PATIENTS WITH RENOVASCULAR HYPERTENSION UNIMPROVED BY SURGERY

| Pat.,Age/Sex | B.P. mm Hg. | Fundi (K-W) | Renal Arteriogram | R.A. ng/10 ml | | | | Surgery | Follow-up B.P. mm Hg. | R.A.† ng/10 ml |
| | | | | Renal Vein | | | Periphe-ral Vein | | | |
				Involv. Side	Uninv. Side	Differ-ence				
D.H.,18/M	220/120	IV	Bilat. Art. stenosis Aortic Coarct.	34*	12*	22*	11	Arterioplasty. Died post op. complica-tions		
R.J.,42/F	164/104	I	Rt. main Art. stenosis	180,492*	351,557*	171,65*	195,468*	Rt. nephrectomy	1 yr. 168/108	282
B.C.,45/F	180/120	I	Lt. Art. branch stenosis	8*			7, 7*	Lt. heminephrectomy	2 yrs. 190/110	5
W.S.,61/M	220/120	II	Bilat. Art. stenosis				585	Arterioplasty. Died post op. complica-tions		

R.A., renin activity.
*Specimen obtained at surgery
†Peripheral venous blood

TABLE 4—RENIN ACTIVITY IN PATIENTS WITH PRESUMPTIVE RENOVASCULAR HYPERTENSION

| Pat.,Age/Sex | B.P. mm Hg. | Fundi (K-W) | Renal Arteriogram | R.A. ng/10 ml | | | | Remarks |
| | | | | Renal Vein | | | Periphe-ral Vein | |
				Involv. Side	Uninv. Side	Differ-ence		
D.Z.,47/F	200/98	0	Rt. main Art. occlusion				3353	Died C.V.A., autopsy
V.A.,52/F	180/106	II	Lt. main Art. stenosis				131	Died C.H.F., autopsy
R.A.,66/M	150/80	I	Lt. main Art. occlusion				145	
M.A.,78/F	190/120	I	N.D.				480	Delayed timed Lt. urogram
A.F.,58/M	150/92	II	Lt. main Art. stenosis	20	17	3	26	
G.F.,76/F	192/104	Bilat. Cataracts	Lt. main Art. stenosis	38	27	11	35	
A.B.,54/F	140/86	0	Rt. main Art. stenosis	24	24	0	23	
	130/85	0		37	35	2	35	

TABLE 4—RENIN ACTIVITY IN PATIENTS WITH PRESUMPTIVE RENOVASCULAR HYPERTENSION (Continued)

| Pat.,Age/Sex | B.P. mm Hg. | Fundi (K-W) | Renal Arteriogram | R.A. ng/10 ml | | | | Remarks |
| | | | | Renal Vein | | | Periphe-ral Vein | |
				Involv. Side	Uninv. Side	Differ-ence		
M.S.,32/F	108/68	I	Lt. Art. branch stenosis	10	6	4	11	
G.K.,64/M	222/114	III	Lt. main Art. stenosis				50.4	
M.G.,39/F	206/110	0	Rt. main Art. stenosis	78	54	24	32	
L.E.,44/F	176/104	II	Lt. main Art. stenosis	139,354*	58,168*	81,186*	68,116*	Lt. nephrectomy, 2 mos. post op.
J.T.,25/F	170/118	III	Rt. main Art. stenosis	1034	693	341	725	Rt. arterioplasty, 2 weeks post op.
B.C.,28/F	220/130	0	Rt. main Art. stenosis	1037*	419*	618*	68,150*	Rt. arterioplasty, 1 mo. post op.
C.S.,55/M	204/146	III	Bilat. Art. stenosis greater Lt.	1926*	500*	1426*	184,650*	Lt. arterioplasty, 2 weeks post op.

R.A., renin activity.

TABLE 5—EFFECT OF DIETARY SODIUM RESTRICTION AND DIURETIC ADMINISTRATION ON RENIN ACTIVITY IN PATIENTS WITH RENOVASCULAR HYPERTENSION

Pat.	B.P. mm Hg. Sup.	Sodium Intake						Remarks
		Ad Libitum		10 mEq/day		10 mEq/day + Hydrochlorothiazide		
		R.A. ng/10 ml Sup.	Up.	R.A. ng/10 ml Sup.	Up.	R.A. ng/10 ml Sup.	Up.	
A.L.	176/94	12.4				211.0	410.0	Rt. Art. branch occlusion Rt. nephrect. Cured.
D.W.	175/115	29.2	70.3	64.4	42.3	478.0	1053.0	Lt. main Art. Stenosis. Lt. nephrectomy. Cured
R.J.	157/114	140.0		924.0	1415.0			Rt. main Art. Stenosis. Rt. nephrectomy. Unimproved.
	158/106	153.0	238.0	212.0	452.0			
L.E.	160/100	68.0	150.0	116.0	222.0	128.0	137.0	Lt. main Art. Stenosis.
A.S.	107/70	10.9	31.7	13.3	39.9	94.0	164.0	Lt. Art. branch Stenosis.
A.B.	140/85	29.0	55.2	50.0	136.0	505.0		Rt. main Art. Stenosis.
	120/72	61.0	56.3		68.0	164.0	150.0	
M.G.	210/108	17.4	29.7	25.0	75.5	681.0	1032.0	Rt. main Art. Stenosis.
Mean		57.9	90.1	200.7	306.3	323.0	491.0	
±S.E.		19.1	31.3	133.1	177.5	93.3	196.0	

R.A., renin activity.   Sup., supine.   Up., upright.

TABLE 6—RENIN ACTIVITY IN PATIENTS WITH DIFFERENCES IN SIZE OF KIDNEYS

| Pat.,Age/Sex | B.P. mm Hg. | Fundi (K-W) | Renal Arteriogram | R.A. ng/10 ml | | | | Remarks |
| | | | | Renal Vein | | | | |
				Involv. Side	Uninv. Side	Differ-ence	Periphe-ral Vein	
C.F.,28/F	124/80	0	Normal	31	23	8	21	Urogram small Rt. kidney
N.S.,35/F	148/96	I	Normal	9	16	7	10	Urogram small Lt. kidney
W.W.,30/F	176/120	I	Normal	216	52	164	41	Urogram hydronephrosis on Lt., surgery
	114/78	0		31	27	4	19	Urogram normal 6 mos. post op.
D.W.,34/F	190/120	II	Normal	39	40	1	30	Urogram contracted Rt. kidney
N.D.,29/F	170/100	I	Normal	32	34	2	29	Urogram small Rt. kidney; biopsy nephrosclerosis
M.M.,51/F	126/76	0	Normal				63	Urogram Lt. kidney smaller Rt.
M.W.,50/M	184/110	I	Normal	194	84	110	67	Urogram Lt. hydronephrosis
V.J.,44/F	164/94	I	Normal	77	70	10	62	Urogram Rt. hydronephrosis obstruction UPJ

R.A., renin activity

TABLE 7—RENIN ACTIVITY OF PERIPHERAL VENOUS BLOOD IN
HYPERTENSION ASSOCIATED WITH RENOVASCULAR DISEASE

| | Renin | | | | |
| | Increased | | Normal | | All Cases |
Reference	*Total*	*%*	*Total*	*%*	*Total*
Barraclough *et al.* (1)	6	86	1	14	7
Brown *et al.* (2)	32	73	12	27	44
Cohen *et al.* (5)	5	56	4	44	9
Fitz & Armstrong (12)	9	90	1	10	10
Genest *et al.* (13)	17	68	8	32	25
Gunnels *et al.* (14)	11	100			11
Itskowitz *et al.* (16)	2	50	2	50	4
Pickens *et al.* (25)	1	3	31	97	32
Warzynski *et al.* (31)			5	100	5
Winer *et al.* (32)	10	45	12	55	22
del Greco and Simon (this study)	16	64	9	36	25
Total	119		94		213
Mean		57.7		42.3	

Data listed include all cases with Renovascular Disease and Hypertension studied
regardless of results of surgery, and relate to renin determinations made on blood
samples drawn with patients recumbent. Percent increase relates to renin levels above
upper range of normal or above normal ± twice S.D. where indicated.

Renovascular Hypertension.

1. *Patients Cured or Improved by Surgery.* Preoperatively during recumbency and on *ad libitum* sodium intake, R.A. of peripheral venous blood was increased above normal in 4 patients (range: 46 to 1264 ng/10 ml) and within normal limits in 3 (range: 12 to 25 ng/10 ml) (Table 2). At the time of surgery, blood was sampled from one or both renal veins, and from a peripheral vein in 5 patients. R. A. of renal venous blood was significantly increased in each case, and in 3 patients with bilateral samples R. A. from the ischemic kidneys was from 2.5 to 8 times greater than that from the uninvolved kidney. R. A. of peripheral venous blood was also significantly increased at the time of surgery (range: 83 to 1870 ng per 10 ml).

However, the levels were lower than those found in renal venous blood.

Preoperatively, 2 patients with normal supine R. A. were subjected to sodium restriction as outined above. In both cases (Table 5), R. A. increased significantly in response to sodium restriction and diuretic administration, to an extent similar to that of normal subjects.

Six to 20 months after surgery, R. A. of peripheral venous blood was normal in 6 patients available for sampling.

2. *Patients Unimproved by Surgery.* Preoperatively, R. A. of peripheral venous blood was markedly increased in 2 patients and normal in the other 2 (Table 3). R. A. of renal venous blood was also normal in the latter 2 patients, but significantly elevated bilaterally in another with unilateral renal artery

stenosis. In this patient (R.J.), preoperative sodium restriction (Table 5) caused a significant increase in R. A. of peripheral venous blood to ranges similar to those of normal subjects.

After surgery, 2 patients died of various complications and 2 remained hypertensive. In one, R. A. of peripheral venous blood is still normal, and in the other still elevated, 18 to 20 months postoperatively, respectively.

3. *Patients with Presumptive Renovascular Hypertension.* In 8 patients (Table 4), R. A. of peripheral venous blood was significantly greater than that of essential hypertensives (range: 50 to 3353 ng per 10 ml). In 4 of these patients recently subjected to surgery, R. A. of renal venous blood was markedly increased preoperatively and the differences between the involved and uninvolved side ranged from 81 to 1426 ng/10 ml.

By contrast, R. A. of peripheral venous blood was normal in the other 6 patients included in this group (Table 4). R. A. of renal venous blood was also normal bilaterally in 4 of these patients, but increased above normal in another patient especially on the involved side.

Four patients were subjected to sodium restriction and diuretic administration (Table 5). In each case, this combination effected an increase in R. A. of peripheral venous blood, which was most marked in 2 patients.

Patients with Kidneys Unequal in Size.
The results are summarized in Table 6. In 4 patients, R. A. was normal in the peripheral as well as renal venous blood from both kidneys. However, in 4 patients, R. A. of peripheral venous blood was slightly to moderately increased above normal (range: 41 to 67

ng per 10 ml). In one of these patients (V.J.), R. A. of renal venous blood was equally increased bilaterally, while in 2 (M.W., W.W.) with unilateral hydronephrosis R. A. was markedly greater on the involved side. In one of these latter patients (W.W.), subjected to ureteroplasty, the blood pressure decreased to normal levels six months after surgery, at which time R. A. of peripheral and renal venous blood was also normal.

Discussion

The findings in normotensive subjects document the importance of physical activity and sodium metabolism in influencing the level of renin activity. The data are in accord with those reported by others (4, 9). The results in patients with essential hypertension reveal that although the response of renin activity to ambulation and sodium depletion was largely similar to that found in normotensive controls, there were notable differences. In particular, in five patients the response of renin activity to ambulation and sodium depletion was decreased or suppressed. The urinary excretion of aldosterone in three of these patients, and the secretory rate in one of them, were all within normal limits during *ad libitum* sodium intake. Thus, it does not seem likely that decreased renin activity after sodium depletion is always attributable to primary aldosteronism. It is notable that in a recent study of essential hypertensives by Kuchel *et al.* (19) 12 out of 29 patients exhibited little increase or no change in renin activity in response to diazoxide injection, or upright posture and sodium depletion. In 5 patients, aldosterone secretion rates were normal, and in 2 subnormal. Helmer and Judson (15) have expressed the view that decreased renin activity in hypertensive patients is probably due to excessive sodium retention and expansion of blood volume, rather than to underlying aldosteronism. Racial and socio-economic factors as shown by Creditor *et al.* (8), may also play a role in the decreased response of renin activity to the stimulus of upright posture and low salt diet. Thus, although the determination of renin activity in patients with suspected primary aldosteronism is of value (2, 6, 7, 9, 21), generalizations are not warranted. As shown by this and other recent studies (14, 15, 19, 20), in the hypertensive population suppression of renin activity seems far more common than primary aldosteronism.

As regards renovascular disease with hypertension, the measurement of renin activity in the blood may prove especially rewarding, provided that the conditions present at the time of sampling are carefully controlled (5, 13). In the course of this study, we found that patients with proven or presumptive renovascular hypertension responded to salt depletion and erect posture with increases in renin activity of the peripheral blood to levels similar to those found in normal subjects and essential hypertensives studied under identical conditions. At any rate, the findings of increased levels of renin activity in the peripheral blood of patients with reno-vascular disease and hypertension on normal salt intake and maintained supine prior to sampling is of value (13) in most cases. Combined with the results of other studies, i.e., renal arteriography and split function (27, 28, 29), increased renin activity can lead to the correct diagnosis. On the other hand, the finding of normal renin activity in the peripheral venous blood does not exclude the renal arterial lesion as being of

functional significance. In two of the patients described previously who were cured by surgery, renin activity was normal in the peripheral blood but greatly increased in the renal venous blood from the involved kidney. In a combined series of 213 patients with renovascular disease and hypertension reported by several investigators (Table 7), 94 were found to have normal levels of renin or renin activity in the peripheral venous blood. In such cases, as initially proposed by Judson and Helmer (17), by Genest *et al.* (13), and more recently demonstrated by Winer *et al.* (32) and Michelakis *et al.* (22), renin activity should be determined in blood sampled from each kidney. This is especially necessary not only in cases with equivocal features of unilateral renal arterial, but also in cases with bilateral arterial lesions. One of our patients (R.J.) listed in Table 3 deserves comment. Preoperatively, renal arteriography and split function studies were consistent with stenosis of the right main renal artery. Renin activity was significantly increased above normal in the peripheral blood, and similar to the level found in the right renal venous blood. However, renin activity was even greater in the venous blood from the left kidney. In view of these findings, the failure of right nephrectomy to benefit the patient's hypertension might have been anticipated.

In four of the patients with presumptive renovascular hypertension, there was very little difference in the levels of renin activity of renal venous blood, although the results of arteriography and split function were consistent with functionally significant renovascular disease. Whether these represent false negative renal renin assays, or indicate that surgery would not be beneficial to these patients, cannot be determined at this time.

In two of the patients with unilateral hydronephrosis and hypertension of recent onset, renin activity was increased in the peripheral venous blood and even more so in the renal venous blood from the involved side. No renal arterial lesions could be demonstrated by arteriography in either of these patients. The dramatic fall in blood pressure along with the decrease of peripheral renin activity to normal levels which occurred in one of the patients subjected to ureteroplasty suggest that the renal pressor system may be involved in the mechanism of hypertension associated with hydronephrosis (30).

SUMMARY

The effect of dietary sodium restriction (10 mEq per day) alone and in combination with diuretic therapy, and of body posture on renin activity of peripheral venous blood has been studied in healthy subjects and in patients with essential hypertension. Eight of 13 patients responded to sodium restriction, diuretic therapy, and upright posture with significant increases in renin activity similar to those of healthy subjects studied under identical conditions. In the remaining 5 patients, the response of renin activity was distinctly less marked. Urinary aldosterone excretion in 3 of these patients, and the secretory rate in one of them, were within normal limits during unrestricted sodium intake.

Renin activity in peripheral venous blood was increased above normal in 14 of 25 patients with renovascular hypertension. Renin activity in renal venous blood was usually increased much more, and the highest values were found in the blood from the involved kidney.

Renin activity in peripheral venous blood was increased above normal in 4 of 8 patients with kidneys unequal in size and hypertension. In 2 of 3 patients with unilateral hydronephrosis, renin activity of renal venous blood was significantly greater on the involved than uninvolved side.

REFERENCES

1. Barraclough, M. A., Bacchus, B., Brown, J. J., Davies, D. L., Lever, A. F., and Robertson, J. I. S.: Plasma renin and aldosterone secretion in hypertensive patients with renal or renal artery lesions. Lancet, *2*:1310-1313, 1965.
2. Brown, J. J., Davies, D. L., Lever, A. F., Robertson, J. I. S., Bianchi, G., Imbs, J. L., Johnson, V. W., Lawrence, M., Fraser, R., and James, V. H. T.: Renin and blood pressure. Proc. III Internat. Congr. Nephrology, Edit. Handler, J. S. Basel & New York, Karger, 1967. Vol. 1: pp. 226-239.
3. Brown, J. J., Davies, D. L., Lever, A. F., and Robertson, J.I.S.: Plasma renin concentration in human hypertension. II. Renin in relation to aetiology. Brit. Med. J., *2*:1215-1219, 1965.
4. Cohen, E. L., Conn, J. W., and Rovner, D. R.: Postural augmentation of plasma renin activity and aldosterone excretion in normal people. J. Clin. Invest., *46*:418-428, 1967.
5. Cohen, E. L., Rovner, D. R., and Conn, J. W.: Postural Augmentation of plasma renin activity. Importance in diagnosis of renovascular hypertension. J.A.M.A., *197*:973-978, 1966.
6. Conn, J. W.: Plasma renin activity in primary aldosteronism. J.A.M.A., *190*:222-235, 1964.
7. Conn, J. W., Rovner, D. R., Cohen, E. L., and Nesbit, R. M.: Normokalemic primary aldosteronism: Its masquerade as "essential" hypertension. J.A.M.A., *195*:21-26, 1966.
8. Creditor, M. C., and Loschky, U. K.: Plasma renin activity in hypertension. Am. J. Med., *43*:371-382, 1967.
9. de Champlain, J., Genest, J., Veyrat, R., and Boucher, R.: Factors controlling renin in man. Arch. Int. Med., *117*:355-363, 1966.
10. del Greco, F., Simon, N. M., Goodman, S., and Roguska, J.: Plasma renin activity in primary and secondary hypertension. Medicine *46*:475-490, 1967.
11. Eyler, W. R., Clark, M. D., Garman, J. P., Ryan, R. L., and Meininger, D. E.: Angiography of the renal areas including a comparative study of renal arterial stenoses in patients with and without hypertension. Radiology, *87*:879-891, 1962.

12. Fitz, A. E. and Armstrong, M. L.: Plasma vasoconstrictor activity in patients with renal malignant and primary hypertension. Circulation, *29*:409-414, 1964.

13. Genest, J., Remblay, G. Y., Boucher, R., de Champlain, J., Rojo Ortega, J. M., Lefebvre, R., Roy, P., and Cartier, P.: Diagnostic significance of humoral factors in renovascular hypertension. In, Gross, F. (ed.): Antihypertensive Therapy. Berlin-Heidelberg-New York, Springer-Verlag, 1966, pp. 518-540

14. Gunnels, J. C., Grim, C. E., Robinson, R. R., and Wildermann, N. M.: Plasma renin activity in healthy subjects and patients with hypertension. Arch. Int. Med., *119*:232-245, 1967

15. Helmer, O. M., and Judson, W. E.: Metabolic studies on hypertensive patients with low plasma renin activity not due to hyperaldosteronism. Circulation, Supplem. II (Vol. *36*): 140, 1967.

16. Itskowitz, H. D., Dudrick, S. J., Doyrda, I., and Murphy, J. J.: Plasma angiotensinase activity in hypertensive patients. Arch. Int. Med., *119*:241-246, 1967.

17. Judson, W. E., and Helmer, O. M.: Diagnostic and prognostic values of renin activity in renal venous plasma in renovascular hypertension. In, Rodbard, S., Sapirstein, L. A., and Wood, J. E., III (eds.): Hypertension, Vol. XIII. New York, American Heart Assoc., 1965, pp. 79-89.

18. Kaplan, N. M., and Silah, J. G.: The angiotensin infusion test, a new approach to the differential diagnosis of renovascular hypertension. New Eng. J. Med., *271*:536-541, 1964.

19. Kuchel, O., Fishman, O. M., Liddle, G. W., and Michelakis, A.: Effect of diazoxide on plasma renin activity in hypertensive patients. Ann. Int. Med., *67*:719-799, 1967.

20. Laragh, J. H., Sealey, J. E., and Sommers, S. C.: Patterns of adrenal secretion and urinary excretion of aldosterone and plasma renin activity in normal and hypertensive subjects. Circulation Research, Supplem. I (vol. *18* & *19*): 158-174, 1966.

21. Lauler, D. P.: Preoperative diagnosis of primary aldosteronism. Am. J. Med., *41*:855-863, 1966.

22. Michelakis, A. M., Foster, J. H., Liddle, G. W., Rhamy, R. K., Kuchel, O., and Gordon, R. D.: Measurement of renin in both renal veins. Arch. Int. Med., *120*:444-448, 1967.

23. Page, I. H., Dustan, H. P., and Bumpus, F. M.: A commentary on the measurement of renin and angiotensin. Circulation, *32*:513-514, 1965.

24. Peart, W. S.: The renin-angiotensin system. **Pharmacol. Rev., *17*:143-182, 1965.**

25. Pickens, P. T., Oxon, B. M., Dustan, H. P., Bumpus, F. M., and Page, I. H.: Measurement of plasma renin activity in hypertension. In Rodbard, S., Sapirstein, L. A., and Wood, J. E., III (eds.): Hypertension, Vol. XIII. New York, American Heart Assoc., 1965, pp. 90-98.

26. Pickens, P. T., Bumpus, F. M., Lloyd, A. M., Smeby, R. R., and Page, I. H.: Measurement of **renin activity in human plasma. Circulation Res.,** *17*:438-448, 1965.

27. Roguska, J., Simon, N. M., and del Greco, F.: Pressor response to angiotensin II in hypertension: Correlation with plasma renin activity and response to norepinephrine and metaraminol. **Am. J. Cardio., *21*:705-713, 1968.**

28. Simon, N. M., del Greco, F., and O'Conor, V. J., Jr.: Differential renal function studies during mannitol diuresis in hypertension. Circulation, *33*:789-795, 1966.

29. Stamey, T. A., Nudelman, I. J., Good, P. H., Schwenker, F. N., and Hendriks, F.: Functional characteristics of renovascular hypertension. Medicine, *40*:347-394, 1961.

30. Vander, A. J.: Control of renin release. Physiological Rev., *47*:359-382, 1967.

31. Warzynski, E., Demirjian, Y., and Hoobler, S.: Method for the determination of "renin" in blood and some preliminary findings. Canad. M. A. J., *90*:225-227, 1964.

32. Winer, B. M., Lubble, W. F., Simon, M., and Williams, J. A.: Renin in the diagnosis of renovascular hypertension. J.A.M.A., *202*:121-128, 1967.

ACKNOWLEDGMENTS

We wish to thank Drs. J. Roguska and S. Steiner for their support and assistance in performing many of the present studies, and Dr. W. E. Wagner, Ciba Pharmaceuticals Inc., Summit, N. Y., for generous supplies of Hypertensin. Misses A. Gomoll and S. Goodman provided skillful assistance in performing the assays of **renin activity.**

Chapter 42

Hypertension in Unilateral Renal Disease

J. M. BRIAN O'CONNELL, M.B., JAMES M. HAYES, M.D., and GEORGE E. SCHREINER, M.D.

The only currently proved pathogenetic mechanism by which unilateral renal disease, i.e., unilateral renal disease with a normal undiseased controlateral kidney, can induce secondary hypertension is through activation of the renin-angiotensin system. The following subjects will be reviewed in this chapter: 1) Assessment of whether or not there is activation of the renin-angiotensin system in patients with unilateral renal disease; 2) Consideration of unilateral renal conditions that have been proved or assumed to be associated with the activation of the renin-angiotensin system; 3) Prognostication as to whether or not unilateral renal disease with proved activation of the renin-angiotensin system will respond to corrective surgery.

Many stimuli (upright posture, salt restriction, volume depletion, renovascular constriction, ureteral obstruction) have been shown to activate the renin-angiotensin system. Common to all such stimuli is an alteration in renal hemodynamics usually but not invariably accompanied by a decrease in renal blood flow (1, 2, 3, 4, 5). This alteration in renal hemodynamics causes or is accompanied by the classical functional changes of renal ischemia, namely, a decrease in urine volume, an increase in the urinary concentration of nonreabsorbable solutes and usually a decrease in urinary concentration of sodium, glomerular filtration rate and renal plasma flow. As a result of the alteration in renal hemodynamics and/or the ischemic renal function changes, there is an increased release of renin usually accompanied by an elevation in peripheral renin (3, 4). If the alteration in renal hemodynamics is severe and of chronic duration, the involved kidney will usually be reduced in size and the contralateral normal kidney will show compensatory hypertrophy.

All current tests for assessing activation of the renin-angiotensin system in unilateral renal disease are based on demonstrating the physiological changes in the abnormal kidney. These tests are listed in Table I. Generally, they will be uniformly positive in main renal arterial lesions, and less so in segmental arterial disease. In the case of pyelonephritic or poorly functioning kidneys, renin measurements may be the only ones of diagnostic value. The intravenous pyelo-

TABLE I—TESTS FOR ASSESSING ACTIVATION OF THE RENIN–ANGIOTENSIN SYSTEM

1. Timed sequence intravenous pyelogram—noting appearance time, renal size, pyelogram concentration, ureteral notching, disappearance time (6).
2. Renal isotope studies—I^{131} Hippuran renogram and sequential scans, Hg^{203} uptake and scans, sequential technetium^{99} scans (7, 8).
3. Split renal function studies—V/min, U non-reabsorb solute (urea, creatinine, inulin, PAH), U_{Na}, C_{IN}, C_{PAH} (9, 10).
4. Renin measurements—Peripheral blood in upright posture on normal salt diet—bilateral renal venous blood before and after acute stimulation of renin-angiotensin system (11, 12).
5. Aortography or selective renal arteriography.

gram and renal isotope studies are used as large scale screening studies. Split renal function studies are used to document more precisely that a renal abnormality is truly ischemic. Peripheral and renal venous renin measurements are made to confirm that there is increased secretion of renin and that the diseased kidney is the source of this increase. Aortography gives little functional information and its greatest value is as a preoperative test to determine the type of surgical intervention, i.e., plastic repair of renal artery or nephrectomy.

The various unilateral renal diseases that have been associated with reversible hypertension are listed in Table II. The vast majority of such cases have been diseases of the renal vasculature, mostly atheromatous disease and fibromuscular hyperplasia, with such entities as renal

TABLE II—UNILATERAL RENAL DISEASES CAUSING REVERSIBLE HYPERTENSION

1. Renovascular abnormalities—varied etiologies.
2. Chronic pyelonephritis.
3. Hydronephrosis.
4. Tuberculosis

aneurysm, renal AV fistula, renal embolism, renal infarction, etc. making up a much smaller number. In a high percentage of these diseases, activation of the renin-angiotensin system has been well documented and corrective surgery has been reasonably successful. Less common causes of reversible hypertension are unilateral chronic pyelonephritis, hydronephrosis and tuberculosis. In these conditions, activation of the renin-angiotensin system is assumed rather than well proven. Most patients with unilateral chronic pyelonephritis and hypertension show a poorer response of their hypertension to nephrectomy (13, 14). Those who have shown a good response, in general, have had more severe degrees of arteriolarsclerosis in the involved kidney. Unfortunately, no renin data are yet available in this group to indicate activation of the renin-angiotensin system and to suggest which patients might benefit from nephrectomy. Unilateral hydronephrosis is an uncommon cause of reversible hypertension but is probably more frequent than is presently recognized. Acute ureteral obstruction has been well documented as a cause of renin release. Thus, in young dogs with experimental unilateral hydronephrosis, a high percentage will develop hypertension (4, 5, 15). Del Greco has recently studied a patient with hypertension and unilateral hydronephrosis and has reported increased release of renin from the hydronephrotic kidney (16). Following corrective surgery for the hydronephrosis, both the hypertension and the increased release of renin returned to normal. These studies support involvement of the renin-angiotensin system in the etiology of hypertension with hydronephrosis but more work needs to be done in this area. Renal tuberculosis is a rare cause of hypertension but it is one cause that has a relatively high cure rate—70%. (17) Classically, tuberculous kidneys are autonephrectomized with severe sclerosis and obliteration of the major renal arteries including the main stem artery. These vascular lesions might be predicted to stimulate release of renin but to date no renin measurements are available on any of these patients.

In spite of meticulous investigation and reasonable documentation of activation of the renin-angiotensin system in unilaterally diseased kidneys, the overall results of corrective surgery in this group of patients is far from ideal. Cure rates in most series range from 50% to 100% with an average of approximately 70% (18, 19). In younger patients, the results tend to be better while in the older age group the reverse holds true. Because of this, and the relatively good results with drug therapy, many centers now try to avoid corrective surgery in the elderly renovascular hypertensive patient.

The currently used prognostic tests for unilateral hypertensive renal disease are listed in Table III. The most generally accepted reason for the lack of response to corrective surgery in the renovascular hypertensive patient is that over a period of time the hypertension has induced disease of the small vessels in the contralateral kidney. At this point, the contralateral kidney will sustain the hypertension even if the diseased kidney is removed and so result in a poor surgical result. Vetes *et al.* have performed renal biopsies of contralateral kidneys in renovascular hypertensive patients and have shown good correlation with poor surgical response and the presence of moderate to severe arteriolar sclerosis (20, 21). Since there is a great risk in the biopsy of a patient's only normal kidney, this technique of prognostication is little used. To provide the same information with a lesser risk to the patient, Stamey has proposed the measurement of renal plasma flow from the normal kidney (22). He showed good correlation of the surgical and biopsy findings with the level of renal plasma flow from the normal kidney. When the renal plasma flow was greater than 200 ml per min, surgical results were good and the kidney showed minimal or no arteriolarsclerosis. When the renal plasma flow was less than 200 ml per min, surgical results were poor and the kidneys showed moderate to severe arteriolarsclerosis. The most exciting recent development in this area is the isolation by Smeby *et al.* of a naturally occurring renin-renin substrate inhibitor (23, 24). *In vitro* this phospholipid blocks renin-renin substrate reaction, and *in vivo* it reduces the blood pressure of renal hypertensive rats. When purified and introduced clinically, this material should be of potential prognostic value in predicting the outcome of corrective surgery. In those patients who are poor surgical risks, use of this compound may be of therapeutic value.

TABLE III—PROGNOSTIC TESTS
IN UNILATERAL HYPERTENSIVE
RENAL DISEASE

1. Biopsy of the normal kidney for evidence of moderate to severe arteriolarsclerosis.
2. Measurement of renal plasma flow in normal kidney.
3. Renin-Renin substrate inhibitor.

REFERENCES

1. Conn, J. W., Rovner, D. R., and Cohen, E. L.: Normal and altered function of the renin-angiotensin-aldosterone system in man. Ann. Int. Med., *63*:266, 1965.

2. Brown, J. J., Davies, D. L., Lever, A. F., Robertson, J. I. S., and Verniory, A.: The effect of acute hemorrhage in the dog and man on plasma renin concentration. J. Physiol., London, *182*:649, 1966.

3. Skinner, S. L., McCubbin, J. W., and Page, I. H.: Control of renin secretion. Circulation Res., *15*:64, 1964.

4. Vander, A. J., and Miller, R.: Control of renin secretion in the anesthetized dog. Am. J. Physiol., *207*:537, 1964.

5. Vander, A. J.: Control of renin release. Physiol. Rev., *47*:359, 1967.

6. Kaufman, J. J., Schanche, A. F., and Maxwell, M. H.: Excretory urography in the diagnosis of renovascular hypertension: methods of enhancing its value. J. Urol., *89*:498, 1963.

7. Winter, C. C.: Renogram and other radioisotope tests in the diagnosis of renal hypertension. Am. J. Surg., *107*:43, 1964.

8. Reba, R. C., McAfee, J. G., and Wagner, H. N.: Radiomercury-labelled chlormerodrin for in vivo uptake studies and scintilation scanning of unilateral renal lesions associated with hypertension. Medicine, *42*:269, 1963.

9. Howard, J. E., and Connor, T. B.: Use of differential renal function studies in the diagnosis of renovascular hypertension. Amer. J. Surg., *107*:58, 1964.

10. Stamey, T. A., Nudelman, I. J., Good, P. H., Schwentker, F. N., and Henricks, F.: Functional characteristics of renovascular hypertension. Medicine, *40*:347, 1961.

11. Cohen, E. L., Rovner, D. R., and Conn, J. W.: Postural augmentation of plasma renin activity: importance in diagnosis of renovascular hypertension. J.A.M.A., *197*:973, 1966.

12. Kaneko, Y., Ikeda, T., Takeda, T., and Ueda, H.: Renin release during acute reduction in arterial pressure in normotensive subjects and patients with renovascular hypertension. J. Clin. Invest., *46*:705, 1967.

13. Crocker, D. W., Newton, R. A., and Harrison, J. H.: Results of surgical management of unilateral pyelonephritis with hypertension. Am. J. Surg., *110*:405, 1965.

14. Birbari, A. E., Howard, F. A., Crocker, D. W., Lauler, D. P., Harrison, J. H., Crane, C., Vagnucci, A. I., and Hickler, R. B.: Comparison of unilateral pyelonephritis and unilateral renal artery stenosis associated with hypertension. Am. J. Surg., *109*:715, 1965.

15. Silk, M. R.: Hypertension secondary to hydronephrosis in adult and young animals. Invest. Urol., *5*:30, 1967.

16. Del Greco, F., and Simon, N. M.: Clinical significance of the renal pressor system.. Chapter *41* of this book.

17. Kaufman, J. J., and Goodwin, W. E.: Renal hypertension secondary to renal tuberculosis. Am. J. Med., *38*:337, 1965.

18. Perloff, D., Sokolow, M., Wylie, E. J., and Palubinkas, A. J.: Renal vascular hypertension—further experiences. Am. Heart J., *74*:614, 1967.

19. Hunt, J. C., Bernatz, P. E., and Harrison, E. G. Jr.: Factors determining diagnosis and choice of treatment of renovascular hypertension. Circulation Res., *21*(Suppl. II):211, 1967.

20. Vertes, V., and Grauel, J. A.: Observations on renovascular hypertension. The role of renal biopsy. Circulation, *28*:536, 1963.

21. Vertes, V., Grauel, J. A., and Goldblatt, H.: Studies of patients with renovascular hypertension undergoing vascular surgery. New Engl. J. Med., *272*:186, 1965.

22. Stamey, T. A.: Renovascular hypertension—1965. Am. J. Med., *38*:829, 1965.

23. Sen, S., Smeby, R. R., and Bumpus, F. M.: Isolation of a phospholipid renin inhibitor from kidney. Biochemistry. *6*:1572, 1967.

24. Smeby, R. R., Sen, S., and Bumpus, F. M.: Naturally occurring renin inhibitor. Circulation Res., *21* (Suppl. II), II-129, 1967.

Chapter 43

Current Concepts of Urinary Tract Infection

ROBERT H. HEPTINSTALL, M.D.

This chapter presents no new advances in concepts of urinary tract infection. Rather, the chapter is a plea to take a closer look at what is being called "chronic pyelonephritis," and to emphasize the importance of the pyelo part of the name (3).

Acute infections of the urinary tract include infection of the pelvis of the kidney, and originally the condition that was—and still is—prevalent among girls and young women was called pyelitis. It soon became apparent to the pathologist that the infection was not confined to the pelvis but that it also involved the parenchyma. For this reason, the name was changed to pyelonephritis. This had the great merit that attention was focussed on the more widespread nature of the infection, but it very soon led to the belief that a pure pyelitis could not exist, and certainly as far as the pathologist was concerned his energies and interests were deviated toward the parenchymal changes. Although the concept of acute pyelonephritis had been enunciated, several years elapsed before the entity of chronic pyelonephritis was appreciated. It is of interest that Wagner in 1882 appears to have separated chronic pyelonephritis off from the main body of contracted kidneys (7), but his observations made little impact. Its subsequent rise to fame (or notoriety) was meteoric, and over the years it became one of the most fashionable diagnoses in the pathologist's repertoire. This enthusiasm was shared by the clinicians.

There are certain reasons why suspicion should be cast upon the apparently great frequency of chronic pyelonephritis. It should be clearly understood at the outset, that in using the term chronic pyelonephritis reference is made to the end result of a bacterial infection of the kidney.

In the first place, a scrutiny of the various papers which have recorded the incidence of chronic pyelonephritis in an autopsy population show considerable variation. This would indicate that different criteria are being used for the evaluation of the diagnosis.

In the second place, the observations of Kleeman and Freedman (5) are most pertinent. They noted that clinically, acute pyelonephritis occurred predominantly in females, yet when they studied the autopsy protocols in their hospital it was found that chronic pyelonephritis occurred just as often in the male as in the female. This was all the more striking when it is considered that they excluded all cases with overt obstruction thereby eliminating the group of elderly men with prostatic obstruction. The inference to be drawn from this study is that there are causes other than bacterial infection for the morphologic picture of chronic pyelonephritis.

Third, a study of the type of renal pathology in patients presenting for renal transplantation indicated that chronic glomerulonephritis was a more common cause of chronic renal failure than chronic pyelonephritis (1). This is a most important study for it gives an indication of the incidence of *significant* chronic pyelonephritis; many of the papers on the incidence of chronic pyelonephritis make no distinction between significant renal involvement and small focal areas of what are regarded as chronic infection.

Fourth, it is apparent on reading many articles and listening to many talks on renal pathology, particularly studies on renal biopsies, that chronic pyelonephritis is being diagnosed with reckless abandon and without any appreciation that other conditions may produce similar parenchymal changes.

CRITERIA TO BE ADOPTED FOR THE DIAGNOSIS OF CHRONIC PYELONEPHRITIS

It would be helpful at this stage to define the changes that are present in the kidney in chronic pyelonephritis.

By virtue of the fact that the great majority of cases of acute pyelonephritis are caused by gram-negative bacilli, and because these almost invariably reach the kidney by the ascending route (the evidence for this is reviewed elsewhere (2)), lesions are to be anticipated in the pelvi-calyceal system and the overlying parenchyma. This focally occurring acute inflammation spreads out into the parenchyma to produce triangular areas of involvement. Renal tissue is destroyed during the acute phase and heals with the production of a coarse depression of the subcapsular surface, the result of a considerable thinning of parenchyma accompanied by a widening and blunting of the affected calyces (4, 6). The resultant picture of a dilated calyx with an overlying scar is quite distinctive and not mimicked by any other process. The numbers of calyces so affected varies, sometimes only one or two situated at one or other pole are abnormal; on other occasions, several may be involved. The pathological diagnosis of chronic pyelonephritis is therefore made on the gross organ. The histological changes in the scars are varied. The main damage is to the tubules which may in extreme instances have disappeared completely, or have become so altered that large numbers of them lie side by side lined by low epithelium with eosinophilic casts in the lumens, an appearance resembling thyroid tissue. The glomeruli show a variety of changes; some are apparently unchanged, others may show a change consisting of a shrinkage of the tuft with a laying down of collagen-like material inside Bowman's capsule, while some show periglomerular fibrosis. In cases attended by hypertension, there may be necrotizing lesions or areas of cellular proliferation in glomeruli. The arteries may show intimal thickening with reduction of the lumen; this is found particularly in cases with hypertension. The interstitial tissue shows fibrosis and variable numbers of lymphocytes and plasma cells. In less severely involved parts of the parenchyma there may be merely atrophy of tubules, such as is seen in ischemic kidneys while many areas show no change at all. The calyceal epithelium has numerous chronic inflammatory cells on its under surface, a change seen also in the pelvic epithelium.

OTHER CONDITIONS SHOWING SIMILAR HISTOLOGICAL PICTURE

a) Ischemia

It will be apparent from the description that virtually all of these histological changes may be seen in the ischemic kidney. The only change that is not seen is the characteristic calyceal dilatation associated with an overlying area of thinned scarred parenchyma. Many of the kidneys diagnosed in the past as chronic pyelonephritis have undoubtedly been of an ischemic origin. This is particularly true of what have been alleged to be chronic pyelonephritic changes in the diabetic kidney. While infections of the kidney undoubtedly occur in the kidney of diabetics, the changes, usually attributed to chronic infection are much more satisfactorily explained on the basis of ischemia caused by the considerable degree of renal arterio- and arteriolo-sclerosis seen in this state.

b) Chronic Insterstitial Nephritis

This is a term that is used to describe a kidney in which there has been extensive tubular loss, interstitial fibrosis and infiltration with chronic inflammatory cells, but with no glomerular alteration of the type seen in glomerulonephritis. There are many causes of this type of change, such as analgesic abuse, hypersensitivity to certain drugs, irradiation injury, Balkan nephritis, certain type of hereditary nephritis, etc. In spite of the fact that these changes are identical histologically with the changes that may occur in chronic pyelonephritis, the

calyceal deformity and its related scar are confined to the latter condition.

c) Obstruction

Histologically, the changes seen in simple non-infected hydronephrosis may be indistinguishable from chronic pyelonephritis. However, gross inspection reveals a generalized dilatation of the pelvi-calyceal system with a uniform narrowing of the parenchyma.

CONCLUSIONS

Much greater caution is required in the diagnosis of chronic pyelonephritis than has been shown in the past. The pathologist is largely to blame for the uncritical and indiscriminate way in which the condition is diagnosed by concentrating too much on changes in the parenchyma and ignoring those in the pelvi-calyceal system. The gross examination of the kidney is of the utmost importance, and a judicious choosing of blocks essential as a preliminary to microscopy. The limitations of the renal biopsy in the diagnosis of chronic pyelonephritis are apparent.

REFERENCES

1. Gault, M. H. and Dossetor, J. B.: Chronic pyelonephritis: relative evidence in transplant recipients. New Engl. J. Med., *275:*813, 1966.
2. Heptinstall, R. H.: Pathology of the Kidney. Boston, Little, Brown, 1966. P. 397.
3. Heptinstall, R. H.: The limitations of the pathological diagnosis of chronic pyelonephritis. In, Black, D.A.K. (ed): Renal Disease, 2nd ed. Oxford, Blackwell, p350, 1967.
4. Hodson, C. J.: Radiological diagnosis of pyelonephritis. Proc. Roy. Soc. Med., *52:*669, 1959.
5. Kleeman, S.E.T., and Freedman, L. R.: The finding of chronic pyelonephritis in males and females at autopsy. New Engl. J. Med.,*263:*988, 1960.
6. Smith, J. F.: The diagnosis of the scars of chronic pyelonephritis. J. Clin. Path., *15:*522, 1962.
7. Wagner, E. L.: Handbuch der Krankheiten des Harnapparates: I. Hälfte. Der Morbus Brightii. In, von Ziemssen, H. W. (Ed.): Handbuch der speciellen Pathologie und Therapie, 3rd ed. Leipzig, Vogel, 1882. Vol. 9, pt. 1, p. 309.

Chapter 44

Renal Complications of Diabetes Mellitus

BENJAMIN H. SPARGO, M.D., and ROBERTA PENKSA

The renal complications of diabetes mellitus may take a variety of forms that differ not only as to the structure involved but also as to the clinical significance. There is little question that despite increased efforts for more extensive screening procedures with a resultant earlier detection of diabetes mellitus and a general emphasis on improved medical management, the severity and frequency of renal lesions has not decreased. The proper documentation of this problem must take into consideration the wide spectrum of pathologic changes included in this category and the clarification of the incidence, pattern and natural history of each. Since it is now generally accepted that the study of serial renal biopsies can illuminate the natural history of disease, reliable identification of specific lesions utilizing ultrastructural observations should clarify prognosis and perhaps improve the evaluation of effects of different therapies on the progress of the organ pathology. Recent reviews by Kimmelstiel, *et al.* (23) and Churg *et al.* (10) include detailed ultrastructural studies and have comprehensive bibliographies.

TABLE I—RENAL LESIONS OF
DIABETIC NEPHROPATHY

1. Glomerular
    Nodular cellular—KW (Figs. 2, 3, 4)
    Diffuse (Fig. 7, 8)
    Microaneurysms
    Nodular acellular—exudative (Fig. 9)

2. Arterial
    Small—afferent and efferent arteriole
        (Figs. 10, 12)
    Medium—arteriosclerosis

3. Tubular
    Glycogen vacuolization—Armanni-Ebstein

4. Interstitial
    Pyelonephritis
    Necrotizing papillitis (Fig. 13)

NODULAR DIABETIC GLOMERULOSCLEROSIS

This lesion, first associated with the clinical syndrome by Kimmelstiel and Wilson (25), is accepted as reliably related to diabetes mellitus (Figs. 2, 3, 4). The nodules which may be either occasional or numerous are round or oval with a central lobular mass. This is distinct from axial extensions of hyaline from the arterioles. Residual nuclei representing mesangial cells may be frequent throughout the

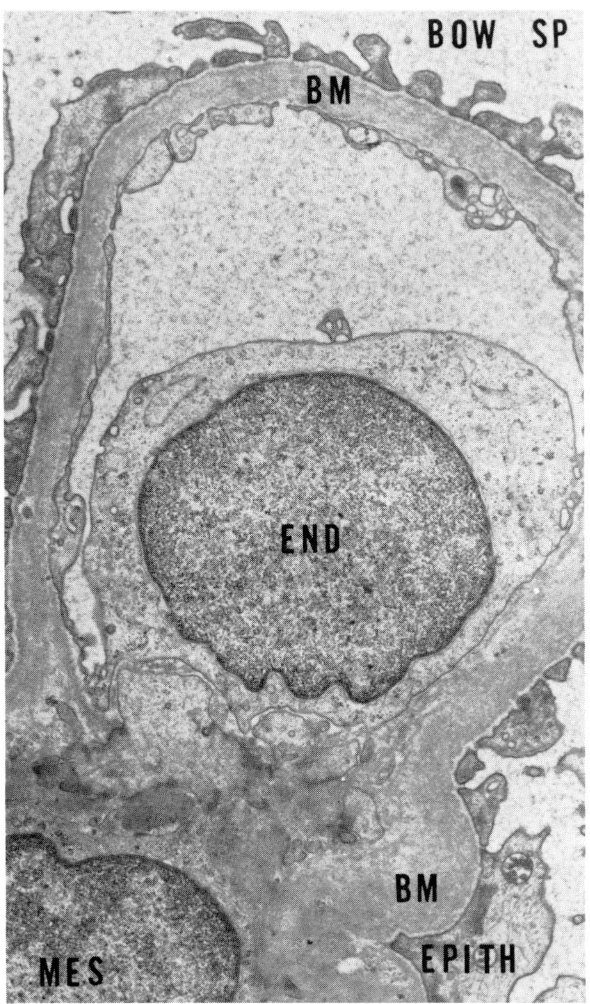

ABBREVIATIONS
BB = brush border
BM = basement membrane
BOW SP = Bowman's space
END = endothelium
EPITH = epithelium
HYAL = hyaline
LUM = lumen
M = muscle
MES = mesangium
MES NOD = mesangial nodule
RBC = red blood cell

Fig. 1. Normal glomerulus. The epithelial foot processes cover the entire outer surface of the glomerular tuft. A slit pore membrane connects the foot processes and may permit the passage of small molecules while the larger ones enter the cytoplasm and appear as droplets. The basement membrane covers the stalk area but does not completely surround the lumen as the mesangial cell is in contact with the endothelial cell in this region. The endothelial cell has a thin inconspicuous cytoplasm lining the entire lumen but has large pores that measure up to 900 Å. The mesangial cell occupies the central lobular area and is occasionally separated from the basement membrane by spongey fibers that are more prominent than the peripheral basement membrane fibrils. Mag. 10,540X

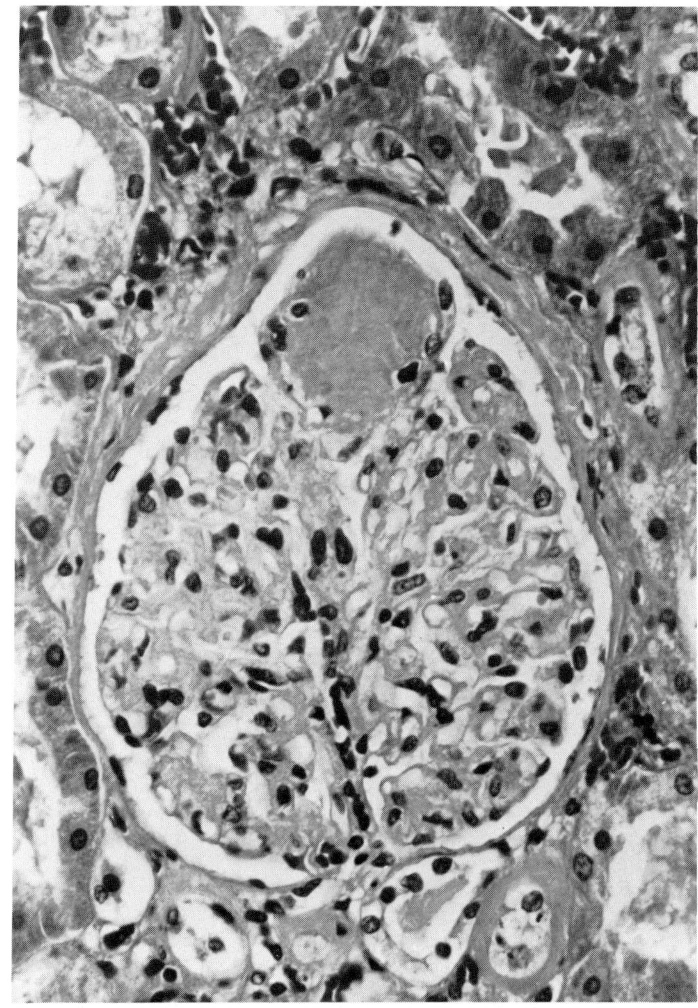

Fig. 2. Nodular diabetic glomerular sclerosis with a poorly cellular mass bordered by patent capillaries in a peripheral lobule. The glomerulus is normally cellular though slightly enlarged. H & E, Mag. 450X

nodule. In the more sclerotic forms, they can be limited to the outer margins or even be scarce, with a lamellar appearance evident in the hyaline material. The degree of cellularity may be increased to the point of confusing the lesion with lobular glomerulonephritis. This is seldom a problem except with limited sampling. The nodular diabetic glomerulosclerosis frequently can be shown with normal cellularity in the remainder of the involved glomerulus and in the adjacent glomeruli. The nature of the sclerosis and hyaline change is not clear. By special stains (26, 31, 33), ultrastructural studies (12) and chemical analysis (8, 29), it can be shown to contain collagen, but not as a major component. Sudanophilic deposits may be interspersed throughout the lesion, but usually these are scattered small aggregates. The nodules are intensely PAS positive but resist tryptic digestion in contrast to the basement membrane (32).

DIFFUSE GLOMERULOSCLEROSIS

Bell (6) distinguished between the nodular and diffuse types of intercapil-

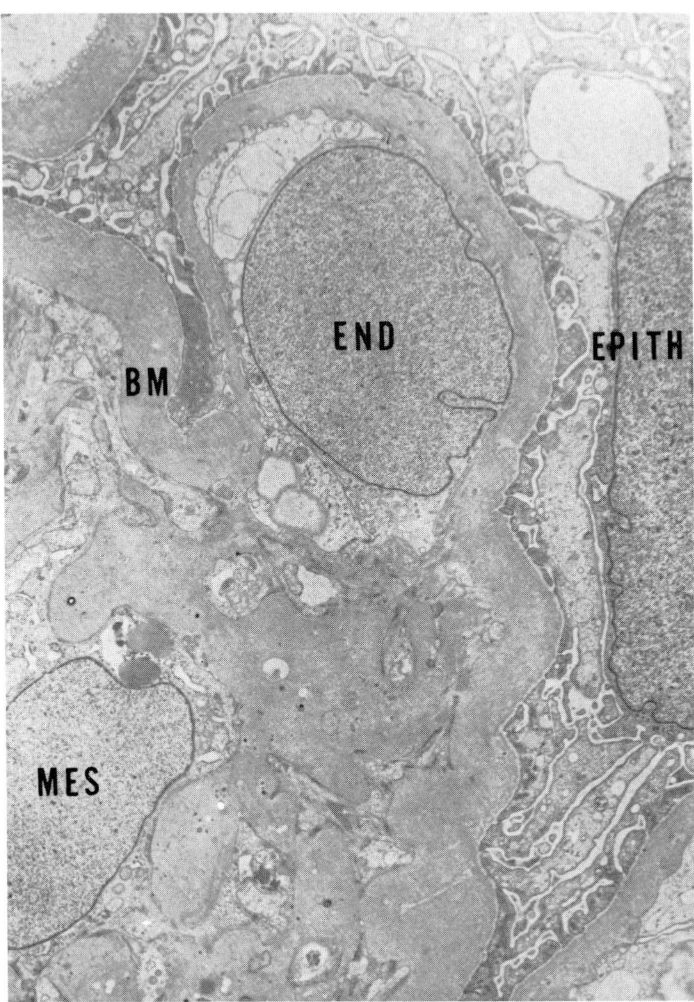

Fig. 3. The electron micrograph of a K-W nodule clearly shows the great increase in basement membrane-like material. The appearance and location of this material are interpreted as indicating an increased formation or decreased destruction rather than a blood borne deposit as seen with amyloidosis. Focal small calcifications within the nodule are shown. The nodule clearly distorts the entire lobule by widening the stalk area and narrows the capillary with only mild thickening of the peripheral basement membrane. The epithelial cell appears normal. Mag. 9,800X

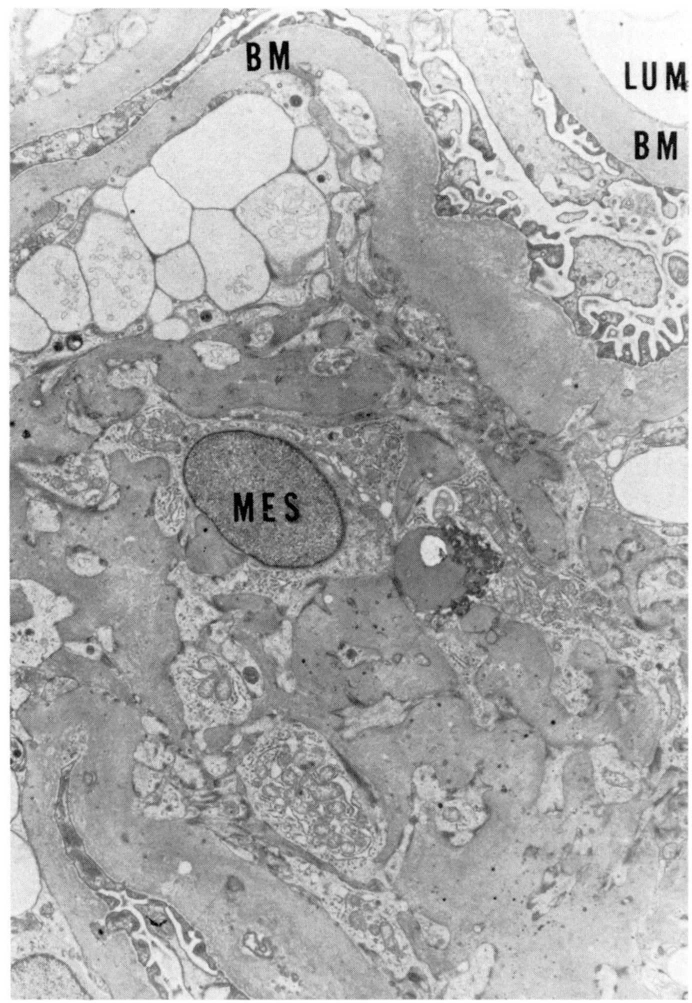

Fig. 4. Larger nodules may have few residual mesangial cells between the irregular tufts of basement membrane-like material which is more dense. Occasional dense bodies appear to be lipid in mesangial cells. Mag. 10,500X

lary lesions. He felt that the nodular lesions formed from the diffuse. There is continued perplexity over the diffuse lesion (Fig. 7, 8). It may be defined as a widespread general thickening or deposition in the mesangium with more or less involvement of peripheral capillary basement membrane (23) or it may be a uniform thickening of the peripheral basement membrane, as emphasized in the early electron microscopic observations (13). Kimmelstiel, *et al.* (24) made elaborate measurements of the basement membranes of diabetics and found that the mean width in the peripheral capil-

lary was within normal limits in diabetes up to ten years' duration of the clinical disorder, but was thickened in the presence of nodular glomerulosclerosis. On the basis of these impressive studies, it appears that the fundamental change in both nodular and diffuse diabetic glomerulosclerosis is the same. The increase in basement membrane—like material in the mesangial or stalk area may be more fibrillar (Fig. 5) in appearance (10) but is associated with variable focal or diffuse thickening of the peripheral basement membrane (Fig. 6, 7). This thickening of the basement membrane has been of

Fig. 5. Higher magnification of the mesangial nodules reveals a fine fibrillar pattern and loose texture that is similar to the spongey material normally present in small amounts between the mesangial cells and the basement membrane. The basement membrane proper, seen on the upper right, has a more compact texture and its feltwork of finer fibrils is not shown. Mag. 60,800X

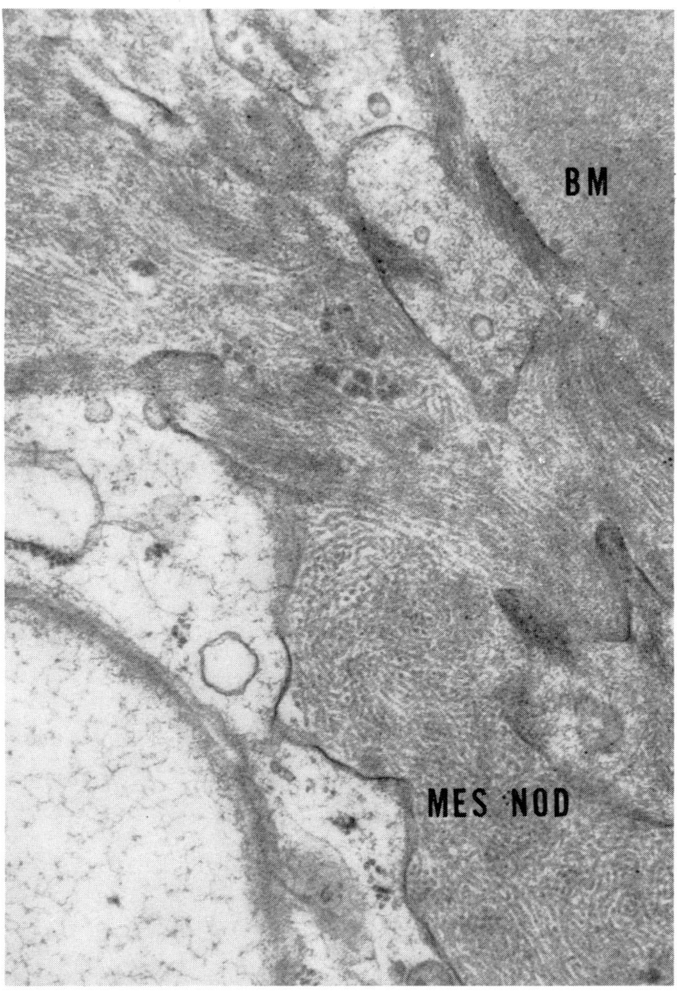

special interest in recent years with emphasis upon this pathologic response in many of the lesions of diabetic angiopathy. Cogan, *et al.* (11) and others (43) have ascertained that with diabetic retinopathy the early changes involve increased basement membrane, loss of mural cells and, with hyalinization, the development of aneurysmal dilatations and subsequent changes. Others have demonstrated marked basement membrane thickening in diabetic patients when measured in the skin (1, 35) and skeletal muscle (42, 44). These general observations have been interpreted as indicating that this and other evidence of a diffuse angiopathy have a bearing on the interpretation of the glomerular diabetic lesion.

MICROANEURYSMS

Two types of glomerular aneurysmal dilations have been described. Anderson (3) described a widening of the axial portion of the glomerular tuft with an extension of hyaline material similar to that of the adjacent arteriole. This lesion is not found only in diabetics and may be related to nephrosclerosis. Allen (2) has described another pattern with widening of capillaries within the lobule

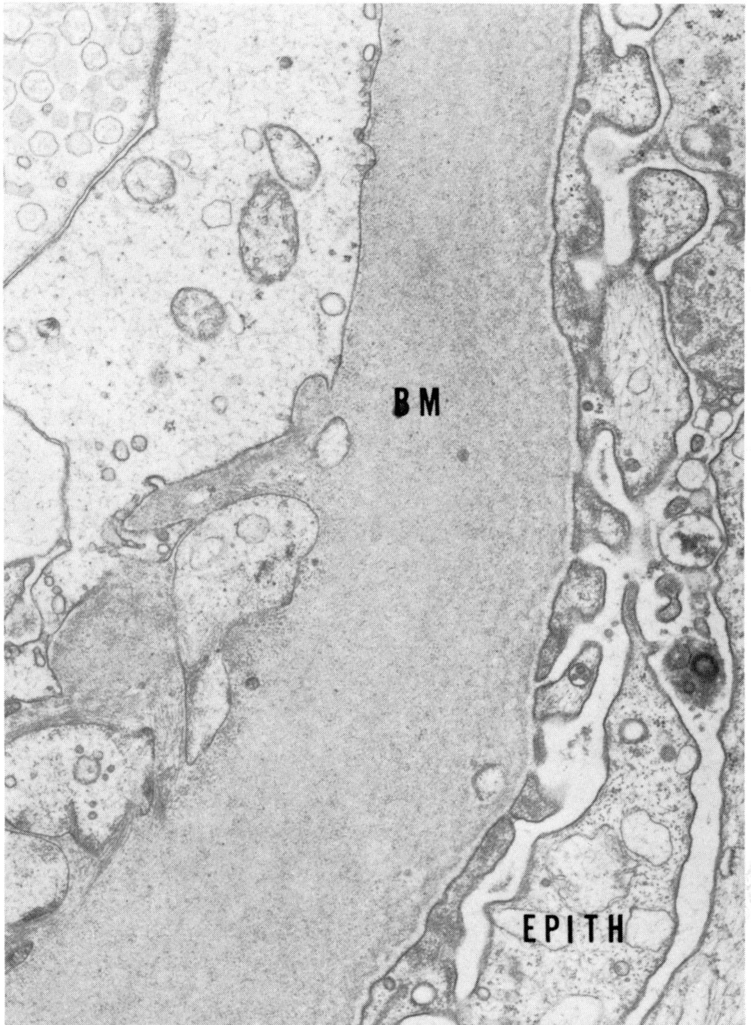

Fig. 6. Diffuse diabetic glomerulosclerosis may have a marked thickening of the basement membrane of peripheral capillary loops. In addition to the thickening this structure, seen as a continuous layer under the epithelial foot processes, is less compact and has a looser texture although the small tufts of spongey material on the left are not prominent. Mag. 22,210X

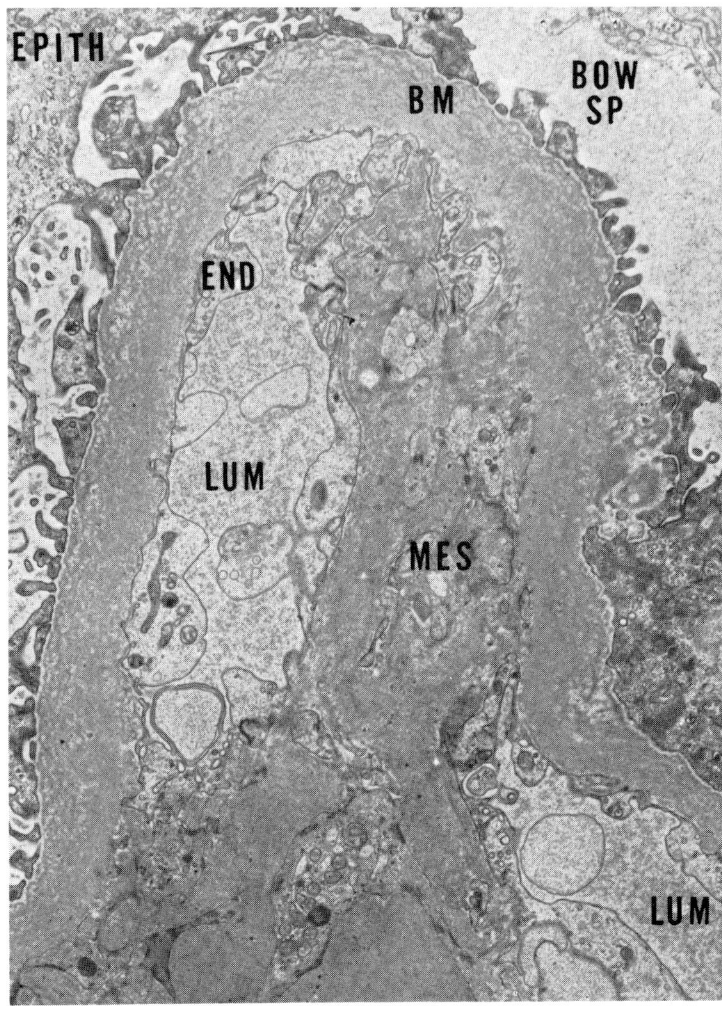

Fig. 7. More frequently, both the peripheral and mesangial basement membrane material is increased in the diffuse lesion. The marked variations in density and texture of the basement membrane are evident. The increased mesangial material is evident but does not appear as a nodule. Proteinuria was heavy with this lesion. Mag. 8,640X

near one of the nodules and he interprets this as secondary to obstruction to blood flow by the nodule.

NODULAR
ACELLULAR – EXUDATIVE

The nodular acellular or hyaline fibrinoid lesion (Fig. 9) is also known as fibrinoid cap, fibrin cap, acidophilic hyaline and exudative lesion (17, 20, 27). This lesion while not specific for diabetes mellitus appears to be more reliably associated with the severity of sclerosis of the preglomerular arteriole. Hyaline material is most often within the capillary lumen but may also be along Bowman's capsule (capsular drop). Muirhead (33) has suggested that these lesions contain plasma proteins and lipids.

The pathogenesis of diabetic glomerulosclerosis is not clear in spite of extensive studies of these lesions. Some of the confusion is related to the uncertainty about the relationship between the diffuse and nodular forms of the glomerular lesions. At the present time, it is widely accepted that the distinctive

Fig. 8. The diffuse glomerulo-sclerosis with diabetes may be difficult to distinguish from other lesions with diffuse membranous change by light microscopy but higher magnifications as in Figure 7 clarify the specific nature of the lesion. H & E, Mag. 400X

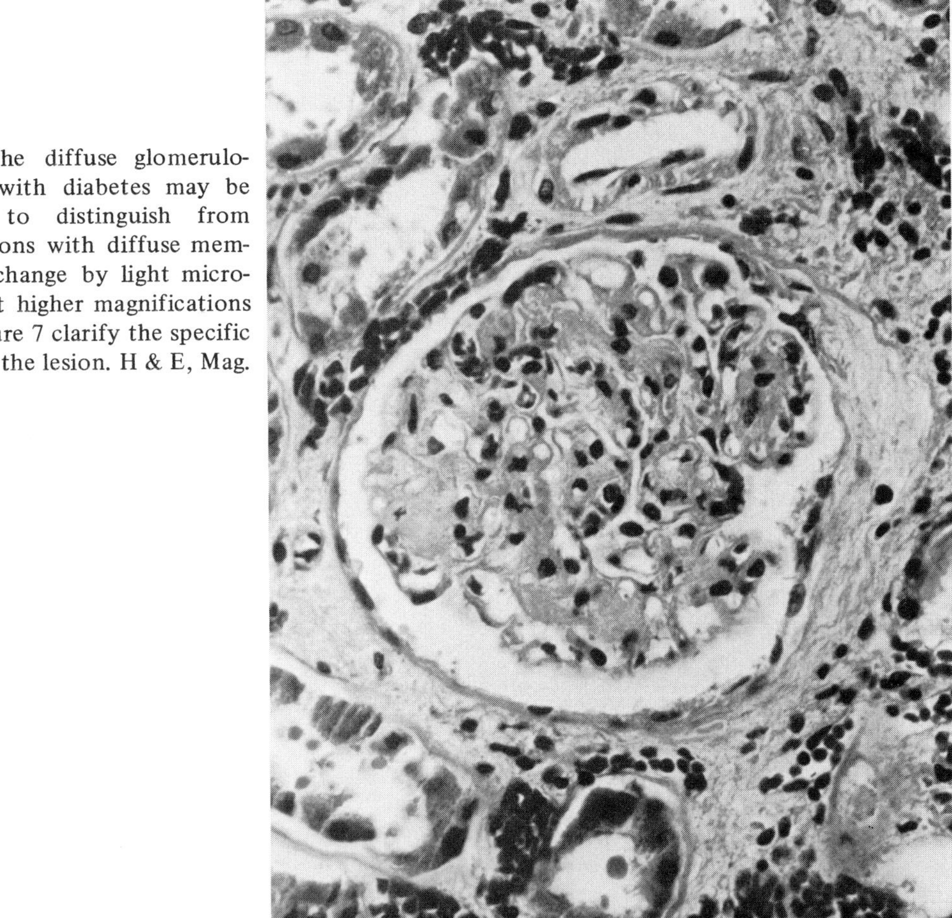

change with diabetic glomerulosclerosis is an increase in basement membrane. Whether this represents an increased production of basement membrane or one of its constituents has not been satisfactorily resolved. Another possibility is that there may be a net increase in basement membrane because of a decreased mesangial cell activity and decreased removal of basement membrane in the axial area (Fig. 3 4). Farquhar (14) from a study of the turnover of ferritin particles has suggested that the mesangial cells have a phagocytic function. Ireland, *et al.* (22)

have proposed a cellular mechanism for the diabetic lesion and describe ultra-structural evidence for increased glomerular epithelial activity related to increased basement membrane and decreased activity of the mesangial cells. Their data is not entirely convincing and more studies are needed to resolve this aspect of the pathologic change.

Despite the problems in interpretation that are related to a separation of the diffuse and nodular lesions, it appears justified in attempting to relate clinical observations to pathologic findings. The nodular glomerulosclerosis is reliably

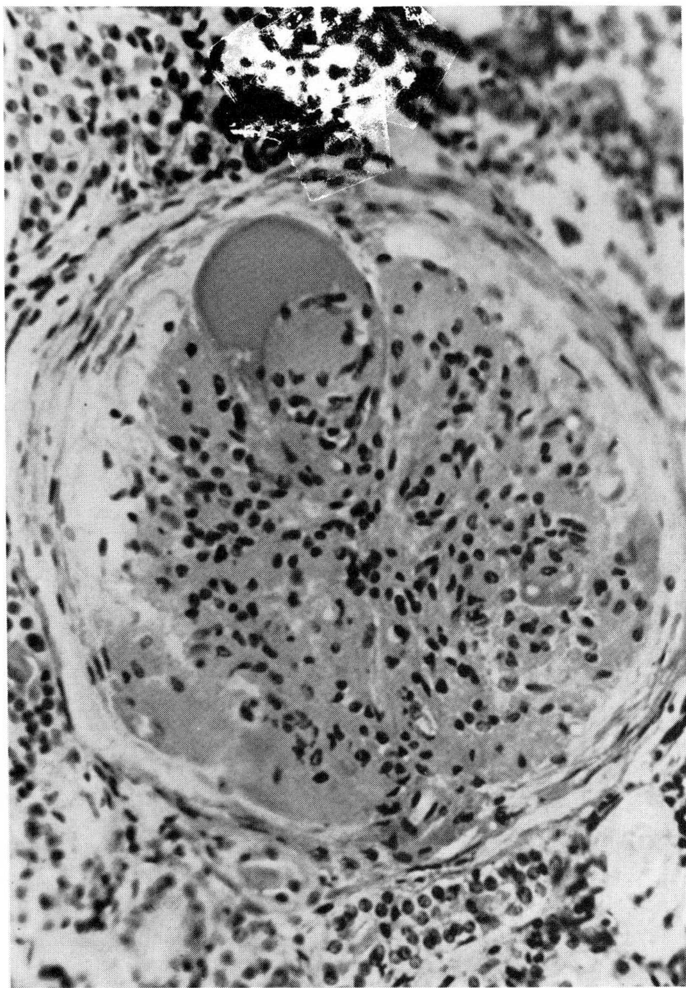

Fig. 9. The nodular acellular or exudative lesion frequently is seen as a hyalin cap over a nodular cellular lesion. The highly refractile, brightly eosinophilic material stains as the lesion of arteriolosclerosis. H & E, Mag. 450X

associated with the diabetic state (10, 23) but clearly does not correlate well with the presence or absence of the nephrotic syndrome or hypertension. The diffuse diabetic glomerulosclerosis does appear to be reliably related to the nephrotic syndrome (15) although its reliability as a specific diagnostic change with the diagnosis of diabetes is less certain. The eventual resolution of the question of the relationship between the diffuse and nodular lesion in the natural history of the disease must await further studies with good quantitative data as reported by Kimmelstiel *et al.* (24).

The incidence of glomerulosclerosis in diabetes increases with the duration of the disease. Muirhead *et al.* (33) examined 1,000 glomeruli in 6 diabetics and found nodules in 20% and hyaline exudative lesions in 7%. Bell (6) reported 1,445 autopsies of diabetics with 12.8% nodular lesions in males and 19.4% in females. When cases showing only diffuse lesions were included, the total incidence was 19.5% for males and 30% for females. While in general nodular involvement is found only after diabetes has been present for a period of years, well documented cases with advanced glomerulosclerosis have been found even before the clinical disease is manifest (4).

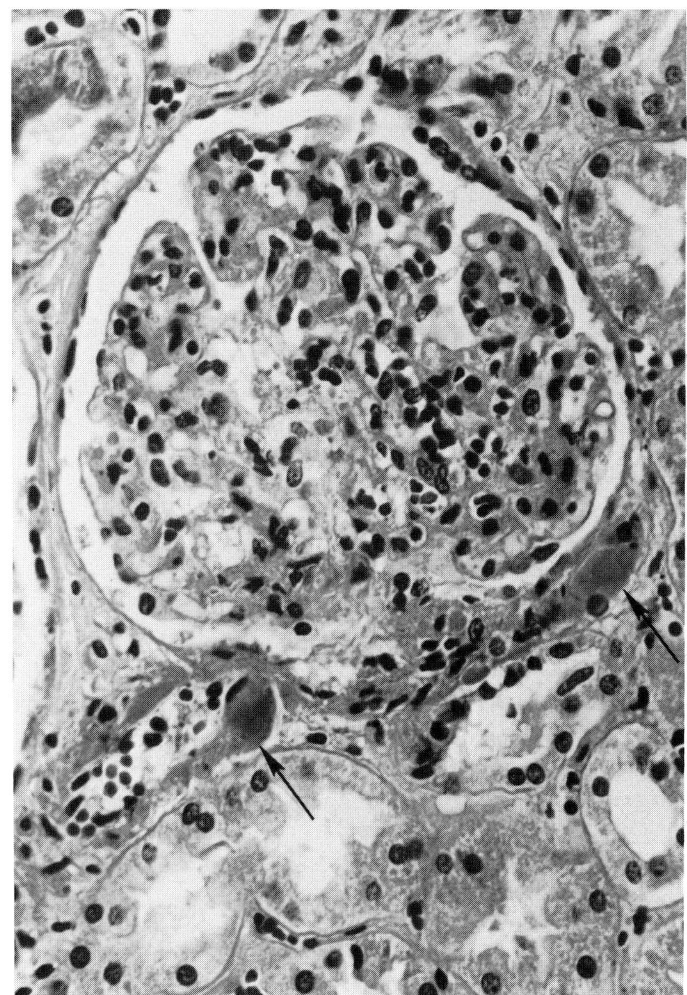

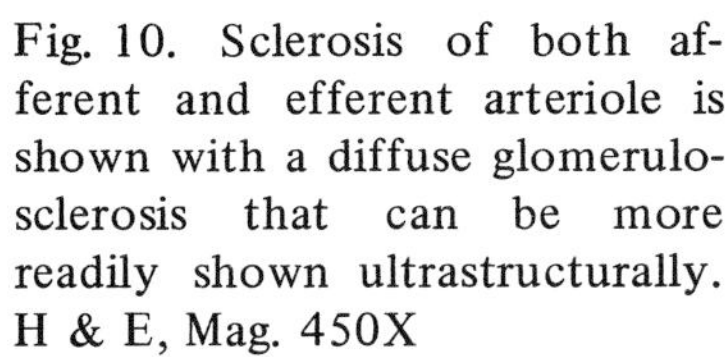
Fig. 10. Sclerosis of both afferent and efferent arteriole is shown with a diffuse glomerulosclerosis that can be more readily shown ultrastructurally. H & E, Mag. 450X

Electron microscopic evidence of diffuse glomerulosclerosis has been reported in patients from diabetic families who had normal glucose tolerances (9, 30, 38).

ARTERIOLOSCLEROSIS

Hyaline sclerosis of both the afferent and efferent arteriole (Fig. 10) are accentuated in diabetes. The lesions are prominent at an earlier age and are more severe. The ultrastructural change resembles that of hypertensive sclerosis and involves a prominent hyaline widening of the intima with narrowing of the lumen (7). Extension of the process is associated with separation of smooth muscle in the media, and loss of these cells with hyaline extension through the entire wall. Dystrophic remnants of smooth muscle cells may be found but this change seems to be secondary to the hyaline accumulation which appears more as a deposition of material from the blood plasma. Electron microscopic demonstration of early stages of the subendothelial lesion are granular (Fig. 12) and no distinctive periodicity has been demonstrated. The hyalinization of the efferent arterioles is generally

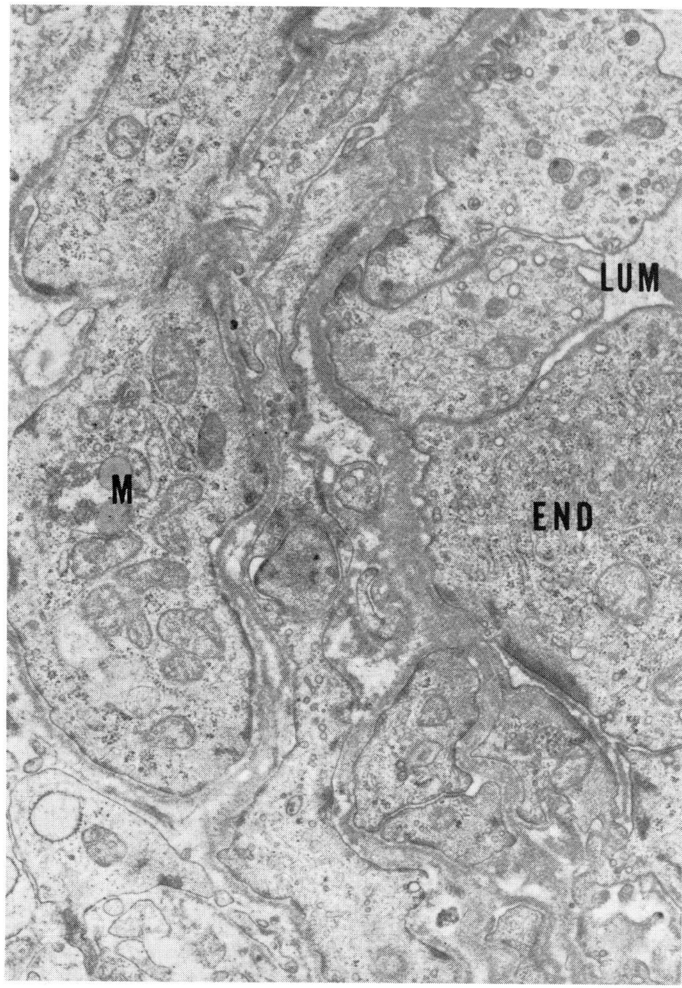

Fig. 11. The normal arteriole has only a small amount of basement membrane material separating the endothelial cells and the smooth muscle layer.
Mag. 13,1000X

considered to be specific for diabetes but this has also been reported associated with glomerular lesions of cyanotic congenital heart disease (39).

TUBULAR

The concomitant tubular changes of diabetes include the Armanni-Ebstein glycogenic vacuolization (36). This proximal tubular lesion appears to be related to the severity of the disease and the lack of adequate therapy. It is seldom demonstrated in current material. The localization of this lesion to the terminal straight portion of the proximal convoluted tubule is now generally accepted but is not adequately explained. A more frequent tubular change seen with severe glomerulosclerosis is basement membrane thickening (Fig. 13) which is reticulated and appears to be a condensation effect rather than sclerosis as seen in the glomerulus.

INTERSTITIAL

It has been generally believed that pyelonephritis and urinary tract infections occur more frequently in diabetic patients than in other groups. In autopsy studies, pyelonephritis has been esti-

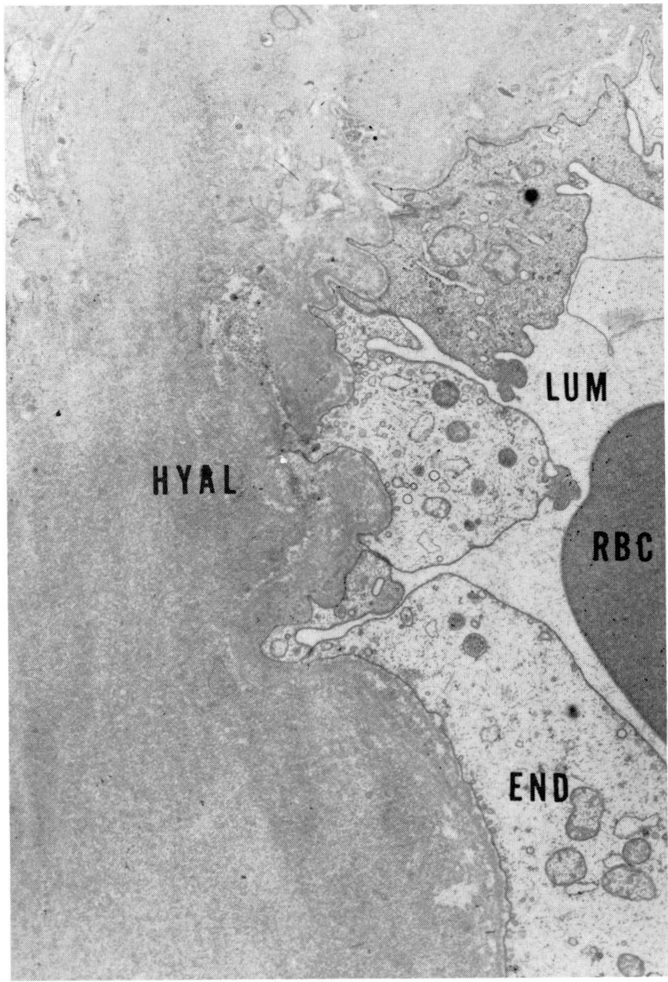

Fig. 12. Sclerosis of the arteriole can be shown as an amorphous deposit of hyaline material between the endothelium and smooth muscle. This material does not have the fine fibrillar texture of the glomerular basement membrane. Mag. 13,770X

mated to be 5 times as frequent in diabetics as in nondiabetics (40). Robbins and Tucker (37) reported acute pyelonephritis at autopsy in 7.3% of diabetics against 1.6% in nondiabetics. These published reports are not directly comparable because of variations in histologic criteria and patient population.

Renal biopsy studies have resulted in different impressions. Gellman *et al.* (15) did not find evidence of pyelonephritis in 65 biopsies of diabetic patients, while Halverstadt (18) reported a 9% incidence in a group of 80 juvenile diabetics. The latter suggested that factors other than the continued presence of bacteria in the kidney may play a role in the pathogenesis of chronic pyelonephritis.

Reports on the frequency of urinary tract infections in diabetic patients have also varied. Huvos and Rocha (21) studying a group of hospital patients

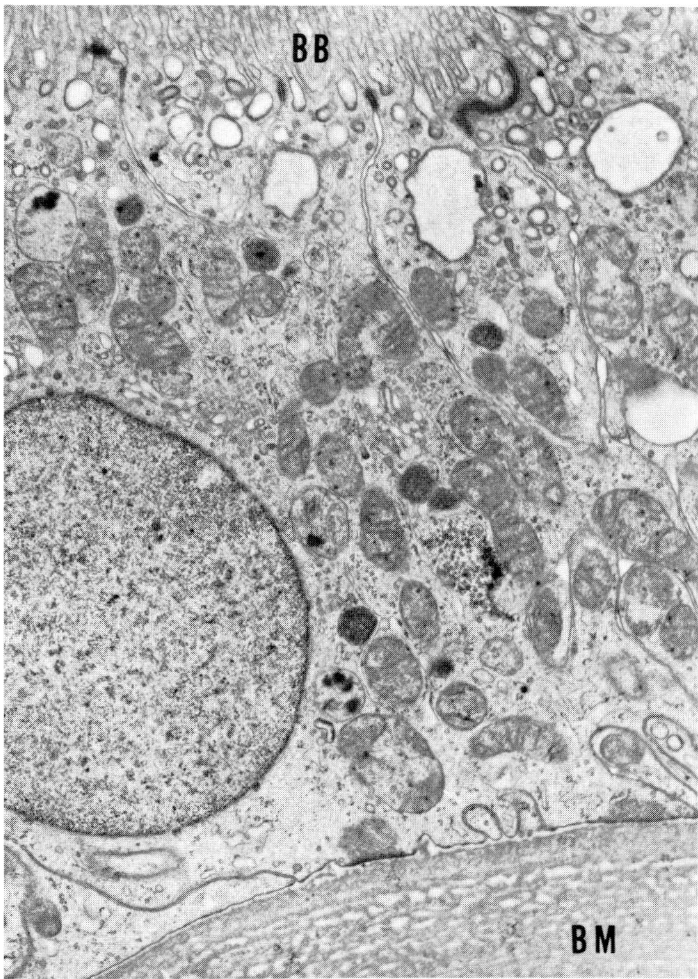

Fig. 13. Tubular changes secondary to glomerular sclerosis include the thickening of the basement membrane appearing as a reticulated condensation with atrophy of the nephron. Mag. 14,750X

found no significant difference in the incidence of bacteriuria between diabetic patients and nondiabetics. O'Sullivan *et al.* (34) with a larger series came to the same conclusion. Vejlsgaard (41) in a study of outpatients found no significant difference for the entire group but felt that diabetic women did show an increased incidence of bacteriuria. It would appear from these studies that the old concept that urinary tract infection is more frequent in diabetics should be revised although the urinary tract of diabetic females may be slightly more susceptible to infection.

PAPILLARY NECROSIS

Acute papillary necrosis (Fig. 14) is an ischemic necrosis most often associated with infections of the urinary tract. Its more frequent association with diabetes mellitus was first pointed out by Gunther in 1937 (16). An incidence of

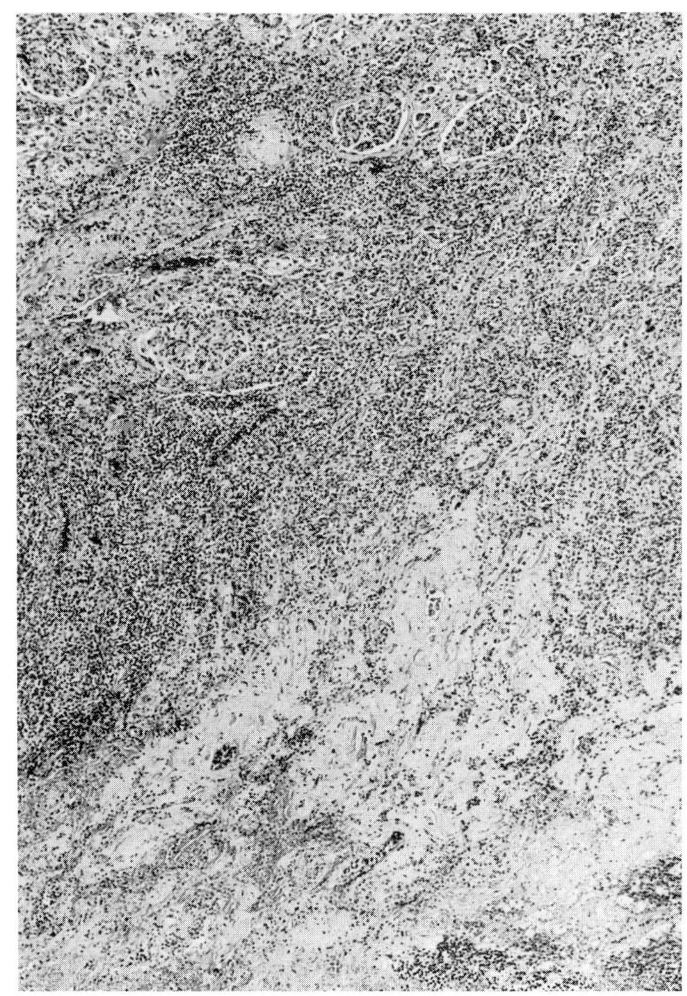

Fig. 14. Papillary necrosis while associated with an acute pyelonephritis has prominent sclerosis of the medullary and papillary vessels. H & E, Mag. 100X

18% has been found in patients with longstanding diabetes in a radiologic study (19) but 2.7 to 7.2% of autopsied diabetics have been shown with the lesion (28). It does not appear that the severity or degree of control of the diabetes is in any way related to the incidence or severity of the papillary necrosis. Baker (5) has demonstrated a dual blood supply to the renal papilla and suggests that obstruction of the spiral arteries to the calyceal mucosa of the papilla results in an ischemic necrosis of the papilla in diabetics.

BIBLIOGRAPHY

1. Aagenaes, O., and Moe, H.: Light-and electron-microscopic study of skin capillaries of diabetics. Diabetes, *10:*253-259, 1961.
2. Allen, A. C.: The clinicopathologic meaning of the nephrotic syndrome. Amer. J. Med., *18:*277-281, 1955.
3. Anderson, G. L.: The pathogenesis of diabetic glomerulosclerosis. J. Path. Bact., *67:*241-248, 1954.
4. Arnold, J. D., Tarlov, A. R., Spargo, B., and Brewer, G. J.: Subclinical diabetes mellitus in patients presenting with clinical chronic "glomerulonephritis." Trans. Assoc. Amer. Physicians, *71:*186-194, 1958.
5. Baker, S. B. De. C.: The blood supply of the renal papilla. Brit. J. Urol., *31:*53-59, 1959.

6. Bell, E. T.: Renal vasular disease in diabetes mellitus. Diabetes, *2:*376-389, 1953.

7. Biava, C. G., Dyrda, I., Genest, J., and Bencosme, S. A.: Renal hyaline arteriolosclerosis. An electron microscope study. Amer. J. Path., *44:*349-363, 1964.

8. Bonting, S. L., De Bruin, H., and Pollak, V. E.: Quantitative histochemistry of the nephron. VI. Hydroxyproline in the human glomerulus. J. Clin. Invest., *40:*177-183, 1961.

9. Camerini-Davalos, R. A., Caulfield, J. B., Rees, S. B., Lozano-Castaneda, O., Naldjian, S., and Marble, A.: Preliminary observations on subjects with prediabetes. Diabetes, *12:*508-518, 1963.

10. Churg, J., and Dachs, S.: Diabetic renal disease: arteriosclerosis and glomerulosclerosis. Pathology Annual, *1:*148-171, 1966.

11. Cogan, D. G., Toussaint, D., and Kuwabara, T.: Retinal vascular patterns. IV. Diabetic retinopathy. Arch. Ophthal., *66:*366-378, 1961.

12. Dachs, S., Churg, J., Mautner, W., and Grishman, E.: Diabetic nephropathy. Amer. J. Path., *44:*155-168, 1964.

13. Farquhar, M. G., Hopper, J., and Moon, H. D.: Diabetic glomerulosclerosis: electron and light microscopic studies. Amer. J. Path., *35:*721-753, 1959.

14. Farquhar, M. G., and Palade, G. E.: Functional evidence of the existence of a third cell type in the renal glomerulus. J. Cell Biol., *13:*55-87, 1962.

15. Gellman, D. D., Pirani, C. L., Soothill, J. F., Muehrcke, R. C., and Kark, R. M.: Diabetic nephropathy. Medicine, *38:*321-367, 1959.

16. Gunther, G. W.: Die Papillennekrosen der Niere bei Diabetes. Munchen. med. Wchnschr., *84:*1695, 1937.

17. Hall, G. F. M.: The significance of atheroma of the renal arteries in Kimmelstiel-Wilson's syndrome. J. Path. Bact., *64:*103-110, 1952.

18. Halverstadt, D. B., Leadbetter, G. W., and Field, R. A.: Pyelonephritis in the diabetic. J.A.M.A., *195:*827-829, 1966.

19. Harrow, B. R.: Nephropathy of diabetes with emphasis on papillary necrosis. Postgrad. Med., *37:*63-69, 1965.

20. Horsfield, G. I., and Lannigan, R.: Exudative lesions in diabetes mellitus. J. Clin. Pathol., *18:*47-53, 1965.

21. Huvos, A., and Rocha, H.: Frequency of bacteriuria in patients with diabetes mellitus. New Engl. J. Med., *261:*1213-1220, 1959.

22. Ireland, J. T., Patnaik, B. K., and Duncan, L. J. P.: Effect of pituitary ablation on the renal arteriolar and glomerular lesions in diabetes. Diabetes, *16:*636-642, 1967.

23. Kimmelstiel, P.: Diabetic nephropathy. Chapter 11 in Mostofi, F. K., and Smith, David E., (eds.): The Kidney. Baltimore, Williams & Wilkins 1966, p. 226.

24. Kimmelstiel, P., Osawa, G., and Beres, J.: Glomerular basement membrane in diabetics. Amer. J. Clin. Path., *45:*21-31, 1966.

25. Kimmelstiel, P., and Wilson, C.: Intercapillary lesions in the glomeruli of the kidney. Amer. J. Path., *12:*83-90, 1936.

26. Laipply, T. C., Eitzen, O., and Dutra, F. R.: Intercapillary glomerulosclerosis. Arch. Int. Med., *74:*354-364, 1944.

27. Laufer, A., and Stein, O.: The exudative lesion in diabetic glomerulosclerosis. Amer. J. Clin. Path., *32:*56-61, 1959.

28. Lauler, D. P., Schreiner, G. E., and David, A.: Renal medullary necrosis. Amer. J. Med., *29:*132-156, 1960.

29. Lazarow, A., and Speidel, E.: The chemical composition of the glomerular basement membrane and its relationship to the production of diabetic complications. In, Siperstein, M. D., Colwell, A. R., and Meyer, K., (eds): Conference on Small Blood Vessel Involvement in Diabetes Mellitus Warrenton, Virginia, 1964. p. 124.

30. Linner, E., Svanborg, A., and Zelander, T.: Retinal and renal lesions of diabetic type, without obvious disturbances in glucose metabolism, in a patient with family history of diabetes. Amer. J. Med., *39:*298-304, 1965.

31. Lynch, M. J. G., and Raphael, S. S.: The nature of diabetic (Kimmelstiel-Wilson) glomerulosclerosis. Diabetes, *6:*488-497, 1957.

32. McManus, J. F. A.: Medical Diseases of the Kidney. Philadelphia, Lea & Febiger, 1950.

33. Muirhead, E. E., Montgomery, P. O'B., and Booth, E.: The glomerular lesions of diabetes mellitus. Arch. Int. Med., *98:*146-161, 1956.

34. O'Sullivan, D. J., Fitzgerald, M. G., Meywell, M. J., and Malins, J. M.: Urinary tract infections, a comparative study in diabetic and in general population. Brit. Med. J., *2:*786-791, 1961.

35. Pedersen, J., and Olsen, S.: Small-vessel disease of the lower extremity in diabetes mellitus. Acta Med. Scand., *171:*551-559, 1962.

36. Ritchie, S., and Waugh, D.: The pathology of Armanni-Ebstein diabetic nephropathy. Amer. J. Path., *33:*1036-1057, 1957.

37. Robbins, S. L., and Tucker, A. W.: Cause of death in diabetes. Report of 307 autopsied cases. New Engl. J. Med., *231:*865-871, 1944.

38. Rosenbaum, P., Kattine, A. A., and Gottsegen, W. L.: Diabetic and prediabetic nephropathy in childhood. Amer. J. Dis. Child., *106:*83-95, 1963.

39. Spear, G. S.: Implications of the glomerular lesions of cyanotic congenital heart disease. J. Chron. Dis., *19:*1083-1088, 1966.

40. Thomsen, A. C.: Significance of renal biopsy for diagnosis of pyelonephritis in diabetic patients.

In, Wolstenholme, G. E. W., Cameron, M. P., (eds.): Renal Biopsy: Clinical and Pathologic Significance, Boston, Little, Brown, 1961, p. 281.

41. Vejlsgaard, R.: Bacteriuria in patients with diabetes mellitus (a controlled study). In, Kass, E. H. (ed.): Progress in Pyelonephritis. Philadelphia, F. A. Davis Company, 1965, p. 478.

42. Vracko, R., and Strandness, D. E., Jr.: Basal lamina of abdominal skeletal muscle capillaries in diabetics and nondiabetics. Circulation, *34:*690-700, 1967.

43. Yamashita, T., and Rosen, D. A.: Electron-microscopic study of diabetic capillary aneurysm. Arch. Ophthal., *67:*785-790, 1962.

44. Zacks, S. I., Pegues, J. J., and Elliott, F. A.: Interstitial muscle capillaries in patients with diabetes mellitus: a light and electron microscopic study. Metabolism, *11:*381-393, 1962.

Chapter 45

Idiopathic Renal Lithiasis

LYNWOOD H. SMITH, M.D.

The formation of bladder and kidney stones has plagued man throughout his existence; yet, the etiology of this problem remains undefined in most cases. Only now is some insight being gained into the many factors in urine that promote or prevent formation of stones. The lack of understanding of these physical and chemical properties has led to misconception in the cause of recurrent renal lithiasis and its treatment. It is the purpose of this presentation to review these properties of urine in the heterogenous syndrome of idiopathic renal lithiasis.

The present classification of idiopathic renal lithiasis includes the recurrent formation of calcium oxalate, calcium phosphate, and hydroxyapatite stones without an apparent underlying cause such as hyperparathyroidism, renal tubular acidosis, or hyperoxaluria. This type of idiopathic renal lithiasis prevails in at least 70% of the patients who have recurrent stones containing calcium, and it has a definite predilection for males. The onset of formation of stones is unusual before the age of 20 years; the peak incidence occurs in the fourth to sixth decade. At least 50% of the patients will have hypercalciuria using the upper limits of normal calcium excretion—250 mg per 24 hr in females and 275 mg per 24 hr. in males on a 700

mg calcium diet (1). Mild hypophosphatemia is not uncommon. A few patients may show a slight elevation of uric acid in the serum similar to that in patients who have hyperparathyroidism. Serum calcium falls within the normal range, but the mean value may be higher than that for a normal population. Formation of stones is variable, ranging from only a few stones within a lifetime in some patients to one or more stones each month in others. Likewise, the presence or absence of hypercalciuria does not correlate with the formation of stones, in that patients with large amounts of urinary calcium may show relative inactivity and others with normal urinary calcium may show considerable activity.

Patients with idiopathic renal lithiasis have been divided into two groups based on the presence or absence of excessive amounts of calcium in the urine. Several differences between the groups have been observed. Patients in whom formation of stones is most active often do not have significant hypercalciuria as would be predicted if the solute load were the primary causative factor. Rigid dietary restriction of calcium in hypercalciuric patients often will lower the urinary excretion of calcium, but this maneuver seems to have little effect in the normocalciuric group. Treatment directed toward reducing the solute load appears to be effective in preventing formation of stones in the hypercalciuric group but not in the group with normal excretion of calcium. This finding suggests that there may be real differences in the etiologic factors in these two groups of patients.

Kidney stones, like calcification anywhere in the body, are made up of matrix and various types of crystals (2). Available matrices are present in all urine, the primary variable in the formation of stones being the factors which influence crystallization. Urine and its ultrafiltrate contain considerably more calcium phosphate that can be held in solution by water. It is the solubility of these potential crystals and the physical and chemical factors causing this solubility which are of primary concern in patients who have idiopathic renal lithiasis.

Factors which influence the potential crystal systems in urine are: 1) pH of urine; 2) concentration of crystalloid material; 3) inhibitors of crystallization (organic acids, magnesium, pyrophosphate, peptides), and 4) counterinhibitors. The formation of calcium oxalate crystals in monohydrate and dihydrate forms is not affected by the physiologic ranges of urinary pH in man. On the other hand, the tendency to form calcium phosphate crystals is progressively increased when the pH is more than 5.5 In patients who have idiopathic renal lithiasis, no defect has been found in the ability of the kidneys to excrete an acid urine.

In patients who have idiopathic renal lithiasis and significant hypercalciuria of 300 mg or greater per 24 hours, the recurrent formation of stones usually can be controlled by significantly decreasing the excretion of calcium. Hypercalciuria, therefore, must be at least partly responsible for the stones. In patients without hypercalciuria, it must be postulated that there is an imbalance of the urinary substances which normally prevent crystallization, to the extent that the capacity of the urine to maintain calcium salts in solution is seriously reduced.

The existence of a basic difference between the urine from patients with idiopathic renal lithiasis and the urine from normal persons was first noted by Howard and Thomas (3) in 1958. Using an *in-vitro* system with rechitic rat cartilage they observed the ability of urine from each group to hold its crystalloid content in solution. Though the calcium phosphate product of urine from each group was comparable and much greater than was usually necessary to mineralize the cartilage system, only the urine from patients with idiopathic renal lithiasis mineralized the rachitic cartilage. These authors did not find any other substance in the urine of either group that would explain this difference. The levels of known inhibitors of mineralization, including organic acids, magnesium (4), and inorganic pyrophosphate (5), were the same in urine from the two groups. These known inhibitors could block mineralization of the rachitic cartilage, but a large amount was required to convert a mineralizing urine to a normal nonmineralizing urine; in fact, the quantity was greater than the kidney could excrete under physiologic conditions. Thus, for unexplained reasons, the physical and chemical properties of the urine from patients with idiopathic renal lithiasis appeared to be altered.

In 1967, Howard and associates (6) reported the isolation from normal urine of two small peptides with extraordinary ability to inhibit mineralization in the cartilage system. The structure and mechanisms of action are not yet known, but preliminary studies suggest the possibility of a decreased amount of these peptides in urine of patients who have idiopathic renal lithiasis. If the concentration of these peptides is actually decreased, it will represent the only difference which has been found so far in the known inhibitors between mineralizing urine from patients with idiopathic renal lithiasis and urine from normal persons.

To complicate further the story of crystallization in urine, it is known that certain polyvalent cations will block or inhibit solubilizers. Usually, only small amounts of some of these cations are found in urine but they may have an effect on the balance of inhibitors. Should such substances prove important subsequently, a category of "counter-inhibitors" would need to be added in the consideration of formation of stones.

To understand better how these factors affecting crystallization are altered in the therapy of patients who have idiopathic renal lithiasis, it will be helpful to consider the forms of therapy that are listed in the Table. Forced fluid intake increases the volume of urine thus diluting the solute load. Rigid restriction of calcium intake in patients with hypercalciuria may cause the same results by decreasing the calcium excretion. An acid load in patients who tend to have alkaline urine will drop the urine pH and increase the solubility of calcium phosphate.

Thiazides will decrease urine calcium in hypercalciuric patients by 50% or more and have proved to be effective in preventing the formation of stones (7). At the Mayo Clinic, thiazides have not been found to be helpful in the treatment of patients who have normal excre-

CURRENT THERAPY FOR IDIOPATHIC RENAL LITHIASIS

Type of Therapy	Mechanism of Action
1. Forced fluids	Decrease solute load
2. Low calcium intake	
3. Thiazides (HydroDIURIL, 50 mg twice daily)	
4. Increased acid load (Ammonium chloride, citric acid, cranberry juice)	Increases solubility of calcium phosphate
5. Magnesium	Increases excretion of magnesium in urine
and	and
pyridoxine	decreases solute load (oxalate)
6. Inorganic ortho-phosphate	Decreases solute load (about 50% of patients)
	Increases inorganic pyrophosphate

tion of calcium and recurrent formation of stones.

Magnesium given orally will increase the level of urine magnesium which competes with calcium at the sites of crystallization. Pyridoxine has been used with magnesium in the hope of decreasing the excretion of oxalic acid in the urine by diverting glyoxylate to glycine. No defect in oxalate metabolism has been demonstrated in these patients, but the stones which they make often contain oxalate.

In idiopathic renal lithiasis, orthophosphate taken orally will convert mineralizing urine into nonmineralizing urine (8). At the same time, stones are no longer formed regardless of the urinary excretion of calcium. In approximately 50% of patients so treated, hypercalciuria was significantly decreased. In the remaining half, an initial drop in the urinary excretion of calcium sometimes occurred but it returned to pretreatment levels whether the patient had hypercalciuria or normal excretion of calcium. This difference is not dependent on the presence of hypercalciuria prior to therapy. All patients will experience a modest increase in urinary inorganic pyrophosphate, but it is not great enough to explain the changes in the capacity of their urine to hold calcium salts in solutions. Preliminary studies have not shown a change in the amount of inhibiting peptides with orthophosphate therapy, so the mechanism of action remains unknown.

Because of the sporadic formation of stones in many patients, the evaluation of effects of treatment depends on the demonstration of active formation of stones before therapy is indertaken. Colic or passage of a stone does not necessarily mean that the stone was recently formed. The recurrent passage of gravel as well as x-ray evidence of formation of new stones are accepted as indications of active idiopathic renal lithiasis. If activity cannot be established, the patient's condition is followed periodically and no therapy is used in order to define the activity of stone formation.

A total approach to the problem of formation of stones has been presented though many questions remain unanswered. It is hoped that such an approach which avoids the obvious hazards of considering only one part of a complex system will result in a better understanding of the causes of idiopathic renal lithiasis and more effective therapy.

REFERENCES

1. Litin, R. B., Diessner, G. R., and Keating, F. R., Jr.: Urinary excretion of calcium in patients with renal lithiasis. J. Urol., *86:*17-23 (July) 1961.
2. Howard, J. E.: Urinary stone. Canad. M.A.J., *86:*1001-1007 (July) 1962.
3. Howard, J. E., and Thomas, W. C., Jr.: Some observations on rachitic rat cartilage of probable significance in the etiology of renal calculi. Trans. Amer. Clin. Climat. A., *70:*94-102, 1958.
4. Mukai, T., and Howard, J. E.: Some observations on the calcification of rachitic cartilage by urine: One difference between "good" and "evil" urines, dependent upon content of magnesium. Bull. Hopkins. Hosp., *112:*279-290, 1963.
5. Lewis, Anne M., Thomas, W. C., Jr., and Tomita, A.: Pyrophosphate and the mineralizing potential of urine. Clin. Sci., *30:*389-397, 1966.
6. Howard, J. E., Thomas, W. C., Jr., Barker, L. M., Smith, L. H., and Wadkins, C. L.: The recognition and isolation from urine and serum of a peptide inhibitor to calcification. Bull. Hopkins. Hosp., *120:*119-136, 1967.
7. Yendt, E. R., Gagne, R.J.A., and Cohanim, M.: The effects of thiazides in idiopathic hypercalciuria. Trans. Amer. Clin. Climat. A., *77:*96-110, 1965.
8. Thomas, W. C., Jr., and Miller, G. H.: Inorganic phosphate in the treatment of renal calculi. Mod. Treat., *4:*494-504 (May) 1967.

Chapter 46

Hematologic Disturbances in Renal Diseases

FARID I. HAURANI, M.D.

Although the hematologic disturbances of renal disease are the subject of this presentation, yet, just as interesting and challenging are the renal complications of certain hematologic disorders. Therefore, comment on some of these conditions will preface the main subject of this chapter.

1. Myelomatosis and the Kidney

Early in the course of myeloma, polyuria and hyposthenuria may be present because of the hypercalcemia (52). A rare complication is a tubular disturbance of the Fanconi type (17). Myeloma cell infiltration of the kidneys seldom impairs renal function (23). The most common complication of myeloma which is responsible for the fatal outcome of the disease is renal insufficiency with acidosis (adult rickets). The nephrocalcinosis, the precipitation of the various abnormal proteins including the Bence-Jones in the tubules (especially in acidic urine) with giant cell reaction and the deposition of paramyloid, are factors considered responsible for this nonhypertensive renal failure. Therefore, dehydration of the patient should be avoided particularly in preparation for an intravenous pyelogram (41).

2. Sickling and the Kidney

In sickle cell disease, trait or the doubly heterozygous sickle cell-C disease, there are two striking renal defects; hematuria and hyposthenuria. The hematuria is due to severe stasis of blood in the peritubular capillaries of both the cortex and the medulla, however in the latter, extravasation of blood is more evident.

Papillary congestion, submucosal hemorrhage and occasional frank papillary necrosis are the gross pathological lesions. Hematuria occurs in about 20% of hospitalized patients with electrophoretic pattern of SS, SA or SC (39) and when it is unilateral it is more frequently so on the left side. This, too, probably reflects vascular conditions favoring stasis of blood and sickling (42).

The other renal abnormality is a defect in the concentrating ability of the kidneys and is usually a constant finding (32). The kidneys can dilute but not concentrate urine. No response is observed following administration of pitressin or water deprivation. Early in life this defect is reversible folllowing exchange blood transfusion (replacing S hemoglobin with A), however, in time it becomes permanent and reflects perma

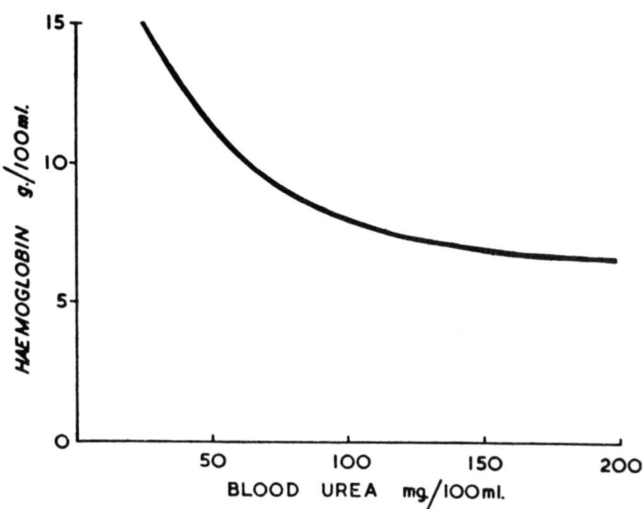

Fig. 1. The relationship of anemia to blood urea nitrogen. (Courtesy of Dr. De Wardener and Little, Brown and Co.)

nent structural changes in the kidneys. There are several alterations that may account for the hyposthenuria but it is outside the scope of this review to list all of them. One interesting theory may be found in the observation that hypertonic solutions promote the sickling phenomenon (45). Thus, the countercurrent multiplier system may be reabsorbing less sodium at the vasa recta level if sickling and sludging occur as the result of a hypertonic surrounding.

3. Intravascular Thrombosis and the Kidney

Renal failure, usually acute with or without hematuria, may complicate thrombotic episodes occuring as a result of vascular or intravascular disturbances in hemostasis. In man, Henoch-Shönlein and thrombotic thrombocytopenic purpura may be considered as examples of Vacular disease with secondary thrombosis. The intravascular thrombosis seems to lead to a morphologically well

characterized (schistocytes and burr cells) hemolytic anemia (4, 6). Thus, the well characterized "microangiopathic hemolytic anemia" (5), often with thrombocytopenia, occurs in patients with thrombotic thrombocytopenic purpura, malignant hypertension, renal cortical necrosis and acute necrotizing glomerulonephritis. In children, a similar process, "the hemolytic uremic syndrome," characterized by similar red cell morphologic changes, hemolysis, thrombocytopenia and acute renal failure may serve as another illustration of the renal disturbance that may complicate a disorderly hemostatic function. The pathological picture consists of patchy necrosis of renal cortex, microthrombi and glomerulitis (37). The disease occurs acutely in a healthy child, usually less than twelve months old but up to four years. The mortality rate is 40% but those who recover do so completely within a few weeks (46).

The pathophysiology of the relationship of intravascular thrombosis to hemolysis and renal failure has been studied in the experimental animal. The infusion of phospholipids containing platelet factor 3 activity in rabbits previously given Thorotrast to block the reticuloendothelial system results in a pathological picture similar to that of the generalized Schwartzman reaction produced with two injections of endotoxin. Grossly, there is bilateral cortical necrosis of the kidneys and, histologically, areas of focal necrosis limited to the cortex with tubular degeneration and hyaline masses are observed. These hyaline masses having the characteristics of fibrin block glomerular capillaries, and other vessels show stasis and congestion. The over-utilization of fibrinogen, platelets, factors II, V, and VIII produces a "consumption-coagulopathy" which in turn causes bleeding (50). A similar pathologic picture with deformities in the red blood cells and increased hemolysis is observed in animals defibrinated by thrombin (6).

4. Uric Acid and the Kidney

Hyperuricemia is a frequent complication of hematologic disorders characterized by marked proliferation of the cells of the bone marrow. As a result of this, nucleic acid derivatives appear in the urine in excess. Leukemias as a rule (perhaps with the exception of chronic lymphatic leukemia (1)), myelomatosis, extramedullary hemopoiesis and polycythemia vera are hemotologic disorders frequently associated with hyperuricemia. In acidic urine, uric acid precipitates causing acute or subacute renal failure with or without renal colic. Myelodepressive therapeutic agents increase the excretion of this compound so much so that hydration and alkalinization of the urine are constantly

employed as supportive therapy. More recently an inhibitor of the enzyme, xanthine oxidase, has been effectively used to prevent further oxidation of purine derivatives to the end-product compound (uric acid) of purine metabolism in man (51a).

5. Iron and the Kidney

Hematuria is seldom the cause of blood loss to produce anemia. One must always look for another mechanism of the anemia if hematuria is present. Color and volume may be misleading. However, the amount of blood lost to the urine can be quantitated (2a). In one severe (Grade IV) hemophilia A patient, whose hematuria lasted 18 days, the total urinary blood loss was 1390 ml and the patient received 1000 ml of whole blood. Another condition, where a drain or iron by the kidneys is a frequent occurence, is nocturnal paroxysmal hemoglobinuria (3 to 10 mg per day). The excessive urinary loss of iron in this disease (even in the absence of hemoglobinuria (8)) does indeed suggest a functional defect in the kidneys. The metal is usually in the form of hemosiderin in the epithelial cells of the tubules or in the urine (hemosiduria).

6. Changes in Hematocrit and the Kidney

In the normal kidney, anemia produces a substantial decrease in renal blood flow, a small reduction in plasma flow, and no change in the glomerular filtration rate (G.F.R.) (14, 35). Increase of the hematocrit causes an increase in the renal blood but the G.F.R. and the plasma flow are not affected until values of 75% or above are reached (14). Then it is sharply decreased (See Fig. 2). In diseased kidney, these adjustments take place more slowly or not at all (see below).

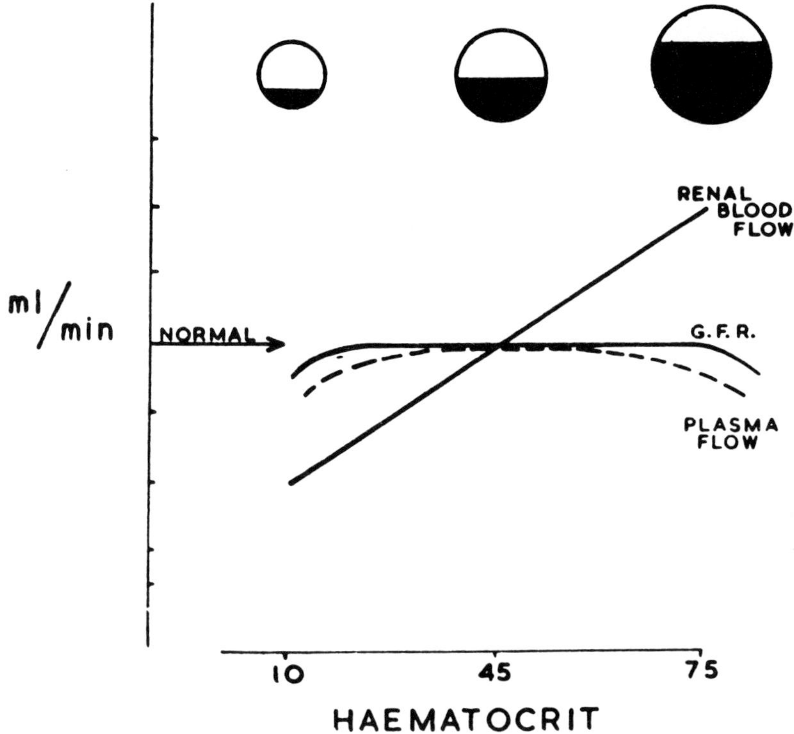

Fig. 2. The relationship of renal blood flow, plasma flow and glomerular filtration rate (G.F.R.) to hematocrit in the normal kidney. The three circles represent cross sections of renal vessels. (Courtesy of Dr. De Wardener, and Little, Brown and Co.)

ANEMIA AND RENAL DISEASE

1. Acute Renal Failure

Dilution anemia could be the first sign of sudden renal shut-down and many a time it is detected before the anuria or the oliguria. A hemoglobin concentration of 14.0 gm per 100 ml of blood falling to 8.0 or 9.0 in 24 hrs. does not necessarily mean an error of the laboratory but should alert one to the possibility of acute renal failure in the absence of a change in the clinical picture.

As the course of the disease unfolds, the mechanism of the anemia changes. The persistence of the anemia through the diuretic phase, even until a few weeks after the recovery from the renal failure, and the return of the blood urea nitrogen to a normal value, is a more puzzling feature of acute renal failure. The mechanism, therefore, of the anemia is not clearly understood but most erythrokinetic studies seem to indicate that a relative failure of the bone marrow is present, i.e., a moderate increase of red cell destruction with incomplete compensation of erythropoiesis (40). This concept of bone marrow failure will be discussed further in connection with chronic anemia. The increased hemolysis is due to premature ageing of red cells. No random destruction is noted (56).

The labelled red cells taken from three oliguric patients had a reduced life span when injected into normal recipients. In contradistinction, the red cells from patients with chronic renal failure usually have a normal life span in normal recipients. The apparent contradiction may be due to a more severe insult to the red cells in the acute oliguric state (56).

The red blood cell in acute renal failure has normal or increased concentration of reduced glutathione and glucose-6-phosphate dehydrogenase activity yet the stability of the reduced gluthathione after exposure to an oxidant is poor (58). No red cell antibodies can be demostrated by the Coombs test. The autohemolysis is not increased and the osmotic and mechanical fragility is either normal or slightly increased (13, 38). The retention of phosphates and ureates in excess of urea (the opposite occurs in chronic renal failure) may be responsible for the vacuolization and then rupture of red cells to form burr cells (56).

Cytologically, the bone marrow shows increased granulocytopoiesis with a high myeloid erythroid ratio. There is a shift to the left in the erythroid series with an increased number of proerythroblasts. Plasma cells are numerous but the lymphocytes are diminished in number. Megakaryocytopenia ia responsible for the thrombocytopenia when present (44). Reticulocytopenia is seen in some patients with acute renal failure (54).

2. Nephrotic Syndrome

Here again, anemia is a conspicuous feature of the disease regardless of whether azotemia is present or not. Just as the physical appearance of those patients is similar to patients with hypothyroidism, so is the anemia.

The anemia is macrocytic yet the bone marrow is normoblastic and not megaloblastic. The pathogenesis of this anemia, again, is obscure. Loss of transferrin (21) and, therefore, of iron into the urine may decrease the level of circulating transferrin but iron stores as a rule are not significantly reduced to cause hypochromia. One nephrotic patient in our series, who was losing 7 gm of albumin in a day, lost only 0.7% of an intravenously administered dose of Fe^{59}.

3. Chronic Renal Failure

There are two main and common hematologic disturbances associated with chronic failure of the kidneys: a) anemia, and b) alterations in the hemostatic function. Changes of the white blood cells besides a mild leukocytosis are not significant. Another complication, namely, secondary polycythemia though a rare occurrence is of a great hematologic significance.

A. ANEMIA

Anemia is a common feature of renal failure. Its severity seems to correlate well with the concentration of the blood urea nitrogen as depicted in Figure 1. Moreover, the mechanism of the anemia changes as the blood urea nitrogen exceeds 150 mg per 100 ml of blood, that is, from relative failure of the bone marrow to absolute. Its presence within certain limits does seem beneficial to the patient. Figure 2 depicts the relationship between the hematocrit of the blood and the glomerular filtration rate. Therefore, patients free of symptoms should not be transfused unless the hemoglobin concentration falls below 7.0 gm per 100 ml of blood and then it should not be raised to a value more than 10.0 gm per ml of blood. The fresh donor's blood is washed and only the packed cells are slowly given watching for any circulatory embarrassment.

The anemia is usually attributed to the effect of the retention of waste products upon the bone marrow interferring with the metabolism of the red blood cell. Although, this concept has not been supported by *in vitro*, yet, some of the transient beneficial effects of hemolysis on the erythrokinetic studies lend support and establish a causal relationship (33).

Another causal but more definitive consideration in the pathogenesis of anemia is the hormone, erythropoietin. Most of the evidence indicates that this hormone which has a proliferative effect on the stem cell of the bone marrow is produced primarily by the kidney (31). (Anephric patient (43a) continues to make reticulocytes.) A feed-back mechanism seems to exist between the kidneys and the bone marrow. In one direction the oxygen supply to the kidneys controls the secretion and/or release of erythropoietin and, in the other direction, the hormone controls the differentiation of the stem cells to erythroid cells (18). The concentration of erythropoietin in patients with chronic azotemia and anemia is much lower than in patients with anemia of comparable severity but without renal disease (43, 19, 7). Uremic plasma does not interfer with the action of erythropoietin (49). Peritoneal dialysis does not change the level of erythropoietin suggesting that renal damage rather than azotemia is responsible for the low lovel of the hormone (51).

The third factor responsible for the anemia and most probably the initiating trigger in the chain of events is increased rate of red cell destruction. The defect responsible for the excessive hemolysis seems to be primarily extracorpuscular

and not intracorpuscular. Red cells of uremic patients have normal survival rate when given to normal individuals (38). This does not rule out reversible and secondary intracorpuscular metabolic defects. In fact, decreased concentration of potassium and reduced glutathione (58) and phosphate esters (48) have been observed and may account for the morphologic abnormalities (burr cell, helmet, tear drop and star shaped) that are constantly (though relatively few in number) seen in chronic uremia. The *in vitro* autohemolysis of red cells correlates well with the severity of *in vitro* hemolysis. The increased autohemolysis is attributed to decreased glucose content and lowered pH of the erythrocytes (20).

The red cell destruction rate also seems to correlate well with the degree of azotemia and in a rare patient could be corrected by dialysis (33, 3).

The interrelationship of these causal factors have been clarified by the introduction of erythrokinetic studies. Two examples will be given.

No. 1. A 15-year-old girl was referred because of weakness and anemia. The presence of burr cells, fragments of red cells and cremated red cells on the peripheral blood smear suggested chronic renal failure and the determination of blood urea nitrogen (BUN) revealed a value of 87 mg per 100 ml blood. The bone marrow revealed "normal" erythropoiesis with normal iron content. The patient was considered to be in the early phase of chronic renal failure.

No. 2. A 36-year-old diabetic man was known to have chronic renal failure (BUN of more than 200 mg per 100 ml blood) for many years. He was studied during the late phase of his illness. These two patients have similar values for hemoglobin concentration yet the total hemoglobin mass is different. Patient No. 2 was more anemic and patient No. 1 was not as anemic as the hemoglobin concentration indicated.

From these two examples, it is obvious that red cell destruction rate did not change as the diesase got worse; however, erythropoiesis did diminish with time and severity. In the first patient, erythropoiesis was stepped up to almost twice the normal yet is was inadequate to compensate for the loss of red cells by increased hemolysis (relative bone marrow failure (40)). In the second case, in spite of a similar rate of hemolysis, erythropoiesis was less than normal (absolute bone marrow failure). In these two patients and also in published cases, there is no convincing evidence of "ineffective erythropoiesis" (25).

To sum up these findings, one can suggest that, in the chain of reactions, an increased rate of hemolysis occurs, although at first, the bone marrow can compensate partly, it eventually loses this capability. This loss of response could be related to a gradual decrease of the output of erythropoietin by the disease kidneys.

Hypoferremia and hypochromia are occasionally observed in chronic uremia. Most of the time the hypoferremia when present is associated with absent or low iron stores in the bone marrow. As a rule, this is due to chronic blood loss (epistaxis and gastrointestinal) which in turn is due to uremic gastritis and/or the various disturbances of hemostatic function that complicate chronic uremia. In a few patients with hypoferremia, the bone marrow content of iron is not low but rather normal or high. The combination of hypoferremia and increased iron stores suggests defective iron re-utilization by the red cells as a result of retention of the metal by the reticulo-endothelial system (RES). The over-activity of the RES may be due to the deranged metabolic defects of uremia. This, however, awaits confirmation by the determination of iron re-utilization following intravenous administration of Fe^{55} tagged hemoglobin solution (24).

Determination	Patient No. 1	Patient No. 2	Normal Values
Hb. conc. (gm per 100 ml)	7.7	7.2	14.0
Hemat. (%)	24.0	20.0	45.0
Absolute retic. (cu. mm.)	62,640	57,000	45,000-75,000
M.C.H.C. (%)	31.5	36.0	32-34
Blood volume (ml)	4200 (2931 expected)	3952 (4263 expected)	- - - - - - - - - - -
Total hemoglobin mass (gm)	323 (425 expected)	285 (639 expected)	- - - - - - - - - -
Fe^{59} T/2 clearance rate (min.)	107	212	60-120
Serum iron (ug/100 ml)	165	161	60-150
Plasma iron turnover (per day per gm of Hb.)	0.116	0.036	0.061
Plasma iron turnover index	1.9	0.6	1.0
Fe^{59} red cell utilization (%)	66.4	41	> 75
Cr^{51} T/2 red cell survival (d.)	19	18.5	28
Destruction rate	2.0	2.0	1.0

In general, the bone marrow is normoblastic in chronic renal disease. The serum concentration of vitamin B_{12} is normal but that of folic acid is low normal. This mild deficiency may account for the appearance of giant myelocytes and metamyelocytes and represents an early megaloblastoid development. Repeated dialysis over a long period of time brings about a further diminution of, again, only the level of folic acid but not vitamin B_{12}. Then megaloblastic anemia is to be expected (22).

B. SECONDARY POLYCYTHEMIA

The discovery that certain renal tumors, renal cysts and hydronephrosis are associated with polycythemia without thrombocytosis and leucocytosis pointed to the kidneys as the source of erythropoietin. However, it should be emphasized that only 3 to 4% of renal tumors (usually hypernephroma) are associated with polycythemia (12) but about one-third of them are presented by anemia (28) (myelofibrosis with extramedullary hemopoiesis or defective iron reutilization (26)). In some cases, erythropoietin was extracted from the cyst or tumor (29). The polycythemia recedes with surgical resection and recurrence of the polycythemia is an early sign of relapse and/or metastasis.

C. HEMOSTASIS

Bleeding is a common occurrence in renal failure whether acute or chronic (9, 15, 16, 34, 36, 47). The incidence is about 30 to 35% in either state. It carries a bad prognostic sign especially in the chronic condition. There have been reported numerous defects in hemostasis occurring as isolated findings or in various combinations. Their appearance does not depend on the level of blood urea nitrogen, potassium or hemoglobin concentration. The most frequent abnormalities are mild to moderate thrombocytopenia (this by itself seldom causes bleeding), prolonged bleeding time, prolonged prothrombin time, an abnormal thromboplastin generation test, and an impaired prothrombin consumption. The concentration of plasma fibrinogen is usually elevated. For screening purposes, measurements of Ivy bleeding time, clot retraction and prothrombin consumption tests seem to be the most reproducible and reliable.

Most of the investigations have pointed to a qualitative defect in the platelets to be responsible for bleeding. Defective platelet adhesiveness with added thrombin or ADP has been demonstrated (53). Using the revolving plastic tube, the platelets of uremic plasma are shown to be incapable of forming a plug (55). The aggregation of platelets and the activation of platelet factor 3 (which participates in the first stage of coagulation) are initiated by the adenosin 5-diphosphate (ADP). An intermediate of urea metabolism, guanidino-succinic acid, but not urea seem to interfere with the action of ADP upon platelets (30) Peritoneal dialysis or extra-corporeal dialysis corrects the abnormalities in the platelet function and stop bleeding. Phosphatides of platelets seem to be normal (2).

A major cause of bleeding should also be sought in the vascular tree. Many diseases of the kidneys are in reality widely spread vascular disorders with only emphasis on the kidneys. Hypertension, acute glomerulonephritis and Henoch-Schönlein purpura are a few examples. The diseased blood vessel becomes more fragile and bleeding ensues.

Azotemia, too, may increase this fragility and/or induces inflammation or the mucosal epithelium. Frequent episodes of gastritis with hemorrhage occur in the end stage of the disease.

A less frequent cause of bleeding has been stressed recently. A heparin-like anticoagulant (thus prolonging the thrombin time) has been observed in association with chronic nephritis. The defect is corrected by protamine sulfate *in vivo* and *in vitro* (10).

BIBLIOGRAPHY

1. Adams, W. S., Davis, F., and Nakatani, M.: Purine and pyrimidine excretion in normal and leukemic subjects. Am. J. Med., *28:*726, 1960.
2. Altschuler, G., Marcus, A. J., and Ullman, H. L.: Platelets and platelet phosphatides in uremia. Blood, *16:*1439, 1960.
2a. Atwater, J., and Tocantins, L. M.: Methods for estimation of blood loss in body fluids and tissues. In, Tocantins, L. M., and Kazal, L. A., (eds.): Blood Coagulation, Hemorrhage and Thrombosis. by New York, Grune & Stratton (c1964), p. 418.
3. Berry, E. R., Rambach, W. A., Alt, H. L., and del Greco, F.: Effect of peritoneal dialysis on erythrokinetics and ferrokinetics of azotemic anemia. Trans. Am. Soc. Art. Intern. Organs, *10:*415, 1964.
4. Brain, M. C., and Beck, E. A.: Relationship of intravascular coagulation and intravascular hemolysis. Clin. Res., *13:*268, 1965.
5. Brain, M. C., Dacie, J. V., and Hourihane, D. O'B.: Microangiopathic haemolytic anemia: The possible role of vascular lesions in pathogenesis. Brit. J. Haemat., *8:*358, 1962.
6. Brain, M. C., and Hourihane, D. O'B.: Microangiopathic heamolytic anemia: the occurrence of haemolysis in experimentally produced vascular disease. Brit. J. Haemat., *13:*135, 1967.
7. Brown, R.: Plasma erythropoietin in chronic uraemia. Brit. Med. J., *2:*1036, 1965.
8. Brule, M., Hillemand, P., and Gaube, R.: Un nouveau cas d'anémie hémolytique avec hemoglobinurie et hemosiderinurie. Presse med., *46:*1329, 1938.
9. Castaldi, P. A., Rozenberg, M. C., and Stewart, J. H.: The bleeding disorder of uraemia. Lancet, *2:*66, 1966.
10. Cetingil, A. I. Ulutin, O. N., and Karaca, M.: Heparin-like anticoagulant occurring in association with chronic nephritis. Brit. Med. J., *2:*38, 1959.
11. Cheney, K., and Bonnin, J. A.: Haemorrhage, platelet dysfunction and other coagulation defects in uraemia. Brit. J. Haemat., *8:*215, 1962.
12. Conley, C. L., Kowal, J., and D'Antonio, J.: Polycythemia associated with renal tumors. Bull. Hopkins Hosp., *101:*63, 1957.
13. Desforges, J. F., and Dawson, J. P.: The anemia of renal failure. Arch. Int. Med., *101:*326, 1958.
14. De Wardener, H. E.: The Kidney, 2nd ed. Boston, Little Brown and Co., 1961.
15. Donner, L., and Neuwirtová, R.: The hemostatic defect of acute and chronic uremia. Thromb. Diath. Haem., *5:*319, 1960-61.
16. Egeberg, O.: Blood coagulation in renal failure. Scand. J. Clin. Lab. Invest., *14:*163, 1962.
17. Engle, R. L., and Wallis, L. A.: Multiple myeloma and the adult Fanconi syndrome. Am. J. Med., *22:*5, 1957.
18. Erslev, A. J.: Hematology: Control of red cell production. Ann. Rev. Med., *11:*315, 1960.
19. Gallagher, N. I., McCarthy, J. M., and Lange, R. D.: Observations on erythropoietic-stimulating factor (ESF) in the plasma of uremic and non-uremic anemic patients. Ann. Int. Med., *52:*1201, 1960.
20. Giovannetti, S., Giagnoni, P., Babestri, P. L., and Cioni, L.: Red cell survival in chronic uremia. Experientia, *22:*739, 1966.
21. Gitlin, D., Janeway, C. A., and Farr, L. E.: Studies on the metabolism of plasma proteins in the nephrotic syndrome. I. Albumin γglobulin and iron binding globulin. J. Clin. Invest., *35:*44, 1956.
22. Hampers, C. L., Streiff, R., Nathan, D. G., Snyder, D., and Merrill, J. P.: Megaloblastic hematopoiesis in uremia and in patients on long-term hemodialysis. New Eng. J. Med., *276:*551, 1967.
23. Harvey, A. McG., Walker, W. G., and Yardley, J. H.: Renal involvement in myeloma, amyloidosis, systemic lupus erythematosus and other disorders of connective tissue In, Strauss, M. B., and Welt, L. G., (eds.): Diseases of the Kidneys. Boston, Little, Brown and Co. (c1963), p. 580.
24. Haurani, F. I., Burke, W., and Martinez, E. J.: Defective reutilization of iron in the anemia of inflammation. J. Lab. Clin. Med., *65:*560, 1965.
25. Haurani, F. I., and Tocantins, L. M.: Ineffective erythropoiesis. Am. J. Med., *31:*519, 1961.
26. Haurani, F. I., Young, K., and Tocantins, L. M.: Reutilization of iron in anemia complicating malignant neoplasms. Blood, *22:*73, 1963.
27. Hensley, W. J.: Haemolytic anaemia in acute glomerulonephritis. Aust. Ann. Med., *1:*180, 1952.
28. Hewitt, C. B.: Renal carcinoma: a clinical chal-

lenge. In, King J. S., Jr. (ed.): Renal Neoplasia. Boston, Little, Brown and Co., 1967, p. 7.

29. Hewlett, J. S., Hoffman, G. C., Senhauser, D. A., and Battle, J. D., Jr.: Hypernephroma with erythrocythemia; report of a case and assay of the tumor for an erythropoietic-stimulating substance. New Eng. J. Med., *262:*1058, 1960.

30. Horowitz, H. I., Cohen, B. D., Martinez, P. and Papayoanou, M. F.: Defective ADP-induced platelet factor 3 activation in uremia. Blood, *30:*331, 1967.

31. Jacobson, L. O., Goldwasser, E., Fried, W., and Pizak, L.: Role of the kidney in erythropoiesis. Nature, *179:*633, 1957.

32. Keitel, H. G., Thompson, D., and Itano, H. A.: Hyposthenuria in sickle cell anemia: a reversible renal defect. J. Clin. Invest., *35:*998, 1956.

33. Kurtides, E. S., Rambach, W. A., Alt, H. L., and Del Greco, F.: Effect of hemodialysis on erythrokinetics in anemia of uremia. J. Lab. Clin. Med., *63:*469, 1964.

34. Larrain, C., Adelson, E.: The hemostatic defect of uremia. I. Clinical investigation of three patients with acute post-traumatic renal insufficiency. Blood, *11:*1059, 1956.

35. Levin, W. C., Gregory, R., and Bennett, A.: The effect of chronic anemia on renal function as measured by inulin and diodrast clearances. J. Lab. Clin. Med., *32:*1433, 1947.

36. Lewis, J. H., Zucker, M. B., and Ferguson, J. H.: Bleeding tendency in uremia. Blood, *11:*1073, 1956.

37. Lickerman, E., Henser, E., Donnell, G. N., Landing, B. H., and Hammond, G.: Hemolytic uremic syndrome. New Eng. J. Med., *275:*227, 1966.

38. Loge, J. P., Lange, R. D., and Moore, C. V.: Characterization of anemia associated with chronic renal insufficiency. Am. J. Med., *24:*4, 1958.

39. Lucas, W. M., Bullock, W. H.: Hematuria in sickle cell disease. J. Urol., *83:*733, 1960.

40. Moore, C.: The concept of relative bone marrow failure. Am. J. Med., *23:*1, 1957.

41. Morgan, C., Jr., and Mammack, W. J.: Intravenous urography in multiple myeloma. New Eng. J. Med., *275:*77, 1966.

42. Mostofi, F. K., Vorder Bruegge, C. F., and Diggs, L. W. Lesions in kidneys removed for unilateral hematuria in sickle-cell disease. Arch. Path., *63:*336, 1957.

43. Naets, J. P., and Heuse, A. F.: Measurement of erythropoietic stimulating factor in anemic patients with or without renal disease. J. Lab. Clin. Med., *60:*365, 1962.

43a. Nathan, D. G., Schupak, E., and Merrill, J. P.: Erythrokinetics in anephric man. Blood, *22:*811, 1963.

44. Pasternack, A., and Wahlberg, P.: Bone marrow in acute renal failure. Acta Med. Scand., *181:*505, 1967.

45. Perillie, P. E., and Epstein, F. H.: Sickling phenomenon produced by hypertonic solutions: a possible explanation of the hyposthenuria of sicklemia. J. Clin. Invest., *42:*570, 1963

46. Piel, C. F., and Phibbs, R. H.: The hemolytic-uremic syndrome. Ped. Clin. N. Am., *13:*295, 1966.

47. Rath, C. E., Mailliard, J. A., and Schreiner, G. E.: Bleeding tendency in uremia. New Eng. J. Med., *257:*808, 1957.

48. Rees, S. B., Scheitlin, W. G., Pond, J. C., McManus, T. J., Guild, W. R., and Merrill, J. P.: Effect of dialysis and purine ribosides upon the anemia of uremia. J. Clin. Invest., *36:*923, 1957.

49. Reissman, K. R., Nomura, T., Gunn, R. W., and Brosius, F.: Erythropoietic response to anemia or erythropoietin injection in uremic rats with or without functioning renal tissue. Blood, *16:*1411, 1960.

50. Rodríguez-Erdmann, F.: Intravascular activation of the clotting system with phospholipids. Blood, *26:*541, 1965.

51. Rosse, W. F., Berry, R. J. and Waldman, T. A.: Some molecular characteristics of erythropoietin from different sources determined by inactivation by ionizing radiation. J. Clin. Invest., *42:*124, 1963.

51a. Rundles, R. W., Laszlo, J., Itoga, T., Hobson, J. B., and Garrison, F. E., Jr.: Clinical and hematologic study of 6-[(1-methyl-4-nitro-5-imidazolyl)thio]purine (B.W. 57-322) and related compounds. Cancer Chemother. Rep., *14:*99-115, 1961.

52. Roussak, N. J., and Oleesky, S.: Water-losing nephritis. Quart J. Med., *23:*147, 1954.

53. Salzman, E. W., and Neri, L. L.: Adhesiveness of blood platelets in uremia. Thromb. Diath. Haem., *15:*84, 1966.

54. Shaw, A. B., and Scholes, M. C.: Reticulocytosis in renal failure. Lancet, *1:*799, 1967.

55. Silver, M. J., Orocofsky, M., Johns, H., and Clark, J. E.: The hemostatic defect in uremia. Fed. Proc., *26(2):* No. 368, 1967.

56. Stewart, J. H.: Haemolytic anaemia in acute and chronic renal failure. Quart. J. Med., *36:*85, 1967.

57. Stewart, J. H., and Castaldi, P. A.: Uraemic bleeding: a reversible platelet defect corrected by dialysis. Quart. J. Med., *36:*409, 1967.

58. Theil, G. B., Brodine, C. E., and Doolan, P. D.: Red cell glutathione content and stability in renal insufficiency. J. Lab. Clin. Med., *58:*736, 1961.

Chapter 47

Pathologic Aspects of "Blackwater Fever"

SEYMOUR ROSEN, M.D.

The term "blackwater fever" was first introduced by James Easmon (5) in 1884. At that time, he recognized the fever to be the result of the malarial infection and considered the blackwater to represent urinary hemoglobin. The disease was later recognized primarily as a complication of falciparum malaria (9). Since autopsy studies are fraught with interpretative difficulties (8) and the only reported biopsy study involves convalescent patients (15), the basic histology of "blackwater fever" remains unclear. In this chapter, "blackwater fever," as illustrated by the malarial infected monkey (16) and hamster (17) will be considered in relation to the more chronic findings in human biopsies (15).

CLINICAL FINDINGS

The clinical aspects are listed in Table I. The infected monkey (Macaca Mulatta), hamster, and human cases, all fulfill Maegraith's criteria (9) for the occurence of "blackwater fever" in malaria: "The basic phenomenon in blackwater fever is a rapid, severe lysis of erythrocytes associated with the passage of hemoglobin or its derivations in the urine." Although the animal models are analogous to many cases of human "blackwater fever," some patients have hemoglobinemia for reasons such as drug toxicity unassociated with extensive parasitemia (9).

MORPHOLOGY

The pathological descriptions will be confined to the kidney; major histological features are listed in Table II.

Rhesus Monkey.

Besides numerous parasitized erythrocytes, the striking abnormality was the many hyaline droplets within proximal tubular epithelium. Some droplets were positive in silver methenamine and periodic acid-Schiff preparations. In spite of prolonged staining, others were consistently negative. Many of these granules evidently stained for hemoglobin (Fig. 1a) and basilar sudanophilic droplets were common in frozen sections (Fig. 2a). Electron microscopy of proximal tubular epithelium revealed numerous relatively homogeneous, circular electron dense bodies (Fig. 1b) and electron lucent inclusions (Fig. 2b) which corresponded to the tubular sudanophilic droplets.

TABLE I—CLINICAL FINDINGS IN "BLACKWATER FEVER"*

	Number	Parasite	Time (Days) from Initiation of Infection to Obtaining Tissue	Maximal Parasitemia (%)	Lowest Hematocrit (Vol. %)	Maximal BUN (mg per 100 ml)	Comments
MONKEY	9	P. knowlesi	7-8	18-69	10-19 (43±3)	51+18 (22± 5)	Rapid, lethal illness
HAMSTER	68	P. berghei	2-16	26-37	9-25 (50±2)	72± 9† (27± 3)	Considerable weight loss; frequently lethal
MAN	6	P. falciparum	14-182‡	1-70	16-29	20-150	Drug hemolysis additional factor; with present therapy minimal mortality

*Variation is expressed as total range or standard deviation; appropriate normal values are listed in parentheses.
†At 10 days.
‡Reference to initiation of clinical illness.

TABLE II—MAJOR MORPHOLOGICAL FEATURES OF BLACKWATER FEVER

	Proximal Tubules			Casts	Fibrosis and Tubular Atrophy	Comments
	Hyaline Droplets	Iron Positive Granules	Fat			
MONKEY	++	0	++	±	0	Many parasitized erythrocytes; most hyaline droplets unstained in PAS and silver methenamine preparations
HAMSTER	+	++	++	±	±	Many parasitized erythrocytes; intra-vascular pigment laden histiocytes especially numerous in small veins; extramedullary hematopoeisis
MAN	±	+#	0	+	+	Glomerular hyalization in two cases; in one of these electron microscopy of a preceding biopsy revealed many glomerular epithelial electron dense inclusions

0 = Absent
± = Occasional
+ = Frequent
++ = Abundant
\#   Refers also to atrophic tubules and interstitial cells

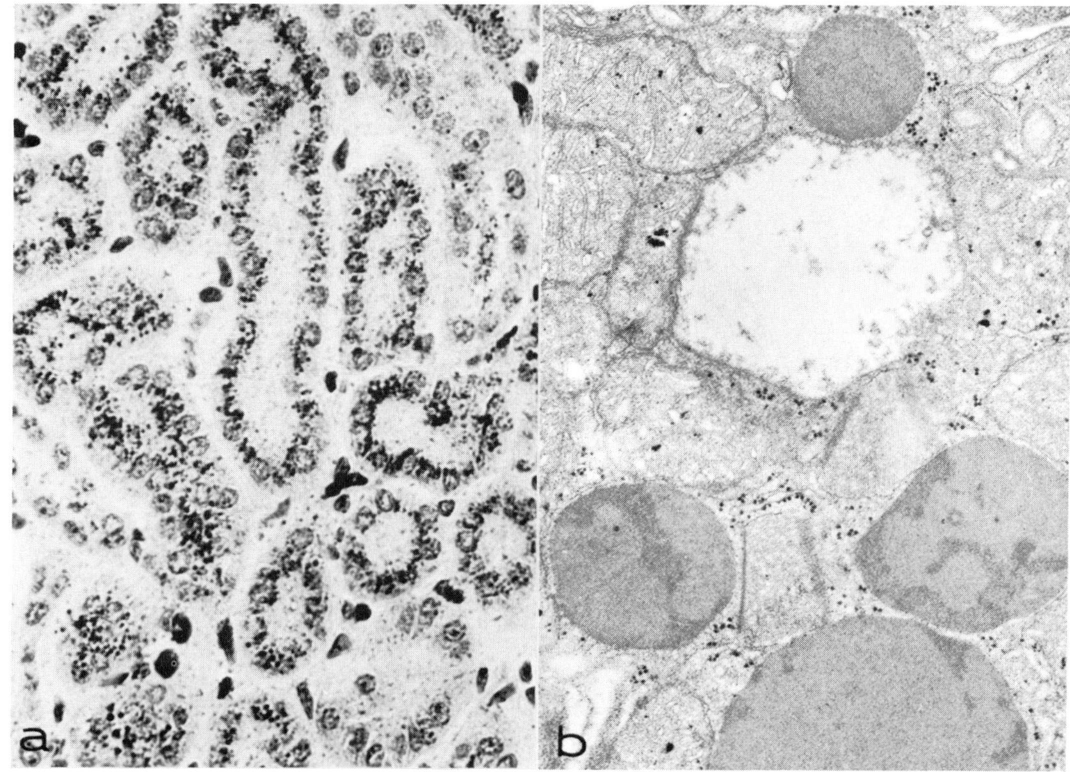

Fig. 1.   Rhesus monkey infected with P. knowlesi.
  a. In this stain for hemoglobin, numerous positive granules are present within proximal tubular epithelium. X 415
  b. Portion of proximal tubular cell. These circular, relatively homogeneous bodies apparently represent absorbed hemoglobin. Electron micrograph X 21840

Hamster.

After a few days of infection, vessels contained many parasitized erythrocytes and pigment laden macrophanges. The latter were especially prominent in interlobular and arcuate veins. At later times, extramedullary hematopoeisis apparently of the erythrocytic variety was present in the inner cortex and outer medulla. The proximal tubules contained extensive apical hemosiderin deposits (Fig. 3a) and in some animals marked basilar deposition of sudanophilic droplets was observed. Electron microscopy of proximal tubular epithelium disclosed extremely electron dense, irregular,

finely granular single membrane limited inclusions (Fig. 3b) and basilar electron lucent bodies similar to those noted in the monkey kidney.

Human.

The most common findings included focal fibrosis and tubular atrophy associated with hyaline and hemoglobin casts (Fig 4a); iron positive pigment was present in tubular epithelium and interstitial cells. Electron microscopy revealed increased interstitial collagen and fibroblasts containing inclusions, some of which were identified as malarial pigment (Fig. 4b). In general,

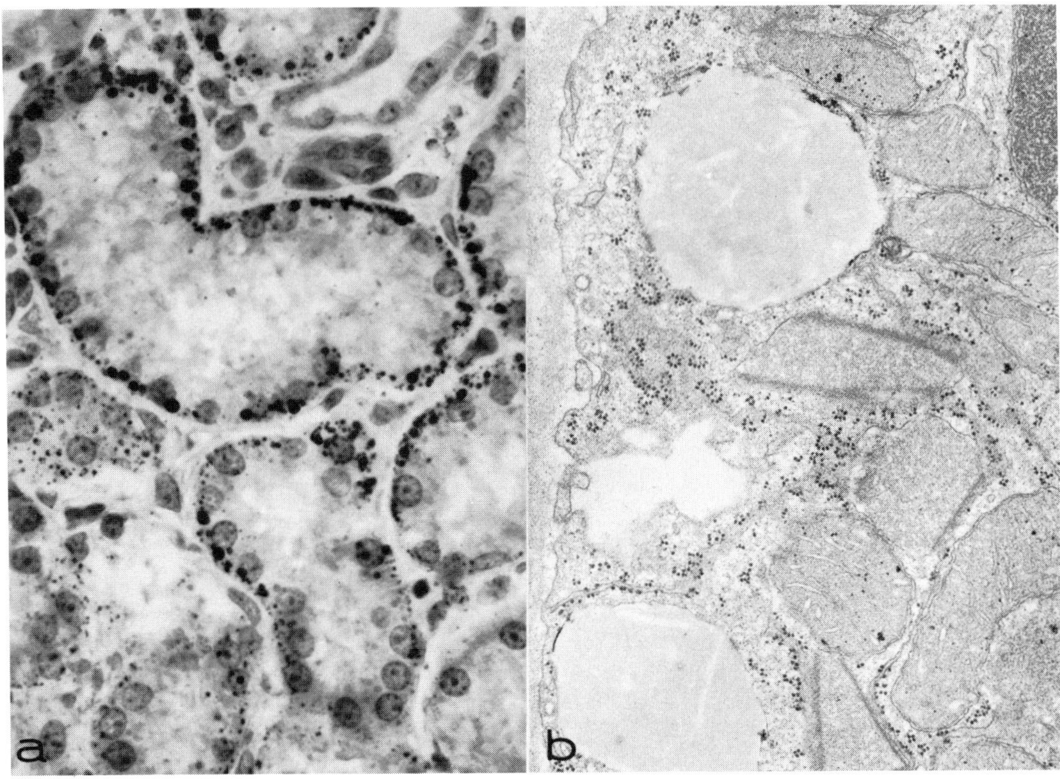

Fig. 2.   Rhesus monkey infected with P. knowlesi.
    a. Basilar sudanophilic droplets are common in many proximal tubular cells. X 550
    b. Portion of proximal tubular cell. Electron lucent bodies are noted near the basement membrane seen on the extreme left. These correspond to the sudanophilic droplets. Electron micrograph. X 17470

tubules were unremarkable; numerous electron dense bodies were present in the proximal tubular epithelium of one patient biopsied 14 days after the initiation of clinical illness.

HEMOGLOBINURIC NEPHROSIS

The nephropathy of blackwater fever is basically a hemoglobinuric nephrosis (1). Nephrosis (12), a classical term used to distinguish a tubular disease from dominant glomerular change is particularly appropriate in this situation where tubular hemoglobin absorption and fatty change constitute the major pathological features. The basic study in this regard is that of Rather (14) who demonstrated, after the injection of hemoglobin, a sequence of proximal tubular hemoglobin reabsorption droplets, hemosiderin formation, and later focal tubular atrophy. Ericcson (6, 7) has examined, in part, these alterations by electron microscopy. He demonstrated pinocytotic uptake of hemoglobin with subsequent sequestation into acid phosphatase containing bodies, a process described by deDuve as heterophagy (4). The fatty tubular change may reflect the high levels of circulating free fatty acids which occur during malarial infection (3, 10, 11).

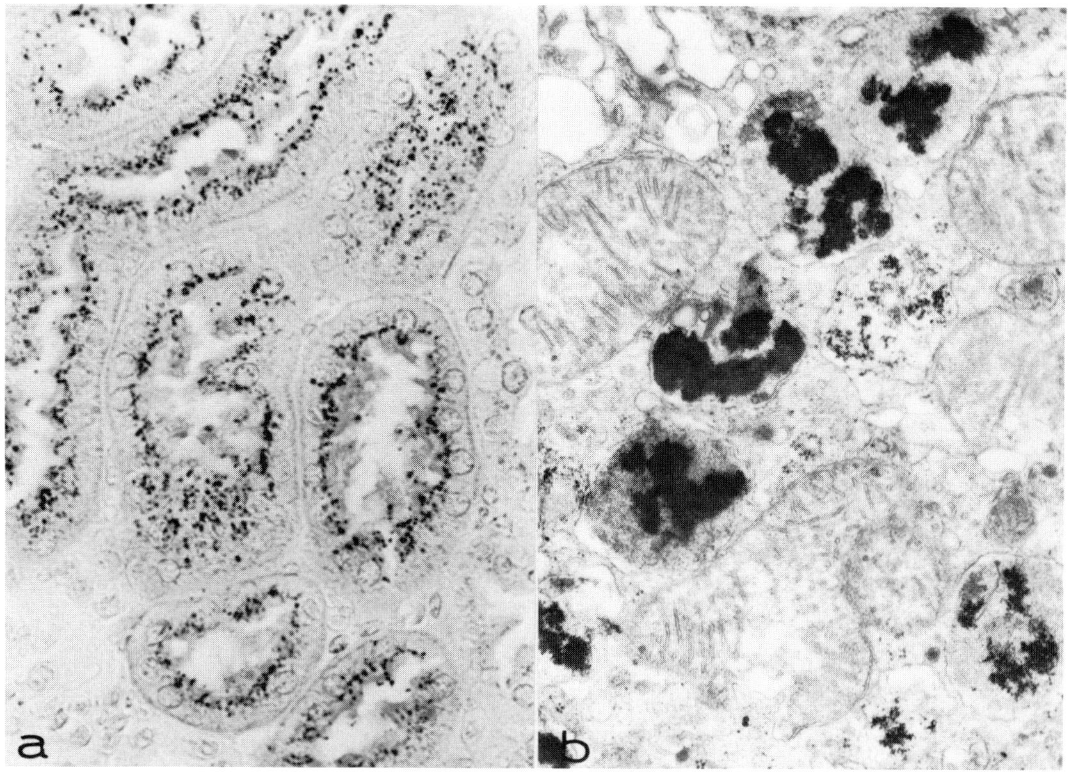

Fig. 3.   Hamster infected with P. berghei.
   a.   The apical portions of these proximal tubules contain many positive granules in the stain for iron. X 530
   b.   These extremely electron dense bodies correspond to the iron positive granules. Electron micrograph. X 21770

PATHOLOGY OF ACUTE RENAL FAILURE

It has become apparent in the last few years that there is little pathological basis for most cases of acute renal failure (2, 8, 13). This disparity was first noted by Brun (2) in a percutaneous renal biopsy study. Other workers (8) using carefully controlled autopsy material could not find histological features which characterize the kidney of renal failure. In an electron microscopic study of renal biopsies taken from patients with acute renal failure, Olsen and Skjoldborg have noted comparatively little alteration (13). There was no correlation with the extent of azotemia and the various pathological features of blackwater fever as described in this communication.

SUMMARY

The clinical and renal pathological features of "blackwater fever" associated with malarial infection are described for Rhesus monkey, hamster, and man. Accompanying the parasitemia, there is a fall in hematocrit and elevation of the blood urea nitrogen levels. In monkey, the disease is rapidly lethal. Its course in the hamster is more indolent and the mortality in man in minimal. Except for fat deposition in the monkey and

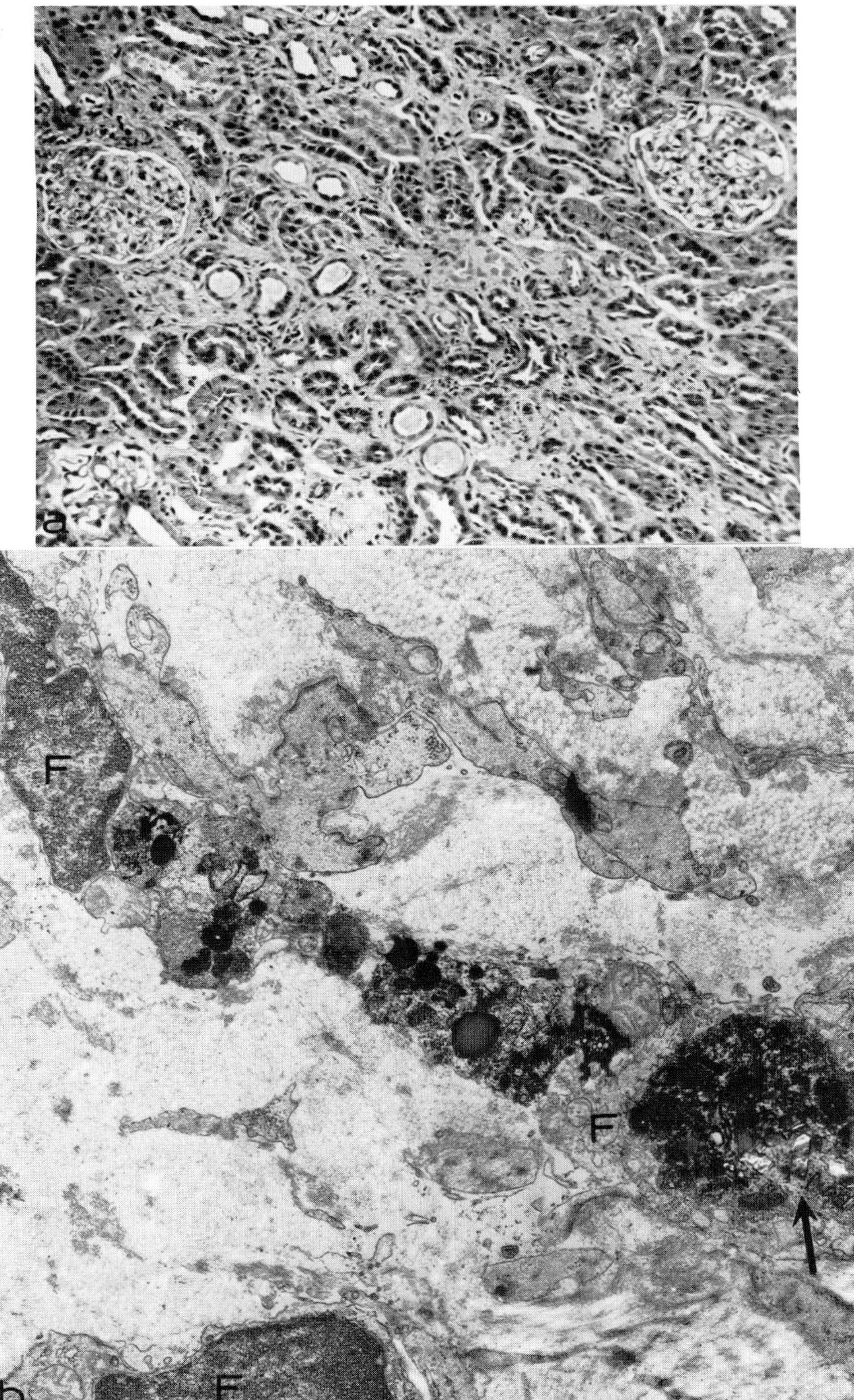
a
b
F
F
F

hamster, the morphological alterations are basically similar to the response occuring after the injection of hemoglobin: proximal tubular hemoglobin reabsorption droplets, hemosiderin formation, and late focal tubular atrophy.

REFERENCES

1. Allen, A. C.: The Kidney. New York, Grune and Stratton, 1963, pp. 479-483.
2. Brun, C., and Munck, O.: Lesions of the kidney in acute renal failure following shock. Lancet, *1*:603-607, 1957.
3. Carlson, L. A., Liljedahl, S. O., and Wirsen, C.: Blood and tissue changes in the dog during and after excessive free fatty acid mobilization. Acta. Med. Scand., *178*:81-102, 1965.
4. deDuve, C., and Wattiaux, R.: Functions of lysosomes. Ann. Rev. Physiol., *28*:435-492, 1966.
5. Easmon, J. F.: The nature and treatment of blackwater fever. Printed for the Government of the Gold Coast, London, 1884.
6. Ericcson, J. L. E.: Absorption and decomposition of homologous hemoglobin in renal proximal tubular cells. An experimental light and electron microscopic study. Acta. Path. Microbiol. Scand. (Suppl. 168):1-121, 1964.
7. Ericcson, J. L. E.: Transport and digestion of hemoglobin in the proximal tubule. II. Electron microscopy. Lab. Invest., *14*:16-39, 1965.
8. Finckh, E. S., Jeremy, D., and Whyte, H. M.: Structural renal damage and its relation to clinical features in acute oliguric renal failure. Quart. J. Med., *31*:429-446, 1962.
9. Maegraith, B. G.: Pathological Processes in Malaria and Blackwater Fever. Oxford, Blackwell Scientific Publications, 1948, pp. 24-26, 215-221.
10. Maegraith, B. G.: Comments on pathophysiology. Military Med., *131*:1112, 1966 (Suppl.)
11. Maunsback, A. B., and Wirsen, C.: Ultrastructural changes in kidney, myocardium and skeletal muscle of the dog during excessive mobilization of free fatty acids, J. Ultrastruct. Res., *16*:35-54, 1966.
12. Mueller, F.: Morbis Brightii. Verhandl. Deutsch. Ges. Path., *9*:64, 1905.
13. Olsen, S., and Skjoldborg, J.: Ultrastructure of the kidney in acute anuria. III International Congress of Nephrology, Washinton, D. C., 1966 (Abstract).
14. Rather, L. J.: Renal arthrocytosis and intracellular digestion of intraperitoneally injected hemoglobin in rats. J. Exp. Med., *87*:163-174, 1948.
15. Rosen, S., Hano, J. E., Inman, M. M., Gilliland, P. F., and Barry, K. G.: The kidney in blackwater fever: Light and electron microscopic observations. Amer. J. Clin. Path., *49*:358-370, 1968.
16. Rosen, S., Hano, J. E., and Barry, K. G.: Malarial nephropathy in the Rhesus Monkey, Arch. Path., *85:*36-44, 1968.
17. Sesta, J., Rosen, S., and Sprintz, H.: Malarial nephropathy in the Golden Hamster. Arch. Path., *85:*663-668, 1968.

Fig. 4. Human with "blackwater fever" associated with P. falciparum infection. Renal biopsies obtained 2 months after the onset of illness and when the patients had normal renal function.

    a. Note the focal fibrosis and tubular atrophy associated with casts. X 190

    b. These fibroblasts (F) containing numerous inclusions are separated by large amounts of collagen. The inclusion in the lower right includes several rectangular, partially electron lucent areas representing malarial pigment (arrow). Electron micrograph X 7480

Chapter 48

Effects of Radiation on the Kidney

F. K. MOSTOFI, M.D.

The kidneys may be affected either by total body irradiation, or by local irradiation. The problem has been discussed in considerable detail elsewhere (7). It is the purpose of this chapter to review briefly the changes induced by local irradiation.

ETIOLOGY

Radiation to the kidney results from therapy for malignant tumors of the ovaries, uterus, kidneys, pancreas, and retroperitoneum. Patients with these tumors are treated either by surgery and radiation, or by radiation alone if the tumor is inoperable.

It is of interest that the largest reported number of cases with radiation damage to the kidneys has been in those with testicular seminoma treated with radiation to the retroperitoneal and hilar regions, either for known metastasis or as a prophylactic measure to prevent the development of metastasis (5, 6).

It has generally been maintained that the kidneys are resistant to irradiation. The increasing frequency of renal involvement seen after radiation, however, has led the radiotherapist to consider 2500 r as a safe level if spread over a period of 3 to 6 weeks. Some maintain that as much as 5000 r may be given in 5 to 9 weeks if only a part of each kidney

is included (4). Tublin and Gambos have called attention to the fact that renal damage may result from doses below 1385 r (11).

Luxton has classified the clinical symptoms into four categories: proteinuria, benign hypertension, chronic radiation nephritis, and acute radiation nephritis (5, 6). From the pathological point of view, there are 2 main categories: a) the chronic renal involvement developing over a period of years, and b) the acute renal involvement developing within a few months. The pathologic features and pathogenesis of each group will be discussed in relation to the clinical manifestations.

PATHOPHYSIOLOGIC PATTERNS AND PATHOGENESIS

I. Most, if not all, the patients receiving radiation therapy to the upper abdomen and the renal area show some proteinuria. Usually, there are no signs of renal disease. Aveoli and his associates, however, have carried out extensive renal-function tests in patients who were being given radiation to the renal region (2). They observed a progressive drop of renal plasma flow during radiotherapy. Transient depression of glomerular filtration rate occurred, followed by an increase at cumulative doses of 2000 to

2400 rads. Although tubular activity was variable, there was a trend to a decrease during and after irradiation. These changes were transient. No biopsies were reported from these patients (2).

In experimental animals exposed to irradiation, however, we have reported the earliest postradiation renal changes to consist of congestion, edema, and transitory tubular epithelial damage (8).

After this initial proteinuria, the majority of these patients apparently show no clinical evidence of renal impairment, and the causes of death in those who die are other than radiation effects on the kidney. Some of these patients do show mild hypertension but whether this is entirely on the basis of renal disease, extra-renal vascular effects of radiation or essential is unknown. Pathologic examination of many of these kidneys, however, will show the tell-tale radiation effects. Although the architecture is well preserved and both the glomeruli and the tubules appear normal, careful examination, especially with reticulum stains, will reveal a shrunken kidney in which the major changes appear to be in the tubules. They are small and collapsed, and there is also mild increase in the interstitial fibrous tissue.

If renal involvement is more severe, the patients will manifest evidences of renal disease. The symptoms consist of proteinuria, anemia, weakness and progressive impairment of renal function, and eventual death in renal failure. The onset of symptoms is insidious, developing slowly over a period of years without any prior warning. In some cases, however, the condition may develop following an acute attack, to be described later.

The end stage in patients who die of renal failure is a scarred kidney, the extent and location of scarring depending on whether only the lower pole or the whole of one or both kidneys had been in the beam. The capsule is thickened, fibrosed, and adherent. The underlying kidney is collapsed, gray, and fibrotic. There is often a sharp line of demarcation between the normal and the irradiated areas.

Microscopically, the changes consist of tubular atrophy, interstitial fibrosis, and sclerosis of the vessels. Most of the glomeruli are normal, but in patients with protracted clinical course there is eventually glomerular involvement with varying degrees of sclerosis and hyalinization, but this is much less severe than the extensive tubular atrophy and interstitial fibrosis. Inflammatory infiltration per se is not a usual component of the reaction, but a few lymphocytes, plasma cells, and monocytes may be seen.

In about half of the patients dying of chronic renal failure, hypertension is present, and this is reflected in the intimal and medial thickening, with or without focal areas of necrosis (6).

The pathogenesis of the lesion is fairly clear. The vascular alteration is a well-known sequela of radiation, and—while the specific mechanism responsible for its development is unknown—it is nevertheless a recognized entity. The tubular atrophy and degeneration could be either due to direct effect of radiation on the tubular epithelial cells or secondary to vascular changes. Based on our studies in experimental animals, we believe that both factors play a role (8). The glomeruli escape injury until late and then show hyalinization, indicating an effect secondary to tubular and/or vascular damage. Interstitial fibrosis may be in response to tubular degeneration and stromal collapse or due to the primary stromal response to radiation.

The term "sclerosing nephrosis" has been proposed for this group in preference to "chronic radiation nephritis" or "radiation sclerosis," since neither term adequately describes the lesion (7).

Sclerosing nephrosis with tubular degeneration and atrophy, sclerosis of the vessels, and interstitial fibrosis constitute the basic and the most frequently encountered effect of radiation on the kidney. A number of patients with mild sclerosing nephrosis who have proteinuria and mild hypertension for many years suddenly manifest malignant hypertension. The mechanism of development of malignant hypertension in these patients is unknown, but it must be considered to be of renal origin. It is quite frequent, as Luxton found it in 14 of his 54 patients (6). The recognition of renal origin of the hypertension is essential, because if only one kidney is involved, split-function studies may pinpoint the side and nephrectomy may be life saving (3).

The clinical course of the patients with malignant hypertension is similar to that of other patients with malignant hypertension of renal origin. The pathologic changes consist of severe sclerosis of arteries and arterioles, endarteritis, and necrotizing vasculitis. Involvement of glomerular capillaries with fibrin thrombi and infarction is not infrequent. Areas of renal infarction and interstitial hemorrhage are frequent, but the inflammatory reaction is not present except in association with necrotizing vasculitis.

II. In contrast to the sclerosing nephrosis which develops over a period of many years and which may be associated with benign or malignant hypertension, irradiation of the kidney may lead to yet another clinicopathologic entity. Designated as acute radiation nephritis, this is manifested as severe renal vascular disease within 3 to 12 months after irradiation (6, 9). The symptoms consist of proteinuria, weakness, anemia, progressive ankle or facial edema, headache, exertional dyspnea, malignant hypertension, and uremia. While the symptoms are basically similar to those of the sclerosing nephrosis, they develop dramatically and within the first year after irradiation, in contrast to the insidious and prolonged course of sclerosing nephrosis, which develops many years after irradiation.

The immediate prognosis is related to the occurrence of malignant hypertension. Eight of Luxton's 20 patients had had malignant hypertension, and 6 of these died in 3 to 12 months; the other 2 recovered spontaneously, but both continued to have persistent chronic renal failure. All but 4 of the remaining patients died of chronic renal failure with or without hypertension (7 patients) or with chronic hypertension without renal failure (1 patient) (6).

Grossly, the kidneys are large and swollen. The cortex is smooth but shows petechial hemorrhages. Microscopically, the glomeruli are severely involved. They are large and hypocellular. There is fusion of capillary loops as well as thickening of capillary walls, leading to the diagnosis of membranous glomerulonephritis (1). Thin sections stained by periodic acid-Schiff (PAS), Masson trichrome, and periodic acid-methenamine silver (PAMS) show that the basement membrane is for the most part intact and that the thickening consists mainly of swelling and vacuolization of the cytoplasm of the endothelial cells and—to a lesser extent— of the epithelial cells. Electron microscopy has demonstrated that considerable amounts of basement membrane-like material are present in the endothelial or luminal side of the capillary. The lamina densa-like material surrounds and sometimes even penetrates the endothelial cells (10). Similar changes are seen in the endothelium of the arterioles and arteries. These glomerular and vascular changes, which are quite prominent, are superimposed on the basic lesion of tubular damage and interstitial fibrosis. Obviously, the latter are not as severe or advanced as they are in patients who die of sclerosing nephrosis years later. It should be emphasized that there may be associated malignant hypertension, with necrotizing glomerular lesions, focal infarcts, and capillary thrombi.

The pathogenesis of the glomerular lesion has been discussed in detail elsewhere. It is due, in part, to damage to the endothelium and in part to the formation or deposition of excessive amounts of basement membrane-like substance. The basic mechanism may well be an autoimmune reaction.

The term "acute radiation nephritis" (6, 9), which has been applied to this entity, is a misnomer, as there is no true nephritis; rather, there is glomerular and vascular endothelial damage. The term "nephroglomerulosis" or "nephroglomerulo-endotheliosis," is preferable (7), but it must be emphasized that this is superimposed on the basic sclerosing nephrosis. The pathological manifestations of the latter, however, are in their earliest stages.

SUMMARY

In a number of patients who have received radiation to the kidney areas, symptoms of chronic renal failure develop years after irradiation. The pathologic picture of radiation damage to the kidney consists basically of vascular and tubular damage. In its early stages, there is damage to the capillaries; in later stages there is subendothelial thickening of the arteries and arterioles similar to that observed in other organs. The tubular epithelium is degenerated and atrophic. The interstitial fibrous tissue shows edema and congestion in the early stages and fibrosis later. The glomeruli are essentially normal until later, when they may be hyalinized and sclerosed. The term "sclerosing nephrosis" has been proposed in preference to the term "chronic radiation nephritis" or "radiation nephrosclerosis," commonly employed in published reports.

Superimposed on this basic lesion, the patients may develop the clinicopathologic picture of malignant hypertension. Recognition of renal origin of the hypertension in these patients may be lifesaving, since nephrectomy has been shown to alleviate the symptoms.

A second and, fortunately, less common entity encountered after irradiation to the kidneys develops as an acute phenomenon within 1 year after exposure and consists principally of glomerular and vascular endothelial involvement. The endothelial cells show swelling and vacuolization, and there is a deposit of basement membrane-like substance in and around the endothelial cells. The term "nephroglomerulosis" has been proposed for this lesion, which had previously been designated as acute radiation nephritis.

Damage to the kidneys may result even from doses below the accepted safe level of 2500 r.

REFERENCES

1. Allen, A. C.: Radiation nephritis. In, Allen, A. C. (ed.): The Kidney-Medical and Surgical Diseases, 2nd ed. New York, Grune and Stratton, 1962, pp. 233-236.

2. Aveoli, L. W., Lazar, M. Z., Coltone, E., Bruce, K. C., and Andrews, J. R.: Early effects of radiation on renal function in man. Amer. J. Med., *34*:329-337, 1963.

3. Dean, A. L., and Abels, J. C.: Study by newer renal function tests of an unusual case of hypertension following irradiation of one kidney and the relief of the patient by nephrectomy. J. Urol., *52*:497-501, 1944.

4. Friedman, M.: Normal tissue tolerance. In, Friedman, M., Brucer, M., and Anderson, E. (eds.): Roentgens, Rads and Riddles. U. S. Atomic Energy Comm., Washington, 1959.

5. Luxton, R. W.: Radiation nephritis. Acta Radiol (Ther.) (Stockholm), *1*:397-406, 1963.

6. Luxton, R. W.: Effects of radiation on the kidney. In, Strauss, M. B., and Welt, L. G. (eds.): Diseases of the Kidney. Boston. Little, Brown 1963, pp. 769-785.

7. Mostofi, F. K.: Radiation effects on the kidney. In, Mostofi, F. K., and Smith, D. E. (eds.): The Kidney. Baltimore, Williams & Wilkins, 1966.

8. Mostofi, F. K., Pani, K. C., and Ericsson, J.: Effects of radiation on canine kidney. Amer. J. Path., *44*:707-725, 1964.

9. Mostofi, F. K.: Acute radiation nephritis. Med. Ann. D. C., *34*:64-68, 1964.

10. Rosen, S., Swerdlow, M., Muehrcke, R., and Pirani, C.: Radiation nephritis, light and electron microscopic observations. Amer. J. Path., *41*:487-502, 1962.

11. Tublin, I., and Gambos, E. A.: Subclinical radiation nephritis. Report of a case. Med. Ann. D. C., *33*:552-556, 1964.

Chapter 49

Association of Renal Disease with Liver Disease

FREDERICK I. VOLINI, M.D., and
GEOFFREY KENT, M.D., Ph.D.

Simultaneous impairment of hepatic and renal function may occur in a variety of pathologic conditions (1). The liver and kidney may be the seat of two independent disease processes or the target of systemic diseases involving both organs. A more direct relationship between the two organs may exist where an established disease process in one organ is followed by disturbances in the other. Thus, renal tumors may affect hepatic function (2), and hepatic parenchymal disease may be followed by renal failure. The last group is of particular clinical significance and is often referred to as the hepatorenal syndrome. Most prominent among the hepatic diseases giving rise to death in renal failure is cirrhosis. The pathogenesis of renal dysfunction in these instances is obscure. Although recent studies have pointed to renal circulatory failure and abnormalities of tubular function as important intermediary mechanisms, the specific factors leading to these disturbances have not been clarified. Morphologically, a host of structural changes may be found in the kidney in these patients. In most instances, however, the alterations encountered cannot be correlated with abnormalities of renal function or with the severity of hepatic disease.

The term hepatorenal syndrome was first applied to conditions in which renal failure developed as a complication of biliary tract surgery or various forms of liver disease (3). Today, the term is used by some to imply a pathogenetic relationship between hepatic and renal disease and by others to include all conditions affecting the liver and kidney simultaneously. Because of the differences in connotation and lack of evidence for a direct or specific functional interrelationship between the two organs, use of the term hepatorenal syndrome is not encouraged.

In this chapter it is proposed to review the conditions which may give rise to combined hepatic and renal dysfunction with special reference to the syndrome of renal failure in patients with cirrhosis.

RELATION BETWEEN KIDNEY AND LIVER DISEASE

The conditions in which renal disease is associated with liver disease may be classified as follows (Table I):

TABLE I—SIMULTANEOUS OCCURRENCE
OF KIDNEY AND LIVER DISEASE

I. Independent diseases of liver and kidney.

II. Disease of liver and kidney caused by the same agent.
   A. Infections.
   B. Drugs and chemicals.
   C. Generalized disease processes.

III. Primary renal disease followed by hepatic dysfunction.

IV. Primary hepatic or biliary disease followed by renal dysfunction.
   A. Biliary tract disease.
   B. Acute and chronic liver disease.
   C. Metastatic neoplasm.

1. Independent Disease of the Liver and Kidney

A pertinent example in this category is the coexistence of cirrhosis with pyelonephritis. The occurrence of these two processes is apparently fortuitous and yet with such combinations as cirrhosis and diabetic nephropathy, the association may be more than coincidence.

2. Diseases of the Liver and Kidney Caused by the Same Agent

Simultaneous injury of the liver and kidney by the same disease process may be seen in infectious diseases (Weil's disease, septicemia), reactions to drugs or chemicals and in such diverse and generalized conditions as periarteritis nodosa, lupus erythematosus, shock, fever therapy and blood transfusion reactions. The best known example of such an injury is seen following exposure to carbon tetrachloride. The latter has direct toxic effects upon the parenchymal cells of the liver and kidney. Hepatocellular and renal tubular necrosis are then prominent features. Incompatible transfusion reactions are well known to affect the kidney. However, they may also give rise to hepatic disturbances as evidenced by central fatty change (Fig. 1), intrahepatic cholestasis, hepatocellular necrosis and the development of jaundice with a large component of direct-reacting serum bilirubin. The changes in the liver may be the result of the combined effects of anemia, shock and antigen-antibody reactions (4). The kidneys are swollen and display dark reddish medullae. Microscopically, pigment casts are seen in the lumen of medullary tubules (Fig. 2), while a remarkable degree of hydropic change is often seen in the cortical tubules (Fig. 3).

3. Primary Renal Disease Associated with Hepatic Dysfunction

The category is illustrated mainly by cases of hypernephroma in which there is evidence of hepatic dysfunction (2, 5). According to the reports in the literature, hepatic function is restored following surgical removal of the tumor-bearing kidney.

4. Primary Hepatic or Biliary Disease Associated with Renal Dysfunction

Renal disturbances may follow acute hepatic disease such as viral hepatitis or massive infarction, or chronic disease such as chronic hepatitis or cirrhosis. Renal dysfunction may also be found in biliary tract disease caused by stricture, calculi or carcinoma despite minimal evidence of hepatocellular injury. The syndrome may furthermore occur in cases of extensive metastatic malignancy in the liver. Of the examples given, cirrhosis is by far the most important condition associated with renal failure and will be dealt with in greater detail.

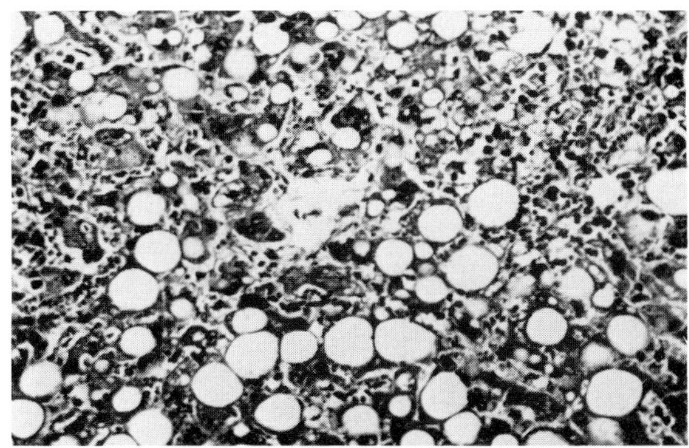

Fig. 1. Centrolobular area of liver from patient after transfusion of incompatible blood. There in moderate fatty change, necrosis of liver cells and inspissation of bile in canaliculi. Hematoxylin and Eosin, X 200.

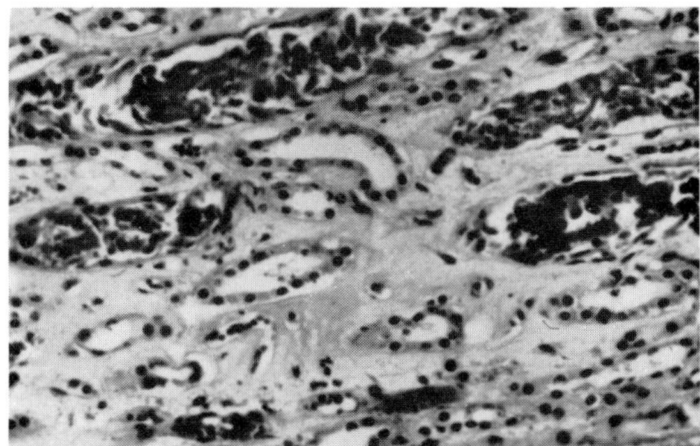

Fig. 2. Medulla of kidney following transfusion reaction. Heme pigment casts are present in several tubules and are associated with necrosis of lining epithelium. Hematoxylin and Eosin, X 430.

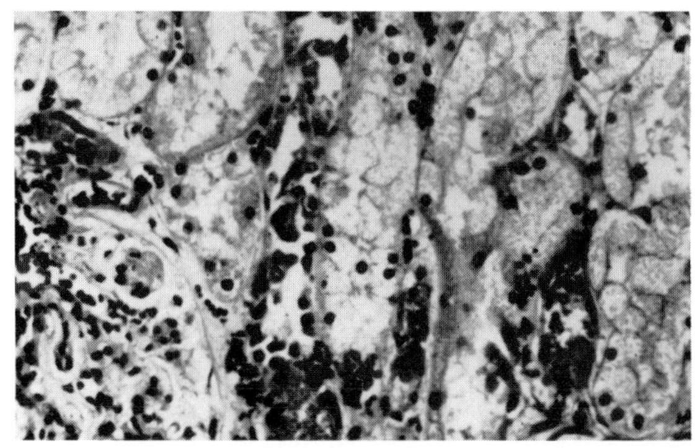

Fig. 3. Proximal convoluted tubules of kidney following transfusion reaction. Note severe hydropic change. Hematoxylin and Eosin, X 430.

CHRONIC LIVER DISEASE AND RENAL FAILURE

The occurrence of a syndrome consisting of progressive oliguria, hyponatremia and azotemia has been recognized for years as a serious complication in patients with cirrhosis. Austin Flint (6) in 1863 commented on the frequency of oliguria in patients with decompensated cirrhosis, especially in the presence of ascites. Similar findings were recorded by Brouardel in 1876 (7). In recent years, the various aspects of renal dysfunction have been studied in greater detail (8–10).

In its most typical form, renal dysfunction in the cirrhotic follows such events as surgery, shock, gastro-intestinal bleeding or paracentesis. However, in one-third of cases, such precipitating events are not a feature (1). Ascites is almost always present, but varies greatly in degree. Jaundice may or may not be evident and coma is present in less than 40% of patients (11). A history of mild decline in blood pressure just prior to the development of renal failure of during the early period of renal failure is common. Renal failure develops rapidly and has generally been regarded as having grave prognostic implications. Survival is rare once the syndrome is established.

The urine is markedly reduced in volume, more acid than normal and often contains small amounts of albumin, hyaline and granular casts and a few erythrocytes. Solute concentration is elevated and often remains high throughout the course of illness until the patient's demise. Urinary sodium is decreased and may appear to be completely absent. Serum sodium concentration is also diminished. Blood urea nitrogen rises gradually, but generally does not reach the extreme values seen with primary renal disease.

The pathologic findings at autopsy may be meager and often show no more severe changes than in controls of the same age (3). On the other hand, the convoluted tubules may display alterations ranging from spotty and mild degenerative changes to extensive necrosis. Additional findings include chronic pyelonephritis, arteriolar nephrosclerosis and cirrhotic glomerulosclerosis (3, 12). Two distinct morphologic lesions not uncommonly seen under these conditions are biliary or cholemic nephrosis and acute tubular necrosis.

Biliary nephrosis is the morphologic lesion accompanying severe jaundice. Grossly, the kidneys are swollen and bile-tinged. The kidney bulges through the capsular surface, and there is marked widening of the cortex with sharp demarcation from the medulla. The bile staining of the medullary pyramids is more striking and the radial markings are generally preserved. Histologically, bile staining of the epithelium of the proximal tubules is often conspicuous and extends to the loops of Henle. This is associated with hydropic vacuolization and, in some areas, with necrosis of the epithelium of the proximal convoluted tubules. Bile casts appear within the distal convoluted tubules (Fig. 4) and in greater amounts within the collecting tubules. This is associated with varying degrees of degenerative change in the lining epithelium and occasionally with interstitial inflammatory exudates surrounding the tubules. The glomeruli are often enlarged and hypercellular (Fig. 5) and occasionally reveal glomerulosclerosis (Fig. 6). Whether or not bilirubin per se has toxic effects is presently not established. The lesion may merely reflect the excessive amounts of conjugated bilirubin excreted by the kidney. On one other hand, there is some evidence that bilirubin may be toxic in the presence of complicating factors (1).

Acute tubular necrosis is analogous to lower nephron nephrosis and is seen especially following massive blood loss or prolonged shock. The morphologic findings consist of segmental tubular necrosis (Fig. 7) with destruction of the basement membrane and reactive inflammation. It has been postulated (13) that these areas provide for an escape of glomerular filtrate, thus aggravating if not causing oliguria. However, none of the morphologic changes outlined are consistent enough to account for the functional disturbances displayed.

From the studies available, it seems evident that renal failure in patients with cirrhosis has no consistent morphologic counterpart.

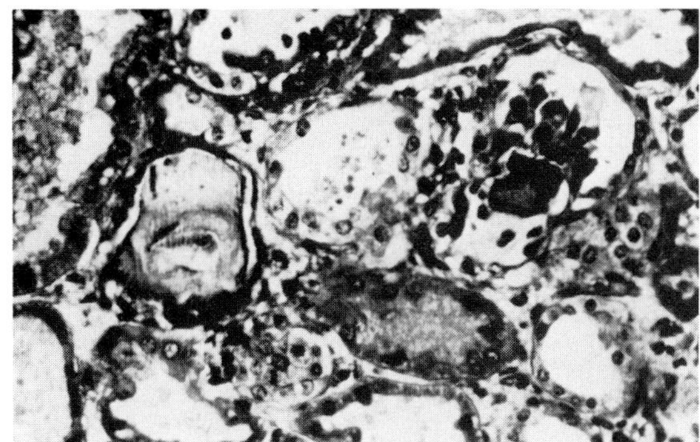

Fig. 4. Sections from kidney in patient dying with liver failure. Note bile casts within tubules. Hematoxylin and Eosin, X 430.

Fig. 5. Hypercellular glomerulus in patient dying with azotemia and oliguria. There is an increase in endothelial and epithelial cells. Hematoxylin and Eosin, X 400.

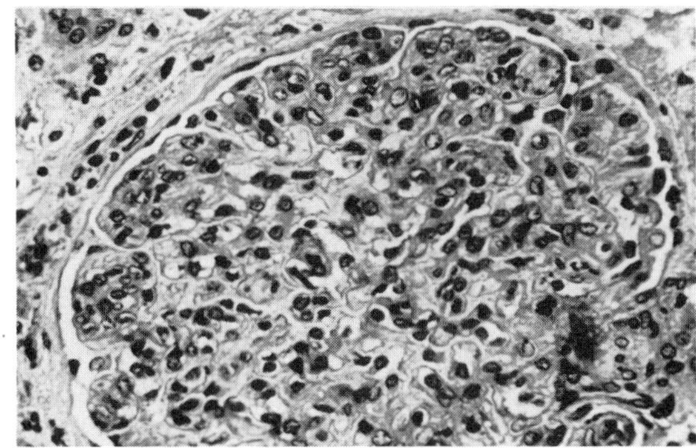

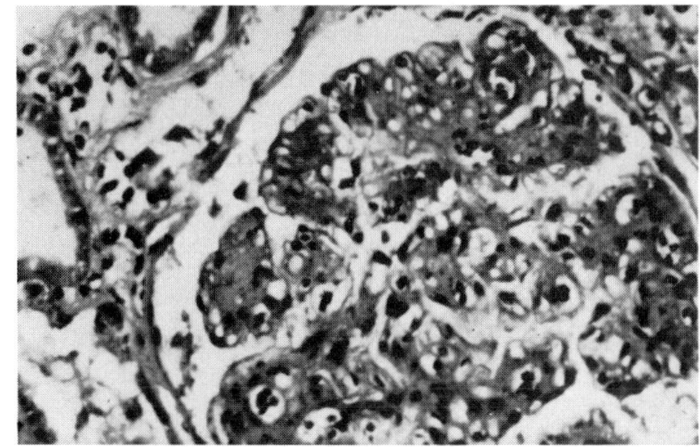

Fig. 6. Glomerulosclerosis in patient with cirrhosis. Hematoxylin and Eosin, X 400.

Fig. 7. Necrosis of medullary tubules in cirrhotic patient following massive blood loss. Hematoxylin and Eosin, X 400.

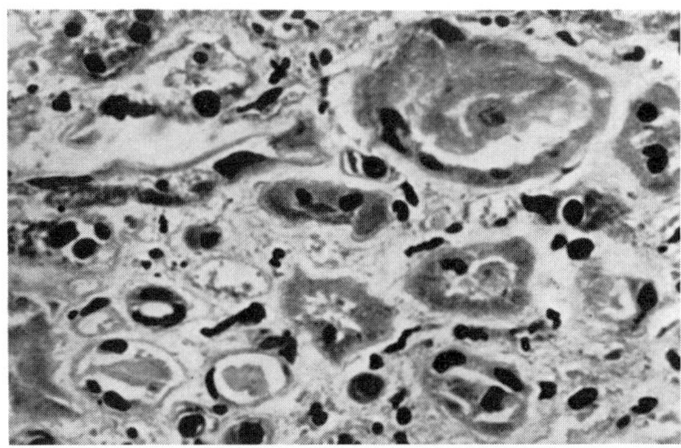

RENAL PATHOLOGY
IN CIRRHOSIS

In the past 20 years, a number of studies have appeared in the literature dealing with the renal changes in cirrhosis, irrespective of the presence of renal dysfunction. These will be briefly reviewed.

1. Autopsy Findings

Baxter and Ashworth (14) described a variety of glomerular lesions in cirrhosis. The most frequent fingings were thickening of the basement membrane of capillaries, vascular sclerosis and mild periglomerular fibrosis. The convoluted tubules displayed granular swelling of epithelial cells, atrophy or regenerative changes. The tubular degenerative changes were thought to be more pronounced in the presence of jaundice. In a study of 100 cases of cirrhosis, Fisher and Helstrom (15) noted diffuse and focal thickening of the mesangium, occasional thickening of the basement membrane of glomerular capillaries and blunting of glomerular lobules in about 25% of cases. The glomeruli were generally hypercellular and contained occasional segmented leukocytes. The changes were interpreted as a type of exudative and proliferative glomerulonephritis. No correlation was found between the glomerular lesions and the presence of complications, such as hepatic coma, gastrointestinal hemorrhage or history of alcoholism. The extent of glomerular lesions moreover was not related to the presence or degree of tubular changes. In another autopsy series, Bloodworth and Sommers (12) reported glomerular lesions consisting of deposits of eosinophilic, PAS-positive material with fibrillar thickening of glomerular basement membranes. These findings did not correlate with the occur-

rence of azotemia. Glomerular lesions in cirrhosis were also reported by other authors. Horn and Smetana (16) described nodular glomerular sclerosis not unlike that seen in diabetics. Similar changes were noted by Raphael and Lynch (17). A proliferative and membranous glomerulonephritis on the other hand, was described by French (18).

2. Biopsy Findings

Renal biopsy material is particularly useful for the evaluation of early alterations. Sakaguchi *et al.* (19) reported a study of 24 patients with acute and chronic liver disease. The series included viral hepatitis, alcoholic hepatitis, Laennec's cirrhosis, post-necrotic cirrhosis and biliary cirrhosis. Glomerular lesions were found in all cases. These showed thickening of the capillary wall with increase in mesangial matrix and electron dense deposits in the subendothelial space of the capillary wall. Diffuse and focal destruction of foot processes was also noted. The changes seemed less severe in acute liver disease, but were essentially the same as in chronic liver disease. Accordingly, the term hepatic glomerulosclerosis was suggested as more appropriate than cirrhotic nephropathy, the description previously used.

3. Experimental Findings

Some observations in experimental hepatic injury and cholemia have provided for a relationship between declining liver function and abnormal kidney function. The early work of Shorr and colleagues (20) suggested the presence in the blood of a substance with antidiuretic effects following liver injury. In more recent work, (21) experimentally-induced cholemia in rabbits following bile duct ligation resulted in alteration of renal tubular morphology. The histological changes, however, were minimal until the liver injury was combined with short episodes of renal ischemia. The combination of bile duct ligation with anoxia produced a greater decrease in glomerular filtration, sodium excretion and urinary output than renal ischemia alone. Other studies (22, 23) were conducted on the effects of hepatic necrosis following ligation of the hepatic artery, with and without renal ischemia. The results again indicated more severe renal functional impairment in the presence of both hepatic necrosis and anoxia. It was concluded that the anoxic kidney is more prone to injury in the presence of liver disease. Dawson and Stirling (24) also found that ligation of the bile duct in the rat severely aggravated the effects of anoxia on renal function and morphology. They found a two to three-fold increase in the degree of azotemia when renal injury was combined with experimentally-induced cholemia. The latter also resulted in more severe degenerative change of the tubular epithelium and exudative and proliferative changes in glomeruli. Administration of Mannitol had a remarkable protective effect, resulting in lower blood urea nitrogen values and less severe morphologic alterations of the tubules and glomeruli.

The marked degenerative change often found in renal tubules in cases of icterus gravis neonatorum has been attributed to the toxic effects of indirect-reacting bilirubin (25). While this interpretation is open to question, there has been some evidence to suggest that bilirubin in itself may have toxic effects (26). Bile acids have received greater attention recently as a factor in the renal injury associated with liver disease. Despite numerous attempts, a nephrotoxic substance of hepatic origin has not yet been identified.

To summarize the renal findings in cirrhosis, both glomerular and tubular lesions may be encountered. The tubular lesions vary widely and show no consistent relationship to clinical manifestations. Cholemic nephrosis and acute tubular necrosis, when present, are some of the more characteristic forms. Glomerular lesions have been found in both acute and chronic liver disease and consist of destruction of foot processes, deposits of electron dense material in the subendothelial space and mesangial fibrosis. In more advanced liver disease, glomerulosclerosis seems a prominent feature. While the glomerular lesions in themselves may not seem clinically significant, they may conceivably become functionally important in conditions of anoxia and diminished renal perfusion and play some part in the causation of the fully developed syndrome of renal failure.

PATHOGENETIC CONSIDERATIONS

While the association between impairment of hepatic function and renal circulatory changes can be considered established, the specific factors underlying these disturbances remain ill-defined. The immediate mechanisms leading to abnormalities in renal function have been defined as changes in renal perfusion and abnormalities of tubular function (27).

Azotemia is the result of increased production, diminished glomerular filtration and increased tubular re-absorption of urea. Increased production of urea often follows intestinal bleeding. The clearance of urea through the glomeruli is diminished and parallels diminished clearance values for uric acid, inulin and PAH. Clearance values decline further as hepatic failure increases in severity (11). Total renal plasma flow and the renal fraction of cardiac output are reduced even though cardiac output is not diminished. The alterations in renal blood flow have been attributed in part to the hydrostatic effects of ascites. However, while some parameters of renal function may improve after the subsidence of hydroperitoneum, glomerular filtration and renal plasma flow seem to improve only slightly.

Hyponatremia appears to be due largely to an increase in plasma water. Total body exchangeable sodium is increased (27), and there may also be an intracellular shift of sodium (28). The decrease in urinary sodium is the result of decreased amounts of sodium in the filtrate and increased tubular re-absorption. The latter is attributed to hyperaldosteronism which is known to be a feature in cirrhosis with ascites (10).

Oliguria in the initial stages of the syndrome occurs despite the increase in total body water and the expanded plasma volume. Diminished renal plasma flow and reduced glomerular filtration together with the increase in ADH activity contribute to the decline in urine volume. The elaboration of free water by the distal portion of the nephron is diminished (27). In the terminal phases of the syndrome, a drop in arterial blood pressure may further aggravate the oliguric state.

Other circulatory changes which may play a role include arterio-venous shunting of blood within the kidney and changes in total renal vascular resistance. Shunting of blood away from glomerular capillaries with increased medullary blood flow could explain the low extraction ratios of PAH (10), decreased filtra-tion fraction and defects in renal concentrating ability (29). However, studies of the oxygen saturation of renal arterial and venous blood have thus far not indicated the presence of significant intra-renal shunts. Increase in renal vascular resistance has also been offered as an explanation for the decrease in glomerular filtration and abnormal tubular function.

While the immediate causes of oliguria, azotemia and hyponatremia are evident, their relationship to primary liver disease is less apparent. In a consideration of this relationship, two factors seem important: 1) primary factors of hepatic origin, and 2) precipitating factors which arise out of the complications of liver disease. The presence of primary factors of hepatic origin is suggested by the observations (1) that renal failure in cirrhosis often develops in the absence of complications. The uniform presence of glomerular abnormalities (19) in liver disease may further support this concept. The substances which may be implicated include bilirubin, bile acids and a host of others. The evidence for nephrotoxic effects of bilirubin is controversial. Although it would seem that less can be attributed to high levels of bilirubin than has been indicated by some authors (23, 24), the suggestion has been made that bilirubin may be toxic in the presence of anoxia or hypotension (21); its toxic effects therefore cannot be dismissed in conditions where reduced renal perfusion is known to occur as it is in cirrhosis. The possible toxic effects upon the kidney of bile acids are presently unknown and require further investigation. The significance of precipitating factors such as blood loss, shock, paracentesis, diuretic therapy and the administration of nephrotoxic drugs in triggering the syndrome of renal failure seems well established for the large majority of cases. These factors may act in conjunction with renal circulatory changes in bringing about progressive renal failure.

CONCLUDING REMARKS

The syndrome of renal dysfunction which follows acute and chronic liver injury (hepatorenal syndrome) is an important clinical problem. In a definite but small percentage of cases, the renal disease is related to obvious complications such as severe blood loss and shock. However, in most instances, the immediate cause of the renal dysfunction is not apparent. Significant factors which predispose to the development of this syndrome include ascites, recent paracentesis, electrolyte deficiencies often associated with diuretic therapy, recent surgical procedures and administration of nephrotoxic agents. The mechanism by which these factors alter renal function is not always clear, but acting in concert, they often lead to the syndrome of progressive azotemia and oliguria. The renal morphologic changes such as the presence of bile pigment casts, tubular degeneration or necrosis and glomerulosclerosis do not correlate with the presence of azotemia. More pertinent are functional changes which include altered hemodynamics, altered tubular function or both. The circulatory changes may explain altered tubular function, mediated in part by substances such as aldosterone. The problems surrounding the complex inter-relationship between liver and kidney function remain a challenge, evidently requiring further study.

REFERENCES

1. Summerskill, W. H. J.: Hepatic failure and the kidney. Gastroenterol., *51*:94, 1966.
2. Lemmon, W. T., Jr., Holland, P. V., and Holland, J. M.: The hepatopathy of hypernephroma. Amer. J. Surg., *110*:487, 1965.
3. Spellberg, M. A., Sandlow, L., Allen, H., and Eshbaugh, D.: Current concept of the hepatorenal syndrome. Geriatrics, *18*:837, 1963.
4. Minick, O. T., Volini, F., Orfei, E., and Kent, G. Ultrastructure of the liver in hemolytic anemia. Fed. Proc., *27*:672, 1968.
5. Stauffer, M. H.: Nephrogenic hepatosplenomegaly (abstr.). Gastroenterol., *40*:694, 1961.
6. Flint, Austin: Clinical report on hydroperitoneum, based on an analysis of forty-six cases. Amer. J. Med. Sc., *45*:306, 1863.
7. Brouardel, P.: L'uree et le foie, variations de la quantite de L'uree eliminee dans les maladies du foie. Arch. de Phys., 2^e Serie, III., 373, 1876.
8. Baldus, W. P., Feichter, R. N., Summerskill, W. H. J., Hunt, J. C., and Watkim, K. G.: The kidney in cirrhosis. II. Disorders of renal function. Ann. Int. Med., *60*:366, 1964.
9. Shear, L. J., Kleinerman, J., and Gabuzda, G. J.: Renal failure in patients with cirrhosis of the liver. I. Clinical and pathologic characteristics. Amer. J. Med., *39*:184, 1965.
10. Vesin, P.: Late functional renal failure in cirrhosis with ascites: pathophysiology, diagnosis and treatment. In, Martini, G. A., and Sherlock, S. (Ed.): Aktuelle Probleme der Hepatologie; Ultrastruktur Steroidstoffwechsel Durehblutung Leber und Niere. Stuttgart. Georg Thieme Verlag, 98, 1962.
11. Papper, S.: The kidney in liver disease. In, Strauss and Welt (eds.): Boston, Little, Brown, 1963.
12. Bloodworth, J. M. B., and Sommers, S. C.: Cirrhotic glomerulosclerosis: A renal lesion associated with hepatic cirrhosis. Lab. Invest., *8*:962, 1959.
13. Allen, A. C.: The Kidney New York, Grune and Stratton, 1951.
14. Baxter, J. H., and Ashworth, C. T.: Renal lesions in portal cirrhosis. Arch. Path., *41*:476, 1946.
15. Fisher, E. R., and Hellstrom, H. R.: The membranous and proliferative glomerulonephritis of hepatic cirrhosis Am. J. Clin. Path., *32*:48, 1959.
16. Horn, R. C., Jr., and Smetana, Hans: Intercapillary glomerulosclerosis. Amer. J. Path., *18*:93, 1942.
17. Raphael, S. S., and Lynch, M. J. G.: Kimmelstiel-Wilson Glomerulonephropathy—its occurrence in diseases other than diabetes mellitus. Arch. Path., *65*:420, 1958.
18. French, A. J.: Glomerulonephrosis. Arch. Path., *49*:43, 1950.
19. Sakaguchi, H., Dachs, S., Grishman, E., Paronetto, F., Salomon, M., and Churg, J.: Hepatic glomerulosclerosis. Lab. Invest., *14*:533, 1965.

20. Shorr, E., Zweifach, B. W., and Furchgott, R. F.: Hepato-renal factors in circulatory homeostasis. III. The influence of humoral factors of hepato-renal origin on the vascular reactions to hemorrhage. Ann. N. Y. Acad. Sci., *49*:571, 1948.

21. Fajers, C. M.: Experimental studies in cholemic nephrosis. Acta Path. et Microbiol., *41*:44, 1958.

22. Fajers, C. M.: Experimental studies in the so-called hepato-renal syndrome. Part 3. Acta Path. et Microbiol. Scandinav., *41*:44, 1958.

23. Fajers, C. M.: Experimental studies in the so-called hepato-renal syndrome. Part I. Acta Path. et Microbiol. Scandinav., *39*:225, 1956.

24. Dawson, J. L., and Stirling, G. A.: Protective effect of Mannitol on anoxic jaundiced kidneys. Arch. Path., *78*:254, 1964.

25. Bernstein, J., and Landing, B. H.: Extraneural lesions associated with neonatal hyperbilirubinemia and kernicterus. Am. J. Path., *40*:371, 1962.

26. Zetterstrom, R., and Ernster, L.: Bilirubin, an uncoupler of oxidative phosphorylation in isolated mitochondria. Nature, *178*:1335, 1956.

27. Summerskill, W. H. J., Baldus, W. P., Feichter, R. N.: Renal function in cirrhosis with ascites: Clinical, biochemical and physiologic changes. In, Martini, G. S. (ed.): Aktuelle Probleme der Hepatologie. Stuttgart, Thieme, p. 90, 1962.

28. Clowdus, B. F., Summerskill, W. A. J., Casey, T., Higgins, J. A., and Orvins, A. L.: Isotope studies of the development of water and electrolyte disorders and azotemia during the treatment of ascites. Gastroenterol., *41*:360, 1961.

29. Vaamonde, C. A., Vaamonde, L. S., Morosi, H. J., Klinger, E. L., Jr., Papper, S.: Renal concentrating ability in cirrhosis. I. Changes associated with the clinical status and course of the disease. J. Lab. Clin. Med., *70*:179, 1967.

Chapter 50

The Diagnosis of Renal Tumors

MEYER M. MELICOW, M.D.

Tucked snugly in the trough bordered mesially by the dense lumbar spine and posteriorly by the firm quadratus lumborum psoas muscles lie the million nephron units comprising the kidney. Set in this secure arrangement, it is protected against the threat of physical trauma, and sudden external temperature changes. But this same "secure arrangement" may harbor a slowly expanding neoplastic mass within the corpus, inaccessable, hidden, non-palpable, painless and not detectable. The mass may metastasize and kill; if diagnosed early, however, it might be nipped in the bud! But how diagnose early? This is the physician's dilemma.

SYMPTOMS AND SIGNS

1. Urology

The classic triad of urologic symptoms and signs caused by cancer of the kidney is:

a) painless hematuria
b) dull ache in flank
c) palpable abdominal mass

These are really not early symptoms.

To cause hematuria, tumors of the corpus—(they comprise 85 to 90% of renal growths), must press against or invade the pelvis. This occurs early in growths near the pelvis; late in those developing deep in the corpus and perhaps never in those arising near the capsule. When it does occur, it is in most cases a late symptom. It is usually painless and may not recur for a long time or it may never recur. Meanwhile, the tumor grows. The episode therefore, must not be ignored. Sometimes, only microscopic hematuria is found. Unless the finding is readily explainable, a thorough investigation of the entire urinary tract is imperative. The incidence of hematuria caused by tumors of the renal pelvis is greater and occurs earlier than in those of the corpus.

Dull ache in flank is caused by the ever-increasing size of the tumor, or invasion, or pressure on nerves. It is not an early symptom.

Finding a palpable abdominal mass depends upon its size and on the thickness or firmness of the anterior abdominal wall. For a mass to be palpable, even in a thin person, there would have been considerable expansion. It is usually smooth or nodular and moves with respiration. The findings should accelerate investigation and be viewed with concern.

In a large number of patients (45%) hematuria is the only symptom. Some patients complain of flank pain only and in some the abdominal mass is discovered during a routine physical examination. The complete triad is found in only a small number of patients and is usually of grave prognosis.

2. Non-urologic

a) Metastases: The expanding intracorporal mass may be urologically symptomless (30), but the patient may seek medical aid because of nonurological symptoms. We have examined patients whose only presenting symptoms were: pulsating lump in the scalp thought to be a cyst (21), ptosis of a lid due to a retro-orbital or brain metastasis or persistent infection of toe (treated as ingrown toe-nail infection), swollen jaw thought to be due to gum boil, or hemoptysis. In all these patients, further clinical investigation (biopsy or radiographic studies) revealed metastasis from a renal cancer (21, 29).

b) Fever of Unknown Etiology: The incidence of fever in renal cancer ranges from 15 to 20% (1, 6, 31). With associated findings, diagnosis is made readily in the majority of cases. In 2.5%, however, fever was the cardinal complaint; its cause was discovered after some delay. The exact mechanism of the hyperpyrexia (100-102° F) is not known; however, it is known to occur often in necrotic tumors.

c) Debility Evidenced by Weight Loss, Anorexia and Anemia is a frequent accompaniment of the symptom complex caused by renal tumors. However, it was found in only 1.8% (1) as the sole manifestation of the malignancy.

d) Persistent Hypertension is seen in certain patients with renal tumors and is reversible following nephrectomy (13, 17). There are three probable mechanisms for the production of the hypertension:

1) Arteriovenous fistula involving the main renal artery
2) Extrinsic pressure on the renal artery
3) Ischemia of renal parenchyma adjacent to tumor.

e) Secondary polycythemia has been reported in 1.8% of patients with neoplasms of the kidney (4, 6, 32). The diagnosis was based on hemoglobin values above 17%, red cell counts above 6.5 mm per cu mm and hematocrits of 55% and higher. It has been observed in other lesions of the urologic tract (Table 1). In most cases, removal of the kidney (and metastases, if present) (2) eliminates the erythrocytosis. The mechanism for producing polycythemia is not understood but it should be pointed out that the juxtaglomerular apparatus is involved in the elaboration of erythropoietin (26). Since renal tumors arise from the nephron unit, such activity may be going on in the tumor (9) (Table 1).

f) Hypercalcemia and hypophosphatemia have occurred in the presence

Table 1—Renal Lesions Associated with (Secondary) Polycythemia

Tumors (4, 32)	Hydronephrosis (11, 15, 20)
Adenoma	Unilateral, bilateral
Carcinoma	
Hemangioma	*Vascular Lesions*
Fibromyxoma	Renal artery stenosis (16)
Sarcoma	Renal hypertension (14, 16)
Cysts (4)	*Nephrocalcinosis* secondary
Simple	to hyperparathyroidism (25)
Multiple	
Polycystic (8)	*Ureter*
	Carcinoma (without
Malformations (3)	hydronephrosis).
Double kidney	

of renal cancer, (7, 12, 9, 33) cancer of the lung, breast, ovary and some of the lymphomas. The patient complains of weakness (myopathy-like features), (18) nausea, vomiting and constipation. There are no bone lesions. The parathyroids are not abnormal. Removal of renal cancer causes a sudden drop in serum calcium and relief of symptoms. Theories as to the mechanism of the syndrome are that the tumor produces: 1) a parathyroid-like substance; 2) a parathyroid stimulating substance or a Vitamin D-like substance; and 3) a circulating calcium bonding substance.

g) Amyloid may be present, either in the resected kidney or throughout the body in some 3% of cases (1). It is rarely diagnosed before the operation (5, 10).

h) Unilateral edema of a lower extremity due to pressure on the inferior vena cava of retroperitoneal extension of the renal neoplasm.

RADIOGRAPHIC STUDIES

When clinical suspicion points to the kidney as the site of an expanding mass, radiographic studies will confirm the suspicion and in over 95% of the cases, will differentiate between cyst and tumor. It must be emphasized that a radiograph is merely a documentation on a sensitive film of the relative densities and lucencies in an organ or in tissue exposed to roentgen rays. Interpretation of the patterns requires a back-ground of experience in comparing radiographic findings in the normal with those in a variety of pathological lesions and of cataloging the latter according to their distinctive characteristics. Most carcinomas of the kidney for example, are honeycombed by large vascular channels into which the radio-opaque fluid flows

producing dense complex patterns in the radiograph: "tumor vessels," "tumor stain," arteriovenous fistula etc. (Fig. 1). In contrast, most cysts are relatively avascular, radiolucent, and reveal a sharp margin in the radiograph along the periphery of the cyst wall (Fig. 2). The exceptions are: papillary and tubular adenomas or carcinomas, papillary and tubular cystadenomas or carcinomas, and some of the stromal growths. All are relatively avascular (23) (Fig. 3).

Radiographic Procedures
a) Plain or "scout" film (KUB). Note the presence of a lump or bump and whether the renal shadow in enlarged, distorted, or displaced.

b) *Intravenous urography:* observe alteration in the pelvic and calyceal outlines (dilation, elongation, compression, distortion obliteration). Absence of function may signify renal vein invasion by tumor.

c) *Retrograde urography:* This procedure is not imperative but is helpful when the findings are inconclusive or when the intravenous urograms reveal absence of the contrast medium in one kidney. During the cystoscopic examination, pathology of the lower urinary tract should be ruled out and ureteral urine specimens should be obtained for Papanicolaou studies. This is particularly important if there is suspicion of a urothelial growth in the pelvis or ureters.

d) *Nephrotomography:* The compounding of glomerular excretion and resultant concentration of the opaque medium in the collecting systems leads to opacification of the renal mass, except in areas where function is reduced or absent (necrotic areas in tumor, cyst, abscess, granuloma etc.).

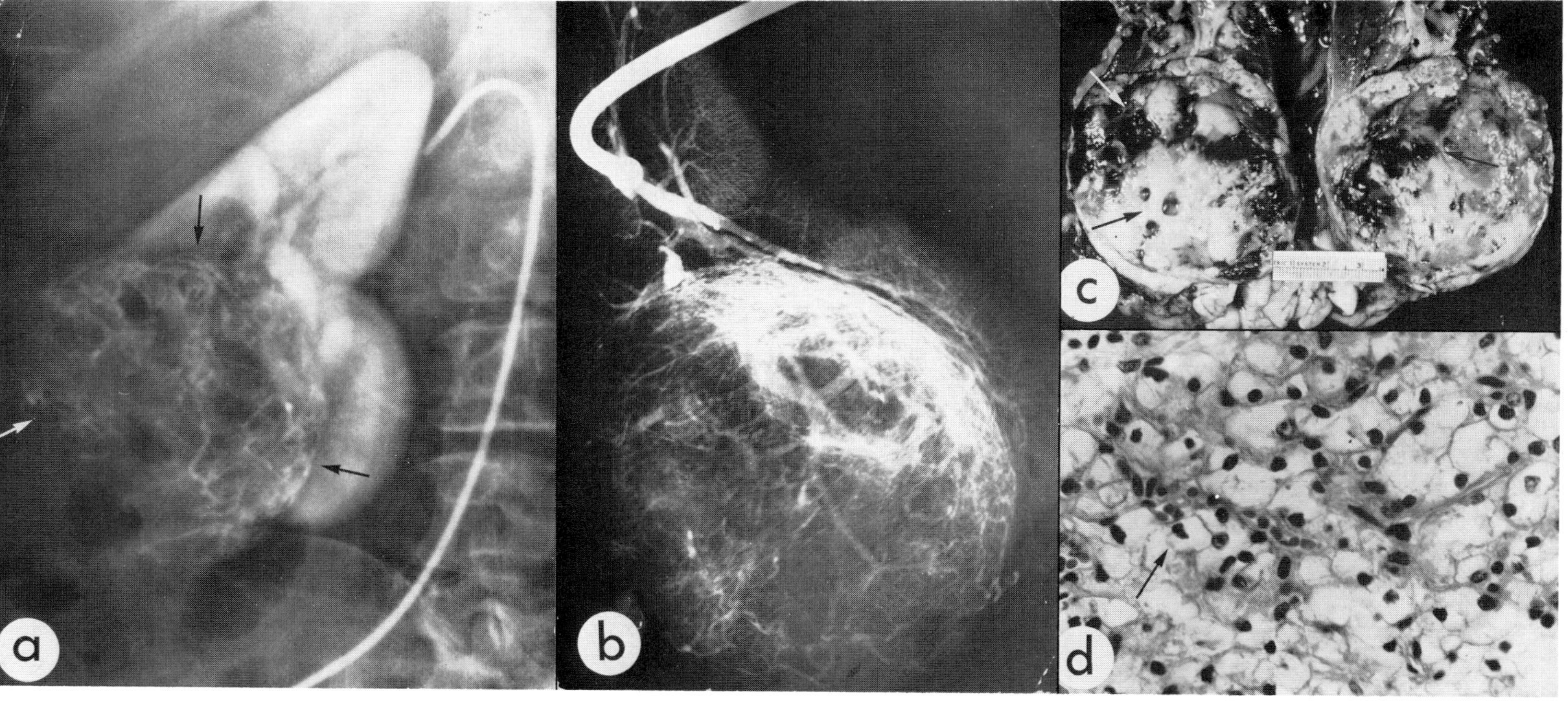

Fig. 1. Usual radiographic pattern in a patient with renal tumor: S. F., 04-33-87, 66-year-old woman; a) delayed arteriogram revealing tumor vessels with "puddling" and "corkscrew" formation and opacification of normal portion of kidney; b) same case, the renal artery has been injected with the opaque medium. Note complex vascular pattern; c) gross specimen: observe large vascular channels (arrows), and d) microscopic section shows the pattern of clear cell carcinoma X-200. (Reproduced by permission of authors and of J. Urol. (23).)

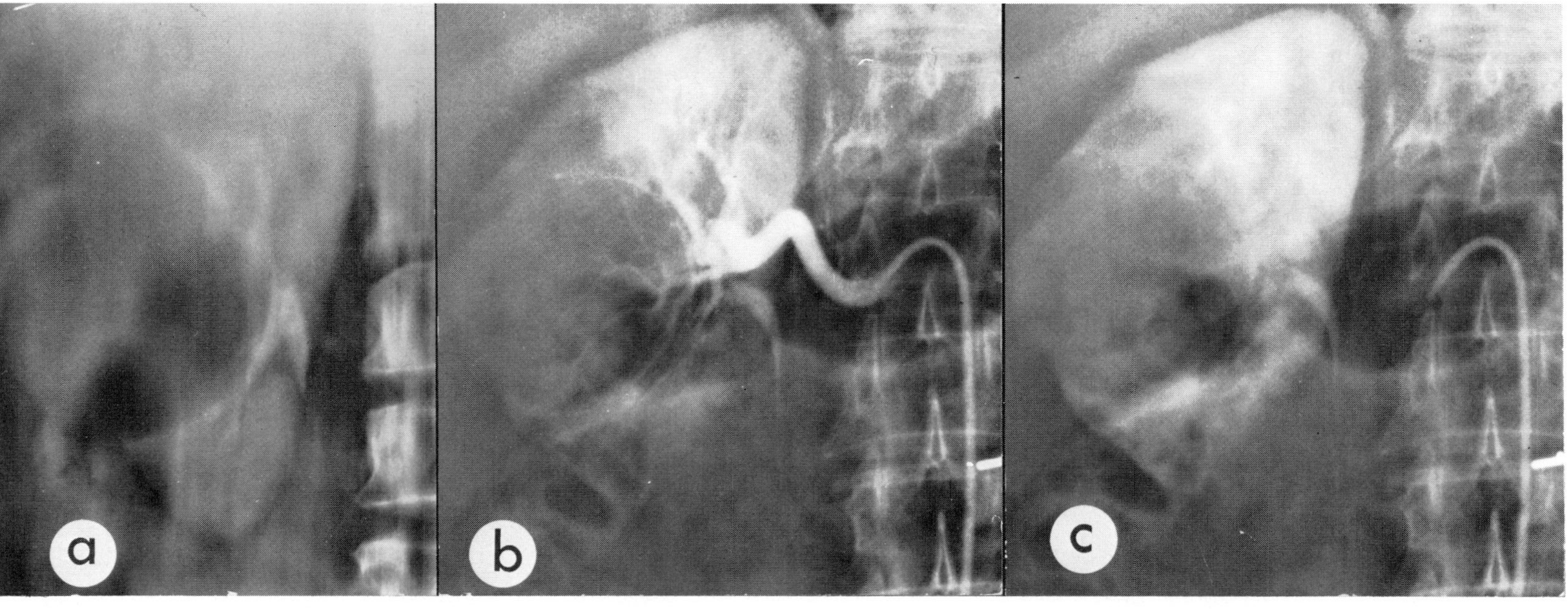

Fig. 2. Usual radiographic pattern in patient with renal cyst: a) spherical lucency at site of cyst; note sharp line of demarkation between it and the rest of the renal corpus which is partially opacified; b) arterial phase of arteriogram: note displaced blood vessels and their absence in the cyst area, and c) nephrogram phase of arteriogram: note opacification of parenchyma and its absence in cyst area. (Reproduced by permission of authors and of J. Urol. (23).)

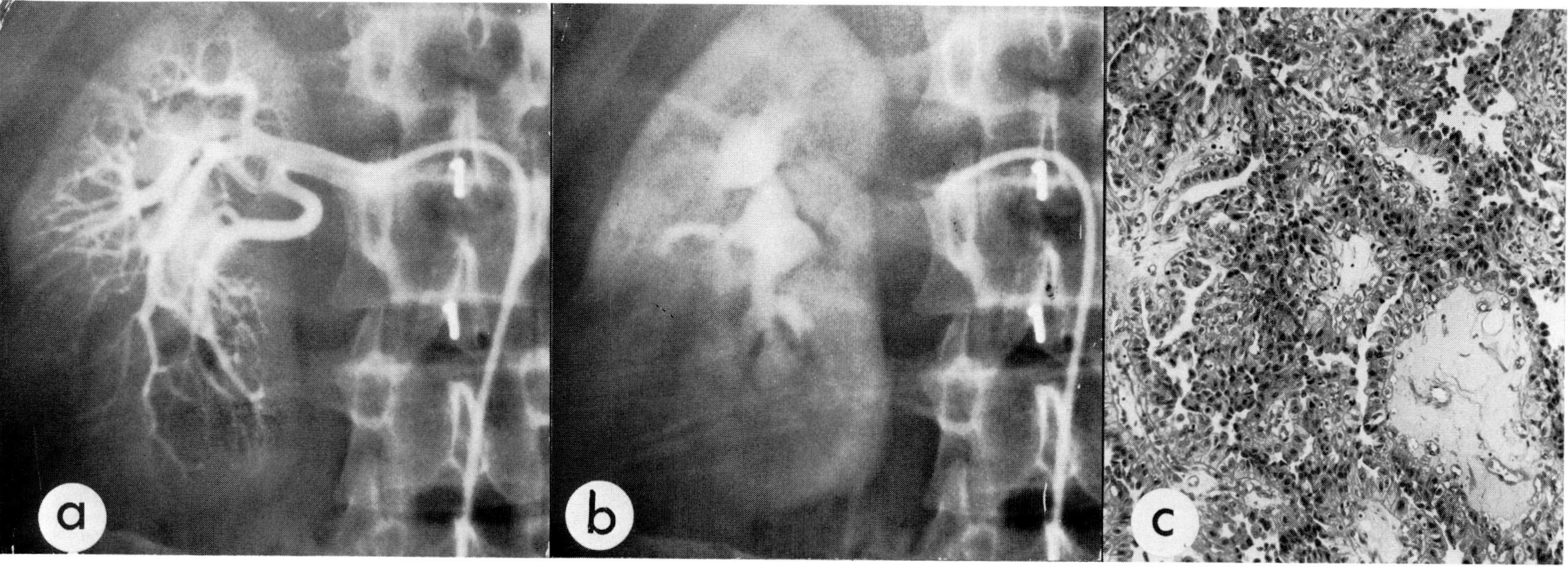

Fig. 3. Arteriogram and nephrogram suggestive of cyst which turned out to be a papillary cystadenocarcinoma following nephrectomy: J. A., 105-99-24, 54-year-old man with palpable right flank mass: a) arteriogram devoid of abnormal vasculature; b) nephrogram: there is an area of lucency suggestive of cyst, and c) the tumor was solid and avascular and the microscopic sections revealed a papillary cystadenocarcinoma X-150. (Reproduced by Permission of authors and of J. Urol. (23).)

e) *Selective angiography:* This will in most instances aid in the differential diagnosis between cyst and tumor, mainly because of differences in vascular patterns. However, on rare occasion, as mentioned, certain solid avascular tumors may resemble cysts:

f) *Renal scan:* Radioisotope scanning is helpful in differential diagnosis. A defect is usually present at the site of a tumor, cyst or abscess and the isotope uptake is reduced in the areas adjacent to it (24).

SUMMARY

The following are the step-by-step procedures in the diagnosis of renal tumors:

1. *History:* a thorough account of events pertinent to the urologic tract should be elicited. Over 30% of patients present non-urological symptoms.

2. *Physical examination:* this must include careful palpation of the abdomen.

3. *Laboratory examination:* complete urinalysis, Papanicolaou smears of sediment; blood studies: hemoglobin, hematocrit, RBC and WBC counts, blood serum urea, calcium, phosphorus, alkaline phosphatase etc. Papanicolaou smears aid in the diagnosis of urothelial tumors, but not in parenchymal tumors arising in the renal corpus.

4. *Radiographic studies:* (in addition

TABLE 2—NEOPLASMS OF RENAL CORPUS

I. PRIMARY
    A. PARENCHYMA, origin: probably from epithelial components of nephron unit
        1. Benign
           a) adenoma: (clear or granular cell, or papillary adenoma)
           b) cystadenoma (clear or granular cell)
           c) (?) metanephroma
        2. Malignant
           a) *carcinoma,* solid: clear cell (renal cell) (hypernephroma), (Grawitz tumer),
               granular (renal cell) (hypernephroid ca), mixed: clear and granular
           b) carcinoma in cyst (often papillary; clear or granular cell or mixed)

    B. STROMA, origin: from supporting framework of kidney
        1. Benign: fibroma, lipoma, hemangioma etc. angiomyolipoma (hamartoma,
           benign mesenchymoma)
        2. Malignant: fibrosarcoma, liposarcoma etc.

    C. MIXED, contains epithelial and stromal elements
        1. Benign: adenomyoma, fibroma,
        2. Malignant: nephroblastoma (Wilms' Tumor)

    D. MISCELLANEOUS:
        1. Tumor of adrenal rest or choristoma ("true hypernephroma")
        2. Endometrioma
        3. Dermoid cyst, teratoma etc.

II. SECONDARY
    A. From adjacent neoplasms (of retroperitoneum, adrenal gland etc.)
    B. From distant neoplasms (stomach, lungs, breast etc.)

to those of the lungs, skeletal system etc.):

a) Flat or scout film of the abdomen

b) Intravenous urograms

c) Retrograde urograms

d) Selective angiography and tomography

e) Renal scan.

A comprehensive classification of tumor of the renal corpus and pelvis is presented. (Tables 2 and 3).

BIBLIOGRAPHY

1. Berger, L., and Sinkoff, M. W.: Systemic manifestation of hypernephroma. A review of 273 cases. Am. J. Med., 22:79 1-796, 1957.
2. Blanshard, G., and Smith, H.: Polycythemia with metastases from carcinoma of the kidney. Brit. J. Urol., 36:66-70, 1964.
3. Boyd, R. V.: Polycythemia associated with congenital duplex kidney. Brit. J. Clin. Pract., 17:409, 1963.
4. Damon, A., Holub, D., Melicow, M. M., and Uson, A. C.: Polycythemia and renal carcinoma. Am. J. of Med., 25:182-197, 1958.
5. Ellenberg, M.: Amyloidosis secondary to malignant Grawitz tumor (hypernephroma) of kidney. Death from uremia due to amyloid disease of the kidney. J. Mt. Sinai Hosp., 10:323-325, 1943.
6. Enders, W., and Friderici, L.: Renale Polyzythämie. Deutsch. Med. Wschr., 88:1512-1518, 1963.
7. Goldberg, M. F.: Renal adenocarcinoma containing a parathyroid hormone-like substance and associated with marked hypercalcemia. Amer. J. Med., 36:805-814, 1964.
8. Gurney, C. W.: Erythropoietin, erythropoiesis, and the kidney. J.A.M.A., 173:1828-1829, 1960.
9. Hewlett, J. S., Hoffman, G. C., Senhauser, D. A., and Battle, J. D. Jr.: Hypernephroma with erythrocytemia. Report of a case and assay of the

Table 3—Neoplasms of Urinary Drainage Tract

(Tumors of urothelium lining pelvis, ureter, bladder, urethra)

I. Primary

 A. of UROTHELIUM
  1. Benign: papilloma
  2. Malignant: (trnasitional cell or urothelial ca)
   a) intraurothelial (Bowen's disease) (carcinoma in situ)
   b) papillary, *commonest*
   c) non-papillary or solid

 B. by SQUAMOUS CELL METAPLASIA
  1. Benign: squamous cell papilloma
  2. Malignant:
   a) intraepithelial
   b) papillary epithelioma
   c) solid (squamous cell epithelioma), commonest

 C. by GLANDULAR METAPLASIA OR GLANDULAR REST
  1. Benign: adenoma (very rare)
  2. Malignant:
   a) in urachal and trigonal regions
   b) in metaplasia from cystitis glandularis

 D. of STROMA
  1. Benign: fibroma, lipoma, rhabdomyomas etc.
  2. Malignant: fibrosarcoma, myxosarcoma, etc.
   "sarcoma botryoides"

II. Secondary Neoplasms

  a) from neighboring organs, rectum, sigmoid, cervix
  b) from distant organs, carcinoma of breast, lungs, lymphosarcomas etc. (rare)

tumor for an erythropoietic-stimulating substance. New Eng. J. Med., *262*:1058-1062, 1960.

10. Hyman, A., and Leiter, H. E.: The association of hypernephroma with amyloidosis of the kidney. J. Urol., *56*:303-309, 1946.

11. Jaworski, Z. F., and Wolan, C. T.: Hydronephrosis and polycythemia. Am. J. Med., *34*:523-534, 1963.

12. Lamberg, B. A., Pelkonen, R., and Frick, M. H.: Hypercalcemia in renal carcinoma. Report of a case. Acta Med. Scand., *176*:187-194, 1964.

13. Lampe, W. T. II, and Crovatto, A. C.: Renal adenocarcinoma producing hypertension: Diagnosis by radioactive renogram and aortography. J. Urol., *93*:673-677, 1965.

14. Lattimer, J. K., Melicow, M. M., and Uson, A. C.: Nephroblastoma (Wilms' tumor). J.A.M.A., *171*:2163-2168, 1959.

15. Lawrence, J. H., and Donald, W. G., Jr.: Polycythemia and hydronephrosis or renal tumors. Ann. Int. Med., *50*:959-969, 1959.

16. Luke, R. G., Kennedy, A. C., Barr Stirling, W., and McDonald, G. A.: Renal artery stenosis, hypertension, and polycythemia. Brit. Med. J., *1*:164-166, 1965.

17. Lytton, B., Rosof, B., and Evans, J. S.: Parathyroid hormone-like activity in a renal carcinoma producing hypercalcemia. J. Urol., *93*:127-131, 1965.

18. MacKenzie, D. W.: Perirenal hematoma primary with polycythemia. J. Urol., *23*:535-543, 1930.

19. Madanagopalan, N., and Saratchandra, R.: Renal carcinoma with myopathy-like features. Lancet, *1*:1351-1352, 1966.

20. Martt, J. M., Sayman, A., and Neal, M. P.: Polycythemia and hydronephrosis. Ann. Int. Med., *54*:790-795, 1961.

21. Melicow, M. M.: Classification of renal neoplasms. A clinical and pathological study of 199 cases. J. Urol., *51*:333-385, 1945.

22. Melicow, M. M.: Tumors of the urinary drainage tract: Urothelial tumors. J. Urol., *54*:186-193, 1945.

23. Melicow, M. M., and Becker, J. A.: Radiographic simulation of certain solid tumors of the renal corpus to renal cyst. J. Urol., *97*:592-610, 1967.

24. Morris, J. H., *et al.* The diagnosis of renal tumors by radioisotope scanning. J. Urol., *97*:40-54, 1967.

25. Murphy, F. J., Mau, W., and Zelman, S.: Nephrogenic polycythemia. J. Urol., *91*:474-477, 1964.

26. Naets, J. P.: Le Role du Rein dans L'Erythropoiese. Acta Clin. Belge., *15*:361-496, 1960.

27. Nixon, R. K., O'Rurke, W. O., Rupe, C. E., and Korst, D. R.: Nephrogenic polycythemia. A. M. A. Arch. Int. Med., *106*:797-802, 1960.

28. Oberling, C., Riviere, M., and Hagueanau, F.: Ultrastructure of the clear cells in renal carcinomas and its importance for the demonstration of their renal origin. Nature, *186*:402-403, 1960.

29. O'Grady, A. S., Morse, L. J., and Lee, J. B.: Patathyroid hormone-secreting renal carcinoma associated with hypercalcemia and metabolic alkalosis. Ann. Int. Med., *63*:858-868, 1965.

30. Plaine, L. I., and Hinman, F., Jr.: Malignancy in asymptomatic renal masses. J. Urol., *94*:342-347, 1965.

31. Shipman, K. H., Downing, S. W., and Bradford, H. A.: Hypernephroma presenting as fever of unknown origin associated with elevated serum alkaline phosphate level. J. Urol., *89*:160-163, 1963.

32. Thiel, G.: Polycythemia in renal tumors. Deutsch. Arch. Klin. Med., *208*:111-134, 1962.

33. Thomson, W. H. G., Karat, A. B. A.: Hypercalcemia associated with adenocarcinoma of kidney without demonstrable bone lesions. Brit. Med. J., *2*:745-746, 1966.

Author Index

Subject Index

H